The Mental Health Professional and the New Technologies

A Handbook for Practice Today

The Mental Health Professional and the New Technologies

A Handbook for Practice Today

by

Marlene M. Maheu, Ph.D.
Pioneer Development Resources, Inc.

Myron L. Pulier, M.D.
University of Medicine and Dentistry of New Jersey
New Jersey Medical School

Frank H. Wilhelm, Ph.D.
Stanford University School of Medicine

Joseph P. McMenamin, M.D., J.D.
McGuireWoods LLP

Nancy E. Brown-Connolly, R.N., M.S.N.
The Iowa Chronic Care Consortium, Des Moines University

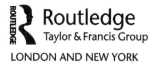

Routledge
Taylor & Francis Group

LONDON AND NEW YORK

First published 2005 by Lawrence Erlbaum Associates, Inc.

Published 2018 by Routledge
2 Park Square, Milton Park, Abingdon, Oxon OX14 4RN
52 Vanderbilt Avenue, New York, NY 10017

First issued in paperback 2018

Routledge is an imprint of the Taylor & Francis Group, an informa business

Library of Congress Cataloging-in-Publication Data

The mental health professional and the new technologies : a handbook for
    practice today / by Marlene M. Maheu ... [et al.].—1st ed.
        p.   cm.
    Includes index.
    ISBN 0-8058-3988-7 (casebound : alk. paper)
    1. Mental health services—Information technology.   I. Maheu, Marlene M.

    RA790.5.M445   2005
    362.2'0285—dc21   2003003997

Cover Design: Kathryn Houghtaling Lacey

This book was typeset in 10/12 pt. Palatino, Italic, Bold, and Bold Italic.
The heads were typeset in Palatino and Berling.

The opinions expressed in the book are the current views of Joseph P. McMenamin, and are not necessarily those of his firm or any of its clients.

ISBN 13: 978-1-138-01269-1 (pbk)
ISBN 13: 978-0-8058-3988-3 (hbk)

For those who suffer from emotional distress and need better access to care

Contents

About the Authors

Marlene M. Maheu, Ph.D., a licensed psychologist with over 25 years of practice experience, is a trainer, speaker, advocate and consultant for technology-based healthcare services. She has served on the American Psychological Association's Committee on Professional Practice Standards (COPPS), co-chaired the Task Force for Media & Telehealth for APA Division 46, Media Psychology, and chaired the Technology Task Force for APA Division 35, the Society for the Psychology of Women. She has also served on the California Psychological Association's Presidential Telehealth Task Force, and been awarded their Division of Media, Technology and Communication, *Jacqueline Bouhoustsos, Ph.D. Award For Contribution to Media Psychology.* Dr. Maheu is Editor-in-Chief and founder of <www.SelfhelpMagazine.com>, an award winning online electronic magazine, with over 7,000 daily readers, and developed of TelehealthNet, <www.telehealth.net>, a networking site for mental health professionals interested in telehealth. The lead author of *E-health, Telemedicine and Telehealth: A Guide to Startup & Success* (2001) she lectures internationally on the ethics and practicalities of using technology in multidisciplinary and psychotherapeutic settings. She also consults with numerous corporations seeking to integrate technology into clinical service delivery.

Myron L. Pulier, M.D., is a board-certified psychiatrist and a clinical associate professor at the University of Medicine and Dentistry of New Jersey—New Jersey Medical School in Newark, NJ, on the faculty of the Mental Health Services Research Fellowship program. He previously worked in county and voluntary psychiatric and general hospitals and in private solo and group practice emphasizing individual and family psychotherapy. He has served as Medical Psychiatric Director for PruCare of Northern New Jersey and for TriState Healthcare Management; he has also founded and operated a multidisciplinary managed care-oriented outpatient clinic. Currently, Dr. Pulier is developing a network of interactive multimedia kiosks to improve clinical communication with severely and persistently disturbed psychiatric patients at the partial care psychosocial rehabilitation unit of University Behavioral HealthCare in Newark. His involvement with computer applications in psychiatry began with projects in the late 1960's at North Shore-LIJ Health System's Hillside Hospital as well as at the Nathan Kline Research Institute of the Albert Einstein College of Medicine and at the Computers in Military Psychiatry program at Walter Reed General Hospital.

Frank H. Wilhelm, Ph.D., is a senior research scholar in the Department of Psychiatry and Behavioral Sciences, and Associate Director of the Laboratory of Clinical Psychopharmacology and Psychophysiology, at Stanford University. Trained in clinical psychology, psychophysiology, and computer sciences, he has ongoing collaborations with a variety of research groups at Stanford and across the U.S. He is internationally known for his high-tech approaches to clinical assessment and has developed a state of the art software system for the comprehensive analysis of biosignals recorded in a psychophysiology laboratory and outside of it. His current work, funded by N. I. H., focuses on psychological and physiological mechanisms in anxiety disorders and the utility of biofeedback as an adjunct to cognitive-behavioral treatments.

Joseph P. McMenamin, M.D., J.D., F.C.L.M., is a partner in McGuireWoods LLP, a large international law firm, and an associate professor in the Department of Legal Medicine at Virginia Commonwealth University's Medical College of Virginia. Trained in internal medicine, Dr. McMenamin practiced emergency medicine before and during law school. He is board-certified in Legal Medicine and his practice focuses on health law, risk management, and product liability defense. As chair of the Committee on Law and Medicine of the Section on Legal Practice of the International Bar Association, Dr. McMenamin conceived and assisted in the preparation of the Draft International Convention on Telemedicine and Telehealth, the first document of its kind. He has written and spoken widely on risk management in health care, particularly in e-health, and advises clients on risk avoidance in electronic health care and Internet activities.

Nancy E. Brown-Connolly, R.N., M.S.N., is a clinical nurse specialist and former consultant and clinical research manager for Blue Cross of California, State Sponsored Programs. She served as a member of the Blue Cross Blue Shield Association (BCBSA) Health Services Research Group and as a member of the Federal Advisory Panel for the Office of Teleheath, developing performance indicators for federal agencies and funding decision-makers. Ms. Brown-Connolly has received awards from the BCBSA National Award Program for Innovations and Best Practices in Medical Management for her project, *"See a Specialist . . . Across the Street or Across the State: A Telemedicine Demonstration Project"*. Frequently invited to speak about telehealth issues and her own work, she has recently completed research on the patient's and provider's perspectives on telehealth care. She has also developed research databases and designed innovative web-based scheduling systems for telehealth applications. She is dedicating this book to the memory of her husband Michael P. Connolly and brother Frank J. Brown, Jr.

Preface

Technology, used for both informational and telecommunication purposes, is becoming one of the most important factors in the future of health care delivery. One can see the oncoming change simply by surfing the Internet and looking at the proliferation of health-related Web sites. The 7 million Web sites uncovered by the Alta Vista search engine using the key words *health care* are actually only a fraction of what is available worldwide. Also discernible on the Web are the international, federal, state, and private sector initiatives supporting the development of an information infrastructure for global, national, and regional health care. For instance, the Healthcare Information and Management Systems Society (HIMSS), the American Telemedicine Association (ATA), and the American Telemedicine Service Providers (ATSP), as well as other private groups, are focused on providing leadership for the adoption of health care information technology and management systems. They help shape health care public policy and industry practices through advocacy and educational and professional development initiatives. Mental health care mirrors these trends of general health care.

By incorporating technologies into various facets of mental health care, from service delivery to practice management, "psychotechnologies"[1] are dramatically changing the field. Even concepts of mental health treatment are affected by the psychotechnologies, as new therapeutic approaches are designed to benefit from technological innovation. When combined with the power of the Internet, the psychotechnologies promise not only increased accessibility and affordability, but also greater acceptability and adaptability in delivering care. This inevitable use of technology means opportunities abound for mental health practitioners who are ready to explore new avenues for service delivery. Mental health professionals need to learn about, and take advantage of, the technologies that have already transformed much of health care delivery.

Some mental health professionals educated in traditional psychotherapeutic modalities worry that the advance of technology may degrade the quality of treatment and threaten their practices. Some professionals may ask, "When should technology be used in mental health practice?" Answers range from "Never" to "We've been using it for 40 years."

To be sure, the introduction of technology into any aspect of a health care practice brings uncertainty and a host of legal, ethical, and risk management issues. Perhaps

---

[1] Jerri Fink probably coined the term *psychotechnology* in the 1990s. See her Web site at http://psychotechnology.com.

some clinicians feel they ought to stay away from technology's risks. However, clinicians and administrators owe it to their patients, their profession, and themselves to make fully informed choices about delivering the best services. They need a working knowledge of what is available now and what is on the way, particularly in light of the legal and ethical issues involved. A large portion of this book assesses these issues and provides suggestions that mitigate risk.

Regardless of our particular perspectives and opinions as professionals, economic forces are inexorably pressing toward the adoption of new technologies. Payers of all types are eager for more technological innovations. Increasingly, administrators and third-party payers will favor professionals who are able to harness technology for their clinical services as well. Either we shape the development of these technologies or we stand by and let the users of these technologies shape us.

OVERVIEW OF BOOK

The Mental Health Professional and the New Technologies is designed as a handbook for professionals. It systematically describes how to expand the reach and quality of mental health services by integrating technology into everyday practice, and it uses case examples for demonstration. It acquaints mental health professionals and administrators with information from think tanks, research labs and legal precedents, as well as from professionals and administrators in the field. It provides them with the nuts and bolts of how and when to consider using the new, rapidly proliferating specialized technologies for behavioral and mental health, and facilitates their thoughtful weighing of the many issues involved in integrating technology into the delivery of care to people with social or emotional problems. We discuss services available to practitioners today, as well as visionary applications of tomorrow.

Chapter 1 reviews the basic concepts, from telehealth and telemedicine to behavioral e-health, and gives examples of some applications of telecommunication technology developed over the past four decades. The trials and errors of early leaders in behavioral telehealth and the insights of researchers offer clues to how practitioners can integrate technology into their practices.

Chapter 2 briefly introduces the essential technical terminology used throughout the book, emphasizing the basic communication methods that mental health professionals use. The chapter is devoted to the beginner. By centralizing the bulk of technological discussion, we can discuss applications without interruption in subsequent chapters.

Chapter 3 allows the reader to explore text-based (e.g., e-mail and synchronous chat) applications of psychotechnologies and suggests how professionals can establish an online presence. To help the reader think critically about when and how to use these relatively familiar telecommunication technologies, we discuss the small body of research literature that has accumulated. "Netiquette" issues are also introduced. Thus, in Chapter 3 we propose a path for learning how to use various text-based communication modalities, progressing from constricted e-mail messaging through more challenging synchronous communications involving groups of people simultaneously discussing highly charged material. The skills needed in these areas are not just technical; they involve new ways of socializing with awareness of new pitfalls and opportunities.

Chapter 4 is devoted to Internet Web sites and related technologies that practitioners might use to expand their services. By the turn of the century, 42% of physicians were already working in practices with Web sites (Harris Interactive, 2001c). Therefore, it is reasonable to think that the Internet will become an ordinary part of the clinical toolbox for mental health professionals as well. The chapter guides the reader through the process of building a Web site, from the planning cycle to Web site building tools and practical considerations for Web site maintenance.

Chapter 5 summarizes fundamental and practical issues in delivering services with audio (telephone) and video technologies and discusses changes in the professional–client relationship created by using these media. Research related to using telephone and videoconferencing technologies is presented, along with special considerations for consumers and professionals using videoconferencing.

Chapter 6 is the first of 3 chapters related to the increasingly important role of computer programs in professional practice. This chapter addresses the benefits and challenges involved in numerous types of computer-aided assessment methods.

Chapter 7 reviews the history of computer-aided psychotherapy and continues with a sampling of desktop, hand-held, and interactive Web-based software developed for adjunctive intervention in specific clinical problems, such as anxiety, schizophrenia, and bulimia. Virtual reality and advanced biofeedback equipment are also discussed. Examples of how professionals can use such computerized aids are drawn from the experiences of practicing clinicians and technology developers to inspire the reader with the innovative technologies available for defined client populations.

Chapter 8 examines technologies that help one manage a practice or operate a mental health clinic. It describes how introducing technology can affect professional–client relationships. After discussing voice recognition software that serves as an automated stenographer, the chapter considers the computerized patient record from the standpoint of potential benefits, impediments to use, privacy issues, and legal and regulatory standards.

Chapter 9 sorts through the myriad regulatory and legislative issues beyond those of computerized patient records. An extensive review of the privacy regulations associated with the Health Insurance Portability and Accountability Act (HIPAA) is provided, as well as references to other important documents and enactments concerning privacy.

Chapter 10 examines ethical considerations related to the use of psychotechnologies. It also further considers standards and guidelines, here with emphasis on issues of professional practice.

Chapter 11 introduces the first of 3 chapters devoted to a 7-step Online Clinical Practice Management (OCPM) model for delivering professional services using psychotechnologies. This chapter focuses on the first step of special professional training for providing psychotherapy online.

Chapter 12 details 3 steps of the preparation phase in the OCPM model. These steps are the development of a referral network, providing patient education about online clinical practice, and obtaining informed consent. Practical considerations and suggestions for each of these steps are given in detail.

Chapter 13 presents the final 3 steps of the OCPM model: conducting an assessment, direct service delivery, and reimbursement for using the psychotechnologies. Chapters 11 through 13 apply much of the technology discussed earlier in the book to each step. Case vignettes give the professional an insider's view into the range of existing practical applications.

Chapter 14 offers a glimpse at the near future of the psychotechnologies—how the next wave of behavioral e-health technologies will change the continuum of care within the next two decades. Chapter 15 takes a longer view to speculate about mental health care by mid-century.

The Epilogue is devoted to immediate action. It outlines steps mental health professionals can start taking to bring the benefits of psychotechnologies into their practice and make them available to patients. It raises ethical issues and suggests promising areas for investigation. It provides lists of organizations to investigate and also discusses potential sources of funding for research.

Appendix A is an annotated list of some of the empirical studies that have shed light on technology in mental health. This list of such studies is neither exhaustive, nor an endorsement, but it is representative of empirical research that is providing science-based guidelines for application of the psychotechnologies in clinical practice.

Appendix B is a charter for an e-mail discussion list. Professionals who wish to develop and host a listserv can used this model charter. A disclaimer is included to help manage the risk involved in such an undertaking.

Appendix C is a compilation of various existing patient consent agreements used in telehealth today. Of course, the reader is encouraged to obtain legal review by a qualified attorney before using any consent agreement with patients.

Appendix D reprints the draft proposal developed by the Committee on Law and Medicine of the International Bar Association to encourage debate and eventual agreement on a multilateral treaty to govern and foster cross-border telehealth services. The International Bar Association is a group of lawyers, including private practitioners, in-house counsel, academics, and jurists from around the world who share an interest in international law. The proposal has been presented to the United Nations and has been the subject of scholarly debate.

Lastly, contact information gathered from this book's many contributors is presented to facilitate direct discussion between readers and leading telehealth professionals.

PERSONAL NOTES

Each author, in his or her own way, has long been entranced by what technology could bring to mental health, and each has been both impatient with and astounded by the rate of progress we have seen. When we signed on with Lawrence Erlbaum Associates to produce a book on this subject, we expected to quickly summarize our ideas and share our enthusiasm with colleagues who had not yet paid much attention to technological developments in the mental health field. We soon realized that we had taken on an enormous, nearly impossible project. Technology was everywhere and growing at a rate that made much of our writings obsolete even before the bytes could be transmitted coast to coast! We had much more to say than could reasonably fit into a book, yet we could not scramble fast enough to keep up with emerging developments. As we wrote, we kept encountering marvelous new applications of technology as well as ominous trends that spelled danger to patients, mental health professionals, and society at large.

This book views psychotechnologies through the eyes of five professionals, each with a different vantage point and all with complementary skill sets. As coauthors, we speak from our combined perspectives as program administrators, managers, researchers, practitioners, professors, litigation lawyers, consultants, and owners of e-health companies. We have received more than 30 independent chapter reviews from colleagues who have challenged and questioned our positions on nearly all issues. The result attempts to strike a balance between pragmatists and enthusiasts on many hotly debated questions and answers.

We realize that in advocating the new technologies we risk being seen as heretical renegades by some traditional practitioners. Such was the case when one author tried to give a presentation about telehealth ethics via a two-way videoconferenced link from California to a European psychoanalytic conference in the mid-1990s. The conference planner sent an urgent e-mail message five minutes before the scheduled video presentation: "Abort, abort! Fist fight about to break out on the conference floor!" Some of the more vocal conference attendees refused to allow the presentation to take place, so it had to be cancelled. While such outrage at videoconferencing of any topic related to psychotherapy may be surprising to us now, it was a reality less than a decade ago. On the other hand, the conservative stance we often present does not make us nay-sayers, rainers-on-parades, wet blankets, or Luddites.

It's just that after witnessing a jury or two, one starts to see things in a different way. All the authors live and work in the United States, the most litigious country in the world. Our views and opinions may therefore be more cautious than those of professionals in other countries. Of course, our national passion for litigation has not prevented innovation, and tinkerers and even governments worldwide are rapidly advancing the psychotechnologies. A tolerably good rule for whether and when to adopt a new technology follows from a piece of wisdom attributed to comedian Steven Wright: The early bird gets the worm, but the second mouse gets the cheese. Running too far ahead of the pack may amount to an invitation for lurking lawyers to single one out for attack; but failure to fulfill ethical obligations to clients by lagging behind and providing substandard care can also attract plaintiffs' attorneys.

To apply a given technological tool, it is important that a health care practitioner understand its operation, risks and benefits. Adopting a communication medium popularized by children and teenagers to communicate inexpensively with each other may well curry favor with the younger set. Such a practice may even permit beneficial therapeutic interventions that would otherwise be impossible without such a medium. On the other hand, if one's younger patient uses hieroglyphics that can be comprehended only by fellow teens, the hapless professional may be linguistically mystified and therapeutically defeated when attempting to conduct psychotherapy with a suddenly suicidal or homicidal patient.

It is important also to think, if only for a moment, like a lawyer. This is less risky and painful than may at first appear. Lawyers think about evidence and about sources of proof. Knowing a fact is all well and good, but proving it in court, within the constraints of the law of evidence, is another thing entirely. A plaintiff must carry the burden of proof by offering evidence sufficient to persuade the finder of fact. In a typical psychotherapeutic environment, how does one show what happened? There is, of course, a medical record and the testimony of the participants. To a large extent, one is likely to accept what the therapist has written and claims to remember. A recording made in the course of delivering treatment at a distance, however, makes it exceedingly easy to prove exactly who said what to whom, when, with what tone of voice, with what turn of phrase, and in what context. For the right defendant—and remember, everyone who reads these words is a potential defendant—this development could be wonderful or catastrophic. The video is a record nonpareil. It can make a case or break it. Professionals who choose to use this technology need to remember that the camera does not blink, and the tape does not forget.

On a broader legal front, battles involve the concept of burden of proof. In order to prevail, one party in a legal proceeding must present evidence beyond a certain threshold. In disputes arising from using the psychotechnologies, legal actions against a mental health professional or provider organization may involve either inappropriate or incorrect use of the technology or failure to have used the technology when indicated. At present, from the somewhat peculiar vantage point of the defense lawyer, the burden of proof weighs most heavily on the early adopters of technology in mental health, but that may change within the next decade.

As we finally commit our edited files to hard copy and ask our publisher to press the virtual "Print" key, we hope that we have achieved what Donald W. Winnicott might have called a "good enough" balance of depth, breadth, detail, generalization, vividness, practicality and idealism while conveying the excitement felt by everyone engaged in expanding the role of the psychotechnologies in the delivery of professional mental health care. We hope our readers will appreciate a balanced presentation and an attempt to introduce innovation, to provide strategies that protect the practitioner from malpractice (real or merely alleged), to encourage professionals to learn how to apply the psychotechnologies responsibly and respectfully, and to promote more accessible service delivery. We believe that, used wisely, the psychotechnologies have the capacity to markedly improve mental health care and greatly expand its pivotal role in all of health care.

GENERAL DISCLAIMERS

The products, programs, policies, Web sites, companies, and organizations mentioned in this book are described solely for the purpose of discussion, demonstration, and consideration, and not as endorsement of any kind. Conversely, failure to mention any entity or product does not imply an adverse decision concerning it. Similarly, reference to a particular Web site does not imply endorsement of its content or of its privacy practices. Readers are reminded that the content and the privacy practices of any Web site may be subject to change at any time without notice to the authors or to the publisher of this work but were current as of May 2003. Readers use any product or program, or surf any Web site herein described, at their own risk. Also, Web addresses may change at any time and without notice. As a result, when we refer the reader to Site X at Address Y, Site X might no longer be accessible and Address Y may have been adopted by a Web site that contains undesirable content or malicious code (such as viruses), or that has damaging effects when encountered by a browser. When referencing a Web site, we guide the reader to the specific Web page whenever possible; but when readers find a link to be no longer valid, they may attempt to search for the document or page referenced by starting from the organization's home page.

Some helpful further hints:

- Reduce the address to its root (for example, http://www.samplesite.com/articles/0201406.html can be reduced to http://www.samplesite.com).
- If an internal search engine is available for the site, conduct a search for the desired document from the site's internal search engine.
- Contact the Web owner or Web manager and ask for the location of the document. Including the previous address of the document in question can greatly facilitate

this search. A link to the Web owner or Web manager should be available from the home page of the Web site.

• Search the Internet using a search engine (for example, Google or AltaVista) for the document in question using author or title. If an e-mail or telephone number can be found for a particular author, write to them directly, and provide the title of the document as well as the non-functional Web site address. That will allow the author to contact the Web site owner to ask about re-routing other readers who may need to find the article in question.

One of the authors is a member of the Board of Scientific Advisors to Vivometrics, maker of the Lifeshirt. None of the other authors has any interest as an agent, servant, employee, officer, director, shareholder, or on any other basis, in any of the companies that provide any of the products or services described in the following list, except where described in the text. Further, this book is not intended to be exhaustive.

The opinions and positions we take are representative of our current views and not necessarily those of our employers, partners, or clients. Similarly, the views and opinions expressed in various contributions, such as personal communications and vignettes located throughout the book, are those of the respective authors only. Such contributions to this work do not necessarily reflect the policies or opinions of the agencies, organizations, or companies that employ these contributors. Some vignettes are reports of actual occurrences; others are fictional stories created to illustrate a point. In such fictional cases, any similarity to a real person, living or dead, is purely coincidental. Also, as used in this work, the term *standard* need not necessarily have the same meaning as it does in law, particularly the law of tort.

Primary sources have been used where possible. Secondary sources have also been used. The newness of the field, the relatively limited scientific literature, and the unavailability of researchers to comment on their proprietary work has forced us to use materials that otherwise might not meet the tests of scientific rigor. We encourage the reader to consider our statements in the faint light of a new day and to make allowances. We have attempted to verify the accuracy of our statements, but in writing about a new and rapidly evolving modality of health care delivery, we are peering through ever changing mists and shadows. For example, statements about reimbursement practices of various managed care entities, although as accurate as reasonably possible when made, could well become outdated by the time the reader encounters them in the text. Accordingly, no warranty concerning the reliability of the information presented can be made.

In addition, we do not create, and do not attempt or intend to create, physician–patient, therapist–client, or attorney–client relationships with readers, nor do we practice or offer to practice our respective professions in any jurisdictions other than those in which we are licensed. Readers desiring professional advice are encouraged to consult appropriate practitioners in their own jurisdictions and not to rely on the content of this work as a substitute for the advice they can obtain by seeking other sources.

With respect to identifying practitioners, professionals, clinicians, or providers, we use all terms interchangeably. Similarly, we make reference to clients and patients interchangeably, except when discussing medical research.

In particular, U.S. readers are reminded that, under current law, many (though not all) of the issues discussed herein are governed by the laws of the several states, and not of the United States. These laws vary widely. Except where noted, no attempt is made in this work to describe the law of any one state (never mind all 50) nor federal law.

Practitioners are advised to confer with appropriate legal advisors about the law applicable to them in their respective jurisdictions. We cannot and do not attempt to speak to practical, technical, ethical, and legal issues worldwide. Rather, we leave that to subsequent writers, who undoubtedly will add their views in light of their own regional perspectives. In fact, we invite any discussion through the Web site http://telehealth.net and the telehealth e-mail discussion list: http://telehealth.net/subscribe/subscribe_all.html.

Acknowledgments

To say that this book is by the authors is an overstatement. Although each author has played an important role, this book is the product of an entire community of professionals, as well as their students and research and office assistants. Contributing various pieces of information at various times, they have shared the vision of advancing the delivery of mental health care through technology. More than 140 individuals were directly involved in developing or reviewing the manuscript, and hundreds more have contributed by discussing core issues on various professional mental health e-mail discussion lists and national convention programs for more than 8 years. We also need to say that there has been, and continues to be, much controversy about the issues. As authors, we hope that we have done a fair job of sifting through the controversy and of constructing a handbook of the remarkable new technologies available to mental health professionals.

If we could give an award for excellence for senior editors, it would most certainly be granted to Susan Milmoe, who has shared our passion and stood by us. With her unwavering support and encouragement, this manuscript survived the vicissitudes of the telecommunications and computer industries, terrorist attacks, as well as multiple injuries and family deaths among authors. Her trust in our professionalism is most appreciated. Special thanks also go to the entire staff of Lawrence Erlbaum Publishers, Inc., for holding true to their reputation of being the best.

Reliable and humble, yet brilliant and discerning, we all appreciate Tim Mount and recognize him for being the research and writing assistant who has carefully crafted this manuscript for more than two years. Without complaint, and filled with wisdom and contributions beyond his years, he has been central to every aspect of developing this manuscript, from outlining to researching, writing, referencing, editing, formatting, printing as well as networking and maintaining several forms of technology to support its development.

Mention of our families and friends is the dearest and deepest of all acknowledgments. Without their inspiration, support, and tolerance, this project would surely have been abandoned long ago.

Among colleagues who have contributed time and energy, we recognize these individuals for sharing their research, experience, and imagination with us:

Michael J. Ackerman	George Alexander
Rosalie Ackerman	Greg Alter
Judith Albino	Frank Anderson
Ace Allen	Page Anderson
Merrick Alpert	Jodi Aronson

Suzanne Ash
Paul Attard
Theresa Baines
Tim Baker
Martha Banks
Azy Barak
David Barlow
Judy Berman
Ellen Betts
Larry Beutler
John Bloom
Cathy Britain
Andrea Seidner Burling
Joanne Callan
Pamela Clark
Conrad Clyburn
Mike Cochran
Linda Cole
Sue Coldwell
Deb Colgan
Yvette Colon
Mary Beth Connolly
Stephen J. Cozza
Susie X. Day
Pat DeLeon
Claude Dennery
Richard Dorsey
Patricia Femiani
Richard Flanagan
Ray Folen
Donna Ford
Todd Foster
Robert V. Franco
Gregory Gahm
Tracy Getz
Richard N. Gevirtz
Dale Giolas
Randy Glasbergen
Robert Glueckauf
Marc Goldyne
Barry L. Gordon
Adam Grant
Mary Gregerson
Kevin Grold
David Haas
Sandra Haber
Linda B. Hallion
Scott Hargrove
Reid K. Hester
James Gil Hill

Shirly Hirschberger
Tim Hodgens
Norm Hoffman
Jennifer M. Hoke
James Hudziak
Carolyn Hutcherson
Paul M. Insel
Larry James
Leigh Jerome
Bond Johnson
Ed Jones
Sherry Jones
Warren Karp
Cleo Keirnan
Justin Kenardy
Paul Kennedy
Erica Kica
Storm King
John Koontz
Sunkyo Kwan
Luciano L'Abate
Scott Laurence
Mark Lediard
Ron Levant
Chao-Cheng Lin
Paul Litwak
Jeff Loomis
Jill Lumsden
Yair Lurie
Michael Mallen
Isaac Marks
Dale Masi
Peter Milgrom
John Miller
David C. Mohr
Peter Murray
Tom Nagy
Paulo Negro
Andrew Nelson
Michelle G. Newman
David Nickelson
Zain Nurani
Monica E. Oss
Stephanie Pacinella
John S. Parker
Les Posen
Colonel Propatich
Dena Puskin
Dana Putnam
Robert Pyke

Jerry Quimby
Fred Rabinowitz
Gene Reich
Harry Rhodes
Skip Rizzo
Nicholas Robinson
Paul Rosenberg
Walton T. Roth
Mark Rothkopf
Holly Russo
Charles Safran
James Sampson
Sherri Scherf
Loretta Schlachta
Mark Schoder
Mark S. Schwartz
Nancy Sharp
Kimberly Shea
Norma Simon
Saul Shiffman
Anna Slomovic
Henry Smith
Sanjay Sood
Duffy Soto
Agnes Spadafora

Rob Sprang
B. Hudnall Stamm
William Stilwell
John Suler
Paul Sussman
Roxy Szeftel
Manny Tau
C. Barr Taylor
David Tener
Tom Trabin
Amy Turkington
Doron Tzur
Star Vega
Mark Verschell
Lenore Walker
Robert Waters
Ken Weingardt
Pam Whitten
Andy J. Winzelberg
Erika Wise
Phillip Witt
Joel Yager
Laura Young
Charles Zaylor

— Marlene M. Maheu, Ph.D.
— Myron L. Pulier, M.D.
— Frank H. Wilhelm, Ph.D.
— Joseph P. McMenamin, M.D., J.D.
— Nancy E. Brown-Connolly, R.N., M.S.N.

The Mental Health Professional and the New Technologies

A Handbook for Practice Today

Introduction

Alice G. went to her second appointment with Dale Giolas, M.D., a psychiatrist who uses his computer desktop as a point of care. In her initial office visit with Dr. Giolas, Alice was given a dual diagnosis of a chemical abuse disorder and another psychiatric disorder; she also received medication prescriptions and a printed description of possible side effects and interactions with other medications.

Dr. Giolas subscribes to InfoScriber, one of several Internet companies that update drug interaction information daily. Dr. Giolas explained, "I use it with every patient every day. It helps me know that I am not hurting them with the medications I am prescribing. I also use InfoScriber as a partial electronic medical record because it tracks a patient's diagnosis, medications, and which diagnosis each medication is targeting. I print this out, handwrite my case notes at the bottom of the page, and put the document in the patient's file.

"If I want to fax a copy to anyone else caring for the same patient, such as a psychotherapist or primary care physician, I get a release from the patient along with the other practitioner's fax number, and I then use a program called WriteFax. If the colleague does not have a secured fax machine, I can give a copy of the InfoScriber printout with my notes to the patient to take to the other practitioner. This is great for building up my referral system, because other practitioners greatly appreciate knowing my diagnosis and any medication changes, and reading my comments on the bottom of the page. It also helps us all if our charts get audited, because there is a complete paper trail of the treatment."

After her first visit, Alice was particularly appreciative of the leaflets Dr. Giolas gave her for the two medications prescribed. She was comforted knowing that her psychiatrist was taking the time to provide her with information tailored to her specific situation. At home, she could read the leaflets at her leisure and come up with questions to ask during her second appointment.

Dr. Giolas said, "There's plenty of reliable information written by other reputable people on the Internet. I don't keep patient information leaflets in my office any more. I print them all off the Internet for each patient."

Within a minute of greeting Alice and both of them getting settled into their respective chairs, Dr. Giolas realized he didn't have her file on his desk. He unobtrusively signaled "Chart" to his office manager through the instant messaging system on his computer. She soon appeared with Alice's chart. Dr. Giolas explained, "I am in immediate contact with any one of several different offices in my facility, so I can send or receive any type of information that I might need during a session with a patient. We have code systems. We all know, for example, that if I type 'chart,' my office manager knows I am missing a chart and she brings it to me. We never use full names on the system but rather the first name and last initial. Everybody knows who I'm talking about because they have my schedule, which is online in a secured Web site accessible only by other staff in my facility."

Once he had Alice's chart, Dr. Giolas reviewed the issues they had discussed during her intake and asked her again about her willingness to attend an outpatient treatment facility for help with her alcohol abuse. She responded that she had given his prior suggestion some thought and would be willing to go, but she was concerned about the cost.

Dr. Giolas told Alice he would check on that and typed an instant message to the manager of the billing department in his facility. The manager was able to look up Alice's insurance carrier, check to see which outpatient treatment facilities it covered, and call the intake coordinator at that facility. The manager obtained an estimate of Alice's cost for a 6-week outpatient treatment program and instant messaged that information back to Dr. Giolas.

Dr. Giolas gave Alice the name of the facility, the name of the intake coordinator, and a rough estimate of costs but informed her that she would need to confirm that information once she went for an intake interview at the treatment center.

Dr. Giolas details other applications of technology in his daily practice: "For $14.95 per month, I use Intranet.com, which allows me to connect with five people from various locations. We can share documents, a chat room, discussion groups, and schedules, and it's all secured so that outsiders can't see what we're doing. For an extra fee, I could add more people. I also use a couple of journal review services. MedLinx has a division called PsychLinx, and for no charge, they will send me the top four or five articles in any area I choose (e.g., addictions, behavioral, geriatrics). I get short blurbs, abstracts, and the opportunity to buy full text. It's great, because I get these for free. Medsite does the same sort of thing, but they charge a fee. You can give them a more specific area of interest, and they will scan over 12,000 articles every month and send you the abstracts. These services make it very easy to keep up with the literature."

Dr. Giolas referred Alice to the alcohol treatment facility but told her he wanted her to keep in touch through his Web site, where he exchanges secured e- mail with patients. "I use this system only with patients whom I've seen and evaluated."

He gave Alice a "skeleton key," which is a password that allows her to enter the Web site to leave messages for him and to read messages he has left for her. She can also read articles he might set aside for her there, too. "Patients can e-mail me from work or home, and whatever answer I send them isn't sitting on someone else's computer; it's at my Web site, instead."

Dr. Giolas has produced a CD-ROM that is self-launching. That is, it starts up by itself when put into a computer's CD-ROM drive. He said, "The CD gives my patients information about my practice and how I work. It also explains the secured Web site, known as an intranet, and how to use it. The software is called PQSafeWeb, and it is designed specifically for secured e-mail and chat messages on the Web. It has lots of other features, and my patients just love it." He added, "These computer-based applications help me deliver better services and help educate my patients in a way that makes them feel more assured of my concern for their specific needs."

—Dale John Giolas, M.D.
CEO
Catalyst Integrations

Alice may be a fictionalized character, but Dr. Giolas is quite real. He is one of a growing number of mental health practitioners who have successfully integrated technology into daily practice. Amid the hum of the computer and the flash of the screen, a patient's personal information is shared, details are revealed, and solace is found—as always, in the time-honored tradition of the therapeutic relationship. As with Dr. Giolas, technological innovation is steadily becoming an enhancement to many different types of health care, including mental health care.

Indeed, unprecedented and inexpensive technologies are already reshaping society, health care, and mental health practice. Laptop computers, mobile phones, personal digital assistants, and portable stereos are permeating everyday experience and steadily building the foundation of a technology-mediated life. Technology will continue to be disseminated throughout the developed world and will become routine, invisible, and indispensable tools for all professions.

The telephone represents one of the first applications of telecommunication technology in mental health. In fact, considerable psychotherapy is already being conducted by telephone and, as detailed in chapter 5, empirical research justifies including expanded use of the telephone in mental health. Appendix A also lists and briefly describes some empirical studies that have shed light on this topic. Although our listing of such studies is neither exhaustive nor an endorsement, it is representative of relevant empirical research. We encourage the thoughtful reader to review appendix A and note the number of research teams that have used the scientific method to examine various topics related to using technology for psychotherapy.

Going one step beyond the telephone, the most immediate promise for mental health care is in *videoconferencing* (two-way communication with moving images). Together with *biometrics* (measuring physiological parameters), videoconferencing technologies will revolutionize health care:

> Each [scientific revolution] produced a consequent shift in the problems available for scientific scrutiny and in the standards by which the profession determined what should count as an admissible problem or as a legitimate problem solution. And each transformed the scientific imagination in ways that we shall ultimately need to describe as a transformation of the world within which scientific work was done.
>
> —(Kuhn, 1962, p. 6)

The spread of telecommunication technologies provides mental and behavioral health care with exciting opportunities in research, teaching, practice, and overall delivery of care. For example, even when used as secondary treatment-delivery vehicles, suitably designed technologies can provide a bridge for continuity of care when the client or practitioner is unavailable for in-person consultation.

Furthermore, as the example from Dr. Giolas shows, technology is making daily practice easier. Clinicians can write reports and make referrals, communicate with colleagues and staff, and retrieve information from records. A worldwide online[1] presence is becoming an ordinary part of the clinical toolbox. An American Medical Association (2002) survey reports that 12% of psychiatrists have a personal Web site. A Datamonitor (2002) report states that 80% of U.S. psychiatrists, 100% of German psychiatrists, and 67% of French psychiatrists polled use the Internet for research. The influential Institute of Medicine, a major quasi-governmental policy-making group in the United States, strongly urges making e-mail more suitable for health care,

---

[1] In this book, the term *online* refers to being in current one- or two-way electronic communication with another entity.

using the Internet for dissemination of information to clinicians and patients, enabling remote access to patient records, establishing chronic care registries, and developing computerized physician order entry systems (Corrigan, Greiner, & Erickson, 2002).

Technology can enhance communication with patients and help them learn about their disorders and their treatments. Tens of thousands of lay-oriented Web sites and electronic discussion groups focus on social or emotional problems (Gross, Anderson, & Powe, 1999; Holden, 2000; Satcher, 1999). These sites have been developed by government agencies, insurance companies, hospitals, universities, foundations, professional associations, consumer organizations, individual practitioners, and laypeople. Beyond discussion of psychiatric disorders is the even heavier Internet traffic concerning psychological and medical self-help, chemical abuse, problems of living, human relationships, and normal human development.

In addition to people seeking information about psychiatric and psychological problems, people with chronic illness and developmental disorders, as well as the burgeoning aging population and caregivers, are turning to telecommunication technologies for contact with peer groups and for better access to health care agencies and professionals (Glueckauf, 2002; Liss, Glueckauf, & Ecklund-Johnson, 2002). The purview of mental health care is thus expanding its range while also blending with less professional approaches, such as "coaching," self-help, "alternative" health care, and spirituality oriented practices. This expansion is creating both a crisis and an opportunity for the mental health professions.

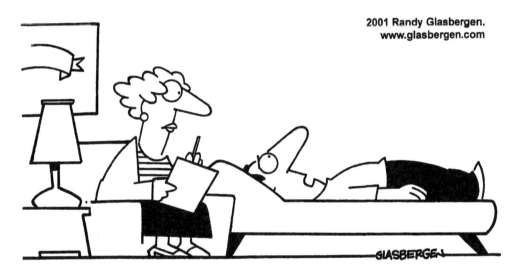

2001 Randy Glasbergen.
www.glasbergen.com

"Opportunity paged me, beeped me, linked me, e-mailed me, faxed me, and spammed me. But I was expecting it to knock!"

Partly because of technology, professional mental health services are coming under increasing commercial control and are at risk of being reduced to a commodity. There are, of course, many good clinical reasons to favor therapy manuals with measurable outcome and a record of efficacy, at least as a starting point for planning treatment. However, practitioners, as well as patients, could come to be regarded as complicated but nonetheless predictable cogs in the wheels of commerce. Already, health specialists are lumped into one category and called providers, or service providers.[2] To the chagrin of many professionals, with business interests and employers dictating health care delivery patterns, health care services are increasingly becoming known as *products* (Oss, 1999). With economic factors driving the health care system, professionals are on a path to continue losing ground to less expensive competitors, particularly those automated by technology.

On the other hand, the technological explosion is helping to shatter some of the greatest obstacles to delivery of behavioral health care—ignorance, stigma, and access. The inevitable advance of technology calls on mental health professionals to find ways to uphold standards of care, to retain their clinical independence, enhance their effectiveness, demonstrate their special value, secure adequate funding for mental health services, and expand the population they reach through the judicious adoption of the emerging *psychotechnologies*.

It is difficult to imagine today's managed care enterprises operating without computers to store information and quickly retrieve it from large databases. The operations of enrollment, verification of benefits, determination of medical necessity, preauthorization of treatment, and claims processing would have been unbearably expensive and error prone without computer networks. Where the adoption of technology will lead is yet to be determined. For now, let's discuss a few key concepts before we describe what we see when we look at the technological waterfront in mental health care.

KEY TERMINOLOGY

We start with the word *psychotechnologies*. At a pace that outstrips the ability of governments or professional associations to regulate, developers of technology are designing powerful new tools to interact directly with mental health patients from a distance. We use the term *psychotechnologies* to denote the many technologies being redirected or specifically designed for delivery of mental health care. We include the telephone because, as we describe in chapter 5, new ways of using and augmenting telephones with new capacities are making significant contributions to mental health care.

The psychotechnologies vary in function, each presenting different potential distortion of communication and relationships when a mental health care professional is interacting with a patient. What we refer to as *psychotechnologies* can be oriented around the professional, the treatment team, the patient, the family unit, the workplace, or the community. We use the term *psychotechnologies* to include:

- Transmission channels (telephone lines or more specialized and high-speed connections).
- Devices (telecommunication devices such as telephones, computers, modems, videophones, etc.). Other technological devices are used for specific functions within mental health care, such as assessment, monitoring, and treatment. These devices include virtual reality biofeedback instrumentation, biosensors, and so on.

---

[2] Health care companies often use the term *provider* or *service provider to denote licensed practitioners* of helping professions and the organizations that employ them.

Overcoming the barriers to using transmission channels and various devices will involve technological innovation, combining various modalities, and developing new therapeutic strategies that will make much current nomenclature obsolete. The general term *psychotechnologies* is proposed for referring to all current and future technologies that are used in mental health.

Specific Definitions

The next sections will describe several terms used by professionals who have adopted various technologies. This discussion is offered as a general guide to the reader and these terms will be used throughout the text.

Telemedicine and Telehealth

"I am often surprised by what the word *telemedicine* elicits when I ask professionals what it means to them. Their visions range from linking metropolitan hospital physicians in a network, to introducing modern medical services into health care."
—(D. Soto, personal communication, July 5, 2001)

Telemedicine is defined by the Telemedicine Information Exchange (TIE, at http://tie.telemed.org) as the use of electronic signals to transfer medical data from one location to another. Although this definition focuses on the communication process, telemedicine has come to refer primarily to clinical or supportive medical practice delivered across distances via telecommunication technology, performed by licensed or otherwise legally authorized individuals. *Tele* is merely a prefix from the Greek language for distance. Of course, some day, this term may seem quaint. Sandy Beinar told us, "I agree with David Balch—the 'tele' will eventually disappear. Telemedicine should be another way of practicing medicine" (personal communication, October 16, 2002). Clinicians experienced in telemedicine consider it a new flavor of medical practice, not an entity separate from "normal" medical services. The following vignette is an example of how such telemedicine services are actually provided in a community.

> *The Arizona Telemedicine Program was created in 1996 by the Arizona state legislature; Representative Bob Burns, chair of Appropriations for the Arizona House of Representatives; and the University of Arizona Health Sciences Center with an initial budget of $1.2 million to establish an eight-site pilot project. Dr. Ronald S. Weinstein, who has been called the Father of Telepathology, was asked to become the director of the telemedicine program. The program is multifaceted, with services provided in more than 55 specialties, including consultations and training in psychiatry.*
>
> *The program has a very active telepsychiatry practice. Clinics are held twice a week in the telemedicine facility. The psychiatry department also regularly sees patients in the clinical area with telemedicine technology. In Tuba City on the Navajo Indian Reservation, the program provides telepsychiatry to two high schools using wireless technology. We discovered that many people in rural sites are reluctant to enter the office of a psychologist or psychiatrist, because of the perceived stigma of having a mental health problem. They are very comfortable entering the telemedicine suite of a rural hospital, because no one knows why they are entering the room.*
>
> *Overall, the program has trained more than 1,000 people in various areas of telemedicine. Employees from each new site that the program brings aboard receive $2\frac{1}{2}$*

days training on telemedicine business, legal, educational, clinical, administrative, and technical practices. Approximately 2 weeks later, telemedicine and technology coordinators are sent to the site to continue training. Training is also provided to Arizona individuals or small groups that are interested in learning about telemedicine. Groups from other states may need to pay a fee for the training services.

—Sandy Beinar
Associate Director
Arizona Telemedicine Program

Design of the Arizona Telemedicine Program is currently the most common model in the United States. It involves a centralized hospital or training facility that offers 24-hour consultation by specialists to general practitioners in outlying and remote areas. Mental or behavioral health care is one of the specialties most often delivered through these videoconferencing networks, along with radiology, oncology, pediatrics, dermatology, and ophthalmology (Myers & Mitchell, 2003; Saab, 2004).

Since 1997, government agencies and legislation have favored the term *telehealth*, but because the older term *telemedicine* persists, particularly for direct service delivery between professionals[3] and clients,[4] we use the words interchangeably in this book. Telehealth has been defined as "the transmission of images, voice and data between two or more health units via telecommunication channels, to provide clinical advice, consultation, education and training services" (NSW Health, 2001). The term now encompasses the use of all electronic technology for health care delivery (Kirby, Hardesty, & Nickelson, 1998). Telehealth ranges from Internet libraries of latest scientific findings for various disorders to satellite connections that transmit interactive video for remote contact with clients to "voice-over-IP" technologies that use computer-mediated audio connections for distance education for professionals. Telehealth also refers to the electronic transmission of physiological data for diagnosis and treatment.

Perhaps looking at a parallel language development for innovation in health care can help us keep the changing terminology in perspective. Although antibiotic medicine was very controversial in the 1930s, it eventually merged with "mainstream medicine" in the 1940s. Similarly, the terms *telehealth, telemedicine,* and perhaps even *psychotechnologies* in behavioral health care will eventually drop out of sight. For now, however, there are important distinctions to be made.

Behavioral Telehealth. *Behavioral telehealth* refers to the use of psychotechnologies to provide behavioral health care services. Making the broad assumption that behavioral and mental health refer to basically the same disciplines, the scientific literature increasingly reflects the use of technology. "Mental health services have been, and continue to be, among the fastest growing applications in [the Office for the Advancement

---

[3] *Clinician* and *practitioner* are other common terms that describe health professionals. For the purposes of this book, however, the more inclusive term *professionals* refers to the wide range of people whose work can benefit from psychotechnologies. The term most often designates licensed practitioners, but in some discussions it designates paraprofessionals.

[4] We refer to people who engage the services of a licensed health professional for treatment interchangeably as *client* and *patient*. Because e-health includes nonprofessional sources offering a broad array of services to caregivers, students, and others who are not seeking treatment, the term *consumer* may be used in place of client and patient, but this term is usually avoided because it is offensive to many psychotherapists who see themselves as delivering a service rather than selling a product. We use *consumer* to refer broadly to carers, patients, friends, family, or the general public seeking health care information.

of Telehealth] telehealth program" (D. Puskin, personal communication, January 8, 2003).

The Telemedicine Information Exchange (2004), an excellent resource for behavioral telehealth programs, lists many programs that involve telecommunication technologies (http://tie.telemed.org/programs/programs.asp). The exact number of behavioral telehealth programs listed on the Web site is difficult to determine because, when searching on the TIE Web site, one can enter the keyword *telepsychiatry* and retrieve a list of 78+ programs. These results, however, may not include programs run strictly for psychotherapy or counseling. Similarly, when searching for resources on the Internet, such keywords as *telemental health* will bring up different results than will *behavioral telehealth*.

Any attempt to survey the field of telecommunications technology in mental and behavioral health will invariably exclude a number of programs. One survey of telehealth programs in 1999 by the Association of Telemedicine Service Providers (http://www.atsp.org) found that 42% included some type of behavioral health care service (Grigsby & Brown, 2000). As stated in the preface, behavioral telehealth offers an abundance of opportunities to professionals willing to take advantage of technology.

One reason for high use of behavioral telehealth is that behavioral services can be delivered using a variety of low-end devices, as well as the more expensive videoconferencing units (described in chapter 5). Also, in contrast to general telehealth, many behavioral telehealth services do not require expensive peripheral devices (i.e., medical instrumentation).

As early as 1959, the Nebraska Psychiatric Institute was using television links for consultations (Benschoter, Witson, & Ingham, 1965; Maxmen, 1977; Wittson & Benschoter, 1972), allowing two parties to view each other interactively, using television sets. "Mental health is one of the most widely accessed services over telehealth systems. This specialty lends itself to interactive videoconferencing technology" (McClosky-Armstrong, 1999).

Today, remote delivery of most mental health consultation is conducted through video links. These links can carry almost every aspect of traditional in-person behavioral and mental health care, including mental status examinations, neuropsychological evaluations, clinical diagnosis, psychotherapy, and crisis intervention. Videoconferencing links also enable education, supervision, research, accessing of client histories, preadmission and discharge planning, administrative functions, staff training, continuing education, case management, court commitment hearings, case conferences, and professional development (DeLeon, Folen, Jennings, & Willis, 1991; DeLeon & Wiggins, 1996; Lamberg, 1997; McCarthy, Kulakowski, & Kenfield, 1994; Smith, 1998; Stamm, 1998; Stamm & Pearce, 1995).

E-Health. E-*health* (or ehealth) is now the preferred term for all clinical telehealth activities delivered through the Internet (McLendon, 2000). Professionals, nonprofessionals, businesses, and clients themselves offer informational, educational, and commercial "products," as well as direct and advocacy services through the Internet. As a term, e-health acts as a bridge connecting telehealth and the Internet (Eng, 2001). In light of the astounding growth of e-health on the Internet, it seems logical for professionals to take advantage of this low-cost and widely accessible medium for many telehealth services (Allen, 1998). E-health continues to be held back, however, by technical limitations of the Internet and by concerns for privacy, confidentiality, security, and data integrity among clients and regulating agencies alike. In chapters 9 and 10, we discuss the legal and ethical issues to be considered.

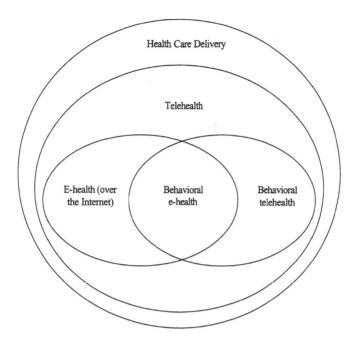

FIG. 1.1. Interactions of terms.

As a subdivision of e-health in general, the term *behavioral e-health* was proposed for using the Internet to deliver behavioral telehealth information and services (Maheu, 2001). Figure 1.1 summarizes the terms introduced thus far.

Even More Terminology.   We need more definitions to pinpoint what is going on in behavioral e-health and in the realm of other psychotechnologies. However, the necessary terminology is in flux, and we can only guess at how definitions might evolve. In this book, the term *online clinical practice* refers to the use of psychotechnologies to deliver therapeutic dialogue at a distance, whether conducted over a direct video link (e.g., telepsychology or telepsychiatry) or over a network, such as the Internet (e.g., therapy online). We include diagnostic procedures, psychotherapy, or any clinical discussion with a client—as well as supervision or case management with trainees or other professionals.

Other terms describing therapeutic contact with clients using psychotechnologies include *e-counseling, cybercounseling, cybertherapy, teletherapy, telemental health, telepsychiatry, e-therapy,* and *behavioral e-care.* More detailed discussions of such nomenclature and terminology are found in chapter 10. In the mass media, articles that refer to online therapy often pertain to e-mail or chat rooms and ignore the use of videoconferencing technology or other research-based combinations of technology to provide mental health care.

Text-based refers to communication media that involves only writing, such as conventional e-mail or chat rooms. *In-person* includes communications where the parties are located in the same room (i.e., one could shake the other's hand). *Face-to-face* is a common term that many use interchangeably with in-person, but it is avoided in this book to reduce confusion when talking about videoconferencing, through which each party can see the face of the other.

During this time of rapid growth and transformation, it is to be expected that new terms will inevitably emerge, that some will persist, and that others will be lost in . . . where else . . . cyberspace. *Cyberspace* refers to the conceptual venue for all computer-mediated electronic communications at a distance over electronic networks, including the Internet. In cyberspace resides the information available on the networks. People "enter" or even "inhabit" this online world. The adjective *virtual* (as in virtual clinic or virtual reality) is used for entities that exist by virtue of technology, as distinguished from *real*.

To clarify, there is a gradient between the real and the technologically created. For example, although computers are increasingly able to approximate reality with better and better video capabilities, there is still a difference in reality among in-person psychotherapy, videoconferenced psychotherapy sessions, and discussing problems with a therapist simulated by a computer.

We are now ready to discuss what makes the psychotechnologies so important and how they are changing mental health care.

INFLUENCE OF THE PSYCHOTECHNOLOGIES

The psychotechnologies are already here, and they are here to stay. Even the relatively conservative Medicare program pays for individual psychotherapy sessions via psychotechnologies (US Department of Health and Human Services, 2001a). Some existing psychotechnologies are clearly cost-effective and are rapidly being improved. As we show, they are proving their benefit for both clinical and administrative applications.

Of course, there are drawbacks slowing the rate at which psychotechnologies are entering mainstream mental health practice. Indeed, there are serious impediments ahead. However, we are on the brink of enormous expansion in the demand for what may be called behavioral services, and the psychotechnologies will be drafted to help meet it. Although economic factors may dominate resulting trends, much will also depend on the efforts of individuals and organizations motivated by idealism and altruism, by scientific curiosity and humanitarian objectives. Amidst the tension between commercial and clinical interests, and between opportunism and responsible practice, the many roles of mental health professionals are being recast.

Benefits to Using the Psychotechnologies

The greatest challenge for the psychotechnologies may be to reach people with severe social or emotional problems who receive no treatment at all; there are an estimated 2 million such people in the United States alone (Hobson & Leonard, 2001). Psychotechnologies have the potential to reach these people because of the five main benefits they provide: accessibility, affordability, anonymity, acceptability, and adaptability. Psychotechnologies have the potential to provide unprecedented access to many people by allowing satellite clinics to be dispersed throughout rural areas. These clinics could then connect with a regional center to provide treatment to underserved populations (Myers, Sulzbacher, & Melzer, 2003; Palmer, Montgomery & Harland, 2003). Similarly, the psychotechnologies may be expeditiously deployed on a global scale in war-torn areas to train and guide local personnel in trauma-response measures. Patients from disadvantaged groups also may benefit (Thomas, 2003). Sadly, those people in the greatest need for access to health care are often subjected to high cost and poor quality of care (Bashshur, 2001).

Behavioral telehealth services may be a solution to this problem. They can now be found in rural clinics, military programs, correctional facilities, community mental health centers, nursing homes, home health care settings, and hospitals. The initial development and provision of these services have been funded largely by grants that have enabled these programs to set precedents for appropriate delivery of mental health services to people with social, behavioral, and emotional problems. At the very least, telehealth services generally reduce the burdens associated with geographic distance (Gibson, 2000; McCarthy, Kulakowski, & Kenfield, 1994; Oberkirch, 2000; Runyon, Han, Hilty, Roberts, Roach, & Connor, 2003; Smith, 1998; Stamm, 1998; Stamm & Pearce, 1995; Whitten, Zaylor, & Kingsley, 2000; Zaylor, 2000).

The following vignette exemplifies how psychotechnologies are making psycho therapy more accessible and are offering novel advantages:

> *A 16-year-old girl was involuntarily committed to the Adolescent Unit of the state psychiatric facility after her parents reported death threats against them. Her diagnosis was oppositional defiant disorder. Over several weeks of hospitalization, the treatment team reported no apparent problems with her on the unit or when the parents came for visits, during which the parents remained casual and nonconfrontational. The patient's discharge was expected shortly. The treatment team decided to use a newly installed videoconferencing system for family therapy sessions in a connection to the mental health center in order to spare the parents a 3-hour drive, one way, to the hospital.*
>
> *In the first videoconference family therapy session, the parents confronted their daughter about the threats that she had made when she was at home. They described their fear of her. The girl reacted violently and angrily, yelling, "I told you I would kill you if you told them about this." She had to be restrained and removed from the room. The parents had previously been afraid to confront her directly, fearing her reaction.*
>
> *This session was the turning point in this adolescent's treatment. In continued family sessions over the network, she came to recognize the destructiveness of her behavior and its effects on her relationship with her parents.*
>
> **—Henry A. Smith, L.C.S.W.**
> **Cumberland Mountain Community Services**

As illustrated in our vignette, videoconferencing offers not only enhanced accessibility but also may improve cost-effectiveness and treatment outcome (McCrone, 2003). This promise is supported by the results of early studies (Troester, Paolo, Glatt, Hubble, & Koller, 1995; Zarate et al., 1997). There is even initial evidence "that telemedicine works well for group therapy as well as individual consults" (U.S. Department of Commerce, 1997, p. 19). The reliability of diagnoses made through videoconferencing has been particularly well established by research (Ball, McLaren, Summerfield, Lipsedge, & Watson, 1995; Dongier, Tempier, Lalinec-Michaud, & Meunier, 1986; Doze, Simpson, Hailey, & Jacobs, 1999; Zaylor, 1999).

It has been asserted that rural and frontier behavioral telehealth programs may benefit mental health clients through cost savings from reduced travel by clients and health care professionals, increased access to quality specialist care, and other factors (Trott & Blignault, 1998). Enter the psychotechnologies, a promising new approach to society's mental health challenges that has something for everyone:

- Improving public knowledge about mental health.
- Directly enabling better mental health care.
- Making treatment more available, more transparent, and more manageable.

- Curbing costs.
- Addressing the needs of an aging population.
- Helping to address drug abuse, crime, and high-risk behaviors.
- Adapting flexibly to the special needs of groups of people worldwide.

Other psychotechnologies can help monitor and document progress, provide professional education, and support practice management. They can link complementary disciplines to provide comprehensive treatment and seamless transition as patients progress from one treatment venue to the next. Furthermore, computerization can make the administration and assessment of psychological tests more convenient, less expensive, faster, and more accurate, leading to wider adoption of an important informational resource for health care practitioners (Randolph, 2002).

The Internet brings an immense volume of current and relevant health information to our fingertips (Ebenezer, 2003). Through a glass fiber no wider than a human hair, the complete Library of Congress can be transmitted in less than a half hour (Alcatel, 2000). By September 2002, more than 182 million people were users of the Internet in the United States and Canada (NUA Internet Surveys, 2003). According to a survey by Harris Interactive (2002), 80% of U.S. Internet users have looked for health care information (Harris Interactive, 2002). With increased access to the Internet, patients can identify potential mental health problems, gain access to insurance benefits, find the names of local practitioners, and initiate treatment more easily.

Internet communication formats, such as chat rooms, e-mail, and discussion boards (see chapter 3), enable people to seek and offer support in novel ways. In these virtual places, people share personal information to a depth unprecedented in the in-person world (Maheu & Subotnik, 2001). People otherwise reluctant to seek out mental health services may find the Internet a desirable and viable place to begin getting help.

More immediate applications of information technology cover automation of billing, obtaining preauthorization, claims submission and processing, reporting, practitioner credentialing, and appointment scheduling. Errors owing to lost paper files may be reduced by electronic systems, and back-office functions may run more efficiently.

One might then ask, "If the psychotechnologies are so great, why aren't we seeing more of them?" Aside from the U.S. NASDAQ crash of 2001, there is a downside to technology. In addition to cost, inconvenience, unreliability, and ignorance, there are potential harmful effects of technology that need to be addressed.

Barriers to Using the Psychotechnologies

> The message of any medium or technology is the change of scale or pace or pattern that it introduces into human affairs.... All electrical appliances, far from being labor-saving devices, are new forms of work, decentralized and made available to everybody.
> —(McLuhan, 1964, p. 153)

Just as the right set of clothes can put a lift in someone's step, adopting psychotechnologies can make subtle but profound changes in the message practitioners give. Applying psychotechnologies can not only empower clinicians but also guide or distract them. Electronic patient record systems emphasize quantifiable and checklist variables. Much that is intuitive in psychotherapy and pharmacotherapy can be pushed aside in favor of "objective" data. Furthermore, automation of procedures can perpetuate the denigration of dynamic aspects of treatment.

Researchers have described many barriers to progress in the telehealth field, including problems within organizations, lack of research, legal and ethical problems, cost, and general resistance to psychotechnologies (Institute of Medicine, 1996; Weil & Rosen, 1997). The lack of applications for efficient integration into practice may have made physicians hesitant to explore behavioral telehealth (Kassirer, 2000). Ironically, though, when a limitation is noticed in an area of technology that has reached critical mass, enterprising individuals usually can be found to capitalize on the limitation. Telehealth technologies have reached critical mass in general medicine, and mental health will soon catch up.

Opportunities abound for individuals and organizations that seek to improve on existing limitations. Organizations that have invested heavily in legacy[5] administrative and clinical information systems may hesitate to scrap their systems (Eng, 2001), but as critical mass is achieved in mental health, these companies may find themselves falling behind those that have sought to improve on behavioral telehealth technologies. Understandably, larger organizations must deal with training and maintaining staff to use the new systems, which may be expensive and frustrating and may slow office operation until the staff becomes accustomed to the new procedures (Institute of Medicine, 1996).

A primary barrier to the widespread adoption of behavioral telehealth is the unreliability of the research methodologies used in early telehealth studies; they suffer from small participant populations, poor design, and a lack of standardization of measured criteria (Whitten & Mair, 2000). Research also has yet to establish reasonable requirements for outcome measurement (Glueckauf, in press; Glueckauf et al., 2002). Although satisfaction reported by both professionals and users with various telehealth interventions is generally high, findings are inconclusive because lack of standardization sometimes leads to contradictory results. Without more high-quality empirical research, there may not be enough definable benefits to justify using many of the psychotechnologies. As yet, only a small fraction of professionals are integrating technology into their practice (Eng, 2001). Most mental health is focused on the individual patient and not on the systems level.

Legal and liability issues also abound. For example, the South Australian Mental Health Services and the South Australian Health Commission began a pilot project connecting two centers using real-time two-way videoconferencing for telepsychiatry. Users expressed support for the medium, and many clients were able to stay in their rural towns. Problems arose when the equipment proved unreliable and prone to breakdown, shifting attention to legal and ethical issues regarding telepsychiatry (Mitchell & Mitchell, 1994).

In the United States, the uncertainties of the legal landscape make it particularly difficult to anticipate legal risks. It is obviously much more difficult to guard against risks that are not yet identifiable. A state may protect itself under the doctrine of sovereign immunity (Cepelewicz, 1998), but practitioners and independent clinics are fair game for lawsuits. To be sure, many of these issues will be addressed in due time. The Health Insurance Portability and Accountability Act of 1996 (see chapter 9 for a further discussion) is a step toward resolving some barriers involved in using telehealth technologies.

Another barrier to widespread adoption of the psychotechnologies for direct care is that penetration of electronic methods into health care delivery is seen as a threat

---

[5] Information technology workers apply the term *legacy* to existing automated or manual information systems that they wish to replace and to the data therein that they may wish to conserve.

to the already dwindling practitioner-patient relationship. Ever fewer patients in the United States have much of a personal relationship with their primary care physicians, and many don't even realize that such a physician has been assigned to them. It comes as a surprise to many practitioners and patients alike that the psychotechnologies can reverse this trend by assisting with continuity of care. Technology can provide links to practitioners through time and geographical distance—through busy work schedules, snow storms, lack of transportation.

Nonetheless, the psychotechnologies are vulnerable to being blamed for depersonalization of health care delivery, especially in mental health. Practitioners as well as patients can experience telecommunication and other technologies as foreign or distancing. Some people prefer in-person contact, even if it means fewer visits or visits with different practitioners over time.

Depersonalization cannot be blamed on technology alone, however. Clients routinely report in psychotherapy that they merely tolerate relationships with health care professionals triaged or chosen by zip code from insurance lists or insurance Web sites. Clients often comply with this arrangement because they see it as the only way to access their insurance benefits. Third-party payers have captured the "locus of control" in treatment. As a result, some health care can be more dangerous than none at all (McCoy, 2002). Mental health professionals are frequently chosen in the same impersonal manner as are other health care practitioners. They can be found through triage from an insurance carrier's telephone access center or at random from a list on an insurance Web site. Private referral still exists but is increasingly outdated. Patients as well as practitioners are feeling the repercussions.

Further barriers to using the psychotechnologies arise from erosion of privacy with the misuse of personal information by numerous entities. There is also serious question about whether telecommunication links can support the intense involvement and intimacy thought essential in some aspects of mental health treatment. All these considerations are cogent and have practical importance, but they will not slow the juggernaut of the psychotechnologies. Rather than either blindly resisting or just grinning and bearing it, the professional community needs research and education to understand the pros and cons of psychotechnology, to explore ways to preserve what might otherwise be lost, and to use technology to deliver higher quality care.

PSYCHOTECHNOLOGIES AND THE DEMAND
FOR MENTAL HEALTH SERVICES

Now is the time for professionals to harness the growing power of the psychotechnologies. Mental illness is considered one of the top health concerns in the world (Gross, Anderson, & Powe, 1999; Holden, 2000; Satcher, 1999). The World Health Organization (WHO, at http://www.who.org) estimates that one in four people worldwide develops at least one mental or behavioral disorder during his or her life (World Health Organization, 2001). The landmark U.S. Surgeon General's report (Satcher, 1999), which emphasized the extent of mental illnesses at all ages, enunciated mainstream professional opinion. It stimulated policymakers at least to acknowledge the disparity between the need for mental health treatment and the availability of services in the United States. Recognition of the need for mental health services, together with continuing progress in viable treatment alternatives, make convincing arguments to increase funding and support from national governments and large employers (Tanouye, 2001).

Economics and Mental Health Care

Even though the growing availability of the psychotechnologies offers ways to secure more support for mental health, it could instead work against professionals. Funding opportunities extend beyond grants for demonstration projects and for setting up videoconferencing facilities. Potentially, the psychotechnologies can help mental health care gain credibility and acceptance, can help show its economic and social importance, and can even allow it to expand its scope and redefine its mission, eventually giving mental health a greater claim on health care expenditures and drawing more commercial investments.

Historically, airtight arguments alone have not sufficed to attract adequate financial backing for mental health research or care. In the United States, success with funding has been typically the result of a confluence of public outcry and a politician's awareness. The public usually reacts to the media's exposure of a dreadful situation. A politician might then champion a cause related to mental health or chemical dependency. We might next see an urgency to channel funds to meet the needs of the identified cause. This happy chain of events has sparked several reforms in mental health. Examples include the development of insane asylums as an alternative to imprisonment of severely mentally ill people and the more recent deinstitutionalization policy, with diversion of patients to community mental health centers. These and other innovations lost momentum, perhaps in part because severely mentally ill people have lacked social power, because mental illness in general has been stigmatized, and because there was no prospect of continued financial profit for any stakeholders who had political clout. Will history repeat yet again?

As for attracting sustained support, the psychotechnologies can enhance mental health service delivery, reduce stigma, and draw a large proportion of the mainstream population into the general "mental health" orbit. They can also streamline operations and reduce expenses for practitioners, patients, and third-party carriers. Specific psychotechnologies may be sufficiently compelling to fire up the bureaucratic imagination and attract political support. The telecommunication technologies that directly support the business side of mental health care may initially receive more attention than do more clinical applications, despite the potentially greater economies of clinical applications as practitioners develop service strategies to work with patients.

Judicious investment in the psychotechnologies will be money well spent—and money will be spent. Third-party payers are interested in involving computers and electronic communications much more in both administrative and clinical aspects of mental health care. Even cautious executives are allocating resources to promote automation through technology. Business-oriented applications of technology are creating an infrastructure on which clinical applications can flourish. Conversely, clinical benefits can hasten professional acceptance and cooperation with administrative needs. In any case, we are seeing the onset of a sea change in how mental health care will be delivered. This change will expose festering problems and create new ones, point to opportunities, present interesting policy questions, and ultimately transform mental health practice.

As technology advances, it may quite suddenly help transform the field into a seller's market. The mental health professions should be prepared to use the psychotechnologies to meet such a rapid increase in demand rather than let a major opportunity slip from their grasp. Instead, this opportunity could fall into the hands of people who would profit from mental health without much regard for patients' welfare.

Fees and payment need to be clarified when using various psychotechnologies. There was a time when the patient actually paid the doctor, whether in cash or in chickens. World War II brought wage and price controls that employers, eager to compete for workers and to appease the unions, evaded by offering health care coverage as a tax-free form of additional compensation for the workforce. Employees now value such benefits on a par with actual pay. European governments increasingly assumed responsibility for health care, and even the United States created its Medicare program in 1965. Geriatric psychiatry has flourished under this program. Lately, however, Medicare funding for mental health services has been cut.

Already by the 1970s, a substantial proportion of payment for mental health services was coming directly from third-party payers in the United States. In the 1980s, the third parties began to control reimbursement schedules and reduced reimbursement rates (Hayes, Barlow, & Nelson-Gray, 1999), to introduce preauthorization requirements, and to encourage subspecialized practice, with one practitioner prescribing medications and another offering behavior modification treatment or psychotherapy. Today, many providers feel that the way to increase their income to previous levels is to treat a larger and more heterogeneous population (Hayes, Barlow, & Nelson-Gray, 1999).

According to the estimates given by Open Minds (http://www.openminds.com), per employee behavioral health benefit costs in the United States decreased between 1988 and 1997 from $151.54 to $69.61 annually (M. Oss, personal communication, October 25, 2002). Reasons for this rapid decline in employer spending have been hotly debated by such futurists as Cummings (1996). Reasons Oss (2001) identifies include:

- Payers seeking "value" by demanding documentation of costs and benefits.
- New technologies creating a market "substitution effect" and new economies of scale.
- Changing supply of programs and professionals, with increasing reliance on paraprofessionals.
- Changing managed health care service distribution channels.
- Consolidation within the health and social service fields.
- Increasing use of privatization, competition, and managed care techniques in public human service systems.
- Changing workplace demographics, causing evolution of private sector services.

More specifically, payers, such as employers and state and county officials, began demanding more accountability in health care spending, particularly in mental health care. Dollars were diverted from traditional mental health specialists to managed behavioral health care companies. In the United States, enrollees using services delivered through managed care increased from 34 million employees in July 1990 to 81 million in July 1999. Kiesler (2000) reports that managed care accounts for the majority of health care delivery in the United States, with 75% of the insured population enrolled in a managed care plan. Of these enrollees, 88% are covered under a managed mental health carve-out program. In a carve-out arrangement management of benefits is contracted out or given over to a division focused on the special issues posed by mental health care. While this can bring more expertise to bear on such matters as so-called medical necessity and can enable insurance benefits to be administered

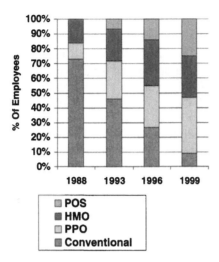

FIG. 1.2. Employer shift to managed care plans. Reprinted with permission of OPEN MINDS, 2002.

more wisely and more flexibly, isolating mental health transactions can obscure how improvements in mental health care delivery can enhance general health and lower overall medical treatment costs.

Medicaid recipients have also been coming under managed care, with the proportion rising from 2% in 1982 to about 61% by 1999 (M. Oss, personal communication, October 25, 2002). The dramatic shift from conventional health insurance to managed care is shown in Figure 1.2. In one decade, managed care had changed the economics of health care.

The largest players in the managed behavioral care world are represented in Table 1.1, with the beleaguered Magellan having the largest market share. However they might jockey for position, such plans will dominate decisions about implementing

TABLE 1.1
Enrollment of Covered Lives for the Largest Managed Behavioral
Health and Employee Assistance Programs

Program	Enrollment in 1000s
Magellan Behavioral Health	69,353
ValueOptions	22,154
United Behavioral Health	20,015
CIGNA Behavioral Health	12,250
MHN, Inc.	9,427
APS Healthcare, Inc.	7,200
First Health Services of Tenn.	6,039
ComPsych Corporation	5,486
FEI Behavioral Health	4,200
PacifiCare Behavioral Health	4,141
Remainder of the market	51,444

1999 enrollment: 193 million
2000 enrollment: 220.1 million

Reprinted with permission of OPEN MINDS, 2002.

automated services for their provider networks, from "back-office" functions such as credentialing and authorizations, to billing and verification of benefits.[6]

Cummings Budman, & Thomas (1998) stated that at the height of solo fee-for-service practice, 20% of patients accounted for 70% of all mental health care expenses. Since then, reallocation of funds by managed care has had profound effects on mental health care. For example, Sanchez and Turner (2003) noted that by providing brief therapy to patients who respond to short-term therapy, the health system may better afford psychotherapy for patients who would benefit from longer-term treatment. It has also been argued that with fewer people using the bulk of resources, mental health decision makers would have the opportunity and the task of finding service delivery methods to reach a broader segment of the population. Practitioners might claim that these are perhaps goals, but the reality is that resources have been hoarded by managed care companies rather than fairly distributed to underserved groups. The use of technology may be a way to redress some of these inequities.

Paradoxically, up to this point, technology has damaged some of the economic climate for mental health care in the United States rather than improved it. Throughout the Western world, the continuing rise in health care costs has forced political bodies and funding agencies to search for cost reduction strategies, with mental health sometimes targeted as being expendable. In addition to economic pressure, maturing concepts of mental health treatment are creating demands for efficiency and "evidence-based" practice and are affecting research agendas, theories of change and intervention, and practice patterns, not always for the good.

Now we are seeing converging client and commercial demand, technological innovation, decreasing equipment costs, increasing competition in the health care marketplace, and both federal and individual state legislative and regulatory support (Bashshur, 1997; Kirby, Hardesty, & Nickelson, 1998). In the United States, the health care revenue stream—close to $1.4 trillion in 2001 and perhaps $2.2 trillion by 2008 (Levit et al., 2000; Smith, Heffler, & Freeland, 1999)—generates much interest. People seeking to improve health care are looking for ways to reduce administrative inefficiencies and waste, estimated by some critics to be perhaps a quarter of this spending (Eng, 2001). As former U.S. Senate Minority Leader Everett McKinley Dirksen supposedly said—a trillion here, a trillion there, and pretty soon you're talking real money.[7]

Reducing the cost of monitoring treatment for even a small proportion of clients could result in substantial savings to the health industry (Mechanic, 2001). Some people feel that telehealth could slash much of the wasted spending in health care, whereas others fear additional costs and complications. The Towers Perrin Health Care Cost Survey follows the average cost of health care for large employers' health benefit plans (Towers Perrin, 2002). Mental disorders (not including those from alcohol and other chemical abuse) account for a substantial proportion of such costs. Seemingly reliable estimates are that 18.5 to 21% of Americans experience a clinically significant mental health disorder during any given year (Narrow, Rae, Robins, & Regier, 2002; Satcher, 1999), resulting in an estimated $77 billion in direct-care costs to mental health services (Johnson, 2001). Treatment for chemical abuse pushes the total much higher.

---

[6] To be sure, in most smaller facilities and private practices the "paperwork" is done in the front office, with back offices reserved for clinical work, but business interests are increasingly taking charge of both treatment and terminology.

[7] This is an urban myth. Senator Dirksen never said anything of the kind (see http://www.dirksencenter.org/featuresBillionHere.htm).

Organizations that foot much of the bill for such services but that fail to identify and incorporate new technologies may find financial stability elusive. A national economy that depends on improvements in worker "productivity" to stave off the next recession or depression can no longer afford to ignore the direct and indirect impact of mental health and chemical dependency issues. Dwindling revenue makes it imperative to identify technologies that reduce costs and improve service (Oss, 2001).

The expansion of the telecommunication infrastructure has temporarily stalled from a spate of frantic overbuilding (Cummins & Spagat, 2002). As predicted by Oss (2001), evaporation of tax dollars is straining local and state budgets. However, these setbacks have not prevented continued suffusion of technologies into the mental health arena. Contractors for behavioral health services are creating lower-cost care management systems, such as those that serve several companies at once. Computer assessment, case matching, service management, and automation of routine trans-actions are being implemented to reduce payer organization payrolls and improve productivity. Wholesale introduction of software for practice management, managed care, and computer assessment of outcome, along with technology-enabled profes-sional services and online interactive client services, is being considered for similar potential.

Investment in technology for clinical services is lagging behind that for adminis-trative activities. Although some studies predict that behavioral telehealth services can be cost-effective (Troester et al., 1995; Zarate et al., 1997), other reports point to the expense of maintaining equipment and the current lack of industry-wide techno-logical standards that may delay the date when the Internet will save enough money and time and sufficiently aid professionals in providing substantially better care to justify the cost (Eng, 2001).

Multidisciplinary Behavioral Telehealth Programs.   Economic and clinical factors increasingly favor a multidisciplinary approach to mental health treatment. Such fac-tors as cost-effective deployment of tasks to the appropriate professionals, workflow issues, and limitations in clinical competence, scope of practice, and licensure call for collaborative, coordinated efforts by team members with complementary skill sets. Using telehealth technology, multidisciplinary teams can address such problems as eating disorders (Goldfield & Boachie, 2003; Myers & Mitchell, 2003), obesity, and substance abuse and can provide counseling related to chronic illness regardless of the physical location of the professional staff. Telehealth technology can also make it easier to draw in a patient's primary care physician, the school nurse, a vocational rehabilitation case worker, and/or other professionals. Family members can be in-cluded on the treatment team, to address social service concerns for elderly patients in long-term care or at home, for example. Of course, the participants would need to sign appropriate consent forms. Perhaps most important, the client can become a more actively participating part of a telehealth treatment team.

Technology and medicine are revolutionizing the delivery of health care. Telere-habilitation, a versatile interdisciplinary tool that can facilitate home- or community-based rehabilitation, is the provision of health care and consultative services to individual patients or family members over distance using telecommunication tech-nologies. Comprehensive, coordinated rehabilitation services can reduce mortality and improve functional outcomes for people who have suffered a brain injury, such as a ruptured cerebral aneurysm. Long-term interventions are usually required to reduce the risk of secondary complications and to achieve optimal physical and psy-chosocial recovery.

The following case example illustrates the collaborative nature of some telehealth programs and the benefits to clients in applying psychotechnologies to serve real needs. Family-centered care using a videophone was provided to Don, who had experienced accident-related neurotrauma and was living in his sister's home. A health psychologist and multidisciplinary team communicated with Don and his immediate caregivers to provide treatment and improve the quality of life for all persons involved.

Telerehabilitation services were provided to Don, a 35-year-old male who sustained multiple aneurysms, and to his caregivers using existing public telephone lines and two-way interactive videophones, which provide audio and video communication. All transmissions were private and accomplished using a home telephone (a plain old telephone system, or POTS, line). While a physical therapist and speech language pathologist worked with Don, I worked with his sister, Sheila, and her husband on family psychotherapy and adjustment to Don's disability.

Don was transferred from a neurotrauma unit out of state to a long-term care facility in the state where his sister and brother-in-law reside. Eventually, he was transferred to an acute rehabilitation unit for about 1 month. When he was discharged, his sister and brother-in-law did not want Don to return to a nursing home facility, so they made every effort to bring him to their home and care for him with the assistance of home health and our telerehabilitation program. Don has been in this home setting for more than a month and a half and has had three to four teletherapy consultations per week.

As a psychologist who works with brain injury, I believe that the telecommunication technology, along with e-mail, has allowed this family to assume a more active role in Don's care and maintenance. Without this support, this young man most likely would be placed in a nursing home with little to no opportunity to receive community-based resources and would have a much reduced quality of life.

Don's sister writes: "I am a little down today. Maybe too much for my emotions this past month. I don't know what I would do without you in Don's corner. I just hope it hasn't caused problems for you and your colleagues. I personally appreciate all the support you have given me over the months. I couldn't have come this far without you and kept my sanity. I'm sure I would have fallen apart by now under the pressure of it all. It has made me stronger, and I do not look at the days the same anymore . . . they are more precious."

—Pamela G. Clark, Ph.D.
Director, Clinical Development
INTEGRIS Jim Thorpe Rehabilitation Center

The support that families and caregivers receive is vital to their emotional health in continuing care for their family member. As members of the human community, professionals need the advantages afforded by technology to reach a broader number of people to provide that support.

The following vignette also illustrates the ease and benefit of using telehealth equipment for multidisciplinary case management. The persons involved have requested anonymity.

An HIV seropositive adolescent presented at the local physician's office with multiple complaints. The young man had been noncompliant with his medication regime. He also had been unwilling to let friends know he was taking medicine, fearing they would learn of his HIV status. When in the physician's office, he reported multiple physical symptoms and emotional issues and a lack of family support. The rural area where he lived offered no specialized HIV services. The patient had been seen by a specialist in HIV care who had traveled to the patient's area for a monthly clinic until the previous year, when the specialist was no longer able to make the 10-hour trip.

Using an interactive videoconferencing system recently installed in one of the examining rooms, the nurse practitioner on duty in the physician's office was able to identify the university medical center where that specialist was on staff. An online consultation was scheduled for later that day. The HIV patient was greatly relieved and intrigued to hear that he would soon be seeing his former specialist by remote technology. The specialist recognized the adolescent, gladly provided the needed expertise, and developed a plan of care with the local practitioner. The communication link provided the opportunity for the patient to receive encouragement to continue his medication regimen, not only from his specialist but also by receiving online counseling and social services from a team of mental health practitioners specializing in HIV and family issues.

With the physician's office used as the local base of operations, follow-up was scheduled and completed on a routine basis by the local clinic primary care provider and the HIV center mental health staff, who were all licensed in the patient's state of residence.

As a result, this young man received good medical support, improved his compliance with his medication regimens, and, along with his family, was given specialized counseling not available through other means. Subsequently, a regular clinic via videoconferencing was organized, providing much-needed continuity and expertise for other local HIV patients. Primary care practitioners were able to benefit by receiving up-to-date education while collaborating with the HIV specialty center.

—**Anonymous**

Home Health Care. The U.S. Administration on Aging projects that the number of U.S. citizens over the age of 65 years will double to nearly 70 million by 2030. The current population of citizens over 65 totals around 35 million and makes up approximately 13% of the entire U.S. population (Administration on Aging, 2001). An estimated 22.1% of U.S. adults over the age of 18 suffer from a diagnosable mental illness within any given year (National Institute of Mental Health, 2001), and 4 of the 10 leading causes of disability for persons 5 and older are mental disorders (Satcher, 1999). According to the National Mental Health Association (2001), 18% of American adults with clinical depression and/or generalized anxiety disorder do not receive treatment for the condition, and many other common debilitating conditions, such as social anxiety disorder or panic disorder, are similarly underrecognized and undertreated. Although some mental or emotional problems tend to subside with age, other conditions, such as Alzheimer's disease, require behavioral interventions and caregiver support. In some cases, the need rises sharply with age.

The implications for the psychotechnologies are staggering. The potential impact of the aging population and the need to provide more services at home are two reasons telehomecare is likely to become one of the fastest-growing market segments. The ability of practitioners to interface directly with clients and caregivers in the home, reliably and frequently, will affect all areas of health care. People desire to make positive decisions regarding their health and the health of family members, and most of those decisions occur where they live—at home.

Telehomecare has been found to be highly acceptable to clients, and it offers cost savings and improvement in the quality of life (Johnston, Wheeler, Deuser, & Sousa, 2000). People who have chronic illnesses, are experiencing depression, need hospice services or counseling, or suffer from agoraphobia and need social services can be accommodated at home. Although the demand for telehomecare has been clearly established, the question of reimbursement for organizations and professionals still remains. Currently, private payment and business models that use telecommunications as adjuncts to other services, capitated models for care, and grant funding have sustained telehomecare programs. A reimbursement model that satisfies the requirement of fair payment but realizes the cost-saving potential is still needed.

A rich source of information in planning telehomecare services is the Web site of the Home Telehealth Community of Care (http://www.informationfortomorrow.com). This Web site provides monthly information on key areas of concern about effective options for the delivery of health care in the home. The American Medical Association (AMA) guidelines for medical management of patients at home (http://www.ama-assn.org/ama/pub/article/2036-2466.html) and the American Telemedicine Association (ATA) telehomecare guidelines (http://www.atmeda.org/news/guidelines.html) are also good resources.

The benefits of home applications in mental health can clearly be seen in the following case example from the Kentucky TeleCare program (http://www.mc.uky.edu/kytelecare). Travel in Kentucky is not always easy. The frontier nurses gained a reputation for arriving on horseback to deliver babies in the "hollers," and some areas still remain remote.

A child psychiatrist who is quite familiar with our telemedicine program inquired if she could use telehealth technology to communicate with a young patient who lived nearly 100 miles away and needed nearly daily therapy sessions. The family was very stressed and could not make daily trips to the clinic. The child had been hospitalized several times for her condition, spending a total of several months in psychiatric care. The location of her last hospitalization was more than 700 miles from her home. She had spent more than a month in the pediatric unit.

Dr. Laurie Humphries, a child psychiatrist in Lexington, Virginia, felt that if she did not have daily contact with the patient and was not easily available for crisis situations, the child would continue to require hospitalization. The family was invited to see a demonstration of a telehealth system that operated on plain telephone lines, and the parents were so impressed that they agreed to purchase a unit for under $500 for their daughter. The system was installed in the child's bedroom, and every afternoon after school, the child psychiatrist placed a video call. A live, interactive videoconference was conducted. The psychiatrist was able to conduct ongoing therapy sessions from her office while the patient was in her room, sitting comfortably on her bed. During the next 18 months, the sessions became less frequent, and eventually the patient required only occasional televisits.

According to the psychiatrist, telemedicine had a tremendous impact on this child's treatment program. In a report, she stated that "easy access to therapy services eliminated additional hospitalizations and reduced the time the child was in therapy." This was a win/win situation. The patient and her family saved money and additional stress by eliminating the need for travel, the child was able to receive the therapy she required for recovery, the insurance company did not have to pay for expensive additional hospitalizations, and the psychiatrist was able to deliver desperately needed services to a child who lived hours away.

This application used a very simple POTS-based (telephone dial-up) videoconference system. Such systems are very inexpensive and very easy to operate. We have used these systems for many physical, mental, and behavioral health applications and expect to continue to use them to reach those patients who cannot afford the initial and ongoing expenditures of traditional videoconference technology.

—Rob Sprang, M.B.A.
Director
Kentucky Telecare

Another innovative use of technology is BabyCarelink, a program designed to provide parents of a premature infant hospitalized for extended periods with a direct video connection to their hospitalized infant (e-Health-Media, 2002). This program is highly successful and has survived on its own after the grant-funding period (C. Safran, personal communication, July 19, 2001). Prematurity and ensuing bonding issues, coupled with family stress and a higher incidence of physical disabilities, are factors that can lead to a higher incidence of abuse and neglect for premature infants.

Disease Management. Considerable resources are being spent on chronic conditions, but little change typically occurs in the health status of the affected populations. A "disease management" approach can reduce cost while improving quality of life. Disease management typically focuses on a particular disorder or class of diagnoses. This approach includes systematic identification of cases (particularly of people at special risk for negative outcomes), notification, and subsequent monitoring and coordination of services.

Often, the best place to manage a chronic illness is at home. A study on the effects of remote monitoring for patients with a chronic illness failure (Bondmass, Bolger, Castro, & Avitall, 2000) indicated approximately an 80% reduction in acute hospitalization at 3- and 6-month follow-up. According to the findings, learning was sustained over time even after the monitoring was discontinued, as the participants continued to make healthier decisions. The benefit to the patients' quality of life and the cost savings to the health care system are readily apparent. The following case illustrates this point:

An 87-year-old woman had recently lost her 94-year-old husband. She was clinically depressed. She also had congestive heart failure and had been given a pacemaker, so her activities of daily living were sharply curtailed. She was dealing with the loss of her husband as well as the loss of function and ill health. She was receiving conflicting advice from family members regarding her health and well-being.

A telephone-based video system was placed in her home, and a health counselor made routine calls to check on the patient's physical status, weight, blood pressure, and general feelings of wellness. In addition, a nurse specialist provided grief counseling. Issues of misinformation were clarified, and a plan of care and a menu of healthy options were discussed and agreed on. The patient's emergency room visits, which had been occurring almost every other week, ceased; she has been able to sustain herself without an emergency room visit for 6-months. Her use of tranquilizers, previously prescribed and taken regularly, has ceased. She has been given enough remote support through technology to mobilize her coping resources.

—Anonymous

Although disease management programs usually focus on chronic conditions, people with episodic conditions, such as bipolar disorders, can be helped remotely and kept in the system of care through in-home video units linked to mental health specialists, Web-based programs, or other modalities.

Disease management programs are also generally more likely to provide reimbursement for online clinical practice than are other health care programs. The programs assume, probably with some validity, that frequent interaction between practitioners and patients will delay or eliminate the need for hospitalization and avoid the attendant costs.

The Next Wave. Currently, funding for mental health seems to have settled into a trough that optimists see as the beginning of the next wave. Much as with the global experience of the Internet, once initial costs are decreased by demand, the rush to install psychotechnologies may outpace our ability to use them wisely. Although back-office functions are on the beachfront of the health care industrialists, clinical functions are slowly swelling behind the scenes. Planners are looking for ways to implement an electronic patient record system that would not only reduce the cost of care delivery but also provide them with more accurate, comprehensive, and timely information. They are waiting for telephone and videoconferencing models to become available through the Internet in a way that complies with legal and regulatory mandates and that approximates current standards of care.

Payers of behavioral health services are researching return on investment (ROI) scales that demonstrate the effectiveness of each service per dollar spent. Organizations may be required to offset the efficiencies realized by technologies with retraining of employees whose tasks are automated. Programs for complying with regulations and the requirements of accrediting agencies and licensure bodies could prove costly as technological modifications are established (Oss, 2001).

Organizations not only will feel the squeeze of their shifting organizational expenses but also must be ever-vigilant against compromising the well-being of the client as they introduce cost-saving technologies. People are beginning to suspect that control of their health care decisions may have fallen into the hands of large organizations that put financial consideration above health needs (Eng, 2001). According to one survey, the majority of members of a health plan report being worried that their health care organization is more concerned about saving money than about providing the best medical treatment (Kaiser Family Foundation, 1997).

Web sites that let managed care enterprises interact directly with their health care "consumers" may become important ways to save money and acquire good will (Bard, 2002). These sites could become communication channels between "participating providers" and consumers or could provide them with information and support in ways that edge out practitioners. Now may be the time for mental health professional organizations to influence the development of such Web sites, channeling the current so the tide will benefit the interests of patients and of professional health care. Commercial trends seem to be favoring employee assistance programs, coaching, and self-help Web sites with the potential to bypass professionals. To understand what technological innovations will mean to the mental health field, one must look at the broader context of behavioral services and what the general public is seeking.

Expanding the Role of Mental Health Care

The introduction of information technology into health care delivery, of improved public access to health information, and a generally widened perspective on mental health issues by policymakers may move the mental health professions from the periphery of the health care field to the center. Toward the end of the 20th century, the major public health agencies began to realize that although the leading causes of death worldwide may seem "medical," nearly all are directly or indirectly caused, triggered, or augmented by behavioral factors. It is now apparent that health outcomes are determined *less* by health care than by behavior patterns, genetic predisposition, social circumstances, and environmental exposure (McGinnis, Williams-Russo, & Knickman, 2002).

Cardiovascular disease, diabetes, HIV/AIDS, suicide, and homicide are linked to tobacco use, poor diet, lack of exercise, excessive use of alcohol, misuse of firearms, unduly risky sexual behavior, and illicit drug use (McGinnis & Foege, 1993). People now recognize smoking and drug abuse as significant contributors to social problems and disease, yet the public remains unaware that most of the other risk factors for cardiovascular disease—the greatest killer in developed countries—also involve habits that can be modified (Robertson, 2001). For example, being overweight, which is associated with increased cardiovascular disease, cancer, diabetes, and other causes of death (Calle, Thun, Petrelli, Rodriguez, & Heath, 1999), is overtaking malnutrition as the greatest influence on health (Kopelman, 2000). Optimal weight control programs combine diet, exercise, behavior modification, and perhaps medication, all guided by a medically supervised interdisciplinary team (Kopelman, 1998). Thus, it can be seen that the bottlenecks in health improvement worldwide, other than war, famine, severe economic hardship, and poor access to care, are mainly behavioral issues, including ignorance, unwholesome lifestyle habits, inadequate self-care practices, treatment avoidance, and noncompliance.

The psychotechnologies encourage interdisciplinary teams to develop common solutions for patients and their caregivers. Interdisciplinary teams go beyond the boundaries of mental or behavioral health, as such. The lines between general medicine and mental health care are beginning to blur. Studies (Mundell, 2000) are showing improvement in clinical diagnosis and treatment when primary care offices undertake more mental heath–related service.

The decoding of the human genome has set behavioral health care on a trajectory that may lead it to a more prominent, if not dominant, role in the health care professions (Eng, 2001). James J. Hudziak, M.D., associate professor and director of child psychiatry at the University of Vermont, College of Medicine, points out that such behavior as smoking cigarettes, drinking alcohol, and eating excessively fatty foods can trigger cancer-producing and other deadly genes. Many of our genes are coded for brain development and function; this leads Dr. Hudziak to predict that behavioral health care professionals will emerge from the shadow of "mainstream" medicine to dominate the field (J. Hudziak, personal communication, June 6, 2001).

To succeed at both patient education and treatment, we need leadership that informs and motivates, economic incentives that encourage change, and science that advances the frontiers. Broadly successful health care depends on convincing and assisting people to change their behavior. It takes more than presenting facts on billboards and handouts to bring people around to healthy lifestyles and optimal collaboration with the health care system. Although a focused chat with a physician can impact a patient's behavior, doctors do not have anywhere near the time it would take to provide even the modest array of preventive services currently recommended (Yarnall, Pollak, Østbye, Krause, & Michener, 2003). A realistic approach to prevention requires the interaction of nonphysician health care workers with patients and their families in a manner that integrates psychoeducational techniques into every aspect of general health care delivery. This is where mental health professionals can be particularly useful in developing and superintending effective approaches using the psychotechnologies.

Mental health professionals now have powerful new communication tools for co-ordinating health teams and for intervening at both the individual and societal levels. These tools include videoconferencing applications (Hilty, Marks, Urness, Nesbitt, Yellowlees, 2004; Simmons, West, & Chimiak, 2003) (where mental health has been a leader), interactive educational computer programs, e-mail, newsgroups, e-mail discussion forums, chat rooms, and sophisticated multimedia presentations on the World Wide Web. Mental health professionals who harness the power of telecommunication media will be in the best position to bridge the gap between patients and the rest of the health care system. Perhaps, then, online behavioral health care, broadly defined, may become the standard "front end" for medical practice.

A smaller but much more dramatic and immediate need for mental health intervention derives from the growing worldwide political use of terror. The primary intent of such terrorism is its psychological impact, and this effect persists beyond immediate reactions of dismay and panic. Several researchers reporting to the New York Academy of Medicine (2003) about adults and children who witnessed the destruction of the World Trade Center, even if only by television, found a high incidence of psychiatric disturbance. Internationally, children in particular are being targeted as victims, forced to fight in genocidal civil conflicts and tortured by repressive governments in efforts to intimidate dissenters (Pearn, 2003). Reparative care may be indefinitely delayed if children require the physical presence of mental health specialists. Mental health intervention should be organized and quickly delivered not only to terror, disaster, and war victims among the general public but also to their family members, to witnesses (often considerably removed from "ground zero"), to stressed and traumatized first responders, and even to the mental health workers themselves. Here is another area in which psychotechnologies can play a vital role.

Virtual reality has taken a gigantic step forward in the recent decade. Stand-alone and Web-based technologies are available for treating a wide range of disorders. Papers, journals, and conferences are proliferating. Interested readers are encouraged to peek at http://graphics.usc.edu/vret for a 360 Degree Panoramic Video Virtual Reality application for anxiety disorders. Much more information is found in chapter 7.

In an ironic twist, in the same way that information, virtual reality, and communication technologists can help behavioral service workers, reciprocal opportunities are developing. For example, Kelly Chessen, formerly a support person on a suicide hotline, has reportedly been hired by a data-recovery company to calm frantic computer users who seek telephone support after having experienced disk drive crashes (Ewalt, 2003).

In addition to strengthening the influence of mental health professionals in general health care, the psychotechnologies can help extend their influence to the realm of self-improvement. A postmodern trend has some physicians abandoning their specialties to perform cosmetic enhancements, such as *Clostridium botulinum* neurotoxin injections and liposuction in anticipation of scads more money, much less hassle, and more pleasing interactions with patients. The dream of forestalling aging seems to have supplemented the "Playboy Philosophy" and repeated bouts of weight loss as the primary and trendy expression of vanity. Assuming that terrorism and wars don't get in the way, another source of economic pressure mental health practitioners are likely to feel will be self-improvement (note: This is different from self-help for a disorder), whereby one can increase IQ, memory, social acceptability, dominance, and other desirable personal attributes with the help of interventions originally developed to treat psychiatric disorders. Some people think Prozac is a step in that direction (Kramer, 1993), and Ritalin for adults already enjoys its own following.

At one time, the field of psychoanalysis was funded to a significant degree by "self-pay" clients whose conditions would not have qualified for DSM-IV Axis I diagnoses but who were motivated to be "in analysis" for its social cachet. To be fair, however, self-improvement should not be derided and can be a truly beneficial area in which to apply professional mental health expertise and the psychotechnologies. As we detail in this book, the psychotechnologies are making psychotherapy and behavior modification methods more accessible. We can expect a large market to develop for a variety of professional self-improvement services as people become more familiar with computers and other technologies. We can expect tremendous growth in the area of Internet-mediated therapy extenders. Its growth will parallel what has been seen in Web-supported classroom instruction (i.e., the interweaving of Internet sites) with intersession "homeworks" and the direct in-person therapy session, as discussed in chapters 6 and 7. These Internet-*supplemented* therapies are likely to be the bridge to Internet-*dependent* therapies.

Psychological self-improvement may become part of a larger wave in which people strive to approach their full health potential. This more comprehensive ideal—being as strong as possible when the inevitable serious disorder strikes, such as diabetes, arthritis, heart disease, or major depression—calls for mental health professionals both to ally themselves more closely with the rest of the health care system and to become more responsive to the needs of people in general, beyond those with diagnosable social and/or emotional problems.

The psychotechnologies are giving patients more power over their health care and improve their communication with members of the health care team. In the "old days," when doctors were less effective and most people didn't live very long, the "wise general practitioner" was close at hand from one's birth to one's death.[8] Technological advances imported from the manufacturing world to the health care field brought economies of scale and other commercial efficiencies, but they have also fragmented treatment delivery and treatment relationships. The introduction of information technology directly into the clinical area of health care is reversing the pendulum swing by enabling patient-centered health care. Patients are gaining substantial control over their own health care, or the care of loved ones, by virtue of their access to vast health information resources and their increasing ability to find and understand the material. Even in the area of mental health, there is both need and opportunity for improved communication and collaboration of clients with their therapists.

Beyond Mental Health Care

Supporters of the psychotechnologies point to the early adoption of technology by professionals who might be considered competitors to licensed mental health practitioners. Outside the realms of psychiatric treatment, psychotherapy, professional counseling, psychoanalysis by highly qualified "lay analysts," and other professional treatment of diagnosed social or emotional problems lie what may be termed *behavioral services*. The vague concept of behavioral services applies to all sorts of advice and guidance offered for a fee or as a benefit. Included in these services are alternative therapies, religious counseling, priestly guidance, awareness training, coaching, personal growth, self-improvement, newspaper advice columns, inspirational texts, self-help groups, and even health and nutrition letters—all in addition to mental health care

---

[8] Actually, in those days, few indigent people received any professional medical attention.

professionals. People who offer behavioral services range from highly trained and competent and part of a defined structure to self-taught enthusiasts to charlatans.

Many people involved in self-help or self-improvement programs may eventually gravitate into formal therapy, just as many in therapy may find it valuable to engage in behavioral services either offered or not covered by their insurance. Funding for such activity is substantial and often out-of-pocket. The point is that this area of service has grown enormously and is positioned to grow at an even faster and more far-reaching rate than traditional mental health care, owing to its rapid adoption of technology. Increasingly, such behavioral services are using technological tools that are also well suited for professional mental health practice.

Although patients' efforts to improve their strengths and resilience would be genuinely valuable in promoting general health and improving or resolving psychopathology, insurers may not cover the costs. Historically, and especially recently, the health insurance industry has been more concerned with short-term goals (i.e., functional improvement and symptom reduction) than with broad preventive measures (Bedell, Hunter, & Corrigan, 1997; Shore & Beigel, 1996). The mental health disciplines need to note these changes, and their use of the psychotechnologies, and respond accordingly.

While researchers and payors move at their own speed, consumers are moving at quite another speed. E-health empowers individuals to make their own decisions about personal and family health care (Spielberg, 1998). Patients have immediate access to worldwide medical databases, libraries, conference proceedings, and, increasingly, their own medical records. By logging on to the National Library of Medicine's MEDLINE (http://www.ncbi.nlm.nih.gov/entrez/query.fcgi), patients can access abstracts of journal articles. Patients can look at textbook collections, drug databases, diagnostic cookbooks, and disease-specific self-monitoring Web sites.

Clients are arriving for treatment seeking answers to very specific questions and already prepared with text-based articles they found on the Internet. In acquiring more information, clients believe that they are creating, and intelligently using, freedom of choice and interpersonal support for judging, selecting, and challenging their health care practitioners. Clients believe that they are helping themselves and each other, with and without the help of professionals. In some cases, clients are correct; in others, they undoubtedly are creating more difficulty for themselves.

Some patients (a minority) want to gather their own information and make their own choices. Some patients want to combine information they glean from the Web and other sources with the knowledge base of the practitioner to make a mutual "best guess" choice. Some patients search for information to reassure themselves but let their practitioner decide their best course of action. Some avoid dealing with the facts and adopt a "you're the doctor" attitude. Each of these adaptive/defensive styles has its merits and should be accommodated. People can even shift from one mode to another. Radio and television talk shows, television newscasts or news magazine programs, print media, or randomly selected Web sites can present health information that is too general, too detailed, too upsetting, too ambiguous or inconsistent, or too inaccurate for certain people at certain times. Some information sources may be large and diverse but feel less intimate.

Table 1.2 lists the types of pathways found on the Web, along with examples of each. Many of these examples are drawn from behavioral e-health sites.

Hundreds of thousands of behavioral e-health Web sites offer information and assistance with mental health topics. These Web sites vary in quality, from the potentially harmful to those with empirically validated content. Few e-health sites and tools have

TABLE 1.2
Main Pathways to Finding E-Health Information

Pathway	Example
Discussion group (professionally moderated or not)	Online Sex Addiction (www.onlinesexaddict.org) SelfhelpMagazine (www.selfhelpmagazine.com)
Commercial (private enterprise, pharmaceutical company)	iVillage (www.ivillage.com) WebMD (www.webmd.com)
Government agency	National Institute of Mental Health (www.nimh.nih.gov)
Professional organization	American Psychiatric Association (www.psych.org)
Health insurance company (managed care sites for consumers and providers)	ValueOptions (www.valueoptions.com) Cigna (www.cigna.com)
Volunteer organization	National Alliance for Mental Illness (www.nami.org)
News enterprise (e-zine, or associated with a newspaper, magazine, or television channel)	MSNBC (www.msnbc.com) abcNEWS.com (www.abcnews.go.com)
Individual (professional or nonprofessional enthusiast)	Telehealth Conferences and Organizations (www.telehealth.net/calendar)
Health care provider (brochure site augmented with articles or newsfeed)	MyTherapyCenter.com (www.mytherapycenter.com)
Professional journal site	British Medical Journal (www.bmj.com) Professional Psychology (www.apa.org/journals/pro.html)
Continuing education sites	HealthStream (www.healthstream.com/hcp/index.html)
General search engine	Yahoo: (www.yahoo.com) Google (www.google.com)
Specialized search service	PubMed (www.ncbi.nlm.nih.gov/entrez/query.fcgi) PsychInfo (www.apa.org/psycinfo)

been evaluated for effectiveness or impact (Science Panel on Interactive Communication and Health, 1999), and most are incomplete or inaccurate (Stone and Jumper, 2001; Suarez-Almazor, Kendall, & Dorgan, 2001). The amazing proliferation of behavioral e-health Web sites clearly points to a previously unmet need, and the weaknesses in so many of these sites amount to a call for more professional participation.

New online self-help and professional educational programs are growing at dizzying speed. Informational Web sites present thousands of articles on psychiatric topics or provide links to such resources on other sites. Direct-service Web sites offer treatment by credentialed professionals by means of e-mail, chat rooms, and interactive video. We describe these applications and discuss their use, risks, and benefits in various chapters of this book (see chapters 3, 5–13).

Mental Health versus Behavioral Services

Aside from behavioral services that collaborate with mental health or address areas most mental health professionals neglect there are some that compete. Many nonlicensed practitioners can actually bring relief, both physical and psychological.

Whether the same holds true for symptoms of psychopathology has not been demonstrated, yet many people seem to have been helped by other behavioral services (e.g., Twelve Step programs or clergy who are not practicing formal "pastoral counseling"). Of course, some professionals are concerned that a patient's progress could be delayed by an ineffective approach attempted by an unskilled or misguided helper.

Just as physicians can pick up valuable lessons from practitioners of traditional and alternative medicine, mental health specialists can learn from others in the behavioral services field. Indeed, although competition for market share and struggles over terminology and the right to practice are inevitable, the mental health field is increasingly emulating some methods of the broader behavioral services or is expanding into them. The psychotechnologies will undoubtedly facilitate and accelerate the trend. As we discuss in subsequent chapters, steering the psychotechnologies into nonprofessional waters can be very tempting and productive, but it entails extra dangers for both the professional and the client (see chapters 3, 5, 11–13). As we introduce the next two sections, we note that employee assistance programs and the growing discipline of coaching are increasingly relying on psychotechnologies to straddle the boundary between professional and nonprofessional personal behavioral services.

Employee Assistance Programs. In general, managed care companies have had a substantial impact on practice patterns in the United States. Many managed care companies are investing significant funding for development and marketing of employee assistance programs (EAPs). These programs were initially designed reduce health care costs by detecting initial mental health or substance abuse problems (Hayes, Barlow, & Nelson-Gray, 1999).

Unbeknownst to many licensed mental health practitioners, many EAPs have expanded their services through technology, using Web sites constructed exclusively for employee audiences. These Web sites are often designed and maintained by affiliated corporations and are sometimes branded with the employer's logo and other identifying information through the employer's own in-house Web site, otherwise known as an *intranet*. In other words, employers contract directly with managed care companies for customized Web site information and backup services, such as telephone or e-mail support for employees seeking individualized responses to their concerns. Many of these EAP Web sites avoid the use of costly licensed mental health professionals to deliver such support. The computerized system can take advantage of the corporation's high-speed connections to include interactive video and other advanced features. These offerings run on the corporation's intranet, using technology similar to the World Wide Web but confined to the employer's own network. Employees are allowed access from their desktops. Such offerings can also have judiciously protected connection with the World Wide Web and can be made partially accessible from an employee's home.

Independent companies are also available to cobrand mental health Web sites. Systems can be integrated with those of other EAP or community health clinics, such as Web sites developed by Centersite (http://www.centersite.net). Administration tools facilitate adding an organization's own content to the resulting Web site to make it more personal for the reading audience.

With some large-scale Web construction companies, aggregated information fed back to the client (that is, to the sponsoring organization or employer) helps justify the expense. In terms of expense, mental health care market analysts have tracked the market share that EAP programs are quickly gaining. In the United States, between 1993 and 2002, enrollment in EAP programs rose 163%, from 86.3 million to 227 million

(Naughton-Travers, 2002). Now, to stay competitive, the EAP market is moving to the telephone and Internet in order to deliver services to workers whose employers have purchased cafeteria-style mental health care packages. The rich array of electronically mediated service is heavily promoted by enterprises offering employers relatively inexpensive solutions to mental health concerns.

The current goal of many employee assistance programs is to maximize employee productivity by minimizing issues that may otherwise detract from time spent at work. The effort to assist with these issues has reached new heights through *work/life* Web sites for employers and their employees. Several industries have joined the push to develop these Web-based EAP-related "products" to help alleviate the pressures caused by unmet practical and emotional needs. These rapidly growing services offer self-assessment and self-instructional activities that may enhance or forestall a quest for direct services. They also offer a range of other assistance, such as:

- Referrals for home care for children, adults, and elders.
- Adoption resources.
- Child-care resources and referrals.
- Adult and elder care information and referrals.
- Pet-care information and referrals.
- Internet wellness libraries.
- Entertainment and shopping discounts.
- Domestic violence resources.
- Workplace violence resources.
- Trauma resources.
- Concierge services (e.g., services that assist in buying theater tickets or taking clothing to the dry cleaner).

Some employees who contact their EAP will engage with self-help groups on the Internet. A portion will make direct contact with a "helper" through e-mail or an Internet chat room. Some will be sent for a professional mental health evaluation and even treatment.

Supporters of work/life products point to high employee and employer satisfaction with text-based (Masi & Back-Tamburo, 2001) or telephone-based mental health care (Masi & Freeman, 1999). People seeking help get convenient and immediate help through these work/life programs. Advocates also see the rising cost of health care in general and claim that alternatives must be found. Some developers of work/life programs seem to be hoping that relatively untrained or unlicensed educators, care managers, or coaches[9] are sufficiently cost-effective for most people. In general, employees may tend to believe this as well.

Indeed, employees seem "ready to go" with work/life programs. For example, of people who responded to a University of Maryland survey of users of the LifeWorks online self-help resource, 48% said they had turned to the computer because of the immediate access available online (Ceridian Corporation, 2002) rather than telephoning for advice or an appointment. Of the 477 respondents, 12% said their concern

---

[9] Pursuing a career as a care manager, counselor, or coach can involve substantial educational backing and professionalism. Yet individuals also can put themselves forth as such without having to meet regulations or obtain certification.

was insufficient to warrant an in-person meeting, and 10% had sought anonymity in getting help because they felt embarrassed about their problem. It may be that many people who appear for mental health care have simple questions that can be answered without the help of licensed mental health practitioners. It is not yet clear, however, how well or poorly these employees or their educators and coaches can identify circumstances and problems requiring more skill and training.[10]

Critics of work/life programs point to the lack of licensed practitioners among the professionals or paraprofessionals offering online (e-mail or chat room) and telephone contact with employees. Critics also claim that some low-cost or no-cost resources recommended by some of these programs may be inappropriate for some of the consumers served. Of further concern is the rampant lack of standards regulating such sites, which are offering referrals to child care agencies or elder care facilities that have never been visited to establish their credibility or the quality of their services (Masi, 2002).

Meanwhile, employees using these services can easily assume that facilities listed on work/life Web sites have been responsibly endorsed and that the work/life company has ascertained the qualifications of affiliated providers. Although there are Web site disclaimers stating that referrals are offered only as information, employees still might assume that because their employers have contracted with the work/life company, these referrals have been investigated and have received appropriate credentialing.

It must be said that some of the work/life programs are offering responsible services. They have licensed professionals at the helm who ascertain the quality of service delivered both through their own paraprofessionals and through vendors. Other programs are certainly aware of these needs but are operating during an unregulated "window of opportunity" while legislation is being developed to regulate their online services. It is incumbent on work/life companies to ensure that their providers and vendors are offering services within the law (D. Masi, personal communication, October 24, 2002). Some mental health professionals fear that this relatively unregulated industry will seize the business opportunity entrusted to them by employers before professional communities exert needed influence.

The Council on Accreditation (http://www.coanet.org) is one of the few organizations that has developed standards regarding the online EAP services (Council on Accreditation, 2002). These standards indicate the importance of having emergency numbers available, as well as having counselors who reside in the same vicinity as the online client when clients are serviced remotely. It is obviously crucial that standards be set and an accreditation process be put in place for all work/life offerings and for their use of technology to deliver their services. For licensed professionals who seek new avenues to develop practice and to deliver services through technology, the work/life model deserves attention. These programs will inevitably be required to hire licensed professionals to provide needed oversight.

Coaching. Managed care is exerting economic pressure on health care practitioners and systems to deliver more efficient and effective services at a lower cost; another factor impinging on traditional practice is the growth of coaching. In the best of circumstances, coaching offers less stigmatized and more forward-looking approaches toward satisfying one's life aspirations (Naughton, 2002). Coaching methods include

---

[10] Some coaches are mental health professionals who have switched careers.

self-assessments, goal setting, self-report checklists, guiding, reminding, and inspiring. Many of these methods are a "natural" for service delivery through the Internet.

Most executive or personal coaches operate on a more modest scale, closer to traditional mental health. As solo operators marketing their services to smaller, select groups, they might work for a single organization or a single type of organization within a particular industry. Other coaches specifically help parents of children with attention deficit hyperactivity disorder or target individuals who need assistance in getting organized at home or at the office.

Fee structures for work/life coaches are particularly interesting. Work/life and EAP programs typically hire coaches for less pay than psychotherapists would receive. At the same time, executive coaches and some personal coaches deliver services to corporate groups and individuals who are willing to pay much more than the average fee for counseling or psychotherapy from a licensed therapist. As a rule, coaches are not encumbered by the training requirements or licensure limitations and sanctions that professional psychotherapists face. Although the coaching movement has its downsides, it has grown rapidly and is increasingly focused on using the psychotechnologies (particularly the telephone and Internet) to deliver convenient interventions.

What of the licensed professional who decides that licensed private practice is too inhibiting and that coaching is a viable way to avoid the limitations imposed by increasingly elaborate training requirements, strict licensure criteria, constricting professional association guidelines, burdensome membership dues, and the daunting specter of malpractice lawsuits? Licensed mental health professionals have not abandoned their legal status by pursuing coaching. Regardless of the title they give themselves, licensed professionals are held to the standards of their licensure. Organized coach training programs, such as Ben Dean's Mentorcoach (http://mentorcoach.com), have made notable strides in recognizing the importance of helping licensed professionals be aware of the continued need to adhere to their state mandates regarding any licensure they hold, the need to maintain malpractice insurance, and the need to maintain client confidentiality, even if they have left the professional associations to which they previously belonged.

Many aspects of coaching can be incorporated into a psychotechnology-enhanced professional practice. Cooperation and confluence of coaching and professional mental health care is an attractive prospect. Issues related to professional training, referrals, client training, consent, assessment, and direct service delivery are likely to be the same for such coaches as they are for any other licensed mental health practitioner using technology, depending on the laws governing one's region of practice. Therefore, we refer interested readers to our Online Clinical Practice model, as detailed in chapters 11, 12, and 13 of this book.

Even professionals who drop their licensure to become coaches can face problems if an unsatisfied client decides to litigate, however. Licensing boards traditionally have frowned on what might be considered a previously licensed professional's attempt to evade oversight. Licensed mental health professionals who decide to offer coaching often try to separate their psychotherapy and coaching services clearly with appropriate service and informed-consent agreements. Such coaches typically use completely different offices, often at different addresses, do not hang diplomas of mental health training on their separate office walls, and avoid use of their titles and credentials as mental health practitioners while describing, marketing, and/or delivering their services. These coaches avoid dual relationships, do not coach their former psychotherapy clients, and typically avoid working with people who have serious social or emotional problems. These coaches also generally avoid working with loved ones of people with severe social or emotional problems if the work involves how to deal with the individual with severe problems. These coaches carry malpractice insurance.

Although the reality is that coaches are potential targets for general or licensing board lawsuits, strict enforcement of state licensure regulations is the exception rather than the rule. Licensing boards rarely act proactively. They more often function to investigate complaints when filed by clients.

Large-Scale Web Site Services

Some large online services have combined technology, behavioral health care research, and coaching to deliver services to employers through password-protected and HIPAA-compliant Web sites. Epotec was one such company. It developed an array of more than 200 online behavioral health programs that were "private labeled" (repackaged to look like the group's own service) and then made available to consumers through another entity, such as managed care organizations, employee assistance programs, health plans, and community health organizations. Epotec's clients created a personalized path to self-improvement by responding to questions and crafting solutions to fit their needs at the Web site created by one of these entities. Epotec's self-help programs helped the user learn a concept and build on previously acquired knowledge. Examples were "Building Coping Skills," "Are You Putting Yourself at Risk?" and "Fear of Flying."

Users could discuss program results with any of a number of coaches and possibly achieve faster treatment, which saved money for third-party payers. Users were given homework and complete written assignments online. A coach participating in an Epotec offering could see all of a user's previous homework, and if the user asked questions of a coach, all coaching questions and responses were available to all subsequent coaches for that user. All coaches were anonymous to the user, and all users anonymous to the coaches. Clinical supervisors could see the responses given to any particular user, as well as the responses given by any given coach over time. Coaching manuals were provided for companies that wanted to train their own coaches to work with the Epotec Web service. Epotec closed its doors on December 31, 2002, as some of the largest managed mental health care companies faced bankruptcy or stumbled to their knees with dropping stock values.

Epotec's model of service delivery is one to note, however. Its innovative use of Web interactivity, coaching, and supervision, combined with its customer base of managed care organizations, hospitals, and other large mental health entities, demonstrated what can be accomplished with the aid of psychotechnology. Whether such companies as Epotec were too early in the cycle of innovation, fell prey to difficult economic times, herald the demise of managed care, or simply fail to adequately win the confidence of those with serious mental health concerns, only time will tell.

E-Counseling Companies. Another breed of primarily text-based Web site service is the e-counseling company, both small- and large-scale. These sites generally offer articles and referrals but typically are developed as income-producing entities delivering direct services through e-mail or chat rooms. These sites may be staffed by one or more licensed mental health practitioners and also may be affiliated with a brick-and-mortar company, but they are usually incorporated as separate entities to conduct business online. Dozens of e-counseling Web sites had sprouted by the year 2000, the majority of which have now filed for bankruptcy (Heinlen, Reynolds Welfel, Richmond, & Rak, 2003).

E-counseling companies typically started with budgets of $10 million to $20 million, obtained most often from venture capitalists from around the globe. Those left standing today typically have a single operations manager or a relatively small panel of practitioners offering services. As many e-counseling companies faced bankruptcy, they approached insurance companies to be purchased and transformed into managed care or work/life Web sites. Some succeeded and were bought; others failed.

Regardless of the status of research, the proliferation of text-based information through private Web sites, work/life Web sites, coaching, augmentation by telephone, university projects, or e-counseling companies, how a professional decides to go online is crucial. The licensed professional must consider such a decision with forethought regarding the potential interpretation of past, present, and future clients, employers, and colleagues alike. By understanding the detours, roadblocks, and freeway fast lanes of developing an online presence, the professional can maximize effect and minimize negative consequences, such as lost time, frustration, public embarrassment, and most important, risk of harm to the client.

Through time, many kinds of mental health service have come from outside to augment and, more fully develop the field of mental health itself. The field of psychosocial rehabilitation has roots among workers in the wards of state psychiatric hospitals, where professionals were relatively scarce. The chemical abuse field has developed somewhat independently from mental health. Developmental disability is another area relatively bypassed by mainstream mental health, but it is certainly closely related.

We are not trying to draw distinctions between these fields; rather, we are suggesting that the boundaries of "mental health services" are vague and fluid, and, more important, we can expect the convenience and low cost of connectivity offered by the psychotechnologies to make these boundaries even more permeable. Our notions of mental health treatment might be outdated and, put simply, are changing with or without the approval of the established mental health community.

Changes in mental health care, as with all of health care, are clearly needed. As we describe in chapter 6, mental health researchers in the area of decision-support software are developing technologies that already enable managed behavioral health care organizations and other third parties to measure clinical effectiveness. Practitioner groups that can demonstrate good results enjoy a competitive advantage. This concern with results, particularly with clinical outcome rather than treatment process, may lead mental health professionals to collaborate, integrate their approaches, and broaden their perspectives.

To the delight of many professionals, some outcome research is looking beyond symptom alleviation and rates of recurrence or hospitalization to take a broader look at the decrease in burden and improved productivity and overall quality of life. These considerations are closer to the behavioral goals people generally have for themselves even when a psychiatric diagnosis is not at issue. Advances in neuroscience, genetics, neurophysiology, learning and cognition; the potential for rehabilitation; the impact of emotional trauma; and other areas aided by technology are likely to swing the pendulum back toward a coordinated view of mental health care. Beyond being merely a tool in mental health, psychotechnologies will help general health care and mental health care converge with self-help and peer support activities, restoring the trend toward unity pursued by Charcot, Freud, and Tourette.

Although some practitioners have veered into coaching, others remain squarely within mental health. Psychology, psychiatry, and counseling sciences have focused primarily on clinical disorders. We apparently know a great deal about human dysfunction and much less about the issues involved in normal development and what makes for healthy psychosocial functioning, even though this is the ultimate goal of much psychotherapeutic intervention. What cognitive and emotional processes and strategies do highly successful people use? How do people regulate their emotions successfully in challenging situations? Much research is currently directed to answering these basic psychological questions (e.g., Barrett & Gross, 2001).

The next few decades will undoubtedly see research about psychological wellness conducted through the Internet. "Subjective well-being" is a concept being advanced by Diener (1984, 1996) to enable measuring psychological health. The shift in conceptualization from mental and behavioral problems to mental and behavioral solutions is the agenda of "Positive Psychology," founded by Martin Seligman at the University of Pennsylvania (http://www.positivepsychology.org). Its goals are to better define, understand scientifically, and help build fulfilling lives and thriving communities in which individuals can unleash their talents and creativity. At the individual level, Positive Psychology refers to character strength, including the capacity for love and work, courage, compassion, resilience, hope, creativity, social skills, integrity, self-knowledge, impulse control, future-mindedness, and wisdom. At the level of community, it refers to the civic virtues and the institutions that nurture better citizenship, such as responsibility, civility, parenting, a work ethic, leadership, volunteerism, and tolerance.

A good example of the movement from traditional mental health training to coach training is Martin Seligman's "Authentic Happiness Coaching Program" (http://www.authentichappinesscoaching.com). His Web pages state that he is offering his newest training program to "psychologists, social workers, psychiatrists and other mental health professionals, coaches, trainers, consultants, educators and all other professionals who want to learn Authentic Happiness coaching skills."

A similar shift in research and practice has also occurred in the field of biofeedback. The journal *Biofeedback* (2001) titled an entire issue "The Pursuit of Optimal Functioning." Biofeedback is most certainly based in technology and is probably the most well known and well established form of psychotechnology. It is recognized not only as a therapeutic technique for medical or behavioral illness but also for improving self-regulation skills in generally healthy individuals who want to attain peak performance in all aspects of their emotional, mental, and physical functioning.

The World Wide Web has already begun to serve as a platform for disseminating the principles of positive psychology and biofeedback as specific mental health focuses to unleash talents and creativity by allowing people of all ages to experiment and develop their own Web pages, create their own discussion groups, and participate in existing communities developed to explore the positive side of the human experience. A Google search for "Positive Psychology" listed 7,150 related links on October 24, 2002, and 22,500 links on March 29, 2004—dramatically demonstrating the power of the Net to develop a good idea and provide avenues for interested parties to participate. The Internet offers many ways to encourage individuals to assume a lot more responsibility for their own health.

The Psychotechnologies in Practice Today. Supporters of services discussed in this chapter might describe any one of them as innovative or groundbreaking. Critics might characterize them as foolishness or quackery. Developers of technology, wherever they may lead, will not stop. Where practitioners find themselves will depend to a large extent on their personal and collaborative choices in the next few decades.

We hope that readers will consider the multitude of possibilities for using the psychotechnologies to expand their practices and improve mental health services.

Individual clinicians who take the initiative to learn about and apply the psychotechnologies in their practices will be in the best position to retain professional control over how they deliver mental health care. Indeed, mental and behavioral health professionals proficient in maximizing the use of the psychotechnologies (such as Dr. Giolas in our opening vignette) may not only flourish in the mental health field but also find their role in general health care and in general behavioral services increasing.

Managed health care organizations are increasingly eager to gain the cooperation—indeed, the collaboration—of practitioners in bringing information technology into mental health practice. To some extent, such organizations will have to accommodate the preferences and values of clinicians in designing computerized systems, meeting government requirements for documentation, and designing work-flow procedures that use automated technologies. Practitioners who learn to use these automated systems already receive quicker payment for claims and may delight in simplified procedures for authorization requests as they quickly enter information into Web sites. As we discuss in subsequent chapters, these processes are just beginning, and many more automated and simplified services are slated to arrive in the next decade.

This first, introductory chapter has given a brief history of the uses of technology in mental health care, delineated key concepts used in this book, pointed to the increasing need for an expansion in mental health service options, and provided an overview of several broad categories of services being aided by technology. Chapter 2 continues to define and explain key concepts and specific terminology related to technology. For the novice, this information will be indispensable. For the experienced, it might serve as a quick refresher and update.

Telecommunication Technicalities

For the unlucky mental health practitioner thrashing about in the swelling sea of technology, this chapter can serve as a "Guide for the Perplexed" (ben Maimon, 1956). It may calm the reader's troubled amygdala, shifting adaptive processing to the ventral and medial prefrontal cortex (Pine et al., 2001).

Spirited professionals who have somehow become familiar with the Internet and other telecommunications networks may want to skip to chapter 3. Other readers may notice that we explain technology only to a degree required to understand the remainder of this book. This chapter does not try to cover the vast world of technology but instead focuses on four general areas:

- The two types of telecommunication.
- Data.
- Transmission channels and devices.
- The Internet, with a focus on the World Wide Web.

Psychotherapy is ordinarily thought of as involving very private and intimate dialogue between two or more people. Technology can connect people to information and to each other, as easily from across the world as from across town. How can psychotherapy and technology be blended? It should not surprise clinicians that the usefulness of telecommunications technology for mental health care rests primarily on extending and otherwise facilitating relationships.

However, common reactions to the notion of delivering mental health services online are to question confidentiality, to mention delays, and to express concern with the elimination of nonverbal behavior through some technologies. Even though such concerns are ripe with merit, exclusively negative reactions to bringing mental health care online ignore important realities. As we explain in the remaining text, some varieties of psychotherapy and support services are well suited to electronic media, and new applications have just begun to emerge from research labs around the world.

Please note the inclusion of the term *support services* in the previous sentence. For the first time in history, professionals are more easily able to develop services that do not involve direct contact with clients. Consider the following example sent by a user of the SelfhelpMagazine.com discussion forums (a type of online bulletin board covering mental health topics), which is not moderated:

> I used your forum for a couple of months when I had lost my therapist. Please know that you are indeed life savers by giving us a vehicle to help ourselves. I thank you.

Telecommunication technology can also assist or supplement much traditional in-person psychotherapy. Furthermore, psychotherapy is not the only service that can be usefully provided electronically.

TYPES OF COMMUNICATION

When used properly, technology may be able to enhance many aspects of clinical practice. Rather than learning to use the new tools by trial and error or at the expense of one's clients, the clinician should take the time to calmly learn the basics. Improper use can add to what Michele Weil describes as "technostress," whereby dealing with technology creates undue anxiety (Weil & Rosen, 1997).

As the Information Age advances, it is increasingly important for clinicians to enhance efficiency by blending practice with technology. For some years, many practitioners have offered biofeedback-enhanced treatments and have used computers for psychological testing or used word processors to write reports. These computerized applications are described in later chapters in great detail, (see chapters 6, 7, and 8) as they are now ready for inclusion in the average clinician's practice. This chapter focuses on current advances in technology involving electronic transmission of information, be it within an office suite or across vast distances.

Synchronous communication describes events that are coordinated in time and is often called *real time*, or *live*. Telephone conversation is an example of synchronous communication. Telephone answering machine messages are an example of asynchronous communication. We begin by looking at synchronous communication.

Synchronous Communication

Synchronous communication, such as the telephone or cable television, requires relatively fast transmission channels that can both send and receive information at the same time. Even synchronous connections are not literally instantaneous. Some delay is unavoidable in all distance communication. For example, the 0.2 seconds it takes radio signals to cross a continent would register as a meaningful pause in an in-person encounter. Some synchronous technologies resemble walkie-talkies in that they blot out transmission from the listener when the other person is speaking, clipping off the little "uh-huhs," snorts, and snickers that provide feedback during local telephone calls. Such transmission devices are not adequate for anything but makeshift psychotherapeutic contact. Similarly, a cellular telephone's often broken signal (in addition to its lack of confidentiality) is inadequate for most remote psychotherapeutic encounters. The end devices are not the problem. The carrier services, or communication channels, are still unreliable compared to standard telephone service.

Videoconferencing, also referred to as interactive television (ITV), is the dominant modality of synchronous communication most often used for delivering mental health care at a distance (discussed further in chapter 5). People hear or see each other during videoconferencing and can interrupt each other. It is particularly useful for directly interviewing and examining a patient (Smith & Allison, 2000), discussing a case with a consultant, and mediating interactive distance learning, or tele-education. The chief disadvantage is that videoconferencing is possible only through transmission channels having sufficient capacity to carry quality video data. Video data with adequate detail and smoothness have been identified in a number of mental health research programs assessing quality of therapeutic contact through videoconferencing (Glueckauf, Fritz, et al., 2002; Schneider, 1999). Videoconferencing can be an expensive and complex modality, particularly when it complies with the security requirements outlined by various privacy laws. However, the price of videoconferencing equipment is decreasing as new devices are developed and market growth intensifies competition.

The following story exemplifies how synchronous videoconferencing can be applied creatively for psychosocial support supplementing medical treatment:

A young woman, critically ill with AIDS, was admitted to the hospital of the College of Georgia in Augusta. Confined to bed, she verbalized her regret at not being able to attend her high school general equivalency diploma (GED) graduation ceremony at a rural high school in South Carolina. It seems that this young lady, in her early 20s, had dropped out of high school as an adolescent. Years later, she decided to go back to earn a GED. She was hospitalized on the very day she was to receive her diploma. A caring physician, hearing the young woman's lament, contacted the telephone company. After the doctor explained the situation, personnel at the company volunteered to run a videoconferencing transmission line into the high school auditorium that very afternoon. The physician himself drove out to the high school, and one of the patient's GED instructors came to the hospital.

That evening, on a videoconferencing unit set up by the patient's bedside at the hospital using the telephone line next to the bed, the young woman virtually attended her high school graduation. The patient's physician placed the videoconferencing unit on the podium in the high school auditorium, and the patient could see her fellow classmates graduate and could speak to them, individually, as they filed past the videoconferencing unit on the way to receiving their diplomas. Finally, the moment came when the high school teacher presented the young patient with her diploma in the hospital room. Her classmates watched the teacher present the diploma to their classmate and cheered. Without the possibilities that videoconferencing provides, the psychosocial needs of this very ill patient, her family, her classmates, her teacher, and her physician could never have been met.

—Warren B. Karp, Ph.D., DMD
Professor Emeritus
The Medical College of Georgia

Synchronous videoconferencing can be supplemented by using an *electronic whiteboard*, which is another type of synchronous communication technology. This feature allows participants on both ends of the transmission to share text or to draw images and make diagrams while they discuss various issues. It is akin to having a whiteboard at the front of a room when participants discuss a topic in-person.

Text-based environments, such as *Internet Relay Chat* (IRC) or *instant messaging* (IM), whereby participants can view a completed text message on their computers almost as soon as it is sent, approach synchronous communication in their sense of immediacy. Fans of IM, especially kids, have developed a cryptic shorthand that reflects this immediacy. Because it is available through the Internet today, videoconferencing can involve noticeable delays for compressing, transmitting, and decompressing its data before it reaches the party on the other end. On the other hand, videoconferencing transmitted through broadband telecommunication channels, and other options discussed in chapter 5, does allow for full real-time transmission.

Asynchronous Communication

As the reader may have guessed, *asynchronous communication* allows two users to communicate with each without being simultaneously connected. This communication type is also known as *store-and-forward*. The user sending the message can direct it to the appropriate destination, where it will be stored until the receiving user decides to access it. Some examples of asynchronous methods used extensively in health care include the postal service (also called *snail mail!*), telephone answering machines (voice mail), e-mail messages, discussion lists, faxes for transmitting clinical test results from laboratory to nurses' desks, Internet-mediated file transfer of radiology images, and distance-learning material posted on the World Wide Web in numerous professional educational programs. To date, most of the world's telehealth systems are based on store-and-forward technology.

Asynchronous communication has inherent advantages over synchronous communication. Moving information at a leisurely pace to a recipient's system, where it can be accumulated and then later played back at full speed, imposes less demand on transmission channels and is therefore less expensive. Further, store-and-forward techniques allow one to retrieve material whenever it is convenient and thus provide more opportunity to research and organize a response.

As with most technologies, however, it also entails some disadvantages, at least in some contexts. By definition, prompt responses to questions or needs are not assured and are in fact unlikely. Asynchronous methods of communication, therefore, are generally unsuited for use in emergency situations.

The Cardiology on the Move project, carried out by the Cardiology Research Lab of the University of Athens School of Medicine (http://users.forthnet.gr/ath/giovas/project), is an interesting application of asynchronous communication. The patient's electrocardiogram (EKG) is transmitted from a moving ambulance in store-and-forward fashion to enable a cardiologist in the hospital emergency department to interpret the EKG before the patient arrives. Similar applications are likely to evolve in the mental health field, where asynchronous communication could allow a client's prior mental health records, psychological tests results and reports, medical lab reports, as well as full medical records, to be accessible to mental health professionals prior to seeing any client.

Of course, in real life, optimal service to the patient may call for both synchronous and asynchronous communication. The following vignette is a description of a project sponsored by the University of Florida. The Alzheimer's Caregiver Support Online (http://www.AlzOnline.net) provides live online classes to caregivers of individuals with progressive dementia. The success of this project may depend in part on the caregivers' perceptions of ease of use, in addition to the clarity of contents and the utility of the Web site. The live classes are conducted synchronously over the World Wide Web, using voice, PowerPoint slides, and written communication instantly shared among all participants. In addition, a number of asynchronous resources are available, such as a bulletin board, online library, and Web site links that are available to facilitate peer support and enrich the learning experience. The reader is invited to decipher between synchronous and asynchronous technologies while reading the following vignette.

Colleen, a 52-year-old shopkeeper in Gainesville, Florida, was caring for her elderly mother, Adele, who had been diagnosed with Alzheimer's disease. After Adele was found by a security guard walking aimlessly in the local Walgreen's, Colleen began agonizing about placing her mother in a nursing home. A friend told Colleen about AlzOnline, and she enrolled in an online class.

Colleen's only online experience involved e-mail. As Colleen tried to connect to a live AlzOnline session, her computer locked up. The AlzOnline had a technician available by telephone for just such contingencies. After speaking with Colleen, the technician made a home visit to assess Colleen's computer capabilities and to show her how to perform basic maintenance on her system. Colleen learned how to access Web applications, to find resource lists for services in her community, and to use e-mail for communicating with the staff of area nursing homes regarding their services and facilities. Colleen was able to make well-informed long-range plans for her mother's care. For the time being, she selected a day treatment service and avoided what could have been a desperate, guilt-provoking, and inappropriate rush to a nursing home.

*   Alzheimer's Caregiver Support Online's experience with problems like Colleen's has led to Web site enhancements and home visits using the telephone to solve computer issues, such as limiting file sizes for caregivers with the slow Internet connections that AlzOnline found in the homes of many of its clients.*

—Robert Glueckauf, Ph.D.
Project Director
Dementia Caregivers Telehealth Support Project

Videoconferencing can be usefully supplemented by asynchronous communication technologies as well, such as by a display of diagrams or slides that may have been stored and forwarded. A text-based chat feature can also be incorporated in a conferencing system that is analogous to an IRC. This evidence of convergence blurs the distinction between synchronous and asynchronous modalities. As we mention in this chapter, this is the nature of getting a short overview of a fast-developing area, such as telecommunication technologies.

Now let us turn to a discussion of data. Data are pieces of information that have been converted into a form that makes them easily stored or transmitted, either synchronously or asynchronously.

THE DATA

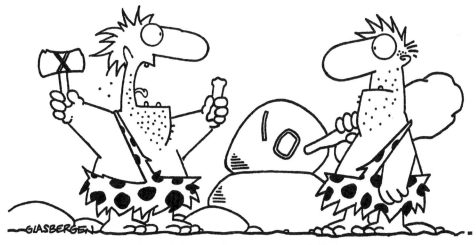

"I JUST INVENTED THE 'ONE' AND THE 'ZERO'.
LET THE DIGITAL REVOLUTION BEGIN!"

Certain data formats have become standard for computer management of text, images, sound, and video, but all formats involve treating the material as *digitized* information. Computerized data are comprised of *bits*, which are the smallest units of data measurement. A group of 8 bits is roughly equivalent to one alphabetic character of data. Standard practice is to group 8 bits into a unit called a *byte*. Bytes may be grouped into *kilobytes*, *megabytes*, and *gigabytes*, each being approximately 1,000 times larger than the previous. To give the reader a feel for these sizes, 1 kilobyte is about half a page worth of text, a megabyte is approximately a 500-page document, and a gigabyte would be about 1,000 copies of Tolstoy's *War and Peace*!

Copying files from one computer to another can be accomplished by physically carrying the storage media (e.g., floppies, ZIP disks, compact disks [CDs], or other removable recording media) between them. *Hardware* involves physical devices. It is distinguished from *software*, which typically involves programs or applications. Broadband access may facilitate greater use of *multimedia* applications in e-health. Multimedia usually connotes some combination of audio, text, pictures, and motion video in a presentation.

As compared to audio and video, text requires very little bandwidth. Speech contains much more information than the printed word, involving timing, pitch, tone, accent, and other features. Therefore, when sounds such as speech must be carried in real time, that is, at the same rate as in conversation, wider bandwidth is required. Sending moving pictures in real time requires even higher bandwidth. Various *data compression* techniques can reduce either bandwidth requirements or the amount of time needed to convey the information through a connection.

Successful data compression may involve compromises. Greater data compression can be achieved to the extent that one is willing to accept loss of data. For example, an image with nonessential areas cropped, that is a bit more blurry than the original, and in which the color scheme is simplified, may require far fewer bytes yet be acceptable. On the World Wide Web, photographic images are typically transmitted using a compression technique, in which one can specify in advance how severe the compression (and data loss) should be. The file may be reduced to less than a quarter of its original size. For some purposes, such as conveying the results of medical tests, data must survive passage fully intact, so that any compression should be *lossless*.

Moving pictures, such as animations and video, involve repeatedly redrawing a still image (or *frame*) so rapidly that the brain bridges the gap between successive frames. If the *frame rate* is too low, we see an unpleasant flickering, or a series of jerky movements. Lowering the frame rate is a very effective way to compress data, but any information that transpired between successive frames is lost. Lost frames can lead to missed information, such as the rapid shifting of the patient's gaze, a long pause, or a facial twitch that can occur when avoiding a particularly discerning question. Similarly, if too much detail is removed from each frame, which results in lower resolution, that is, in less picture clarity, information vital to clinical needs may be lost.

Of course, the higher the quality of video speed and clarity, the better—especially for diagnostic interviews, psychotherapy, or medication consultation (Squibb, 1999). Depending on the purpose that videoconferencing is to serve, the mental health clinician may need to insist on a specific level of transmission quality (and, hence, the compression method and bandwidth). Where ease of use is the overriding concern in connecting an inpatient to family and picture quality is relatively unimportant, a rentable *videophone* installed at the patient's home may suffice. Videophones are devices that connect existing televisions and telephones to provide videoconferencing over telephone services. Readers who may have watched the war in Iraq have a sense of the capacity of these videophones. Several reporters embedded with U.S. military forces used videophones to transmit images of themselves, other military personnel, and equipment back to U.S. television. Even though such images were grainy (poor resolution or clarity), they were certainly adequate to give us a sense of what was occurring in real time, on the other side of the globe.

Mental health applications for videophones are discussed further in chapter 5. Now that we have established a basic understanding of transmission channels, bits, and bytes, let's examine a technology that has already transformed many aspects of modern-day communication.

TRANSMISSION CHANNELS AND DEVICES

Explaining technology in today's ever-changing world is a serious challenge. We ask the reader to imagine a continuum with two poles. At one pole is *telecommunication transmission channels,* and at the other pole is technology *devices* (see Figure 2.1). We use these terms to clarify this process.

Telecommunication channels provide telephone lines, cable television wires, fiber optic cables, wireless satellite connections, and a number of other communication lines. These lines are segmented and repackaged for sale to the public by *carrier services.* The carrier services then lease telecommunication channels to consumers who, for example, seek to purchase Internet access. Typically, contracts with telecommunication service carriers involve *monthly subscriptions* for such services as telephone, cable television, Internet connections, or other specialized services (e.g., videoconferencing). Telecommunication transmission channels transmit data sent by a particular telecommunication device, such as a telephone, fax machine, computer, modem, videophone, or video monitor. Telecommunication devices are usually *purchased.*

Let us now take a moment to suggest that the continuum of transmission channels and devices is one of convenience; it does not necessarily reflect the real world. Developers of technology are striving toward *convergence,* that is, the attempt to combine technologies into an experience that is accessible to everyone. We thus have transmission channels that carrier services are repackaging to include access not only to specialized cable television lines but also to devices. An example of such a combination can be WebTV, which pipes the World Wide Web into a slightly modified TV set from a regular telephone line.

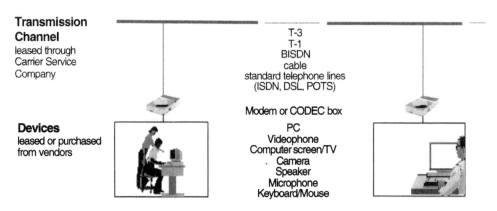

FIG. 2.1. Telecommunication channels and devices.

Confusion can occur in the difference between services and devices, as people have not been taught to think of telephones (devices) as being distinctly different from telephone services. In fact, original telephone service included a telephone. A telephone company extended its services, provided black, rotary-dial telephone devices for each room "extension," and charged a monthly rental fee for each extension, as well as for the telephone service itself. Then, for a little extra charge, one could rent a *Princess phone* that lit up.

After the U.S. government divided the AT&T monopoly into a brood of "Baby Bells," there was a massive unbundling of devices from services. Various enterprises (including telephone companies) began vying in strip malls to sell novelty phones (Felix the Cat, etc.), cordless equipment, and increasingly complex answering machines. The separation of transmission channels and devices changed even further when people owning personal computers were sold modems and leased monthly Internet services. Convergence between telecommunication service carriers and telecommunication devices led to the sweetening of personal computer (device) purchases with a substantial discount if one subscribed to a particular *Internet service provider* (ISP). An ISP is a carrier service company that provides subscribers with access to the Internet.

The same scenario happened with mobile phones. In the early telephone era, the emphasis seemed to be on devices, but the real profits were in providing and leasing telecommunication carrier services for monthly charges. In the new cellular phone market, purchase of the latest device is often bundled with a subscription for a year or more of carrier services that may include voice mail, electronic paging, e-mail, stock quotes, and the World Wide Web.

Similarly, today's personal computer is a blend of devices and can deliver the services of a telephone as well as a CD player and a television set. Convergence, then, allows people to carry fewer devices and to take underlying carrier services more or less for granted.

Although convergence seems to threaten our attempt to simplify this discussion, we maintain our initial distinction between telecommunication channels (along with their repackaged carrier services) and telecommunication devices. The next sections add further detail to our general distinction.

Transmission Channels

Currently, the characteristics and limitations of the transmission channels strongly influence the mental health professional's range of service to clients. When considering the use of telecommunication technology for transmitting a connection suitable for psychotherapy, the professional needs to think about such issues as transmission rate; time needed to establish a connection for each session; reliability, cost, availability, and installation issues; and security.

Bandwidth refers to the amount of data that can flow through a transmission channel each second. The rate at which a transmission channel transmits data is measured in *bits* (not bytes) per second, even though everyone commonly refers to the size of data in bytes (as stated previously). For example, most connections running over telephone lines may be rated as capable of transmitting 56 kilobits per second (written as 56 *kbps*).

Note that the actual transmission rate attained is usually considerably lower than the maximum rating. Devices receiving information can be limited in their rate of data reception as well, which slows down transmission speeds. It follows that buying a high-speed device to transmit data over a slow transmission channel is a waste. Our best suggestion is to determine the need of a project, and then to buy equipment and other devices to match the capabilities of the communication channels available in one's community. With this background, we now turn to the most common type of transmission channel.

Plain-Old Telephone Service. Ordinary telephone technology—*plain-old telephone service* (called, believe it or not, POTS)—is the slowest service used for on-line communication. Its maximum speed for transmitting data is 56 kbps. Of course, telephone technology is almost omnipresent and remains the least expensive, most affordable, and most widely available and reliable transmission channel. When accessing the Internet through POTS, a user makes a *dial-up connection* by dialing the telephone number of the ISP (or letting the modem do so). The telephone line may be shared by several devices (such as a telephone, fax machine, and/or computer modem), or one telephone line can be installed exclusively for any one of these devices.

A low-bandwidth transmission channel, such as a dial-up telephone line, is adequate for most asynchronous communication, such as sending an e-mail. Anything that allows the transmission of data to be much faster than a regular telephone is considered *broadband*, or *high bandwidth*. When transmitting large amounts of data, such as in video communication, broadband transmission channels are more practical for mental health purposes, as discussed in chapter 5.

To give you an idea of the difference between low and high bandwidth transmission speeds, Figure 2.2 compares the transmission rate of POTS with other forms of transmission. In the diagram, the lowest transmission rate, labeled "Modem" is available through POTS.

Broadband Transmission Channels. Each type of broadband transmission channel has its own strengths and weaknesses. In addition to transmission speeds, which can vary widely by type of broadband transmission channel, other considerations are present. Each consideration should be carefully weighed in relation to the type of mental health service being delivered. Selecting the optimal transmission channel for a given application depends on projected needs for transmission speed; system

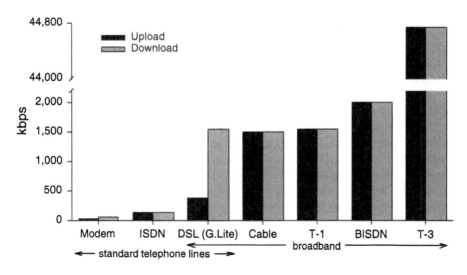

FIG. 2.2. Comparative speed of common transmission channels.

configuration (including number of users accommodated); requirements for encryption, security and confidentiality, availability, reliability, convenience, ease of use, technical support, mobility, anticipated improvements in features; and current and future costs. All these considerations are discussed throughout the book. For now, we offer a brief introduction to the most common types of broadband transmission channels.

The three relatively inexpensive options for broadband transmission service generally available in highly developed countries are *television cable lines, integrated services digital networks* (ISDN), and a *digital subscriber lines* (DSL). In 2002, approximately 24 million U.S. users had high-speed residential Internet connections (Pew Internet and American Life Project, 2002). Estimates of the future prevalence of broadband transmission channels project connections to approximately one third of U.S. households by 2005 (Jupiter Communications, 2000). The following sections briefly introduce the most common types of broadband transmission channels and outline some pros and cons of each.

Television Cable Lines. Originally developed to cover areas with poor television reception, *television cable lines* operate much like telephone party lines. Cable also presents extra security vulnerability because all the customers are linked together. If a particular cable system does not *encrypt*, or encode the information within the local transmission route, than the information is even more susceptible to hackers or others in the network. In the United States, pricing for broadband cable service is usually about $49 per month. User-satisfaction rates are very high. Most users report that they would find it very difficult to return to POTS (Newton, 1998).

Integrated Services Digital Network. An *Integrated Services Digital Network* (ISDN) offers point-to-point transmission speeds of from 128 to 356 kbps over ordinary telephone lines.[1] Because newer technologies are more popular than ISDN (and more profitable), telephone companies have assigned ISDN low priority to date. As a result, the end user may experience installation and service difficulties. Despite this, ISDN is favored in the United States for clinical videoconferencing. Facilities can connect with each other directly with ISDN, minimizing the security vulnerabilities and the disruption of the transmission stream that plague Internet-mediated communication. Furthermore, unlike digital subscriber lines (discussed in the following section), ISDN can serve areas that are far from a central telephone office, albeit at considerable expense. The U.S. government supports ISDN video linkage for health care with grants, special rate-setting regulations, and tax advantages. *Broadband ISDN* (BISDN), with speeds upward of 2 Mbps, could become a particularly useful clinical transmission channel (SearchNetworking.com, 2001).

It takes less time to connect an ISDN call than with POTS (provided the called line is also an ISDN), and ISDN lines can carry higher quality audio. However, subscription fees are high and the equipment is expensive, particularly if the higher transmission rates are to be achieved. It is wise for a practitioner to keep a regular telephone line available for any type of communication emergency, even if investing in ISDN for data transmission. A valuable tutorial on ISDN is available at http://www.ralphb.net/ISDN.

---

[1] Up to three ISDN lines can be yoked together into a 384 kbps transmission channel that allows real-time access to video for individual practice sites on a point-to-point network for quicker Web browsing than dial-up modem connections.

Digital Subscriber Lines.   Like ISDN, *digital subscriber lines* (DSL) use telephone wires between the end user (subscriber) and telephone companies. The difference with DSL is that it offers transmission rates from 128 kbps to 6.1 mbps (Whatis.com, 2001b). For most DSL service, the user must be within 4 miles (and, preferably, 2 miles) of a telephone company's central office because DSL signals degrade with distance, making DSL unsuitable for most rural applications. Indeed, the National Telecommunications and Information Administration (2000) estimates that 56% of U.S. cities with a population of 100,000 or more have DSL service, compared to fewer than 5% of towns with a population below 10,000.

Basic DSL service for home use, costing about $40 per month in the United States, does not allow one to connect directly to other subscribers but instead runs to an ISP. Thus, at least one middleman is involved when communicating through DSL.

Basic DSL is not optimal for two-way videoconferencing. Basic DSL supports downloading (bringing data into the computer) at a higher rate than uploading (sending data out). This is usually acceptable to people not intending to use it for two-way videoconferencing, because they usually want fast downloading of Web pages but do not often send out large files.

For people wanting symmetry between upload and download rates for two-way video communication, other varieties of DSL with faster transmission rates than basic DSL are available at a higher fee if the telephone wiring is adequate. Details and links are available at http://www.everythingcablemodem.com.

Telephone Trunk Lines.   For a relatively high price, an institution can subscribe to a *telephone trunk line* service. From the user's point of view, a trunk line is like yoking many POTS lines together. As seen in Figure 2.2, high connection speeds are possible with "T-1" and "T-3" telephone lines, but for such rapid communication between two devices, each must be connected to a trunk line. This requirement and their expense put them beyond the reach of most mental health practitioners and certainly out of the question for home use.

Devices

Although they are increasingly adept at handling an ever greater variety of tasks, devices are also becoming routine and integrated into the infrastructure of home and office. In the technologically-developed areas of the world, for example, telephones are taken for granted. It also seems that for online activity, Web services will soon become dominant, with most information storage and data processing being effected on supercomputers distributed all over the world. Personal computer devices will act mainly as interfaces and may eventually become essentially invisible. For most computer use, it is no longer necessary to acquire more than rudimentary knowledge of how devices work. It is enough to know that a computer computes and a printer prints.

As for communication technology in general, the current bottleneck lies in connectivity—that is, in the cost, availability, and service provided by telecommunication carrier services. Of utmost relevance to mental health professionals interested in remote delivery of direct services will be the data transmission rate in support of interactive videoconferencing. This is the most rapidly expanding area, offering practitioners the greatest potential for risk management in online delivery of direct mental health care. As we describe throughout much of this book, numerous adjunctive service delivery forms are also poised to move into daily practice.

THE INTERNET AND THE WORLD WIDE WEB

For our purposes, we discuss the Internet as a combination of transmission channels and devices that which enable synchronous and asynchronous transmission of data. When several *devices,* such as computers and modems, are connected through transmission channels, one speaks of a *network.* The largest network of networks is the *Internet.* The Internet enables computers from around the world to share information. The Net carries the bulk of e-mail and other services, of which the World Wide Web is the next most commonly used. The World Wide Web is discussed later in this chapter. To a computer, a network is like an outside world. The set of all existing electronic data networks may be thought of as a kind of world of its own, especially to the extent that the networks are connected to each other.

Connecting to the Internet

A common way to connect to the Internet using a POTS connection is with a *modem* (modulator/demodulator). A modem converts signals from the form produced by the computer into sounds that can readily be carried by conventional telephone lines and that, on the receiving end, can "demodulate" the sounds back into computer-compatible signals. The modem can either be attached externally to a computer or be built in as an internal modem. Today's telephone modems not only transmit data but can also dial out or answer the telephone and help establish a connection with a distant computer.

To connect to the Internet, one must go through an Internet service provider (ISP). Large organizations can act as their own ISPs, but most businesses, clinics, and individuals subscribe to one of the many ISPs available. The ISP connects to the Internet with a high-speed line, but it serves most of its subscribers by telephone or broadband.

Many ISPs offer a one-month free trial and an e-mail account, as well as basic software needed for e-mail and Web browsing. In about 20 minutes or so, an inexperienced user can install and configure the software. America Online (AOL) hosts its own e-mail service and has other offerings via its own network in addition to acting as an ISP.

Using an ISP as a communication intermediary introduces a security problem. Both human beings and computers can link to each other through POTS, the former using telephones and the latter with modems. It takes special effort and wiretap equipment to eavesdrop on a direct point-to-point telephone-to-telephone or modem-to-modem interchange, and such interception could expose the listener to severe legal penalties. In contrast, communications that are routed through a network, such as the Internet, go through intermediary computers, which are quite vulnerable to intrusion and require considerable expertise and continuing vigilance to keep secure. The ISP is privy to whatever passes through it; it is a favorite venue for legitimate law enforcement agencies, as well as for less than legitimate hackers, to acquire information. Hence, many professionals have argued for years that psychotherapeutic contact between a practitioner and client should not be conducted through the open Internet. Rather, if conducted at all in text-based environments, contact ought to be protected by encryption techniques (as discussed in chapter 10). As we see in chapter 9, the U.S. government has agreed to this protection and is mandating compliance with the new Health Insurance Portability and Accountability Act (HIPAA).

The World Wide Web has become so prominent that people often confuse it with the Internet. Actually, the Web is only one of several communication channels implemented within the Internet. E-mail, now one of the most popular communication methods, is for the most part carried by the Internet and is independent of the World Wide Web. Instant messaging, chat, streaming media, newsgroup, "voice over IP," and other services being used for mental health care delivery are also mediated by the Internet. These are described in other chapters that focus more on utility than on technicalities. (see, for example, chapters 3–8.) To encourage familiarity with the World Wide Web, we now glance at how it can be "surfed"; more details about the Web appear in chapter 4.

The World Wide Web

The *World Wide Web* is a scheme for conveying, over the Internet, a specifically requested "page" of material from a central computer. A *Web browser*, a program on the user's computer, displays Web pages and issues demands for other pages. The most popular Web browsers are Netscape and Internet Explorer. One duty of the browser is to receive the coded file that represents a Web page and to render it on the computer screen so that it looks more or less like a book or magazine page.

A Web page can be a very complex and active entity. Many Web pages include not only text but also pictures, animation, sounds, computer programs, and other features. Web pages may be assembled from several files that are stored on separate servers located all over the world. Just as a Uniform Resource Locator (URL), which is the address of a particular file on the Internet (e.g., http://selfhelpmagazine.com/resources), can summon a text file or a picture file from a remote computer, it can also summon a file of sounds, video, or any other kind of data, including computer programs that can run on the user's machine. Indeed, the Web is becoming a universal interface to everything that is available through the Internet.

Theoretically, users can take complete control of remote computers through their browsers, and, conversely, the Web can give remote computers complete access to users' equipment, such as disk drives, printers, cameras, home security systems, and physiological monitoring devices. Although much thought has gone into protecting machines and people from unwanted intrusions via the Web, it developed so quickly that it now has security flaws of particular concern to mental health applications.

You can get practically anything you want on the Web. A *search engine* (such as Google.com) is a program that operates through a Web site to comb the World Wide Web for other Web sites that meet criteria specified by the person "visiting" the search engine site. Search engines point users to Web sites or other Internet channels but do not contain much information in themselves. Search engines are comparable to advanced Rolodexes and point the user to other resources.

Mental health resources are well represented in such engines. For Web surfers, the uncensored gush of information that fills the computer screen in response to an innocent search request can be dismaying. For mental health topics, however general or specific, search engines can link to thousands of online resources. Expertise, persistence, patience, and luck are often required to glean a few grains of value from the tons of chaff retrieved by a search engine. Even professionals sometimes have difficulty finding reliable information on the Web. Future generations of these technologies will undoubtedly become more useful and accepted as they improve their ability to digest a user's request and present results in a more precise manner. Nonetheless, in their current state, search engines are an unparalleled resource for mental health consumers, clients, and professionals.

The following Web search engines can quickly find pages about almost any desired topic (Let the surfing begin!):

- Altavista (http://www.altavista.com).
- Excite (http://www.excite.com).
- Google (http://www.google.com).
- MSN (http://www.msn.com).
- Yahoo! (http://www.yahoo.com).

The most straightforward use of this technology is for clients to acquaint themselves with their psychiatric disorders, their manifestations, prognoses, treatment alternatives, and associated issues, as well as sources of help, by clicking on the results displayed by a search engine. The Web sites selected not only can help clients and consumers gather information about any general or specific disorder they experience, but they can also locate resources for caregivers. For professionals, search engines aid in gathering and placing clinical data into an electronic medical record. This information can then be used for designing and implementing a treatment approach, for assembling handouts, for creating assessment instruments and homework tasks, and for sifting through subjective reports and physiologic data monitored during ongoing treatment. In the future, insurance companies might use search engines to triage services.

This chapter offers the reader a basic understanding of the terms and concepts related to telecommunication services that are further discussed in this book. If additional definitions or explanations are desired, please refer to one of many online resources. We have found these sites to be particularly helpful:

- Alliance for Telecommunications Industry Solutions (http://www.atis.org).
- eHealthCoach. (http://www.ehealthcoach.com/Glossary_ehealth.asp).
- National Telecommunications and Information Administration (NTIA) Institute for Telecommunications Sciences (http://www.its.bldrdoc.gov/projects/t1glossary2000).
- Telehealth.Net (http://telehealth.net/glossary.html).
- Whatis? (http://whatis.techtarget.com).

How to function as mental health professionals in the new field of psychotechnologies, devices, services, direct and indirect, is the focus of the remainder of this book. In the next chapter, we start with direct suggestions and examine how to begin establishing a professional presence online using text-based environments.

$$3$$

E-Mail, Chat Rooms, and Other Text-Based Environments

Moer's truism: The scenery changes only for the lead dog.

Involvement with digital electronics is becoming a prominent part of people's lives. Children's video games, adolescents' instant messaging, adults' e-mail and searches for health information, and the widespread indulgence in Web-mediated pornography consume a considerable proportion of cognitive and affective life in Western society (Cooper, 2002). Mental health professionals need at least a working knowledge of the technological world their clients inhabit. In addition to providing direct service online, mental health professionals will be consulting, continuing their educations, conducting research, and providing supervision and oversight to students and colleagues. Mental health professionals need to become adept at the mechanics of various online modalities and to understand how the new communication systems affect the process of receiving care and the outcomes of care received. Finally, and most important, mental health professionals need to know how people relate to the electronic health care system, to other clinicians, and to clients online.

Clearly, in appropriate circumstances, mental health professionals should be going online. This means not only availing oneself of the information resources present on the Internet but also actively using current technologies to care for and provide service to clients. Getting online is easy. Before investing in a virtual office, however, mental health professionals may first scout the territory, heed the tales of the pioneers, purchase and install the right equipment, and test their online skills on family, friends, and colleagues.

Once professionals venture into cyberspace, their worldwide image is as important as their offline demeanor, dress, office decoration, business-card design, and stationery. The online identity of mental health professionals is an expansion of their offline selves, not an alternative. An online presence can influence one's reputation, ability to deliver service, and other aspects of a career. Displaying a presence anywhere means that onlookers will scan for signs of competence, self-esteem, power, sensitivity, and other characteristics (Miller, 1995). Consumers are particularly concerned about the ethical practices and reliability of the professional behind the image.

Cyberspace began as a lawless frontier with unlimited opportunity and unfamiliar hazards. It is now rapidly integrating with the physical world. Purely virtual dot.coms are fading into the mist of romantic legend, to be replaced by hybrid "bricks and clicks" enterprises spanning both cyberspace and Einsteinian space. The usual requirements for professional skills and credentials, comportment, ethics, and protection of the client are particularly important when applying any largely unexplored yet powerful new technology. Cyberspace abounds with initiatives arising mainly from fads, emotion and intuition, vague expectations of good luck, and hopes for profit, in addition to combinations of altruism and science. A professional image is a necessity in order to stand out from the many commercial enterprises and self-appointed healers clamoring for the attention of health-oriented consumers (Harris Interactive, 2001b). Maintaining one's professionalism is essential.

Going farther than putting a toe into the water calls for learning about how the online world—in which communication and relationships develop differently— diverges from and expands the dimensions of current practice. This chapter briefly explains the history of computer communications and defines the more common text-based communication venues that mental health practitioners use. We then give pointers for how professionals might conduct themselves in these environments without compromising professionalism. We also describe how this new conduct includes perspectives not currently considered in the daily routine of today's practice and how such conduct is not necessarily as easy as one might imagine. We then present professional literature related to working with patients and suggest proper Internet etiquette for text-based communication.

TEXT-BASED COMMUNICATIONS

On the Internet, thousands of low-cost and convenient supportive communities have emerged (Maheu, 1997b; Rheingold, 1993; Turkle, 1995; Wellman & Gulia, 1995). On-line communities are large groups of people connected by the Internet, usually in text-based environments, such as e-mail, newsgroups, or chat rooms. Many such groups allow anonymous participation that facilitates the open discussion of often stigmatized and embarrassing behaviors and issues. Individuals struggling with bulimia, self-inflicted violence, or sexual fetishes can find others who share their experience, offer support, and suggest resources.

In fact, many Internet users rely on Internet communities for emotional support as well as for self-help. After some weeks of membership in a compatible and mature Internet-based community, clients often learn who is reliable and how to ask for assistance. At the very least, this grassroots approach can allow a community member to have a voice, to express an unmet need, and to receive feedback. The social support experienced in Internet-based discussions can itself be an important factor in overcoming a personal problem. Because online peer groups are inexpensive to develop and maintain, are easily accessible, and often are anonymous, many people can now use such communities before starting formal treatment. Let us start by explaining how these communities began and how some of the more common text-based communications happen online.

Just Add Modem and Mix

The original electronic computers, such as Univac I, were controlled by external devices called *terminals* that could input data to the computer (usually through a *keyboard*) and that could display the computer's output, such as by printing it out. At first, old teletypewriters were used, and then began the sprawling proliferation of continually improved devices.

When electronic chips intended for use in electronic games evolved into use in personal computers, they soon were used as "smart" computer terminals, communicating with large central computers over short cables. These early personal computers were soon able to exchange messages with other personal computers remotely by telephone using crude modems. Modems communicate data as tones for telephone transmission. Such communication was point to point (i.e., one to one).

Modems soon dialed the telephone on their own and then began to answer calls automatically. Graduate students and hobbyists set up online *bulletin boards,* some of which are still in operation today. The user can view the contents of the bulletin board file and can append a new message for future visitors to see. Soon bulletin boards added such features as password requirements to bar unwanted visitors. As bulletin board *traffic* (message flow) increased, the owners of some bulletin boards installed telephone systems and software capable of accepting several calls simultaneously. A strong spirit of altruism and mutual support developed among users attracted to the many specialized bulletin boards. This spirit still pervades parts of today's Internet, as does attraction to decentralized governance, distaste for anything commercial, and often admiration of hackers who subvert organized systems.

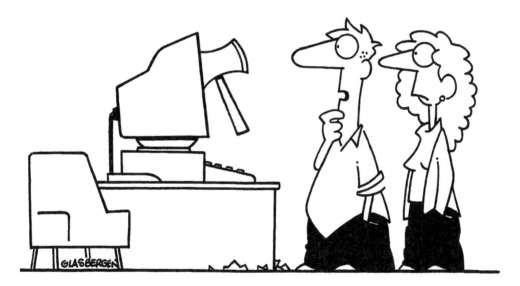

"Somebody broke into your computer, but it looks like the work of an inexperienced hacker."

The Advent of E-Mail. As computer bulletin boards were being elaborated, computer users were also beginning to use e-mail services. Instead of sending a message directly to the computer of the intended recipient (requiring that the computer be kept on to accept calls), one could post the message at any time to an e-mail service. Unlike the bulletin board paradigm, e-mail involves personal *e-mailboxes* that store incoming messages. A subscriber can then connect to such a service when ready to retrieve the stored messages.

At first, owing to technical incompatibility between different services, each e-mail service transferred messages only between its own subscribers. Standards gradually emerged, fostering development of sophisticated e-mail programs that can be used by subscribers from different services, such as America Online (AOL) and CompuServe, as well as local Internet service providers, found in almost every city.

Interpersonal Communication Modalities. Other aspects of the Internet developed alongside bulletin boards and e-mail. The basic original World Wide Web started as pages of text. It grew to include images, sound, and other aspects now found on the Internet. In fact, Web pages now include the ability to house many of these features simultaneously, allowing Web sites to become virtual offices by connecting users with one another through text, images, sound, and low-resolution videoconferencing.

Connection by E-Mail

Electronic mail, commonly known as e-mail, is perhaps the most extensively used application of the Internet. The cyberstreets are expected to be lined by more than 1,000 million e-mailboxes by the year 2005 (Lake, 2000). Nearly half of the 165 million Internet users in the United States already don their virtual slippers everyday to pad over to their e-mailboxes and scan through their 10 billion messages (Pew Internet & American Life Project, 2001a). Ninety-three percent of Internet users send e-mail, at least occasionally (Pew Internet & American Life Project, 2001b). Traffic in nonspam e-mail (or nonjunk e-mail) is projected to swell to more than 65 billion messages daily worldwide by 2005 (Lake, 2000).

One can use e-mail to send messages carrying text, images, video clips, sound files, or virtually anything in digital form. E-mail is asynchronous; people receiving e-mail can read it at their convenience. They do not need to be present while the message is being written. This attractive feature avoids the frustrations of telephone tag and the delay of standard, surface mail.

One can use a program such as Eudora (http://www.eudora.com) (see Figure. 3.1) or Microsoft Outlook Express to post a letter with an attached picture or document and electronically transfer the message to the address(es) of the desired recipients. Some Web sites, notably Yahoo! (http://www.yahoo.com) and Hotmail (http://www.hotmail.com), offer free e-mail accounts accessible through the Web without other software.

An e-mail address looks like this: info@telehealth.net (pronounced as info at telehealth dot net). The first part of the address, "info," defines the name of the person or department to which the mail is to be delivered. It is also called the user name, or the log-in. This part of the address to the left of "@" identifies the person to some extent. The part of address to the immediate right of "@" refers to the host computer (i.e., the name used by the Internet service provider [ISP] where the person has an account and, therefore, an e-mailbox). The extension "com" defines that the address belongs to a commercial organization.

Although e-mail is ordinarily thought of as one-on-one messaging, the programs used for e-mail also permit sending a message automatically to an entire list of addresses. The sender can privately create and modify such lists. If everyone on a list maintains an identical list on his or her own computer, a group of people can share their communications with one another.

In contrast to duplicated private lists maintained on the computer of each group member, *e-mail discussion lists, e-mail discussion forums,* or *listservs* (these terms are used

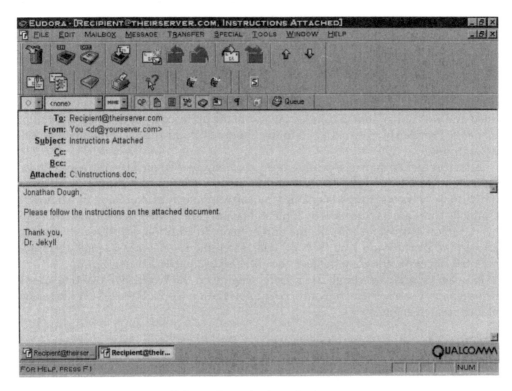

FIG. 3.1. Example of e-mail software.

interchangeably) involve creating a single centralized list on one main computer. This practice makes it easier to enroll and remove group members and allow people to subscribe to or leave a group individually without intervention by the group's leader. In an e-mail list, a member e-mails a message only once to the central server computer, which then forwards the message to each subscriber.

Like e-mail, listservs predate the Internet. The proprietary 1986 mailing list manager program Listserv (http://www.lsoft.com/listserv.stm) came first, and as a result of heavy use, its name soon became as generic as the name Kleenex.

Professional e-mail discussion lists are an excellent arena for mental health professionals to explore and debate issues of concern with colleagues from around the world. Consumer e-mail discussion lists are similar, except that the participating audience is primarily nonprofessional. Each e-mail discussion list has one or more owners. Owners set and enforce the list's password policy and decide who is permitted to review archives of past messages, who can join the list, and who is to be expelled. The owner can designate one or more *forum moderators* to center conversation on the group's core topic and also to ameliorate interpersonal conflicts in the group. *Forum administrators* generally maintain the technical functioning of the list, remove names of people who violate forum rules, send guidelines, and sometimes contribute information to the list, but they do not take responsibility for moderating discussion. Listservs tend to be more private and controlled than are newsgroups, another discussion modality.

Newsgroups

Newsgroups are a way of communicating with like-minded people over the Internet regarding hundreds of thousands of topics, ranging from psychoanalysis to Yorkshire pudding. Newsgroups were one of the first systems developed on the Internet. The system enabled users to post announcements that anyone could read by using special software. Posted material was sorted into major topic areas, with special interest groups developing around each topic. People were exchanging encrypted files, pictures, and programs, as well as text. Overall, supervision of the *Usenet* (the main system loosely coordinating newsgroups) is by informal consensus of anyone interested and was rather anarchic, in keeping with the philosophy of most early Internet pioneers. Previously, one had to go to the Usenet through special software to access newsgroups.

Advertisements, quarrels, pornography, and mischief began crowding in with legitimate material, but valuable and serious activity continues. Reading postings of individuals on newsgroups is enabled by software, such as Netscape or Microsoft Outlook. There are a wide variety of mental health care-related newsgroups that can be important sources for information and opinion. In addition, many search engines also on the World Wide Web (WWW) will search the Usenet and display a subject-oriented directory, allowing the user to subscribe to a particular newsgroup.

Nowadays, one can simply use a search engine on the World Wide Web to access newsgroups. For a sense of how to access a newsgroup through the WWW, go to one of these search engines:

- Altavista (http://www.altavista.com).
- Google (http://www.google.com).
- Yahoo! (http://www.yahoo.com).

Next, type the word *newsgroups* into the search engine, then click on any one of the links offered by that search engine. For example, when using Google, the first offering is all the Google communities. By clicking on this link, one will be taken to another search engine, where one can then type *depression*. The reader will then find a number of newsgroups related to depression.

Now try Google again (http://groups.google.com), but this time, rather than just searching for current Usenet Newsgroups to read and post new messages, look for specific material among its 650 million archived newsgroup postings dating back to 1995. Perhaps a search for factitious disorders will lead to interesting bits of professional or consumer conversation in a newsgroup, either current or past. Google also serves as a remarkable warehouse for pages that were originally captured by this extraordinary search engine but have since been removed from Web sites by their owners.

By now, you will have accumulated a set of promising search terms. Use the same search engine to find a few newsgroups devoted to the chosen topic. Read a series of postings to get a feel for the culture of each group. This acculturation process is an important part of getting to know how to use the Internet.

Note that one does not formally join a newsgroup. Because there is so little commitment demanded, newsgroups are a frequently used place to begin participating in online discussions. If one asks for assistance with a specific problem, surprisingly informative replies will appear within hours if the group is large. People love to help.

Newsgroup postings include announcements, questions and answers, useful lists, and references to Web sites. Participants tend to share social and informational support and seek to improve one another's self-esteem (Muncer, Burrows, Pleace, Loader, & Nettleton, 2000). Note the common acronyms and shorthand ways to communicate and the textual argot that is integral to online society. These shortcuts are important to know in order to avoid misunderstandings. They are found in every form of text communication (e-mail, e-mail discussion lists, etc.). Before actually posting a message, be familiar with the description of online jargon and principles of etiquette and cyberspace citizenship (as described later in this chapter).

Even though nearly all the newsgroups function without a leader, many involve lively discussions and exhibit recognizable group dynamics. The usefulness of an expert's presence and contributions also comes in question. Some users consider the presence of a leader to be a disruption of the group process, drawing attention away from consumer-to-consumer interactions or interfering with people's attempts to establish legitimacy and authority through their communications (Galegher, Sproull, & Kiesler, 1998). A few minutes' searching will make it easy to see how a consumer might feel confused and overwhelmed.

Some bulletin boards and newsgroups have also migrated directly to the World Wide Web; they can be found on private Web sites as in-house discussion forums, which are accessible through Web browsers. Convergence of technologies is improving access to these communication forums for people with limited knowledge or access to the older portions of the Internet. These in-house discussion forums are often protected from hackers who can collect e-mail addresses from bulletin boards, e-mail discussion lists, and newsgroups, and sell these e-mail addresses to commercial groups. Such commercial groups can use large numbers of e-mail addresses for *spamming* (the sending of unwanted e-mail, often for advertising). Specialized programs called "bots" may ferret out and copy listserv archives into huge databases, often without the knowledge of list members or owners. Professionals logging onto newsgroups or encouraging existing clients, friends, or colleagues to find information in public newsgroups may benefit from being forewarned that some people use these groups solely to troll for e-mail addresses or private archives that they copy and sell.

Privacy protections are typically listed on a Web site. For clients seeking free, easily accessed support, more than 100 Web-based discussions are available in *Selfhelp-Magazine* (http://www.selfhelpmagazine.com), operated by one of this book's authors. This and other Web sites owned by individuals and professional associations attend to the mental health information consumer's desire for online communities, while providing privacy protections, including anonymity of varying degrees. As consumers develop skills to interact with one another online, such supportive communities may tend to grow in safety as well as participation, bringing to each mental health issue (e.g., child abuse) an international forum for participants to discuss the problem, treatment, and the impact on their lives and the ones they love.

Internet Chat

In addition to the asynchronous methods of bulletin boards, e-mail, e-mail lists, and newsgroups, people can converse synchronously over the Internet using text-based *chat rooms*. Even though chat rooms originated as another part of the Internet, known as Internet Relay Chat (IRC), most people now use chat rooms available through Web sites. Regardless of their location on the Internet, people can then "enter" a chat room, using a password and appropriate software. Messages posted to the chat room are immediately displayed on the computers of everyone else logged into the room. When a new member enters or when someone leaves, a message is displayed informing the group of the arrival or departure. Chat room facilities often allow a leader to control the flow of messages to prevent confusion (and to expel people who abuse the facility).

More than 27 million Americans have visited a chat room, and more than 3 million people do so daily (Pew Internet & American Life Project, 2001a). Chat rooms have become favorite places for people to engage in serious personal discussions. Most users in medically-oriented chat rooms gather information or share life experiences with one another, such as a divorce or parenting situation (Lavoie, Borkman, & Gidron, 1994). In health care contacts, chat rooms pose complex questions. Chat rooms also can entail significant risks, especially confidentiality and privacy. Ethical questions can be important as well; they are discussed further in chapter 10.

Rapidity of response is the rule in this text-based environment. Delays in crafting a comment can easily render one's belated offering lame or as evidence of stubborn resistance, intended to block the flow of conversational traffic. Chat rooms contain many seemingly off-topic postings, the frequent expressions of greeting, leave taking, bonding, acknowledgment, reassurance, affirmation, or smart-aleck challenge reminiscent of the continual honking of a gaggle of geese flying overhead. This activity is part of the social glue that holds the group together. Paradoxically, the same can be said about the fact that often several separate conversations may occur simultaneously. A group is continually splitting and reforming. Despite the more rapid interpersonal feedback of the chat environment, the rude comments, flaming, and obscenities that sprinkle other text-based communication venues can also be found here.

The informal tone of most chats belies the fact that material may be archived or copied by group members and become etched in the permanent memory of cyberspace. As a result, whatever a professional may post to a listserv becomes a permanent part of his or her online presence. Any insults, expletives, and accusations leveled at the professional by other users may also be retrieved in association with the professional's name.

Chats need not involve multiple participants. Two participants can meet in a variant on the chat room format where no scheduling is required and two people can have a back-and-forth textual conversation. This milieu is known as *instant messaging* (IM), and it occurs in a private type of chat room, where only those invited can appear. Some such systems also support voice conversations. Instant messaging has become very popular with American teens and is now considered vital in business communications.

Chat rooms can also incorporate visual elements. *Visual chat rooms* have also been called multimedia chat, graphical multiuser conversations (GMUKS), and habitats. Visual chat rooms create the illusion of movement and space in a two-dimensional world. Visual chats include two distinct visual elements. First, the room, or backdrop, acts as a virtual environment (described in more detail in chapter 7) in which participants of the chat can move around. For example, multiple users can meet, say, in a wood cabin overlooking the Sierra Nevadas or at an oceanfront cottage to participate in a group therapy session. Entry into these rooms can require a password or other security measures.

The second element is an *avatar*,[1] or "av" as some users call it. An avatar is an iconic (i.e., visual) representation of oneself in the virtual environment (Quimby, 1999). By using software programs users can customize an avatar to make them appear however they wish—as a different race, with different hair and eye color, or with other characteristics. The program then allows the face of the avatar to exhibit emotional and behavioral signals anytime during a conversation—happy, sad, angry, winking, sleeping or bored, blushing, head-nodding, or head shaking (Suler, 1999b). Some programs even allow the facial movements to be synchronized with the text typed in

---

[1] The term *avatar* comes from the Hindu religion in which it refers to the various forms that gods chose to manifest themselves in the human realm (Suler, 1999a).

the chat room. A common visual chat room is the "Palace," which has hundreds of virtual environments and thousands of participants.

Visual chats may help integrate in-person skills with text-based environments by enabling therapists and clients to interact in a virtual space together. Supporters of the use of visual environments in therapy have noted that therapists may gain previously unknown insights into their clients by examining the characteristics of the avatar clients present (Suler, 1999a). In addition, visual chats may allow for therapeutic interpretation or reenacting of fantasies and dreams, role playing and reverse role playing of life situations, and working with transference and countertransference in novel ways (Suler, 1999b).

Clients participating in such new and unproven environments should be made aware of the experimental nature of the therapy. Critics may feel that visual chats could become a distraction or game detracting from the goals of therapy. If and when data emerge demonstrating harm from use of visual chats in a health care context, the principle of informed consent may at some point oblige therapists to advise would-be participants of such risks.

Now that the reader is familiar with the main pathways to communicate and find support using online text-based environments, we can focus on how the reader can engage other professionals through these pathways. The next section outlines how a professional can join or develop an e-mail discussion list or newsgroup. Additionally, we outline some problems with these online text-based groups in order to help avoid common barriers.

PROFESSIONAL PARTICIPATION IN TEXT-BASED DISCUSSION

This section proposes a systematic process by which a mental health professional can become familiar with online discussion milieus over a span of a few weeks. We begin with e-mail in a limited way and then proceed to newsgroups, e-mail lists and forums, and chat rooms. Actually, the first thing to do is to establish one's Web feet. Pick a relatively obscure yet controversial social or emotional problem, such as Munchausen syndrome by proxy, and research it with the aid of a search engine.

Which search engine should one try? Readers who feel lost are experiencing what many patients go through. Accept on faith that the Web holds abundant material about any disorder one can imagine, that there is at least one organization dedicated to it, and that there are several lay discussion groups one can join. This exercise demonstrates how the Web is the pervasive background for much online discussion about health matters and an essential component of online practice.

Joining, Developing, and Maintaining E-Mail Forums

E-mail is where nearly everyone first goes for online interaction. A professional new to the online world had best begin by exchanging e-mail with relatives, friends, and colleagues who will forgive mistakes and interpret ambiguities favorably. Once one is comfortable with e-mail exchanges, the next recommended step is to join (and possibly develop) an e-mail forum. This is more of a commitment, because the process involves submitting one's e-mail address to a public and therefore easily accessible databank. It is safest to start with one or two e-mail discussion lists that are restricted to professionals. Interpsych (http://www.fus.edu/~trauma/ip.html), founded by psychologist Ian Pitchford of Sheffield, England, organizes many excellent professional discussion forums. This site is now administered by other professionals and contains instructions for applying to the various discussion forums. Among the dozens of descriptions, one is certain to find one or two lists of special interest. This comment offered by Berlin psychologist Sunkyo Kwon, an experienced manager and leader of professional online forums, gives a behind-the-scenes view of Interpsych:

I have managed more than twenty mailing lists. One, transcultural psychology (TP), is an InterPsych forum. Discussion on it has been lively and stimulating. Since I took charge of it in 1994, TP has changed servers five times. I have had to handle innumerable requests for information, subscriptions, and changes of subscription, including requests to sign off or to suspend and then resume mail because of vacations. I have had to screen for corrupt addresses, monitor technical glitches, post news and new threads for discussion, and promote the list. Most of this activity goes unnoticed by the average subscriber.

At one point, it became clear that the content of many discussions had departed from the announced aims of TP. Accordingly, in 1995 I established a second list, C-psych (CP) for cross-cultural psychology. TP was redefined as a forum for the study of cultures, particularly with a focus on clinical and counseling psychology, as well as "generic" issues. CP was dedicated to discussion of cross-cultural topics within the "traditional" psychological disciplines (personality, social, developmental, etc.), with the exception of clinical therapy or counseling, and with an additional emphasis on qualitative and quantitative methods. I had even recruited advisory boards with competent scholars in the field, and I invited coordinators.

Although well meant, the changes did not harmonize with actuality. Subscribers kept confusing the purposes of CP and TP, some double-posted their messages to both lists, and some considered the forums to be their private chat rooms. This situation peaked when five members were posting 90% of all exchanges on CP, very often off-topic.

Although useful information and constructive comments were traveling through the lines, the signal–noise ratio was almost intolerable. Many long-term subscribers unsubscribed. The final solution: CP is now a "moderated list," which means that all postings are screened by the coordinator for appropriateness to ensure quality (even more work). TP has become a forum for a wide range of topics and contributions.

Conclusions:

*   *The dynamics of mailing lists are difficult to control.*
*   *Purposes of mailing lists develop and change according to the needs of the subscribers.*
*   *For the coordinator, it means, work, work, work.*

In contrast to CP and TP, the newsletter PsychNews International *(PNI), which I have edited since 1994, involves mostly one-way communication. That is, PNI is a read-only newsletter to which subscribers can respond only by way of "letters to the editor" that might be published in a subsequent issue. Some of the technical work multiplies in serving thousands of readers as compared with mere hundreds in a discussion forum, but one is spared many of the tasks of the e-mail list leader. The tough issues for a newsletter editor are soliciting articles and the actual editing and formatting tasks.*

PsychNews *was launched as the* InterPsych Newsletter *(IPN), covering mainly topics of interest to the InterPsych community (mental health–related issues). We started with heroic ideas, like peer-reviewed articles, a regular distribution schedule, and lots of interactions with our initially more than 10,000 subscribers. However, reality soon reared its ugly head. Because everybody involved in producing IPN was a volunteer, we had to lower our aspirations.*

After 3 years, IPN was renamed PsychNews International (PNI) to reflect that its aims had grown beyond those of service to InterPsych. Now, PNI has some 5,000 subscribers. Present plans involve increasing the international audience and focusing more on the interface of mental health issues and technology, particularly the Internet. Currently, PNI runs three associated Web sites, a separate table-of-contents-only service based on the latest edition of PNI, and a discussion list for staff members.

Just running and maintaining a newsletter can be a lot of work. As for list coordinators, they need to be clear about their goals, how much time and energy investment they can sustain, and how much outside help they can get. After all, sometimes all one really needs for a professional presence on the Net is a humble home-made personal Web site.[2]

—**Sunkyo Kwon, Ph.D.**
Greifswald University
Institute for Psychology, Germany

Some universities have opened their technological doors and supplied the mental health field with free hosting. One of the largest of such pro bono programs is sponsored by St. John's University in Queens (part of New York City), which has many professional, as well as consumer, e-mail discussion lists (http://maelstrom.stjohns.edu/archives/index.html). Similarly, AtHealth (http://www.athealth.com) hosts a number of professional and consumer lists.

Privately held and administered e-mail discussion lists also exist for professionals. Since the early 1980s, New York City psychiatrist Ivan Goldberg has been adeptly leading excellent online discussions on psychopharmacology. A qualified professional can subscribe without charge to Psych Controversies or to his other listservs by e-mailing psydoc@psycom.net. One of this book's authors has founded and administers several professional discussion lists that individuals can join (http://telehealth.net/subscribe/subscribe_all.html).

Most professional mental health associations have their own in-house electronic discussion lists for discussion of general and specific topics. For example, the American Psychological Association (APA) has a Practice Listserv. Call the APA's Practice Directorate to obtain information about this discussion list and many others. Discussion group leaders may require new members to provide evidence of appropriate professional credentials.

After joining a list, new members may be asked to announce themselves briefly. Professionals can openly identify their disciplines, licensure, and affiliations and can explain their reasons for joining. A new member can then lurk silently for a while, observing how people interact and learning what is acceptable for discussion. Ideally, one will encounter some groups at an early stage in their development, a group or two in turmoil, and a few solid but quiet lists.

If the list is quiet, send an open-ended question about a subject relevant to the title of the list. A well-worded and sensitive question will usually draw an answer from

---

[2] To subscribe to TP, send e-mail (subject line empty) to: listserv@lists.apa.org. In the message body put "subscribe transcultural-psychology First name Last name" (substituting your names, respectively). To subscribe to CP, send an e-mail (subject line empty) to listserv@maelstrom.stjohns.edu. In the message body put "subscribe c-psych First name Last name" (again with name as indicated).

long-time subscribers who support the life of the list. Just because a question does not get a flurry of responses does not mean the list is dead. A succession of questions may be needed to spark a discussion. Early questions might not have been read by the very person who has the best answer. "Newbies" might get discouraged, but the reality is that "old timers," who have been reading e-mail for almost a decade, often do spend a night watching television. Nonetheless, mailing lists are a rich source of collegial information, and persistence pays off. Find a way to ask the question again, in different words. Above all, if leaving a list devoted to a topic of interest, do not blame the list for failing to address a specific topic without having made several short but direct inquiries regarding that topic. As with all information, weigh what is read and give it only such weight as it deserves. The fact that someone has expressed a view in electronic form or has a recognizable name does not mean that the advice is sound, the information correct, or the analysis accurate. Even in professional listservs, the signal-to-noise ratio may be low.

Even on professional lists, regression is rampant (Holland, 1996). Group dynamics on the Internet show features of small, large, and fishbowl groups (Weinberg, 2001). It may take a few weeks to experience the psychodynamic shifts that occur in some of the more active groups. As for the list as a whole, Table 3.1 shows the anonymous, tongue-only-halfway-in-cheek description of the developmental phases of mailing lists that is now part of Internet lore. Over the next few decades, these professional discussion groups will grow in number, develop additional communication features, and increase their international audience.

TABLE 3.1
The Natural Life Cycle of E-Mail Discussion Lists

1. *Initial enthusiasm:* People introduce themselves and express gratitude for having found kindred souls.

2. *Evangelism:* People moan about how few folks are posting to the list and brainstorm recruitment strategies.

3. *Growth:* More and more people join, lengthy threads develop, and occasional off-topic threads appear.

4. *Community:* Lots of threads, some more relevant than others; a lot of information and advice is exchanged; experts help other experts as well as less experienced colleagues; friendships develop; people tease each other; newcomers are welcomed with generosity and patience; "newbies" and experts alike feel comfortable asking questions, suggesting answers, and sharing opinions.

5. *Discomfort with diversity:* The number of message increases dramatically; not every thread is fascinating to every reader; people start complaining about the signal-to-noise ratio. Person 1 threatens to quit if other people don't limit discussion to Person 1's pet topic; Person 2 agrees with Person 1; Person 3 tells 1 and 2 to lighten up; more bandwidth is wasted complaining about off-topic threads than is used for the threads themselves. Everyone gets annoyed. Seasoned list owners use a variety of strategies to pull the troublemakers out of the discussion, encourage subscribers to cease responding to off-topic threads, and spark new on-topic threads. Unskilled list owners sit by, and watch their lists wither as disgruntled users unsubscribe.

6. *Smug complacency and stagnation:* The purists flame everyone who asks an "old" question or who responds with humor to a serious post. Newbies are rebuffed; traffic drops to doze-producing minor issues; all interesting discussions happen by private e-mail and are limited to a few participants. Purists privately and self-righteously congratulate each other for keeping off-topic threads off the list.

Or

Maturity: A few people quit in a huff; the rest of the participants stay near Phase 4, with Phase 5 popping up briefly every now and then; many people wear out their second or third "delete" key, but the list lives on contentedly, occasionally coming to life to discuss an interesting issue. Mature lists are similar to familiar library stacks: they exist quietly, are brought to life when something is needed, but much of the time, one forgets about them.

Everything Is Public

We now pause in our tour of online text-based discussion venues to discuss encountering consumers, potential patients, current patients, and possibly even future employers. Participation as a professional in a forum for mental health care consumers calls for a level of awareness beyond what is needed for dealing with colleagues. Any statement may be challenged, misinterpreted, or exploited for someone's personal or political agenda. Then again, that might happen in a professional e-mail discussion list as well, but such responses occur less frequently. Even closed mailing lists may include members who have improperly slipped through the list owner's screening process. Events that are unlikely to occur in relation to any one person are much more likely when hundreds or tens of thousands of individuals are involved.

A professional seen as having joined consumers in any text-based, interactive discussion may need good online skills to initially overcome being stereotyped as a rigid drug dispenser, charismatic healer, pompous money grubber, spiritual guru, or quack. If one is misunderstood or mistreated online, the incident will not necessarily be over when one signs off. It may not be resolved even after clarifying misunderstandings and exchanging apologies or reassurance, and the sting of a negative response can sometimes be felt for hours afterward, if not days.

The following story recounts an early learning experience of one of this book's authors:

In late 1994, having developed the self-help Nicotine Freedom System, I uploaded a few of my smoking-cessation articles onto a Web site. I added pictures of the stop-smoking materials along with advertising language and an order page. To promote this system further, I dropped announcements about my program into all the seemingly relevant newsgroups I found through search engines and Web site links.

Before I knew it, scathing messages began arriving in my e-mail. One contained vulgar expletives and threats to complain to my ISP. It was followed by another, of the same ilk. It seems I had blundered into one of the newsgroups dedicated to celebrating tobacco with a worldwide discussion of taste, aroma, and tips for acquiring the most exotic and luscious leaves at the lowest international price.

I kept my cool and responded both publicly and privately directly to the most vituperative of the e-mails with an explanation of my error and an apology. I quickly got back a private reply expressing understanding and forgiveness, yet sternly admonishing me for not respecting the community by reading their messages before posting mine and for not combing through the earlier posts for the group charter.

Anxiety stricken, I politely asked to be sent a copy of the charter, and yes, indeed, the document clearly stipulated that anyone posting to this list must refrain from attempts to negate smokers' rights to convene and discuss topics of their choice and specifically must not offer tobacco-cessation advice. I repeated my apology and received a courteous and grateful reply.

Returning to the newsgroup after a few days to see how the other group members had responded, I was startled to see that my courteous and grateful guide had proudly posted his original abusive admonishment to me and was now triumphantly and emphatically claiming he had put me in my place. There was no reference of either my public or private apology or his seemingly warm forgiveness of his second private reply. Other group members had not made any reference to my original post or my public apology. I learned my lesson and chose to quietly go on my way rather than attempt further communication.

The newbie becomes hardened to these seemingly abusive distortions of one's intentions, and outright misrepresentations, but not until spending considerable time agonizing before an invisible audience. What must they think of me? How could I be so irresponsible as a professional?

The Internet folds these errors into its massive cyberwaves, where they might turn up again, or might not. Fortunately, the unpleasant experience described in this vignette had no further repercussions. Fortunately, too, the giant Google archive (http://groups.google.com) does not reach back to 1994, so this early learning experience won't necessarily be accessible by patients or future employers. Reports of similar mistakes, however, have included descriptions of how such errors can easily lead to harassment by more intrusive telephone or fax messages from outraged and anonymous users.

Not to discourage professionals from using these communication networks but rather to help them prevent similar blunders, we continue our discussion of perils associated with newsgroups. First, however, we mention that professionals can avoid many of these problems by simply using an alternative e-mail address, easily obtained from one of the several companies offering free e-mail addresses. When formulating messages to be posted to any of these newsgroups, avoid including telephone numbers, fax numbers, street addresses, or other identifying information. That is, travel incognito and enjoy the benefits of newsgroups without the potential risks. Once a particular search for a specific type of information or support is complete, the e-mail address can be discarded and repercussions of using these resources thereby removed.

Let us now and see how these discussions can easily get out of hand. If not treated as the potentially explosive time bombs they are, group discussions over a distance can readily deteriorate into "flame wars," where animosity quickly escalates into personal attacks, name calling, and threats that can even lead to prolonged personal harassment, stalking, and physical assaults. An extensive compilation of typical "flame warriors," complete with caricatures, is available on the Web (http://www.wInternet.com/~mikelr/flame1.html).

A bit of psychological theorizing might be beneficial. It is not clear to what degree psychopathology underlies flame wars and how much the eruptions spring from the asynchronous nature of online text-based discussions and from the anonymity and physical distance between participants. Even a brief sequence of e-mails with friends and relatives reveals how typographical errors produce marked distortion or even reversal of meaning. Witticisms often fall flat. In the health care arena, witticisms posted electronically can be dangerous. Jurors are likely to view with suspicion health care professionals who seems too lighthearted about their business, however well intentioned they may be. In general, it is best to avoid humor, at least in writing, in these settings. Although some people respond almost instantly to e-mail, others do not check their mailboxes or newsgroup messages for weeks. It can be difficult to clear up a misunderstanding by e-mail. This is why it is best first to get one's feet wet with familiar people who are inclined to be forgiving before venturing into general online communication and to deal with colleagues before entering discussions with consumers or patients.

In contrast to interacting with the physical world, as we do on a daily basis, one's ability to comprehend the cyberspace environment is curtailed, and feedback from one's actions is delayed or nonexistent. Thus, an appropriate sense of danger may be absent. In driving a car, otherwise timid, gentle, or dignified people readily take offense, trade obscene gestures, cut each other off, and engage in road-rage behaviors.

Online, some people are even more likely to lash out impulsively from behind a screen of anonymity. Ordinary forum group members do not hold one another to the same standards of accountability for their statements in a discourse as the criteria they impose on special members, such as identified professionals. Scapegoating and other interpersonal maneuvers aimed at discrediting a particular forum member can lead to a virtual online lynching.

Avoiding the Scorch. Experienced list members realize that discussion list flames are usually handled discreetly by list owners rather than escalated publicly. Other list members are left to wonder what happened and often send questions or smart-aleck responses back to the irritating list member. Such posting is not helpful and serves only to escalate the number of off-topic and irritating posts sent to a forum. Some forums have been overrun by such negativity and forced to close if the list owner does not take swift and definitive action. If the situation gets out of hand, the list owner has the option to remove the angry list member from the public forum (assuming the correct name and e-mail address have been registered) and then to offer other disgruntled forum members reassurance that the situation has been handled behind the scenes. This approach is often a last resort and is used primarily as an attempt to salvage a damaged forum by sparing its members further exposure to angry messages. Members often do not understand that it is best to keep quiet at such times and let the list owner handle the situation.

One of this book's authors founded large e-mail discussion groups, to which thousands of people have submitted their e-mail addresses. The consumer in our next example was unable to decipher how to unsubscribe from one of the e-mail discussion list and complained publicly. The list founder steered the conversation to the *back channel* (private one-on-one e-mail) and did not discuss any of this communication publicly:

Monday, public request from consumer, posted to the entire list: I did not subscribe to begin with, someone who I pissed off in a chat room subscribed me to annoy me, I have since discovered that they pick your group because YOU WON'T FUCKING STOP SENDING ME FUCKING E-MAILS NO MATTER HOW MANY TIMES AND IN HOW MANY WAYS I HAVE DEMANDED AND ASKED AND BEGGED THAT YOU FUCKING STOP.

Monday, private back-channel response from the List Founder: Joen, I'm happy to help you unsubscribe from the Cyberaffairs Discussion list but will need your help. The computer isn't recognizing your e-mail address. Please think about what e-mail address someone might have used to subscribe you.

Tuesday, back-channel, from consumer: I really don't understand why, if I am getting e-mail's at joenah@mlp.com, that you can't stop sending them. If they used a fake name like Fucko Shitnuts at joenah@mlp.com, then ignore the name Fucko Shitnuts and just go by joenah@mlp.com. Explain to me why, if I am getting the e-mails from you at that address, that you can't stop sending them?

Tuesday, back-channel, from the List Founder: Joen, I am a psychologist, and I'm doing my best to try and help you. So please send me any other e-mail addresses you have had in the past.

Wednesday, back-channel, from consumer: I'm sorry, that is the only e-mail address I have had, it is with my company and they assigned it to me and it has never changed, this is where I am receiving e-mails from your company. I have BPD if that helps.

Wednesday, back-channel, from the List Founder: Joen, if this is the only address you have ever used, I can't figure this out. I will send a note to the system administrator. He sometimes takes days to respond. (Meanwhile, please know that I am doing everything I can. I apologize for your inconvenience).

Wednesday, back-channel, from consumer. OK, thank you for all your efforts. Hopefully they will stop soon.

This unhappy list member felt it necessary to wax emphatic in order to be heard, but he responded to a professional approach, which included addressing the other party by name and signing all notes. Both the use of vulgarity and the fact that the discussion extended over 3 days were accepted by both correspondents as being sufficiently ordinary for e-mail as not to warrant comment or apology. Although the previous conversation was with a consumer, list owners have found that professional colleagues can be equally difficult.

A hidden aspect of this exchange involves using a worksite e-mail address for personal correspondence. The rapid escalation of vulgarity occurred without considering that all e-mail posted to and from a work address is legally the property of the employer and subject to inspection at any time (Schwartz, 2001).

This exchange with a disgruntled consumer illustrates other points:

- It is possible to "spoof" someone else's address and to "subscribe" him or her to stigmatized mental health groups. In addition, consumers can forget having responded to a notice inviting their participation and can be surprised when they begin receiving messages from a new group.
- "Unsubscribing" requires a message from the registered e-mail account. Consumers are often unaware of the effort it takes for a list owner to remove them if they registered with a false name or a now forgotten e-mail address.
- Consumers can become rude in demanding removal from a discussion list or when communicating with other relatively anonymous online services. Even in direct one-on-one e-mail, some people manage to be markedly discourteous, often unintentionally. Many requests for information are just that, with no salutation and no signature, so that one is tempted to reply to the sender's e-mail address with a snide "Dear whoever you are." E-mail involving a discussion group can be distributed inadvertently to every group member rather than to the single intended recipient. It may then be archived and can become, via search engines, available to the entire world for all posterity, visible to future employers, potential marriage partners, loan officers, law enforcement, licensing boards, and other entities. E-mail posted from the workplace is often archived on the corporate or agency computer and available for inspection by the administration. The prospect of having one's bad manners widely exposed does not seem to daunt some people, but it should at least keep professionals on the straight and narrow.
- The patience and courtesy of a professional can dramatically alter the tone of a consumer's messages. Once trust is established with a professional in a back-channel conversation, a consumer may become comfortable sharing a personal diagnosis, such as borderline personality disorder. In cyberspace, an erstwhile stigma can become a badge of identity.

Exchanges similar to the previous example, complete with arrogance, flat-out demands, expletives, and tantrums are common, even between colleagues on mailing lists restricted to professionals. Although such exchanges can occasionally lead to vindictive electronic sabotage and physically dangerous behavior, such as real-world stalking or violence, the lower degree of verbal restraint characteristic of some Internet communications may permit an intensity of emotional expression that some professionals would consider therapeutically useful, and others would consider traumatic.

Watch for the Guerillas. Another aspect of running e-mail lists is to be aware that a small group of people (even professionals) may decide that they intentionally want to destroy a forum with guerilla-like maneuvers. By posting and responding to messages with angry and often vulgar retorts, they can drive away other members, who simply unsubscribe themselves to avoid receiving such mail (and perhaps avoid exposing their children or other computer users from the profanity and ugliness being exchanged). The challenge for the list owner, then, is to take immediate action. Such action might involve removing the entire group of attackers and blocking their further participation.

For specifics on how to operate e-mail lists commands, potential list owners are encouraged to recruit experienced volunteers to help them understand the inner workings of list management. In all cases, it is wise to have a list charter, or set of forum rules. Members are typically asked to agree to the rules as a requirement for list membership. An example of such a charter appears in appendix B.

Readers may wonder why leaders of online professional discussion lists maintain these volunteer and seemingly thankless jobs. Disseminating information to professionals and consumers alike has its own rewards—thankful messages, open hearts, and open arms. When such discussion forum leaders and members attend a convention of their peers, they are typically greeted with enthusiasm. Such reunions of list members affirm the strength of these professional communities. For example, one of this book's authors and colleagues have hosted annual reunions of psychologists participating in various professional lists since 1997 (http://telehealth.net). These meetings occur annually at the American Psychological Association convention. Similar reunions for psychiatrists have been held at annual American Psychiatric Association conventions.

Online groups are known for displays of admiration and compassion, going out of one's way to be helpful, and lighthearted clowning. Sometimes, having the courage not to respond to a consumer's communication is the better part of valor. Managing a professional online presence includes doing damage control when others are misbehaving. Because the truth can so easily be obscured, reality is defined largely by the raw number of impressions received. If an erroneous accusation is transmitted and correcting it once doesn't work, give it up. Make sure to provide readers with a way to view what is in dispute, either by citing where the material is to be found or by quoting relevant snatches of it. However, rather than protest too much when one's response to a falsehood is met with further distortions, just allow readers of such communication to see the truth for themselves. Destructive uses of e-mail to discredit others have been termed "guerilla Net warfare" (Maheu & Subotnik, 2001).

Even well-meaning members may violate explicit confidentiality agreements deliberately or inadvertently, forwarding messages from one list to another. All posted material can show up on searches conducted years later, perhaps torn from its context, marred by misquotes, and embellished by unflattering remarks. Remember, everything posted on newsgroups and listservs should be considered public, no matter what the group's confidentiality rules and security safeguards may be. The already developed lore of online wisdom warns, "If you wouldn't want to hear it repeated in a courtroom [or by your grandmother], don't post it online."

Although text-based environments present their own set of opportunities and challenges, a completely new set of behaviors can be identified wherever numbers of people agree to share mail or gather to discuss a specific topic. A practitioner who attempts to organize such a group for clients might find the pitfalls both numerous and surprising. Members can demonstrate unprecedented behaviors developed solely as a function of the technology. In other words, the technology makes possible new ways of interacting that can be helpful or harmful. The task of the professional, then, is to harness the helpful aspects of discussion groups while blocking harmful aspects. It can only be hoped that applied research in computer-mediated counseling and therapy will result in ways of diverting more of the growing stream of potential clients away from poorly administered discussions to properly administered ones.

The following section first introduces the professional literature related to text-based environments. It then provides practical pointers for clinicians engaging in e-mail discussions with one another, as well as with patients.

PROFESSIONAL LITERATURE: TEXT-BASED COMMUNICATION

Given the popularity of chat rooms and e-mail with Web users, it is understandable that mental and behavioral health professionals would experiment with them for delivering services to clients (Sampson, Kolodinsky, & Greeno, 1997). Services delivered in e-mail or chat rooms are often called other names, not psychotherapy. We refer to these services in the generic, that is, text-based online clinical practice. Indeed, text-based online clinical practice from professionals is now available, and some patients are responding. These services are so new that there has not been much time to conduct empirical research or garner experience to evaluate the full value or cost of such a service or to determine which aspects are helpful and which may be harmful.

Skeptics think that these new services should be tested through approved research protocols before being offered to the public by mental health professionals. These skeptics usually think that such experiments ought to be forced to comply with the safeguards of internal review boards or human subjects committees. Some skeptics point to the fact that legal systems are traditionally slow to respond but that licensing boards are already paying particular attention to online health care services (R. Waters, personal communication, September 11, 2002). They suggest that the lack of legal sanctions to date does not suggest that professionals ought to jump into e-mail-based psychotherapy or counseling. Until the court rules on the safety and legitimacy of these protections for mental health communications transmitted through the Internet with distraught mental health patients, each practitioner must use clinical judgment to consider these risks on a patient-by-patient basis.

Supporters of such services point to the benefits being given to hundreds, if not thousands, of people who otherwise might never access mental health services, the lack of legal precedents making them illegal, and the lack of ethical complaints against such services. Accordingly, many professionals have discussed the pros and cons of delivering services in text-based environments (Baur & Doering, 2000; Bloom, 1998; Mitchell & Mitchell, 1994; Murphy & Mitchell, 1998; Suler, 2000c). Hsiung (2002) also covered a variety of related topics. Other empirical studies of note are reported primarily in the professional literature on social information processing (e.g., Lea & Spears, 1995; McCormick & McCormick, 1992; Walther, 1996; Walther, Anderson, & Park, 1994).

There clearly is an important role for text-based information and communication with mental health clients. However, all authors in this area must offer a balanced view. It is notable that publications by some advocates of text-based treatment may succeed at conveying enthusiasm by outlining early projects, but cautionary viewpoints are sometimes given short shrift (e.g., Laszlo, Esterman & Zabko, 1999). When the licensed professional looks at all of the information related to online delivery of services through text, it seems wisest to move slowly and to continue urging the development of balanced research and balanced reports. See chapters 11, 12, and 13 for a model that might be useful in meeting the needs of both professionals and their clients in the United States (and perhaps elsewhere).

Relationships formed in text-based environments have been compared to relationships formed in person (Suler, 1998; Wellman & Gulia, 1995). Extending interpersonal relationships is the primary reason household members give for using the Internet (Stafford, Kline, & Dimmick, 1999). One might expect newsgroups to be the least hospitable medium for the development of interpersonal ties, yet in a survey of 176 newsgroup users, approximately two thirds reported having formed a personal relationship with another member of the newsgroup and that the relationship developed in a fashion similar to in-person relationships (Parks & Floyd, 1996). Walther, Anderson, & Park (1994) explained that the "intensification loop" theory may explain why text-based interactions are so appealing for many users. In addition, not having to maintain a social appearance when writing and reading text-based messages may attract users.

Issues of online intimacy abound between members of support groups or between clinicians and patients. From a clinical perspective, intimacy can relate to the therapeutic relationship online. In a discussion of online intimacy, Schnarch (1997) challenged the notion of the "baby step" approach to relationships, that is, the belief that overcoming the anxiety associated with a sequential series of smaller behaviors leads to eventual success with the bigger "real event." Schnarch states:

> Whether or not online baby steps eventually lead to real life giant steps remains to be empirically validated. In the interim, let me offer two observations: First, one overlooked problem with the baby steps rationale is that it focuses on anxiety reduction rather than anxiety tolerance (differentiation), which is vital to keeping sex and intimacy alive in long-term relationships. Second, consider what sociologist William Simon (1989) noted about the failure of the 1960's modern sex therapy: We thought we could discover the secrets of eroticism on the dissecting table the same way we smashed the atom. Some clinicians are ready to make the same mistake three decades later.
>
> The trouble with the relationship skill and baby steps argument is that they perpetuate our mythology that an ongoing emotional relationship is reducible to simple skills, stylized patterns of communicating, or successive approximations of face to face contact. One problem with uncharted territory like the Internet is that it encourages broader application of the shibboleths in our field. A related problem is that these rationalizations are readily received by consumers because they reinforce what people want to hear. I shudder to think about well-adjusted information-age techies who think computer flirting and access to more sexual information than at any point in history prepares them for the trials of marriage—even if they go online and read about them!
>
> —(Snarch, 1997, pp. 16–17)

Research shows that propinquity, rapport, similarity, and mutual self-disclosure were rated especially high for text-based over in-person interactions, perhaps because of the lack of physical presence (Cooper, McLoughlin, & Campbell, 2000). One study categorized discourse in a selection of AOL bulletin boards into help-seeking interchange, informative interchange, supportive interchange, growth-promoting interchange, and punitive interchange (Miller & Gergen, 1998). The results showed that self-disclosure interchanges were most frequent, followed by informative interchanges and supportive interchanges. Indeed, increased self-disclosure seems to be characteristic of computer use, even for such activities as filling out questionnaires (Weisband & Kiesler, 1996). Kiesler (2000) made significant contributions with respect to the topic of culture on the Internet.

In a recent study, Mallen, Day, and Green (2003) explored the differences between synchronous chat and in-person communication without looking at mental health issues. Although working within a mental health framework, rather than focusing on mental health applications, the researchers were concentrating on basic communication effects to develop a foundation for future studies in mental health. The researchers divided 64 participants into two equal groups. The participants were paired in either the synchronous chat or in-person environment and communicated in their respective medium for a total of 20 to 30 minutes on a single occasion. Each participant was then telephoned a week later and asked a number of questions related to the experiment. The researchers, findings indicate that the in-person participants achieved a greater level of closeness and interconnectedness with their partners and self-disclosed more information as compared to the online group. In addition, findings indicate that participants in both groups were equally capable of judging emotions of their partners, and processing of information was the same for both groups. Findings also suggest that conflicts may arise in online communications between counselors and clients during confrontations, possibly because online communications lack the cues found in in-person communications. Other pilot projects are still emerging (e.g., Nagoski & Froehle, no date). Although it is too soon to draw conclusions from these preliminary studies, it is encouraging that graduate students and their faculty are paying attention to this topic.

Other researchers have attempted to show the social advantages or disadvantages of Internet use. For example, in a report of the Internet's influence on parents of special-needs children, Michaelson (1996) stated that subjects' use of online, text-based support groups corresponded with times of conflict in their family was helpful. In contrast, Kraut et al. published a report (1998), that examined the social and psychological impact of the Internet on 169 people in 73 households during their first 1 to 2 years online. The researchers found that greater use of the Internet was associated with declines in participants' communication with family members in the household, declines in the size of their social circle, and increases in their depression and loneliness. Critics of this study point to its lack of methodological rigor. Other studies have looked at various other aspects of social and psychological advantages and disadvantages (Barnett, 1982; Colón, 1999; Finn, 1995, 1996; Frabotta, 1998).

Studies of text-based groups are beginning to surface in such areas as eating disorders (Robinson & Serfaty, 2001). A study by Winzelberg et al. (1998) reviewed 300 messages from an online eating disorders group. The researchers found that many of the text-based interactions resembled patterns found in in-person groups. However, 12% of the messages contained what was considered poor quality information. Miller and Gergen (1998) analyzed messages from an unmediated online suicide support group and concluded that they provided effective support but rarely included information that produced notable change in the recipient of the information. Other researchers have reported on use of text-based environments with posttraumatic stress and grief (Lange, van de Ven, Schrieken, Bredeweg, & Emmelkamp, 2000; Lange, van de Ven, Schrieken, & Emmelkamp, 2001).

Although their early study had a very small subject population, Weinberg, Uken, Schmale, and Adamek (1995) conducted a study of an online support group for six women with breast cancer. The researchers suggested that an active leadership style may be needed to address some of the more serious issues, which went unattended when the women operated without leadership. For instance, a member's postings about fear of death went unaddressed by other group members. Galinsky, Schopler, and Abell (1997) offered an early model for online group practice that advocated active intervention by the group leader. They also called for structured methods to track communication patterns, as well as assessing various types of silence, such as anxiety-based silence.

Michaelson (1996) and Kraut et al. (1998) were early supporters of text-based communities to enhance geographic communities, such as schools and neighborhood groups. Kling (1996) suggested that research focus on how the social design and organization of electronic forums influence workplace and community groups. Finn and Lavitt (1994) offered the opinion that sexual abuse survivors seeking help online could receive support and information from a wider variety of individuals than might be present in face-to-face support groups. Lebow (1998) expressed caution, stating that online support groups may reinforce problematic or mistaken belief systems as well as helplessness its members feel. Rather, this article advocated using text-based environments for psychoeducation or as an adjunct to in-person treatment.

Not all therapy models or clinician personalities will be optimized in all technologies, thought Suler (1999c). Some supporters of narrative therapy advocate the use of text-based environments for narrative therapy (Freedman & Combs, 2002; Morgan, 2000; White, 2000). Research on text-based online clinical practice is sparse, and many professional journal articles are theoretical or anecdotal (Barak, 1999; Childress, 1998; King & Moreggi, 1998; Suler, 1996a, 1996b, 1999c). Theoretical discussions tend to focus on the uses and abuses of text-based environments for mental health care. Although they are too numerous to detail, and some are of questionable use, the more significant contributions include views of how chat rooms differ from the office for counseling (Suler, 2000c). Additionally, the media have touted the benefits, as well as some concerns, of chat room-based counseling (Blair, 2001; Elias, 2001; Imperio, 2000; Kalb, 2001). Impatient for scientific analyses to be published, some popular magazines have carried out their own informal surveys. For example, *Maxim*, a popular men's magazine, conducted a tongue-in-cheek review of three online counseling Web sites offering services in chat rooms. Overall, the article's author reported that the Web sites had scheduling problems, technological failures, and hit-or-miss information (Lerner, 2001). Future studies will undoubtedly also help clarify which types of patients will benefit the most from which type of technology, at which point in their therapy, and with which types of therapists. Some organizations have begun giving direction or financial support to mental health–related research of text-based environments. One such organization is the International Society of Mental Health Online (ISMHO). Meanwhile, opinions by enthusiasts who present their views with a notable lack of empirical support are to be taken as such.

The remainder of the section reviews some of the relevant literature related to text-based environments being used for the delivery of therapy.

In a series of studies conducted at the University of Maryland, employees being given employee assistance services by telephone or over the Web not only were motivated to seek such services but also found them to be very helpful (Masi, 2002; Masi & Back-Tamburo, 2001; Masi, & Freeman, 1999; Masi & Jacobson, 2002). The Masi studies clearly demonstrate that employees prefer Web-based e-mail consultation services that allow employees to engage in anonymous e-mail discussion of emotional problems. This research points to fundamental concerns about the idea of conducting a professional relationship without having first met and screened a potential client, as is often required in traditional behavioral telehealth treatment programs and as an integral part of the Online Clinical Practice Management (OCPM) model we advance in chapters 11, 12, and 13 of this book.

Polauf (1998) suggests that Crisis Intervention Theory could be an effective framework within which to intervene via e-mail. Although we do not support the use of e-mail in emergencies, the essence of how crisis workers have been trained for decades to respond to brief telephone calls may have direct implications for practitioners who wish to seek to respond to nonemergency situations with mental health clients. As a framework for developing an e-mail response, Polauf suggests adherence to a crisis intervention formula. We agree with Polauf's suggestion regarding use of this formula, not because it is adequate for e-mail crises but because the formula is used in situations that are similar to e-mail in the need for a brief response.

Polauf suggests that in response to an initial e-mail from a client, the clinician might use a brief response formula to explore the problem and reframe it in such a way as to instill hope, reduce anxiety, develop trust, and allow for emotional venting. The goal of these steps is to allow the client to feel understood. The next steps would involve the development of concrete and reasonable goals. Collaboration is necessary to achieve these steps and to foster the client's sense of autonomy and competence. Selected goals might focus on symptom reduction, restoration of functioning, insight into stressors and/or an enhanced repertoire of problem-solving skills. A time frame for goal implementation can then be agreed on, along with possible follow up.

It has been observed for some time that a person's online identity, even if an assumed name is not adopted, may differ markedly from identity in "real life" (Rheingold, 1993; Turkle, 1995). People may also assert one or more different online identities (each with a new screen name, perhaps involving a gender change), and it is not clear whether the individuals have actually developed a new self, whether they are for the first time openly exposing a previously hidden one, or whether the very concept of self retains any meaning in the Internet's "culture of simulation" (Turkle, 1995).

Suler has also noted that a shift in identity manifested in text-based communication messages might prove to be valuable in therapy, if properly processed by both the therapist and the client. For example, an alteration in mood or affective tone might be apparent in an e-mail or chat room and, once captured in text, become easier to examine and process as an unconscious expression of self. Suler has commented that this alteration may have a countertherapeutic effect on the relationship between the client and the counselor (Clarkson, 1996; Suler, 2000a, 2000b).

The limited information available in text-based environments may lead each party to develop misleading impressions of the other (Powell, 1998; Sussman, 2000). The greater the number of assumptions the client makes, the more likely he or she is to manifest transference phenomena (Laszlo, Esterman, & Zabko, 1999; Suler, 2000d). Online norms may artificially alter an individual's tendency to offer enough information for a practitioner to conduct an adequate assessment. For example, in the corporate environment, e-mail messages have become status signifiers comparable to those in in-person meetings. A person's social status is found to be reflected in e-mail length, spelling, grammar, and tone, with higher status employees issuing short, curt e-mails, and lower level employees being longer winded and argumentative (Headlam, 2001).

Professionals seeking to use e-mail and chat rooms for contacts related to the psychotherapeutic relationship may benefit from a review of the research involving the use of telephones for client contact (Haas, Benedict, & Kobos, 1996). Such a review may be useful because research related to text-based environments has not yet been adequately developed. Most notable is the similarity between the two modalities with respect to the client's control over the interaction. Both technologies allow the immediate termination of a therapeutic contact with the simple movement of a finger. In other words, telephones, e-mail, and chat rooms allow clients to remove themselves more easily from a therapeutic interaction than when they are in a psychotherapy office. In a moment, clients can hang up the telephone, trash an e-mail, shut off their computers, and focus on the evening's dinner options. Given the diagnosis of the client and assuming that the therapist is not being abusive, this ease of turning off the intentioned therapeutic encounter is not advantageous to the client.

The clinician who chooses to communicate in a text-based environment with patients before research findings have clearly identified appropriate uses of such technologies should read the next section carefully. It takes only one bright, Internet-savvy, hostile consumer to scorch the benevolent clinician with a searing flame or even worse, with a series of destructive posts that can besiege a once thriving discussion list and leave it covered in cyberdust. It takes only one hostile personality-disordered client to find creative ways to torment the benevolent online clinician in the real world—regardless of reports that legal sanctions have not been a problem to date, that security is adequately handled by passwords and encryption, or that risks to text-based treatment are outweighed by benefits offered to would-be patients who otherwise would not receive treatment (Fenichel et al., 2002).

Regardless of the professional literature and its evolution, a professional deciding how to go online must consider the potential interpretation of past, present, and future clients, employers, and colleagues alike. By understanding the detours, roadblocks, and passing lanes of developing an online presence, the professional can maximize effect and minimize negative consequences, such as lost time, frustration, public embarrassment, and most important, risk of harm to the client.

NETIQUETTE: WALKING THE WALK AND TALKING THE TALK

Text-based communications with colleagues, and certainly with patients, should be transacted with special care. To the writer, e-mail seems less ambiguous than speech, and one tends to assume that the recipient will go back over anything that didn't come across clearly when first read. E-mail messages are therefore often blunt and succinct and may lack amenities ("Dear So-and-so" or "Sincerely") that are standard in surface mail. Readers of such terse missives, however, may feel disrespected, criticized, alienated, and misunderstand. For example, what a supervisor or team leader intends as a simple request for a status report for routine monitoring of progress may come across as mistrustful checking-up or nagging. It is good policy to include reassuring social niceties and some description of context in each e-mail.

Proper Internet etiquette can avoid embarrassments and misunderstandings. Online culture has developed its own norms, mores, and taboos. The smart professional will look both ways before stepping into this traffic. Being a good professional *netizen* (citizen on the Internet) includes providing adequate identification through *signature files* in one's messages and observing proper *netiquette* (Internet etiquette).

The Signature File

Anonymity is unacceptable as part of a professional presence. Setting oneself forth as a professional carries an obligation to provide full identification equivalent to displaying diplomas on one's office wall. Typically, this is done with a brief signature file that is automatically appended to outgoing e-mail, the equivalent to a letterhead on office stationery. The signature can show one's name, professional degrees, and license numbers and can often include a personal Web site address or quote that one lives by.

Remember that a return e-mail address may appear automatically in the message of any posting. Other elements of a signature file are optional, but files exceeding six lines may draw criticism for self-indulgence, abuse of bandwidth, listserv clutter, or other factors. Some people include a famous quotation. Displaying one's Web-site address can lead readers to more information about a professional's services and qualifications. Caution about placing too much information on such Web sites is warranted, however, because angry clients can wreak havoc with the material they can gather online about their practitioners. Similarly, a telephone or fax number may bring unwanted calls, whereas e-mail messages can impose thorny duty-to-warn dilemmas from clients seeking treatment. There is also the risk that the practitioner may find himself or herself subject to jurisdiction in other states or even countries. The practitioner's goals will determine which elements to include in a professional e-mail "letterhead."

Charles Dickens Syndrome

There are no Pulitzer Prizes for online discourse. Messages can be short and to the point. Some people receive hundreds of e-mails a day and do not relish receiving a dissertation on the many perils of nicotine dependence. Think of e-mail as a telephone conversation, not a classroom lecture. Keep sentences less than 13 words in length and vocabulary to 8th-grade level. In chat rooms, most postings are phrases, not even sentences. Use both generic and trade names for drugs, eschew obfuscation, and remember that people who can't speak English very well may have difficulty understanding slang, subtleties, and elegant turns of phrase.

The Loudmouth

Although construction sites and drive-through windows often require a matching decibel level, normal conversations need not tax the human larynx. The same goes for text-based communication. E-mail use of all capital letters implies SHOUTING and is typically considered offensive. Conversely, proper capitalization and punctuation enhance readability and are a kindness to the reader. As noted, they also convey an air of professionalism that may be of value if you later need to defend your comments in court.

Ad Out

Commercial postings to online discussion groups can spark *flames* whereby outraged members severely chastise offenders, sometimes choking their private e-mailboxes with hundreds of angry protests and threats. Alerting people to an event or service consonant with group goals is acceptable, especially when done by a bona fide group member, but repeatedly mailing anything deemed exploitative can forever mark the perpetrator as a *spammer* to be added to the list of the banned that is circulated among leaders of online discussion groups. Yes, even leaders of online discussion mail lists have online mail lists to discuss how to manage mail lists.

Lusing the Speling Be

REeding na emial fyll og misspelld wirds canbe frustating, adn embaraassing. Nearly all e-mail programs include spell checkers, and some even check grammar. A misspelled word here or there is tolerable, but when it takes a code-breaking machine to decipher a message, the reader may lose some respect for the writer. As messages will be short and to the point, a quick once-over before clicking "Send" should be no problem.

A Pointless Note

Whether an e-mail or message board note is read or clicked straight to trash may depend on its subject line. An odd phrase in the "Subject:" line, such as "I LOVE YOU," could spark fears of an e-mail virus that will crash a person's computer. An archived message is often recognized by the subject line, and a response is more likely to be elicited if the recipient can identify the content of the note from the subject line. When responding to a message, using the same subject line maintains continuity of the conversational "thread."

Calligraphy Turns Ugly

E-mail is no place for calligraphic excess. Some programs let a user change font, *bold words*, *italicize*, and underline in the body of the message. A *"highly recommended* book entitled E-Health, Telehealth, and Telemedicine: A Practical Guide to Start-up and Success by Maheu, Whitten, and Allen," may appear on the recipient's screen as a "highly recommended book entitled <u>E-Health, Telehealth, and Telemedicine: A Practical Guide to Start-up and Success</u> by ^* #!&, ϶ϛΩℵ ↓ □⊗, ⊃=+ ∇⌋ϖ Ξψ." If it is necessary to send eye candy, use a word processor attachment, such as Microsoft Word.

Always the Last Word

Because receipt of an e-mail cannot be taken for granted, it is often a good idea to return a short reply to the sender. Of course, not every posting needs a response. Two compulsive responders can find themselves in an exhausting string of acknowledgments: "Can we meet at 2pm?" Re: "Ok, I'll be there." Re:Re: "Roger that, I'll see you then." Re:Re:Re: "Copy, I acknowledge receipt of your confirmation." Re:Re:Re:Re: "I confirm your confirmation of my confirmation, out." At some point, enough is enough.

Road Hogs

The information superhighway is not 20 lanes wide; it can support only so much traffic. Unnecessary attachments, multiforwarded mail, unedited lengthy quotes of all previous messages on a topic, lists of other recipients, pictures, and video clips all take a lot of space to transmit and extra time to download, especially with dial-up modems and an older computer. In much of the world, where Internet service is slow, receiving bloated messages is sheer agony. In many countries where Internet service is not competitively priced, bandwidth excesses can cost one's recipient a pretty penny to download. Foisting such excesses on an entire list of recipients can make one widely unpopular.

Lists of Names

You may relish the thought of efficiently sending your message to dozens of people at once, but if you place your recipients' names in a long list on your e-mail note's "TO:" line, savvy Web folks can easily copy those long lists and use them later for junk mail. Being discreet with e-mail addresses is a courtesy to your e-mail recipient. In a health care context, it is more than that: It is vitally important for the sake of privacy. Your Patient A has no right to know that B is also your patient, and vice versa, and no right to know what B's diagnosis might be or how you are treating him. If you want to send mail to a group of unaffiliated individuals, send them to a few people at a time, or use the "BCC:" (blind carbon copy) line of the e-mail program. Be careful with this last function, though, because experienced hackers can crack the secret code and capture your long list anyway. When writing to clients, always write privately and use encryption. Security and encryption are described in chapter 10.

OUCRA

Only Use Commonly Recognized Acronyms. FYI, not everyone has memorized the acronym dictionary. Many acronyms are used in online messaging and in ordinary professional discussions, but most people recognize only the ones used in everyday speech. The Internet has also developed its own argot. Although it is cool to be up on the latest lingo, it is more important for the receiver to understand it.

Professionals are better off using plain speech, especially in deference to readers who may not be fluent with the writer's language. If the communication is later read to a jury, the professional's exposure of liability is probably likely to be diminished if he or she is not perceived as a smart aleck. No one will have much sympathy for a treatment team that fouled up because someone wrote about switching the patient from CPZ to CBZ instead of BZD while continuing with their CBT.

Don't Be a Robot

Some people manifest little-known reactions called emotions. Raised eyebrows, a smile, or a giggle can completely change the meaning of a sentence. Smiley faces and other *emoticons* (symbols that represent different emotions) are the closest approximation to these visual and auditory cues and can be used to emotionalize a written message. "I'll be waiting ☹" is more informative than a plain sentence. Easier on an Internet newbie would be "I'll be waiting <frown>." Even clearer yet for the newbie is, "I'll be waiting <hands on hips, foot tapping>."

Attempts at humor are particularly easy to misinterpret, particularly when related to sensitive topics. Humor usually merits an emoticon in the event that it misfires. (Of course, sarcasm should be used exclusively with severely disturbed clients who know where your children go to school ☺). Murphy and Mitchell (1998) have developed more precise techniques to express emotions in text for psychotherapeutic purposes.

The next chapter helps the reader decide whether to take the next step: developing a professional Web site. Examples of existing mental health sites are discussed, along with the nuts and bolts of how to build such Web sites, the pitfalls to avoid, and the benefits to be expected.

4

Professional Web Site Considerations

Much Internet traffic[1] is directed toward psychological and medical self-help, problems of living, chemical dependency, human relationships, and normal human development. In addition, people with chronic illness and developmental disorders and the ever-growing aging population and its caregivers are turning to online technology for access to peer groups, health care agencies, and professionals. To address these needs, Web sites have been developed by government agencies, insurance companies, hospitals, universities, foundations, professional associations, consumer organizations, individual practitioners, and laypeople.

In 2001, 42% of physicians were working in practices with Web sites (Harris Interactive, 2001c). Today, nearly every large mental health organization maintains a Web site. Consumer use of hospital and health plan Web sites is burgeoning (D'Angelo, 2002). A worldwide online presence will soon become an ordinary part of the clinical toolbox for mental health practitioners as well.

The public strongly favors integrating Web sites into health care practices. The Jupiter Research Center reported in February 2001 that 63% of consumers would switch to a physician whose Web site offered "solid content, appointment scheduling, or secure communication channels" (Florey, 2001b, p. 13). More than half want to make appointment requests, 48% would ask for prescription refills, and 38% favor seeing their laboratory test results online. One third of general health care consumers with a chronic condition said they would participate in an online disease management program on their physician's Web site.

This chapter describes how professionals can develop their own Web sites. It discusses how to best integrate a Web presence with an existing mental health practice or a mental health association's mission. This chapter demonstrates how a Web site can augment a paper office, preserve professionalism, and serve the interests of clients. The chapter briefly discusses some of the legal risks associated with the creation and maintenance of a Web site and steps to take to decrease those risks. This chapter can help the reader plan and outline realistic goals, organize necessary technical and human resources, and recycle to another round of planning. Operating simultaneously with this structured method for constructing and maintaining a Web site is a more organic approach to accommodate various practical considerations. Also included is an example of a successful Web site development project.

---

[1] The activity of a Web site is called *traffic*.

WEB SITE PLANNING

Planning a Web site is much like developing a treatment plan for psychotherapy. Especially for managed care, planning a course of treatment starts with assessment and education. In planning both online activity and treatment, mental health professionals often specify attainable goals and break them down into measurable objectives, selecting for each objective methods and contingency plans based on effectiveness, resources, and risk. Many professionals agree on how to monitor progress to correct the plan as results unfold and then, in both treatment and online work, arrange for necessary resources, line up the team, and commit to action.

In parallel with this formal, systematic approach, Web site owners benefit from proceeding holistically, feeling their way and mixing "art" into science. (In this light, curious readers may enjoy peeking ahead to a later section in this chapter entitled "Web Site Components" before returning here for the methodical approach we advocate.) Flexibility and creativity may be inhibited by being too systematic. In the end, however, enthusiasm alone cannot fully replace coherent planning.

Indeed, although the Internet continues its exponential growth in power, scope, and accessibility, most e-health companies are failing because they did not research the marketplace and match their business-to-consumer strategy to health care realities (Harris Interactive, 2001c). For example, advertising as the main revenue source for a health-related Web site has been disappointing. The public has been unwilling to pay for personal subscriptions to commercial, unspecialized health Web sites. Instead, consumers believe that the general information forming the bulk of the large commercial medical sites should be free (Poensgen & Larsson, 2001). Health care consumers are usually seeking in-depth information on a specific subject, and one fourth of the time, this concerns mental health (Pew Internet & American Life Project, 2000). Furthermore, consumers trust university and medical associations above commercial sites (Grossman, 2001; Poensgen & Larsson, 2001) and tend to regard dot.com firms as run by inexperienced managers who are too interested in fast money (Pew Internet & American Life Project, 2001c). As a result, numerous niches exist for reputable behavioral health care practitioners and for respected mental health associations to develop a successful presence on the Internet.

The best-known giant e-health sites seem to do all things for all people, covering wide areas of health and normal development, selling products, and offering free assessments. Rather than go head to head with these floundering giants, mental health professionals can pursue specific online activities that may enhance their existing practices. Rather than be all things to all consumers, online initiatives might offer a few good things for a defined audience.

What can professionals offer that doesn't already exist on any of the 20,000 health care Web sites? The personal touch. Web site planners who apply technology to a specific clinical need can be more assured of long-term success (Dakins & Jones, 1996).

Some behavioral e-health Web sites have attained success by concentrating their energies narrowly to become the preferred destination for consumers with a clear notion of what they are seeking. A specialized site may expand from its original concept along many dimensions. Professional organizations going online might focus on their core competencies and specialize in problems or treatment approaches in which they have commitment and expertise. Associations that already maintain Web sites may wish to periodically reassess their purposes and retune their online strategies. Small practices may be best off with modest but unique, well-constructed Web sites that describe one particular practice. In addition to being a virtual "shingle," such a

Web site can become the core of office computer functions, such as keeping accounts, obtaining authorizations, and even clinical record keeping. The process we describe applies to upgrading existing online enterprises, as well as to starting new initiatives. It begins by asking, "Why?" Once that question is answered, the general goals of a practitioner or organization can be discovered. Then, more practically, milestones and methods can be set, and the planning cycle can begin.

Overall Goals

Successful online activity requires a clear sense of purpose. Each element of an online presence should contribute to an explicit set of goals. A study conducted by Cap Gemini Ernst & Young Health Practice reviewed 97 Web sites to determine the trends of health related sites. The conclusions of this research may help an organization determine the goals for its Web site:

- "HIPAA regulations are affecting Web sites' design and functionality.
- Strategically, payers are positioning their Web sites as a replacement for customer service.
- Customization is the long term vision, but a mass market approach is today's reality.
- Payers are expanding both the breadth and depth of their Web offerings.
- Payer Web sites have yet to demonstrate a financial return" (Cap Gemini Ernst & Young U.S. LLC, 2002, pp. 6).

Practitioners goal can best be addressed through careful website planning. A storyboard is often used in the planning process. On a storyboard, separate pieces of paper describe individual pages. The designer then decides how each page is to link to the other(s). It is wise to focus on just a few storyboard pages (seven or eight) to meet a few general goals, such as those listed in Table 4.1. Setting a limit of three or four goals can prevent the "feature creep" that typically bedevils initial Web site developmental efforts.

TABLE 4.1
Possible Overall Goals of an Online Presence

√	Overall Goals
	Recruit/retain clients/members/research participants
	Enhance association members' involvement
	Promote a concept (theory, approach)
	Encourage referrals from other professionals/agencies
	Facilitate existing services (intake, assessment, treatment, follow-up)
	Implement new professional services
	Improve operational efficiency (billing, scheduling, authorizations, etc.)
	Create new revenue streams (merchant, clinical services, advertising, etc.)
	Assert organization's brand (maintain brand awareness, loyalty, confidence)
	Enhance self-care
	Enable peer support
	Create a community of consumers or colleagues
	Access underserved population (rural, autistic, foreign language)
	Test a product, opinion survey
	Other (specify)

TABLE 4.2
Goals-Oriented Planning Cycle

Phase	Activity
1	Select overall goals.
2	Describe methods for reaching goals.
3	Concretize methods:
	Tasks (deliverables and deadlines.)
	Resource requirements.
4	Delegate tasks and assemble resources.
5	Measure progress.
6	Modify plans based on results.
7	Critique and improve the planning process.

Because adding extra capabilities may eventually prove valuable, you can establish for the next developmental cycle a special file to hold anything that will not materially contribute to current goals. Do not add a new goal to the current set just because it seems easy to implement. An advantage of good planning is avoiding the urge to do everything the first time.

The Planning Cycle

For each goal, set explicit, objectively verifiable attainment criteria and assessment dates. Each milestone should have at least one associated method, but a method may address more than one goal and may continue across several milestones. The methods are broken down into tasks, deliverables, and deadlines. Each method is then delegated to oneself, a staff member, a consultant, or an outside Web developer. A time line can be drawn displaying the milestones, which can then be expanded into a schedule showing on/off times of the tasks and when specific resources must be ready to add to the Web pages represented in the storyboard.

Before each major expansion of online activity, organize the accrued results, bring out the file of deferred extra features, reconsider the overall goals of the Web site, and rework the entire plan. This is also a time to study the effectiveness of the overall planning process. Table 4.2 outlines the steps of the planning process.

Each cycle of expansion should be attainable. A cache of unanswered e-mail or an overly ambitious Web site riddled with "under construction" notices, broken links, scripting errors, and obsolete information can be a worldwide brochure advertising one's level of professional disorganization. A clinical practice, and particularly a professional organization, needs sustained support of its online presence.

The Web site start-up budget should probably have funds to support operations for the initial 6 to 12 months of operation (Institute of Medicine, 1996). Web sites can range in price, depending on whether a practitioner wants to spend the time and energy to develop a personal site or to have the site professionally developed. Costs for developing a Web site will include an Internet service provider connection, server space, and Web site construction software (to be discussed later in this chapter under "Web Site Construction").

WEB SITE DEVELOPMENT

A carefully designed personal or organizational Web site can eventually become the hub of the electronic infrastructure for all professional activity, both online and offline.

Various issues have become apparent for both the individual and the small-group practitioner, as well as for the organizations seeking to develop Web sites. A Web presence should project stability, energy, and dignity. Ideally, these goals should be accomplished with a minimum of legal risk. This means continuing to keep the Web site updated and relevant. It also means negotiating a reasonable Web contract that allows access for updates and knowing the essential requirements for functional Web sites. Although the most cautious approach may be to start with a simple online brochure, the long-term perspective can be kept in mind. A Web site can be designed to be expandable and should include proper security and risk management protection from the ground up.

Writing contracts with Web developers is crucial. Also important is writing contracts with Web vendors, such as those delivering merchant charge card services through a Web site. All contracts must clarify who owns the Web site, copyright, programming code, variations on scripts developed for a particular purpose, algorithms, artwork and graphics, and traffic generated. A developer who creates special material for one organization can easily adapt the same material to sell to a competitor at a lower cost. Thus, a contract should include a broad noncompete clause that defines the restrictions on contractors hired to develop special material.

Many buyers fail to review a developer's agreement in detail and do not question confusing or unclear terminology. Web developers often have prewritten contracts with hidden costs and unneeded fees. To the uninformed individual or organization, these fees can go unnoticed and prove costly down the road. You may wish to look specifically for clauses that attempt to impose on the owner liability for statements made or omitted or for images projected on sites. In fairness, a development company that did not draft the text used or select the images projected may be able to argue that it should not be liable for adverse consequences flowing from such decisions. To a degree, however, such matters may be negotiable. Ideally, a construction company that refuses to indemnify the owner and contract to procure insurance in an amount sufficient to cover any exposure thereby generated might still be willing to shoulder some part of the burden. A lawyer familiar with such contracts may be asked to look over any Web site development contract entered into.

Good Web site developers understand the specialized needs of health care professionals and will agree to reasonable modifications to their standard agreement. Contracts (or agreements) should have a reasonable termination clause to prevent easy dismissal of vendors that are not performing to the expected level. More specifically, the agreement ought to clearly stipulate how termination will occur, any expense involved, penalties to be paid, how a new vendor might obtain passwords and copies of files, and the time line involved in getting this crucial information to the new vendor. When signing an agreement, practitioners may want to ensure that termination does not lead to prohibitive costs or delays in accessing the Web site if the arrangement is no longer satisfactory.

Developer contracts usually consist of three parts: a master agreement, a license agreement, and a maintenance agreement. Legal considerations, explicit guarantees, ownership of content and coding, unforeseen cost protections, and support issues must all be addressed in these three contract sections to protect the purchaser. Before finding a developer, the specific need for a Web site and related technology should be identified by the professional or organization. It is important to match the requirements of the company to the capabilities of each developer as closely as possible, keeping budget restrictions in mind. Seek the names of reputable developers from satisfied colleagues who are online or in a particular geographic region.

Negotiating and signing an agreement with the developer are the next steps. Extensive reviews of pointers needed when signing a contract are found in the literature (Maheu, Whitten, & Allen, 2001). Review all existing licenses and licensing contracts for specific mention of electronic rights now and in the future.

If friends, colleagues, or other professionals agree to write an article on a particular topic for a Web site, be sure to sign an agreement with them with regard to licensure or direct ownership of copyright for that article. In the agreement with authors, consider obtaining the right to use the article in future electronic venues, the nature of which you may not yet know. The premise is that the types of technologies used may not be known in 10 or 15 years. They may go beyond Web sites. For example, many video companies filming groups of children 10 years ago asked participants to sign permission slips stipulating that the film would be used in educational videos. When the CD-ROM industry evolved, many well-produced video segments could not be purchased for use in CD-ROMS or Web sites, because some participants in the videos could not be reached for authorization to use the same film in another venue. Without explicit permission by all participants, group shots could not be reused. This principle is true of video clips now reproducible for Web sites as streaming video. Be prepared for the future by obtaining all electronic rights to be used in all venues.

Ensuring Security

If you are collecting information from or delivering information or advice to clients through a Web site, be sure that the site is reasonably secure and that the confidentiality of the user is protected at least at the level required by applicable law. Standards for such security are discussed in chapter 10. Do not expect a well-paid Web manager to point out where site performance is poor, especially in the area of security. Instead, follow these simple suggestions:

- Hire someone or ask a well-informed friend to spot-check the Web site (programming code, Java, and CGI scripts) for vulnerability to security breaches.
- Have all internal server error messages sent either to both the Web manager and another trusted staff member or directly to the Web site owner.
- Protect any information intended specifically for the Web owner, including private communications from colleagues, so that information cannot be intercepted or diverted by the Web designer.
- Ask someone to use various browsers to intermittently try to access your Web pages, to review the organization of your files, and to examine the programming code on Web pages.
- If information is received or collected from clients through a Web site, hire an expert to periodically attempt to crack the Web site's security.
- Be aware that the greatest risk to security comes from inside—sloppiness, an accident, or a vengeful employee involved in a dispute.

Even a single security breach can be very costly, both from damage to reputation and actual financial exposure. Along with direct revenue loss, client confidence, employee wages for correction of the problem, and legal fees may inflate the bill. The expenses must be balanced with the costs of in-house expert personnel and technology implementation and upkeep. But in-house security can be expensive, and outsourcing may be one option for providing cost-effective security to psychotechnologies because it reduces staff and lowers maintenance costs.

Other suggestions include the following ideas:

- Register trademarks with the U.S. Patent and Trademark Office. This can be done relatively inexpensively.
- If you are planning to sell services or products through a Web site, it is wise to be apprised of the e-commerce issues that other professionals have faced and to make provisions to prevent any such problems.
- Confirm licensure of practitioners affiliated with the Web site. Diagnosis and other services may require that the practitioner be licensed in the jurisdiction of the client.

Individual or Small-Group Web Sites

A professional online presence can lead to a simple brochure Web site or a virtual office, replete with a library, intake department, and consultation room. Some professional Web sites offer bookstores, self-help services, referrals, or an informational site. An example of a simple Web site that establishes a professional presence is that of Myron L. Pulier, one author of this book. He runs a self-funded personal project at http://www.umdnj.edu/psyevnts. The predominant purpose of this site is to help mental health professionals attend training and research events. The Web site is designed to allow the professional to easily review many upcoming events, including search options for browsing by date and location of an event. The site's purview has expanded to encompass meetings and organizations related to telehealth. As the audience for this Web site has grown, hundreds of other sites have linked up, and visitors have started contributing material. Although this site is tremendously helpful, it does not detail the sources of information and does not guarantee the accuracy of the site's content. Of course, the content of the site is not life threatening if misinterpreted. The visitor will notice that no banner ads appear on the site and that no pitches are made for consumer products. The site is also free to use. The site's owner provides an e-mail address for contact with any suggestions or concerns. The casual, personal feel to this Web site reflects its benevolent motivations.

However, most professional Web sites are simple brochure sites. The individual or small-group practitioner can develop a brochure Web site to:

- Describe specialized services or populations treated.
- Offer maps to the office.
- Answer commonly asked questions.
- Detail age groups of populations served and areas of special training.
- Offer articles of interest to the clients served.
- Make available such documents as intake and consent agreements.

Small or regional clinics may also wish to develop a Web site for these purposes. For instance, The Woodland Centers, Inc., a mental health clinic in Gallipolis, Ohio, offers psychological, drug, and alcohol services to more than 3,500 residents, both adults and children, from three counties in Applachia. Executive Director David Tener explains that as a result of recent growth, "We wanted to communicate with other practitioners and agencies, as well as the public, about the services available at Woodland and the happenings in the mental health world. We decided to implement a Web site to reach the community"(personal communication, October 9, 2002).

The clinic hired CenterSite, a company that offers a service to behavioral health agencies by cobranding a Web site with a clinic's individual domain name (see http://www.centersite.net). For a monthly fee, Web sites created by CenterSite come complete with thousands of pages of behavioral health and wellness content, as well as news feeds. Other features might include access to a question-and-answer column, editorials, advice, thousands of reviewed links, mental health glossaries, medication information, self-help books, book reviews, monthly customized newsletters, or polls. The Woodland Centers Web page provides its community with up-to-date information about the clinic's news and events. CenterSite augments the Web site with thousands of articles about mental health from a database originally organized as MentalHelp.net.

Says Tener, "We struggle with a number of barriers in our community, including lack of technology, but as we focus more on serving children and families, using the Web as a tool is important. As we move in the direction of technology, the costs become another challenge" (personal communication, October 9, 2002). Tener was able to get funding from local businesses and the United Way. Pleased with the results, Tener remarks, "After only a couple of months, our Web site has generated positive feedback from clients, staff, and members of the community." The following vignette exemplifies one such story that received positive feedback:

> *Toby's family was referred to Woodland Centers by the local school system when Toby displayed a number of troubling behaviors in the classroom. After obtaining the necessary releases to protect Toby's confidentiality, an initial assessment was completed by the staff at Woodland Centers. The assessment identified that Toby suffered from obsessive compulsive disorder (OCD).*
>
> *The professionals at Woodland Centers felt that the treatment team would work more effectively together if Toby's parents and teacher received education about OCD and the various treatment options available. They accessed Woodland Centers' recently developed Web page* http://www.woodlandcenters.com, *which contained a wealth of information selected by clinicians from national, state, and local publications about obsessive-compulsive disorder. Toby's parents and teacher all felt that they were able to better understand the problem being addressed. The positive feedback from Toby's parents and teachers included an appreciation for the opportunity to take a more active role in Toby's treatment process.*
>
> —**David Tener, M.B.A.**
> **Executive Director**
> **Woodland Centers, Inc.**

Individuals also offer similar services to mental health professionals and organizations. For example, psychologist Manny Tau has developed such a service. Located at http://www.Psywerx.com, his service is an e-mail and HIPAA-compliant Web hosting and Web design solution developed specifically for mental health practitioners. His expertise in technology has benefited several professional associations in search of Web sites over the past decade. He now runs his own server and is providing services for colleagues.

Suggestions for Brochure Web Sites. It is in the best interest of the mental health care professional to project a positive, yet conservative, image in all Web sites and other online venues, no matter how informal the immediate goal. The need for a disclaimer[2] still exists for small brochure Web sites, but what is disclaimed will be somewhat less extensive than what which is necessary for a larger organization's site. For example, any site, of whatever size, can disclaim promises of absolute reliability and liability for claims arising from use of the content. Unless the owner has made a conscious decision to provide e-health services, the site can disclaim the practice of medicine, nursing, psychology, and/or other health care services via the site and can deny any desire or intent to create a professional–client relationship. The owner might also disclaim creating warranties of merchantability or fitness for a particular purpose, as well as other warranties generally.

Many individuals or groups in the mental health field have not protected themselves with corporate structures and therefore have not considered the advantage of such armor when setting up their Web sites. Common structures include a limited liability company, a partnership, and a professional corporation. Each of these models leads to different tax ramifications and exposes the owners to different types of risk, so choosing a structure with the help of a tax adviser or attorney, or both, is strongly recommended. A full discussion of this topic is beyond the scope of this book.

Professionals tend to forget the worldwide nature of the Internet, as well as the varied motives of potential Web site visitors.[3] A first priority must be the safety of the professional(s) mentioned in the Web site and their loved ones. The professional should not put personal information, especially pictures of family or pets, on the Web. Think carefully about posting fully detailed curricula vitae with names and partial addresses of past educational institutions and employers. What could a malicious client do with such information? The countervailing considerations are the marketing benefit that could be gained by posting such information. The "correct" solution will vary with the circumstances and the needs and risk tolerance of the practice or site owner.

Details of the MyTherapyCenter.com Web site (http://www.mytherapycenter.com) exemplify an individual professional Web site, previously discussed as a brochure Web site. The entire MyTherapyCenter site consists of 12 Web pages. The expense for setting up this site was less than $500, paid to a professional Web designer. The site took approximately three weeks to develop, with daily interaction and supervision from the Web site owner. Web site addresses such as this can be put on office forms to advertisements, or business cards direct clients to updates, and enhance a professional practice.

The home page (see Figure 4.1) has a simple design that visually introduces the viewer to Dr. Marlene Maheu. The home page is not loaded with graphics or flashy scripts, thereby allowing it to appear quickly when a user tries to access its Uniform Resource Locator (URL). A brief introduction explaining the site is presented in large type, and a number of links bring the viewer to other pages on the site. Anyone having trouble viewing the page because he or she is using an old Web browser is provided with a link to a free upgrade to a newer browser program.

Other pages on the site explain the services offered. Note that current clients are instructed not to e-mail Dr. Maheu but rather to use the telephone. This request accomplishes two goals. First, it keeps costs for developing and maintaining the Web site to a minimum. Second, because much more expensive password-protected and secured Web coding is not used, it prevents patients from using unsecured e-mail to

---

[2] A "disclaimer" is a statement that purports to deny legal responsibility for another statement or act, or that attempts to repudiate a legal claim or right. Whether a disclaimer is valid, and accomplishes what it is intended to do, it is often disputed.

[3] People who look at, and perhaps interact with, a Web site are called *visitors*.

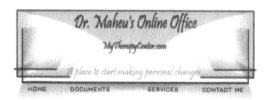

This online extension of my office is designed to help you learn more about my psychotherapy practices and policies. It will also give you convenient access to the documents you'll need to bring to our first meeting. You will find other documents and information that might be useful to you during therapy.

I look forward to working with you, and would appreciate your feedback about your experience with my services.

Marlene M. Maheu, Ph.D.

FIG. 4.1. MyTherapyCenter.com

contact the clinician. It is to the benefit of all concerned to protect patient privacy and confidentiality until the Internet becomes more secure and users[4] are more familiar with encryption programs or until security costs for Web sites accepting text messages from patients are lower.

Dr. Maheu could have organized a secure messaging center at the site, compliant with the Privacy Rule promulgated pursuant to the Health Insurance Portability and Accountability Act (HIPAA) and could have asked current patients to send their mail to her through the site. Such elaborate techniques to contact Dr. Maheu as an individual practitioner seem premature, however, when making contact is easier for her to manage and less expensive by telephone. Dr. Maheu also prefers to hear a client's tone of voice when receiving urgent messages and tends to check voice mail more often than e-mail. For her, the telephone system is more reliable than the Internet,

---

[4] The general term *user* refers to any person interacting with a computer or involved with an electronic device.

for now. Such decisions are based on practitioner preferences, community standards of care, and type of clients served. As for Dr. Maheu, she eagerly awaits the day when text messaging and videoconferencing capabilities are cost-effective and secure through the Web. Meanwhile, patients wishing to make contact are encouraged to pick up the phone and leave a voice mail message if she is not available.

Clearly, this brochure Web site is designed primarily for new patients and for patients who wish to obtain revised copies of office policies and other forms. Privacy laws in the United States may require policy updates, so during the informed-consent process, patients are given this Web address and encouraged to check this site for updates. The Web site also contains other important forms for patients to complete before meeting Dr. Maheu, a map to the office, the privacy policy of the site, and a feedback page asking users and past clients to give their thoughts about both the Web site and the services they have received from Dr. Maheu. The site contains a picture of the site owner; a vitae, or biography, for a prospective patient to read; and mention of languages spoken, awards received, and publications. The user can navigate at any time anywhere on the site through links at the bottom of each page. The site has a set of Terms and Conditions, suitable disclaimers, and a copyright notice. This type of Web site might be appropriate for the average practitioner.

Professional Organizations' Web Sites. Some professional organizations fall into a compromise position based on denial and avoidance. They passively allow an enthusiastic member or two to set up and maintain the association's Web site but provide no support. After the volunteer members leave, no one picks up the ball. The result is blatantly amateurish and out-of-date Web pages, blithely inviting site visitors to annual meetings that were held a year ago. Consider the following personal experience.

> Because of its rocky financial situation, one professional association was unable to come up with the exorbitant fees its Web site designer demanded for even minor changes. Updating the site's address book or posting new information about meetings had to wait until the contract with the designer expired and the necessary access codes and alteration permissions were released.
>
> Another caution... paying for a high-end Web site, only to learn that one's members cannot access the site without specialized software to read the home page.

The leaders of a professional association will readily appoint a committee to report on the advantages, costs, and risks of going online or of substantially expanding an existing presence. Subsequent high-level council meetings then trim such proposals. This procedure may achieve a good balance. However, leaders may be reluctant to approve Web site features that would-be developers properly consider crucial. Lack of knowledge, misunderstandings and personality and turf issues can bring progress to a disappointing halt. Professionals in a group practice may experience similar difficulties.

Overcoming the many obstacles that impede the development of an initial Web site requires diligent preparation. If organizations or group practices must approve the process, getting online might also involve adept politicking and repeated succinct and convincing presentations. The disheartened forerunner in such organizations might take heart in knowing that in mental health practice, professionals have learned by experience to shun initiatives that threaten confidentiality, interfere with therapeutic relationships, disrupt predictable practices, and drain time and money. Such reasonable misgivings can be allayed by showing examples of existing Web sites that demonstrate the kinds of features and services that could be installed. One may wish to outline a sequence of small, achievable steps, each offering rapid return on investment. Efforts to win acceptance from various segments of an organization's membership can involve

holding a leadership retreat, placing announcements and feature articles in the association newsletter, recruiting people to serve on planning committees, and generally
explaining how members can contribute. Do not neglect involving the office staff.

The Web site may appeal to professional association members by listing their names
on a roster, by giving them individual Web pages for describing their own practices
and expertise, and also by inviting them to contribute articles, to help with "Ask-the-
Doctor" features, and to announce special workshops or other events that might be
of interest to the professional or consumer. The site might list books published by
association members and announce awards given to particular members.

A professional association providing features such as these, however, should give
careful consideration to the risk exposure. Generally, a well-drawn disclaimer will go
far toward distancing the association from individual members, and thereby provide
the former a measure of insulation from liability exposure. Typical "terms and conditions" language will also be needed, of the sort that practitioners need to post at their
own individual sites, to protect against risks common to virtually all sites concerned
with health care, collective or individual.

Institutional inertia should not be ignored. A solid presence in cyberspace should
emerge from the sometimes painful processes of democracy and organizational development rather than result from passive acquiescence to the will of a few individuals.
Indeed, an "appreciative inquiry" (Bushe, 1995) can clarify the future vision of the
organization and help the entire organization evolve.

Web Site Construction

Some professionals may prefer to create and edit their own Web sites. This process,
although not complicated, may be time intensive. Creating one's own Web site is a
good way to get a feel for the possibilities and the limitations of Web site construction,
should one decide to deliver more elaborate services in the future and require the assistance of an outside developer. The tutorial at http://www.w3.org/MarkUp/Guide,
offered by the semiofficial World Wide Web Consortium, shows how to use simple
word processors, such as Notebook on Windows systems or SimpleText or TeachText
on a Macintosh, to write HTML files and save them to a disk. The HTML Primer
Web site (http://www.htmlprimer.com) lets the user experiment with elementary
HTML directly from a browser and view the result immediately.[5] Other popular
self-instruction sites include:

- Introduction to HTML (http://www.cwru.edu/help/introHTML).
- NCSA Beginner's Guide to HTML (http://archive.ncsa.uiuc.edu/General/Internet/WWW/HTMLPrimer.html).
- Webmonkey (http://hotwired.lycos.com/webmonkey).

[5] To go beyond experimenting with HTML coding most Web authors turn to authoring programs to more
easily format pages via a WYSIWYG (what you see is what you get) interface. Excellent authoring features
are available as part of certain standard browser and word processing programs.

The Netscape browser package (http://home.netscape.com) includes a word processor-like interface
for entering and formatting text, inserting pictures, and creating tables. Microsoft Word readily converts
ordinary word processor documents into Web pages with the "Save as Web Page" command in its "File"
menu. Numerous HTML editors are available, many without cost or as "shareware" (where the supplier
requests a small, usually voluntary, contribution). These editors can be located via the Yahoo! search
engine by searching for keywords "HTML editor". America Online (AOL) offers a more direct solution
for its subscribers—an online program for creating pages that are automatically posted on the AOL server
(see http://hometown.aol.com).

Many software programs are available to help maintain an overall style, create easy navigation between pages, add embellishments, and get the pages online. A dedicated Web authoring program facilitates keeping an entire Web site organized, updating its content and upgrading its features.[6] With high-level authoring software programs, an amateur can create Web pages, but these pages may not be readable by all Web browsers. It is important to realize that a page will look different to various visitors, depending on their computer hardware and software, as well as on their monitor and browser settings. Even without the author's knowledge, an authoring program may include features that will produce unintended effects when a visitor accesses the Web page. Companies that create commercial Web sites know how to test each Web page for compatibility with various operating systems, browsers, and Internet connections.

Outsourcing. For best results, hiring a professional Web designer is the way to proceed. Guidance by an expert is advisable to create the best impression on visitors, just as one would turn to a professional to design a business card or office shingle. Various designers specialize in such matters as site organization, page layout, graphics, navigation, text style, information capture and databasing, and special program features, each of which requires a different skill set.

Web development companies may charge organizations anywhere from $500 to $10,000 or more to construct a Web site, depending on the features desired (Baldwin, 2001). Many freelancers can do an excellent job with an elementary brochure-style Web site and can keep costs to a minimum. Fees can range from $50 to $1,000 for a basic site, depending on the number of features and pages desired. Individual and group rates are often available from these wholesalers of mental health and related information. Some national and state organizations offer such services to their members.

Some organizations may even offer Web site construction for free. For example, Medem (http://www.medem.com), jointly founded in 1999 by the American Medical Association and specialty medical societies representing more than two thirds of U.S. physicians, sets up and hosts free Web sites for physicians and provides content deemed reliable by the sponsoring organizations. A doctor simply enters office address and phone numbers on an online form, adds a paragraph about care philosophy, and chooses a color scheme. Medem's automated Site Builder Wizard quickly constructs an attractive multipage presentation offering consumers the latest medical articles and patient education resources from medical specialty societies. The Wizard can also post curricula vitae[7] of every therapist in the office and any desired practice announcements, handouts, and documents. Medem discretely avoids many pitfalls involved in maintaining dignity, ease of Web site use, security, privacy, consent, trust, quality of information, liability, and publicity. Medem does not, however, purport to

---

[6] Some of the most popular general-purpose Web design software packages are Microsoft's FrontPage (http://www.microsoft.com/frontpage), Adobe System's GoLive(http://www.adobe.com./products/webcol), and Macromedia's Dreamweaver (http://www.macromedia.com/software/dreamweaver). FrontPage is the least expensive and best integrated with PowerPoint, Access and other Microsoft Office offerings. GoLive is part of Adobe's Web Collection and works well with PhotoShop and Illustrator. Dreamweaver MX can bundle with Macromedia's Fireworks 4 Studio and Flash to bring a less stodgily business-oriented and more artistically capable and industry-compatible development environment. Unlike the others, FrontPage is not available for the Macintosh.

[7] Practitioners may want to carefully consider whether they want their curricula vitae posted on a Web site. Most vitae contain information that a severe personality disordered patient could use to harm a practitioner.

engage in risk assessment or management, nor is it customized, except as noted, to the needs of an individual practitioner.

An individual Web site may be part of an online access package of one's Internet service providers or e-mail host, such as Yahoo! (http://www.yahoo.com) or America Online (AOL; http://www.aol.com). Other Internet service providers offer free personal Web sites built from information one submits via online forms. Many professionals have taken advantage of such resources to set up a basic online presence.

Before hiring any outside Web manager or other developer, do the homework. A company with experience building health-related Web sites is more likely to give adequate attention to the special needs of health care professionals. Ask for a current and past client list, and contact the clients to ask questions about the developer's services. More specifically, ask questions about the developer's ability to deliver needed services and to offer training in how to use whatever hardware and/or software it provides. Hardware and Software can range from equipment to fully integrated systems that can include multiple modalities, that is, private consultation and online services for the Internet. Most important, assessing risk issues will most likely require a careful examination of other Web sites created by the contractor or developer in question.

Ask the developer to supply references and examples of work previously performed for a mental health audience. An expensive disappointment can result from depending on a Web designer who lacks specific expertise with serving mental health clients on psychotropic medication or hampered by cognitive defects.

Potential clients may also run their own search to see whether they can find Web sites designed, constructed, or maintained by the developer. Search engines, such as Yahoo!, may help in such a search, because some Web site construction companies insist, as part of their remittance, on putting their name at the bottom of the pages they construct. Some of these companies also place links to their own terms of use or privacy policies near their names. Rarely do these documents provide any comfort or protection for the site owner; they protect the site-constructing entity alone. The Web site owner needs its own legal armor and ought not rely on what the design company has posted for itself. If Web sites are found, owners can be contacted directly, and satisfaction with the developer can be explored.

Several good Web sites provide technical assistance and information or links to developers for various types of Web site construction:

- American Telemedicine Association (http://www.atmeda.org/news/newres.htm).
- American Medical Association (http://www.ama-assn.org).
- Association of Telehealth Service Providers (http://www.atsp.org).
- Telemedicine Information Exchange (http://tie.telemed.org/vendors) or (http://tie.telemed.org/links/consultants.asp).
- National Library of Medicine National Telemedicine Initiative (http://www.nlm.nih.gov/research/telemedinit.html).
- The List (http://www.thelist.com/index.html).

Additional directory Web sites are described in chapter 12.

If the bulk of site development is given to an outside developer, the Web site owner needs to protect its legal position, monitor the construction process, choose content, and generate and edit material to stock the Web site. Content can be purchased from some organizations constructing Web sites or individually by Web site owners. Individually maintaining the content requires a way of recruiting and training contributors and a reward structure that induces people to complete assigned tasks on time. No one person or developer should become irreplaceable. If the developer drops out, the Web site owner should ask whether anyone is willing and able to pick up the slack. If not, the Web site owner sets aside funds to retain emergency outside help.

When attempting to develop an organization's Web site, investing in a high-priced consultant or developer substantially commits the organization to action. Understandably, the executives and volunteer leaders of professional organizations feel more secure paying outside experts and developers than putting resources directly into the hands of enthusiastic members. Amateurs may have considerable expertise, be more meticulous, understand the organization's needs, devote a great deal of energy, and do a better job, but hiring a paid professional developer may give a more serious air to the activity, at least in the minds of some board members or other leaders. Ideally, the outside developer could collaborate with the organization's own volunteers and talent.

WEB SITE COMPONENTS

> Concern for man and his fate must always form the chief interest of all technical endeavors....Never forget this in the midst of your diagrams and equations.
> —Albert Einstein
> (Simpson, 1988)

When it comes to components, chasing the "more is better" rainbow can lead down an expensive dead end. A common error is excessive reliance on Web designers who do not understand the mental health profession, the populations typically served by mental health Web sites, and the need to address cultural and linguistic diversity, differing socioeconomic groups, disabled communities, and people in underdeveloped regions. Web developers often focus on the newest technology they have learned rather than on the needs of the clients who will frequent the Web site. When a low-end browser crashes while attempting to launch a high-end Web site, the user may avoid the offending site from then on. Confusing technological glitz that is irrelevant to consumers' needs and insensitive to their limitations hardly fosters trust. Well-conceived programming and design can result in attractive pages without alienating users.

Contrary to the tacit assumption of most Web site designers, consumers tend not to upgrade their browsers or adjust their settings after installation, and many consumers are still using the software that came with the computers they purchased 4 or more years ago. Just as new cars can't run on leaded gasoline, new Web pages can't run on old Web browsers. Even if the newest software release of browser or plug-in is located on a professional Web site for the user to download, the user may not to make the download or know how to use a file once it is downloaded. Slow communication channels, such as "Plain Old Telephone Service" (POTS) lines, may take extraordinary amounts of time to download a file.

Despite the previous caveats about burdening a Web site with too many features, overall planning is certainly enhanced by fantasizing about Web site components and by glancing at the competition.

Domain Names

Catchy, easily spelled domain names are essential to any Web site (e.g., Yahoo.com). Users who use a search engine when surfing the Web must choose from among several sites, and a catchy domain name makes a site more appealing and easy to remember for return visitors. Avoid domain names that are easily misspelled (e.g., psychoanything), that contain words that may be mistaken, have alternative meanings (e.g., "therapist" and "the rapist"), or are very long (e.g., the hypothetical http://www.thementalhealthprofessionalandthenewtechnologies.com). Companies such as VeriSign (http://www.networksolutions.com), DNS Central (http://www.dnscentral.com), and InterNIC (http://www.internic.net) sell domain name registrations for various amounts and time periods. When buying a domain name, type it into a Web browser to verify that a domain name is available. Once the domain name is purchased, it is important not to let its registration lapse and enable cybersquatters to take the name over.

Common domain classes other than .com are .gov (for government entities), .org (for noncommercial organizations), and .edu (for colleges and universities). Domains can also refer to nations, such as .ch for Switzerland. As interest in the Web has grown, other domains have evolved. It may be a good idea to register domain names with similar spellings and extensions (.com, .net, .org) in order to avoid losing users who spell the name incorrectly or inadvertently access a similarly named site.

It is recommended that a spreadsheet be kept on each domain name's registration information, including which company the domain name is registered through and any user names and passwords the company requires. The spreadsheet also records the expiration date of each domain name. The market for domain name registration is very competitive. Some companies attempt to steal customers away from other companies by sending renewal letters months in advance of the expiration date. One author of this book learned this lesson the hard way and spent hours on the phone speaking with two companies to correct multiple registration errors. Domain name owners are advised to look for unscrupulous policies by these registration companies before buying a domain name and also to register all domains through only one company.

Home Page

A *home page*, the official entry point for a Web site's visitors, can provide orientation and easy access to the site's main features. Waiting for pictures to download or for an opening video or animation may turn people away, especially visitors with low-bandwidth connections. A well-done animation, on the other hand, can be very engaging and entice visitors to return. Showing nothing but a logo and expecting visitors to know they must click to proceed can confuse viewers and immediately turn them away. However, an opening *splash page* can effectively display special announcements along with a logo and *tag line* and then can automatically carry visitors to the actual home page with an enter-this-site button.

The tag line should present at a glance what the Web site is for, what makes it unique, and why the visitor should look into it (Nielsen, 2001b). The home page should assertively display the name of the sponsoring practice or association, a link to the site's privacy policy, terms and conditions for using the site, and main areas within the site. The title or logo of an organization should be prominent and catch the viewer's eye. Additionally, some state licensing boards are bolstering consumer rights by publishing new guidelines that require professionals to list their license numbers on directory Web sites (e.g., Board of Psychology, 2002).

Navigation

A basic Web site table of contents will aid navigation from the home page to other sections of the site. The simplest feature to bring visitors from one page to another within a Web site is hypertext that links to the "next" or "previous" page. Adding further links can let visitors view pages in other than serial order. A table of contents can keep the trails between pages from becoming a confusing maze. Tables of contents can be hierarchic, so that clicking on "Psychotherapy" can summon a page offering subtopics under the Psychotherapy heading. One alternative scheme (for example, PsychSite at http://kenstange.com/psycsite) provides a special navigation page, or site map, accessible from any page.

The Web site should have a hypertext link that brings the user to a contacts page that lists e-mail address and other contact information of the *Web master,* or more politically correct albeit rarely used, *Web manager* of the Web site. The Web site owner's address should be accessible. Standards developed for health Web sites require provisions to allow users to provide feedback to the site and to register complaints. Standards also require site owners to have policies for resolving these complaints in a timely manner (American Accreditation HealthCare Commission, 2001).

Site owners should bar the posting of information that may be defamatory, obscene, or copyrighted by another party. Other restrictions may also be appropriate, depending on the site owner's needs and desires. The site owner should also give careful thought to how to field inquiries and complaints. The people charged with doing so should realize that in the eyes of the visitor, the person "speaking" is the "voice" of the practice or sponsoring association. These individuals must be trained to act accordingly and to use caution in their responses, particularly to inquiries that may be hostile in character.

Another common feature on a home page is an internal search engine that searches the entire Web site for a keyword. The home page also contains the date that the Web site was last updated. Some of these features are explained further in the next section.

Content

Many decisions, as well as much time, money, and energy, can go into developing content for Web sites. To help the reader be mindful of some underlying issues, this section focuses on the practicalities of developing Web site content. We discuss how to establish trust in the reader, develop editorial policies, write for Web sites, and maintain accessibility with one's readership, as well as basic legal issues.

A Basis for Trust. Making a good first impression is a key to establishing trust. Displaying privacy policies in a highly visible area of the home page can reassure visitors who might be leery of using the services being offered (Reents, 1999). More important, the U.S. Federal Trade Commission (FTC) is taking the position that a failure to post and to abide by a posted privacy policy is itself an unfair trade practice. Failure to post a privacy policy may allow a Web site to fly below the radar of the FTC, but professionalism demands that privacy assurances be made and that the policy be readily available to visitors (preferably by a link on every page in the site).

The bottom of the home page is a good place to display honors, seals of approval, and links to organizations that promote standards. Be cautious about labeling a given organization's recommendations as standards, however. The word *standards* has a very specific heavy meaning in the law of tort. Once a particular recommendation has been publicly labeled a "standard," it may be difficult to overcome a claim that in allegedly failing to comply with it on a given occasion, one has violated a "standard" and hence is subjected to liability that otherwise might have been avoided.

Professional organizations should state whether they are nonprofit, clarify their missions, explain who their members are, and supply complete contact information. A new visitor should quickly be able to grasp the mission of the organization, see how to reach organization officers, and understand what will happen to any information that the Web site might glean from the visitor. An association dedicated to public service may wish to prominently differentiate itself from private or for-profit groups that call themselves institutes or societies. Hospitals and commercial Web sites often reveal their ownership and corporate ties and identify their top executives and board members. Although there are advantages in offering this information, such postings should be considered against the modestly augmented risk of claims made against the local affiliate and also against the parent organization. Professional associations can also post their criteria for membership, their membership categories, their by-laws, and perhaps an application form. It is best to disclose any potential conflicts of interest of the Web site sponsor and leadership.

The site should also distinguish clearly between advertising and editorial content. Even if it does not accept frank, paid-for advertising, the site may subtly or blatantly promote a particular agenda. There is nothing inherently wrong with that, but a critic might contend that the readers should understand when they are being pitched to and when they are reading material that is or at least purports to be objective, scientific, and nonpromotional. This approach can avoid misunderstandings, enhance the reputation of the site and hence of its owner, and decrease the likelihood that someone will allege fraud.

A clinical question can be raised of whether it is wise to use advertising at all on brochure or practice-promotion Web sites. Aside from magazines (containing ads), does the typical therapist have product or service advertisements in his or her waiting room? What will potential or existing clients and patients think about a practitioner promoting a product through a practice Web site?

Apart from obvious paid-for advertising, more subtle forms of product promotion may be possible using the Web. Although not yet amounting to a legal obligation, there may be an ethical question whether, in discussing the risks and benefits of a particular drug, a site owner must disclose holding an equity position in the drug's manufacturer or whether the manufacturer has provided grant support to the sponsoring organization. Obviously, more research on the effects of advertising on visitors is needed. In the meantime, professionals are reminded to use their own clinical judgment regarding the clients they wish to refer or draw to the Web site and to consider seeking legal advice about the risks and benefits of advertising, especially for brochure Web sites.

The quality of content posted on health Web sites is often disappointing (Berland et al., 2001). The fact that thousands of Web sites propagate advice on every conceivable personal problem makes credible Web sites difficult to find. Many Web sites of non-profit professional mental health organizations have gone untended and display obviously out-of-date material. Resources posted by gifted amateurs and lay organizations exist on the Web side by side with material published by faddists and fringe groups. Clinics tend to issue self-serving statements. The line may be thin between advertising the latest snake oil remedy and scientific findings interpreted for a lay audience.

Already surfacing are proprietary-content developers who sell specialized packages of quality information amassed from various respectable sources to specialty practitioners, associations, hospitals, and other health care groups for rebranding and placement on their Web sites. Many Web sites include content created by public relations firms or outsourced to Web developers but presented as the official position of a health care organization. Some Web sites even distribute articles with misleading or incorrect headlines and content, presumably for the sake of capturing the reader's interest.

Fortunately, such organizations as the American Medical Association and the American Accreditation HealthCare Commission (URAC) have been quick to respond with guidelines to help professionals make the proper distinctions when identifying issues and developing their own Web sites. As Web consumers become more familiar with these and other credible organizations, it will become more important to display such credentials via logos on their home pages to assure readers that the content of the Web site is reliable.

Regular updating of content can keep consumers returning to the site (Hagel & Armstrong, 1997). It is difficult, however, to continue to generate new, readable, credible, and accurate material. To make a site attractive, lively, and timely, some professionals or groups turn to a reliable external source of news and features. Such suppliers include HealthGate (http://www.healthgate.com), LaurusHealth.com (http://www.laurushealth.com), and drkoop.com (http://www.drkoop.com), but they typically demand a hefty fee and require cobranding.

Instead, a Web site may simply post links to consumer health care portals (Wilson-Steele, 2000). However, the FTC states that if a consumer comes to harm as a result of unfair trade practices at Site B and got to B via a link from Site A, Site A may be held liable for B's conduct. This position may be vulnerable to attack in court; but until it is successfully challenged, Web sites wishing to create links should proceed with caution.

On all pages providing links, it is important that the reader find a suitable disclaimer of responsibility for control of the content and privacy practices of the link. A link to the host site's terms and conditions does this nicely. A site failing to create this link, however, should post a disclaimer relevant to links at all pages from which links can be accessed.

Another effective feature is a pop-up screen expressly advising the users that they are about to leave the host site, coupled with a warning to proceed at risk. Even without the pop-up warning, it should always be obvious to the visitors that they are leaving the host site for another.

Editorial Policies.   Easily accessed editorial policies are another important feature. Perhaps more than anything else, editorial policies determine the credibility, trustworthiness, dignity, and professional aura of a Web site. Such policies range from what will and will not be shown, through language usage, and to general look and feel. In addition, they determine the peripheral information that accompanies presentations, such as who put the material together, what sources they used, what potential biases they reflect, and how current the material is. Empowering the visitor to evaluate, select, and reject Web site information (and do the same with a doctor, treatment, or both) would be to ride the crest of the current wave of patient-centered health care, perhaps the most important benefit of electronic communication technology for mental health.

Contrast a current editorial policy to one quoted from the 1901 *Journal of the American Medical Association*:

> A newspaper in an Eastern city changed hands about July 1, and the new proprietor, who has a large practical experience in legitimate journalism, at once formulated a set of rules for the conduct of the paper under its changed management. Among the rules were the following suggestive prohibitions: "No medical advertisements"; no advertisements that a self-respecting man would not read to his family; no advertisements of immoral books, of fortune tellers, of secret diseases, of guaranteed cures, of clairvoyants, of palmists, of massage; no advertisements of offers of large salaries, of guaranteed dividends, of offers of something for nothing; no pessimism; no prize-fighting details; no personal journalism; no private scandal. Here is a program that involves the removal of most of the objectionable features in so-called modern journalism. If its details could be conscientiously carried out for newspapers, medical men would find less objection than at present to the promiscuous reading of the daily press, which is working such great harm. Two prohibitions should be added to the list: no details of suicides; no details of homicides, especially such as are committed under circumstances that point to the mental disequilibration of the active agent in the tragedy. ("The newspaper as a pathological factor," 2001, p. 278)

Writing for Web Sites. Many professionals involved in clinical practice or association Web sites could be tempted to write articles. Writing for the Web requires understanding the Web audience and how technology makes the experience of reading online different from reading a magazine or newspaper. The World Wide Web brings its own opportunities and difficulties to the writer.

Much like channel surfing on television, people rapidly scan a Web page for interesting material and click off if not immediately hooked. An author or designer often has less than 1 second to make an initial impression. If read, articles are usually scanned rapidly. Furthermore, writing content for consumers is more challenging than for colleagues, who will be familiar with most relevant concepts and vocabulary. The prospective author may benefit from a visit to the Web site of the National Association of Science Writers, Inc. (http://www.nasw.org), and from reading its *Field Guide* (Blum & Knudson, 1998).

Much of the space available on a Web page is often occupied by the Web site logo, navigation links, and distracting promotional material. A computer screen shows no more than the top third of a sheet of paper $8\frac{1}{2} \times 11$ inches, which is less than one sixth of the space available in many print journals. The special challenges in Web presentations are capturing and maintaining the attention of a reader who is essentially glancing at the material. The restricted field of view makes it difficult for a reader to feel oriented, especially when the screen shows nothing but paragraphs full of text.

The absence of nearby clutter can make a catchy article title more noticeable. The author's name should immediately follow the title and separate the title from content. A vignette with emotional overtones or an abstract showing the article's importance and its main point are effective openers.

Numbered or bulleted lists pack more punch than does text. A checklist promotes engagement, especially if it is interactive and calculates a result for the viewer. Amplifying text with illustrations, such as graphs, animations, and video clips, is appealing, and an interested reader will usually wait for the download. Putting the first image well into the body of the article allows the visitor to begin reading while the picture downloads.

Topics should be introduced by headers, which should appear frequently, introducing each new topic. The discipline involved in writing with headers can have useful side effects, including helping an author to define the objectives of the presentation, to determine the key points to be conveyed, and to organize the topics in ways useful to the reader. It may be wise to spread an article over several pages linked by Next and Previous buttons and to include no more than four concepts per page.

Approximately 10% of readers do not realize that they must scroll down to keep reading an article that extends past the bottom of their computer screen. Readers may get more from an article if reminded to scroll or given buttons to click on to continue. In any case, two screens of text per page is a reasonable limit. Paragraphs should be brief, newspaper style.

Take judicious advantage of hypertext. Among useful features are links to related articles and resources, explanations of terms and concepts, sidebars with extra detail, and links between article sections. Readers with a serious interest in learning how to be proficient at writing for the Web might consult one of several chapters and texts devoted to human factors and Web development (Omanson, Lew, & Schumacher, 1998). The relevant keyword is *usability*, and an excellent corresponding resource is on the Web at http://www.usability.gov.

Intended Audience. Proceeding without clearly assessing the potential audience's culture, goals, and resources is a business plan for disaster. A rule of publishing is to design every presentation to the needs and interests of the audience. Online communication can flexibly meet the diversity of its audience, greatly expanding the range of who can be reached. Prime-time network television is obliged to appeal to the lowest common denominator, and even independent cable channels try to broadcast to a defined demographic. In contrast, a Web site can simultaneously narrowcast to numerous small populations and can even tailor communications to individual visitors. On the Web, one speaks not of a target audience but of target audiences. Keep in mind such attributes as age, sex, ethnic origin, and life circumstance, which may specifically relate to the services being offered.

Many Web sites attempting to appeal to multiple audiences segment their visitor groups very clearly at the home page level. For example, the American Psychological Association (APA) home page (http://www.apa.org) immediately offers three choices: psychologists, public, and students, with quite different content for each group. Like many other membership organizations, the American Psychiatric Association home page (http:// www.psych.org) houses a password-guarded "Members Corner." Some Web sites are divided into areas for visitors who speak particular languages; other Web sites have special sections for children.

Glancing through a list of potential audiences may stimulate some ideas about behavioral e-health services that might be delivered to each. Some potential audiences include:

- Professionals: psychologists, psychiatrists, nurses, social workers, counselors, teachers, technicians, students, pharmacists, clergy, correctional facility personnel, law enforcement professionals, chemical dependency specialists, academics, researchers, and managed care personnel, as well as vendors for each of those groups.
- Consumers: potential clients, general information seekers, parents, children, teenagers, minorities, foreigners, and family and friends of anyone with an illness.

A survey of audience characteristics, knowledge, attitudes, and practice conducted through a Web site can clarify the characteristics of visitors. Such surveys have their limitations, though. People responding to an online survey will not necessarily represent the general makeup of the entire audience; nor are they likely to represent potential new visitors. Focus groups and individual audience interviews can also be valuable but are usually expensive.

Sophisticated personalization software can automatically track a user's behavior (clicks, dwell time on particular pages, responses entered into online forms, etc.), construct a profile, and thereafter shape presentations and select content estimated to best meet the user's needs and wishes. Hundreds of companies are now selling Customer Relations Management (CRM) software and services. CRM can help a visitor formulate inquiries and can generate such responses as Web page presentations or brochures and pamphlets or can help staff prepare for a telephone call to the visitor. The considerable benefits of ever-closer automated adaptation to individuals (Kreuter, Strecher, & Glassman, 1999; Skinner, Strecher, & Hospers, 1994) come at the cost of ever-greater penetration of privacy and correspondingly increased risks and duty to inform, obtain consent, and protect the data (Orleans, 1999).

The broadest audience, crossing ethnic, class, and language boundaries, will have limited literary skills. About 47% of the U.S. population has low literacy (Kirsch, Jungeblut, Jenkins, & Kolstad, 1993; National Work Group on Literacy and Health, 1998). For example, in an analysis of medical information Web sites, Graber, Roller, and Kaeble (1999) reported that most Web site content was written at a 10th-grade level, which is above the comprehension level of most users. Trial lawyers are trained to present information at a 7th-grade level on the theory that this is an average among a typical jury pool. Even educated people who are not fluent in the language used in a presentation tend to interpret material literally. Emotionally laden images may be an important adjunct for people with below-average literacy. Another time to consider lowering the literacy level is when the content is inherently intimidating or potentially upsetting to the reader. More adept readers however, may appreciate the availability of material efficiently presented in higher level language.

The Digital Divide. The digital divide refers to the gap in Internet access by people with differing incomes, races, ages, education levels, and disabilities. It is another important concept to consider (*Falling through the Net*, 2001; Wood & Smith, 2001). People with high incomes are likely be early adopters of technology, with other groups following (Miller, 2001). Although more people are continually accessing the Internet, focusing a Web site on impoverished populations may prove unreasonable. Conversely, many Web sites may focus on the largest Internet populations, as minority populations on the Internet may be underserved and an untapped audience.

Providing Interactivity. A Web site should provide a way of sending feedback (a checklist for rating the article and a place to write to the author or editor) and a link to a discussion group on the article's theme (see Figure 4.2). Also popular are buttons for e-mailing the article to a friend, for adding it to a list of favorites ("bookmarking"), or for printing. References ought to follow the article if it isn't an opinion piece. The date of the article (very important), how to cite it, reprint and copyright information, and a picture of the author (or at least a brief biography) also are key elements to include.

If publishing articles from colleagues, the issue of whether to include their e-mail or private Web site addresses at the end of their articles may be a problem. Many

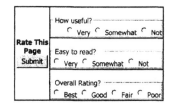

FIG. 4.2. Participation features following a Web page article.

authors like to have their own Web sites and e-mail addresses linked from the bottom of articles they write. Even though this practice may be advantageous to the author, it may not be advantageous to the site owner, who could be held responsible by a consumer dissatisfied with an author's services provided after contact has been made with that author through the hosting Web site. Host Web site owners may not be aware of any such contact between authors and readers, but they are nonetheless often perceived as a deep pocket by a litigious consumer who seeks services directly from the author through such Web links.

Our suggestion is that the reader err on the side of caution and omit links to authors from articles they contribute. Such a cautious approach may be wise, at least until this risk management issue is clarified in the court system. On another note, when formally referencing someone else's work online, the APA has suggestions for citing electronic references and proposes special citation formats to use in a Web document located at http://www.apastyle.org/elecref.html.

Figure 4.2 shows a survey and a mail-to-a-friend feature. The survey also includes an invitation to provide more extensive feedback, which leads to a page offering several options, including joining a discussion group that relates to the article.

Beneath the rating checklist in the figure is a brief description of the author, a mention of his publications most relevant to the article, and how the author's books can be purchased. The author's picture (at the top of the Web page and not shown in the figure) adds warmth to the invitations.

A Web site owner may choose to develop an official affiliation with one or more large online bookstores, such as Amazon.com or BarnesandNoble.com, as these companies pay a small commission on products sold through their affiliates. Book sales for mental health professionals certainly can help defray the maintenance costs of a Web site.

Readability. Readability and reading-level software can provide a rough estimate of the appropriateness of one's writing style for the intended audience. Two popular word processing programs, Microsoft Word and WordPerfect, can calculate a Flesch-Kincaid Grade Level and a Flesch Reading Ease rating based on vocabulary and polysyllabic words. The perplexed reader might refer to the user's guide of the specific program purchased to find out whether and how this can be done. Guidelines are available for creating health articles suitable for readers with low literacy ("Clear and simple," 1995).

Some browsers cannot display images. Pictures are also a burden for users with impaired vision. Web page designers can accommodate the diversity in their target audience by using the accessibility provisions in HTML. For example, all pictures should be tagged with a text alternative that browsers can present instead of the picture itself. Some browsers can read such alternative text aloud or render it in Braille. Users can purchase special programs that read and analyze HTML to evaluate and correct problematic code, such as Bobby http://www.bobby.watchfire.com/bobby/html/en/index.jsp.

Multilingualism. In some circumstances, readers who will be working on Web sites should consider trying to post information in a long more than only the English language. Presenting health care material in a visitor's primary language can be advantageous competitively (Broadhurst, 2000). Even in the United States, the large number of people for whom English is a second language should make a Web site owner consider the role of language in meeting the preferences of the site's target audience.

Although commercial translation services are expensive, some skilled translators may be willing to work at no or a low fee to help a particular group gain access to mental health information online. The Web site owner may want to determine whether the translators are doing an adequate job when discussing complicated or sensitive mental health issues, however. Seeking a second and third reader may prove essential, at least until the first-choice translator has proven to be competent. Perfectionism, of course, has its limits, and polishing prose in a foreign language may be unnecessary for readers who are seeking answers. On the other hand, the fact that users do not speak English need not mean that they are unaware of the opportunities for fun and profit that our tort system may provide. As an example, if one's Spanish is not adequate for professional use and one is doubtful of the skills of a particular translator, beware the perils of discussing health-related matters in a manner insensitive to nuance. Silence may be preferable to "Spanglish," especially when working with people who have social or emotional problems.

Accessibility. Even technology wizards with high-speed Internet access, large display screens, and 20/15 vision find themselves flummoxed by massive, ill-fashioned, and tangled Web sites. User friendliness is a matter of navigation aids, conventions of placement and design, and other principles. Beyond ordinary user friendliness are so-called accessibility measures to accommodate people with slow Internet connections, dyslexia, visual difficulties, or other limitations. An estimated 8.5 million potential viewers with disabilities may be lost if a Web site is inaccessible (Royal National Institute for the Blind, 2000). Accessibility is considerate and a way of enlarging one's audience; it's also the law (Architectural and Transportation Barriers Compliance Board, 2000).[8] U.S. government Web sites are required to be accessible to the visually handicapped. The government has pressured its contractors to do the same with their Web sites as well.

A gratuitous introductory Flash movie or soundtrack can be an obstacle even for visitors without special limitations; for sites devoted to mental health issues, this practice is seldom good technique. Sometimes, however, an animation or streaming video segment is absolutely necessary to get certain information across deeper in a Web site. For people with hearing problems and who lack speakers on their computers, whose privacy would be threatened by audio material, or who are using a text-only browser, a synchronized text equivalent similar to closed captioning should accompany a video presentation. This presentation should include indications of sound effects ("bam," "whoosh," "creak"), tone of voice, and other audio elements. The visitor should be able to pause the action and resume so as to absorb the material at a personal pace.

Don't use color to convey information, although color may serve as a supplementary orientation cue for people with adequate vision. A surprisingly high percentage of men are color blind (approximately 8 to 10%). Check how a page may appear to a person with red–green color blindness (a "deuteranope") by submitting the page to Vischeck (http://www.vischeck.com). Keep electronic forms short, and make them navigable with the keyboard. Some users will require extra time to complete a form and will be stymied if one automatically times out too soon. The Web site should provide an e-mail address or feedback page to allow users to point out any barriers they encounter. The site should also contain links to accessibility instructions and relevant information.

PROMOTIONAL ACTIVITIES

One's Web address can be mentioned not only in telephone answering machine messages but also on business cards, office stationery, billing statements, general correspondence, telephone book advertisements, client handouts, and under the authorship line in published articles. Organizations may include their URL on every flyer, newsletter, and announcement. On the other hand, depending on theoretical orientation, type of clientele, and comfort with the technology, some clinicians may decide not to make their e-mail addresses known to potential clients. Newcomers are encouraged to wade slowly into these waters. Withdrawing e-mail privileges from a client and setting appropriate boundaries may be fraught with even more hazards than setting telephone limits for people with severe social or emotional problems.

---

[8] Assistance is available from the Access Board (http://www.access-board.gov), an independent U.S. federal agency. Further guidelines developed by the nonprofit World Wide Web Consortium are described at http://www.w3.org/WAI. Automatic verification of compliance with standards is available from such vendors as HiSoftware (http://www.hisoftware.com). The former has a useful resource of white papers on accesibility. The latter suggests excellent accessibility techniques on its Web site. Paciello provides an in-depth discussion (Paciello, 2000).

Certain principles can markedly enhance accessibility without undue effort or expense. Keep Web page size below 30,000 bytes, including images, to avoid prolonged waits for downloading. Avoid graphics and graphical representations of text—they consume extra time. Where graphics are worthwhile, favor small, simple monochrome images that can be compressed into .gif format over large, multicolored and detailed .jpg pictures.

Visibility to Search Engines

Much is made of enhancing consumer loyalty to a Web site (so that visitors return often), but 77% of patients looking at the Internet for health issues do so only when they have specific questions, and 65% use search engines rather than going to a particular site (Internet Healthcare Strategies, 2001). It is therefore crucial that one's site be easily accessible to Web crawlers—search engines that automatically seek out new sites to add to their databases (Harris Interactive, 2001c). Judicious choice of keywords in a hidden meta-area of each Web page helps some search engines index a site under appropriate topics.

Many search engines show the user the opening lines of Web pages that they retrieve. Therefore, pages designed so that the top lines convey a good sense of the overall contents may attract more visitors. A shocking statement, cute paradox, or opening quotation aimed at grabbing a visitor's attention could be a serious deterrent to new visitors who might be put off by seeing only that statement reflected in a search engine's description of a Web site.

Aside from relying on Web crawlers, sites can be registered manually with search engines, although services that authenticate requests can take up to 6 months to list a new Web site. Services that promise to list Web sites in numerous search engines at once are usually a waste of money. It is best to submit Web sites for consideration individually, that is, by going to each search engine and completing its specialized form. Hiring a skilled search engine promotions expert can be worth the required time and expense. At present, there does not appear to be an ethical or legal obligation to indicate that a professional's site has been prioritized by a given search engine as the result of such promotional effort. Such an obligation may arise eventually, however. Bard (2000) estimated that only 13% of online health consumers know which sites to visit. This shows that strong advertising campaigns are needed to direct them to one's Web site.

Other Attractions

Quizzes inserted before or after an informational article can arouse curiosity and induce people to pay more attention to a Web site's content. Including a poll on a Web page is an easy way to let visitors express and share opinions: The visitor responds to a question, then sees statistics on how previous visitors have responded. A free poll resource is available at http://www.Pollwizard.com.

Special e-mail features encourage return visits or can encourage visitors to bring in new users by word of mouth. For example, a visitor can provide an e-mail address in order to receive an alert whenever a particular Web page is updated or material on a selected topic is added on the Web site. This practice is particularly relevant to people interested in specific kinds of information.

Some Web sites strive to present comprehensive lists of other Web sites that fall into categories of interest, whereas other sites serve as anthologies, appending evaluations to a listing of preferred Web sites. Having one's own Web site listed in such sites can bring in many new visitors. In fact, acquiring linkage from other Web sites is the best and most successful form of Web promotion. After determining which sites most resemble one's own, a Web site owner can search for all the sites that link to them. (Some search engines, such as AltaVista, have this ability as a special feature of their "advanced search" capabilities.) An e-mail to the Web master of these sites to ask for a link is often obliged and matched by a request for a "reciprocal" link.

A policy of forging reciprocal links should entail seeking written agreements with the cooperating sites. Such agreements define the rights and responsibilities of those people concerned, avoiding misunderstandings and decreasing the risk of litigation. Although one-size-fits-all approaches are not appropriate here, linking agreements may address such topics as technical specifications, intellectual property rights, safeguards against libel, liability for claims, indemnification, dispute resolution, and applicable law.

Web rings are of groups of sites that each recommend the "next," with the links eventually leading back around. Posting announcements and remarks about one's Web site or its features in newsgroups and listservs can also attract visitors. Write articles for newsletters and newspapers, and ask Web sites visitors to join an e-mail newsletter list. Such e-mailing lists are easy to develop by using a listservtype program. These programs can be set to send but not receive e-mail. If such a list is collected from a Web site, be sure to provide the e-mail address of the sender and instructions for unsubscribing somewhere in the newsletter. It is advisable to send e-mail only to people who have requested such mail. On the other hand, some Web site owners also send announcements to everyone on lists of e-mail addresses purchased from commercial vendors. Although push advertising to newsletter subscribers respects their privacy, sending unsolicited e-mail ("spam") degrades one's professional image.

Simply stated, push technology reaches out to the consumer and delivers messages to their browsers (as in pop-up advertisement windows) or directly to their e-mail boxes. This form of information delivery can be considered either a convenient means of receiving important information the user may not otherwise know exists or an unwanted, intrusive, and possible ruse or lewd message delivered to the user's desktop, without warning. An example of a legitimate use in health care is push mail from a hospital pharmacy to house staff advising them of changes in the hospital formulary. For advertisers, this evolving distribution technology is substantially changing how users interact with information, particularly in the time-sensitive financial services arena. For consumers, particularly of mental health information, it can be an embarrassing reminder that they have a problem or an unsolicited invitation to once again engage in problematic online behaviors, such as gambling and cybersex. For professionals who choose to use spam as a means of advertising their services or products anyway, the law requires that unsolicited mail give recipients a means of removing themselves from such mailing lists. Our suggestions are that all professionals respect the privacy of e-mail recipients and intentionally send mail only to individuals or groups that have requested it, such as from a professional brochure Web site.

Retaining Visitors

Public demand and marketplace pressures have nearly swamped the cautionary principles developed a century ago to restrain the excesses of so-called modern journalism. Today, awash in the vast sea of media hype, there persist islands of legitimacy: television productions and newspaper articles characterized by accuracy and restraint. A similar natural history is evolving in the realm of e-health. Today's Internet user discovers many behavioral e-health Web sites—strange, wondrous, colorful, fascinating, and even dangerous, yet of uncertain value. One often associates each novelty with some familiar memory ("It tastes like chicken"). Most people end up clinging safely to a few favorites with which they feel comfortable ("I get my car fixed there because that's the service center my brother used").

Making a Web site *sticky* means using tactics that keep people from straying away during a visit. Where consistent with the mission of a site, links to other Web sites can be replaced with links to content within the present site. If visitors must be referred out, it may help first to remind them that they can return by using their browser's Back function.

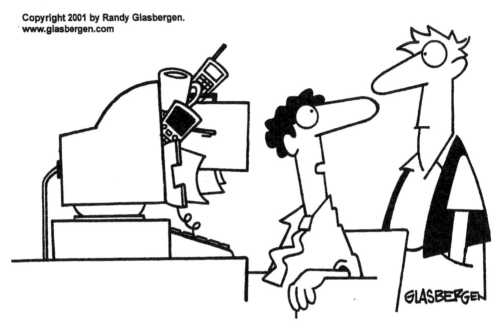

Copyright 2001 by Randy Glasbergen.
www.glasbergen.com

"You made our web site too sticky!"

Visitor engagement and sense of community enhance Web site stickiness and consumer loyalty, as well as its effectiveness. Surveys, contests, and polls can help break the ice, encourage readers to be interactive, and induce them to join the Web site's community, thereby enticing them to return. In 2000, Sheryl LaCoursiere of the University of Connecticut conducted a study of 265 participants who used online health care sites. She found five factors to be most important to clients: community and news (by far the most important factor), physical and psychological outcomes, trusted information and advice, self-efficacy in evaluating information and intention, and disclosure (LaCoursiere, 2001).

The affordability of constructing professional Web sites and their ease of access by consumers make them ideal for offering services addressing many social and emotional issues (Bruckman, 1996; Jones, 1995; Rheingold, 1993; Shields, 1996; Turkle, 1995; Wellman & Gulia, 1995). People who "belong" at a Web site return more consistently, remain on the site longer, use more features, and bring others around.

SelfhelpMagazine (http://selfhelpmagazine.com) supports a large community of volunteer contributors and discussion forums, including the one devoted to cyberaffairs shown in Figure 4.3. As seen on the left side of the page, participants can start their own "threads" (discussion topics), and the software lets forum participants know how many responses each topic has drawn. Participants are allowed to give themselves pseudonyms ("screen names"), as seen in the Author column, so that forum participation can be anonymous.

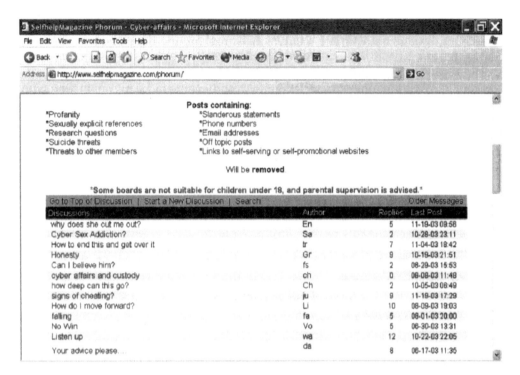

FIG. 4.3. Topics posted to a Web forum.

Actively participating in a discussion or contributing in any way increases a visitor's sense of investment in a Web site. Members can become very involved, such as by volunteering to inform the Web site owner of any postings that violate the code of conduct established for a forum (or in legalese, terms and conditions). It is helpful if such rules are outlined at the top of every forum page and further detailed in several legal documents made available by links on all forum pages.

Highly emotional topics have generated up to 15 KB of responses within a single day on the *SelfhelpMagazine* Web site. Readers might also be interested to note that this Web site's traffic is limited by the owner because of the cost of processing additional visitors. Otherwise, traffic could be considerably higher. Forum members know that not only can they post anonymously but also that inappropriate responses will be removed. The kind of cathartic release involved in writing has been shown to alleviate inner torment and to improve physical health over time, even when the description of a stressful event involves as little as 20 minutes of writing and is initially distressful (Pennebaker & Beall, 1986; Pennebaker, Hughes, & O'Heeron, 1987; Pennebaker & Susman, 1988, reviewed in Smyth, 1998). Although the efficacy of describing stressful or traumatic experience in online discussion forums has not been documented, the amount of traffic generated suggests that people receive considerable benefit.

Volunteerism: By the People, for the People. Some valuable and elaborate Web sites are powered almost entirely by volunteer labor. The previously mentioned *Selfhelp-Magazine* Web site is completely designed, constructed, and maintained by a volunteer staff. Readers who offer Web site improvement suggestions are recruited for a wide array of activities. Ads for various job openings are posted in the affiliated

SelfhelpMagazine Newsletter, which is sent by e-mail to readers who subscribe to the newsletter through the Web site. Professionals from around the globe offer their expertise as volunteers in writing articles in any of 20 topic areas.

The following vignette describes *the SelfhelpMagazine* Web site as an example of the benefits of careful planning, development, and maintenance in conjunction with coordination of community response to the Web site.

Established in 1994 as one of the first mental health sites, SelfhelpMagazine (http:// selfhelpmagazine.com) *immediately developed a reputation. It has grown and maintained its position as 1 of the top 10 mental health Web sites online ever since. Its features and traffic rival Web sites built by companies with $10- and $20-million budgets. Yet, with careful planning and management of resources, it has cost less than $1,000 per year to develop and operate for almost a decade.*

SelfhelpMagazine *does not offer direct access to clinicians for psychological service. Rather, it is an educational publication, aiming to help consumers understand and deal with issues ranging from mental illness through problems of living to normal psychology. Its goal has been to translate scientific information into plain English for a worldwide readership. The Web site is offered only in English, yet it receives traffic from more than 120 countries every month.*

Even though it receives some support from sponsors and advertisers, the Web site relies principally on the contributions from hundreds of volunteer professionals. These unpaid writers and editors may benefit from exposure in print, but they and the nonprofessional volunteers handling technical matters for the Web site seem motivated mostly by an altruistic desire to serve the public. As is often the case, finding willing helpers is easy, but keeping them well organized and happy is difficult.

SelfhelpMagazine *regularly recruits volunteers by advertising in various locations, especially its e-mail newsletter. Design volunteers sign agreements donating their work, giving ownership of all code and content developed for the magazine. They also agree to protect the confidentiality of any information they might come across on the server. They agree to alert the Web owner of any irregularities they find on the server, such as evidence of attempted disruption of code, hacking, or destruction of files.*

A five-level internal management system has been developed for the design staff, upper-level management supervises new recruits and shows them the ropes. Recruits receive duties only after signing an agreement that stipulates the time commitment they are to give, the weekly reports they are to submit, the ownership of all work they donate, and the staff person to whom they report. New recruits receive limited server access only after they have proved themselves by honoring their initial agreement for at least 3 months. Staff members graduate through the ranks, and about 1 in10 survives to the second level.

On the other side of the house, the authoring staff of SelfhelpMagazine *also is comprised of volunteers. Their work is peer reviewed and edited before publication. Volunteer authors sign agreements giving limited license to the owner of* SelfhelpMagazine, *that is, to Pioneer Development Resources, Inc. This corporation, which owns the magazine, provides an added layer of liability protection. Press releases from a variety of professional organizations are occasionally used for contact. Completely managing such a volunteer organization through e-mail is tricky and demands daily attention, especially when volunteers are located around the globe, with many speaking English as a second language.*

All of SelfhelpMagazine *is freely available to any visitor, and only visitors making a written request are put on the e-mail newsletter's mailing list (the Web site's privacy policy prevents sale of the subscription list). Although some reprints and artwork are obtained with permission from other Web sites and publications, much of the material in* SelfhelpMagazine *is original and specifically tailored for its readership.*

The articles convey varied science-based perspectives on psychological issues and usually include guidelines for working on problems. The articles also encourage readers to join a discussion about their topic. Any professional can submit articles to the editor in chief. One of its most significant contributions to the mental health community is the vast number of discussions it operates in-house. Protected by the Web site's dedication to privacy and an option to post anonymously, visitors are allowed to post messages on any number of bulletin boards for support and guidance by other visitors. More than 95 discussion forums have been successfully maintained with a minimum of cost since 1996. Benefiting from worldwide traffic, the boards are very active.

Terms of conditions of use make the rules very clear. Participants who do not follow the stated rules have their posts removed by the staff. It is clearly stated that professionals associated with the Web site will not answer consumer questions and that users are to proceed at their own risk with any advice they obtain from other people who post in any discussion forum. SelfhelpMagazine *disclaims intending to or creating a professional–patient relationship between lay questioners and professional answerers.*

Complaints about posts violating the stated rules are directed to the Web manager for consideration. The manager then forwards them to the appropriate staff for removal when appropriate. Messages found to violate of the stated rules are deleted or edited, without further explanation through the forum. Terms and conditions are clearly stated, including this consequence for violations. Explanations of rules have previously proved fruitless with some anonymous forum members. Such explanations seem to invite argument about the sites terms and conditions, so such explanations are completely avoided in the open forum. Members with complaints have a link on each page to contact the Web manager, if they wish. Individuals sending complaints receive a response if their complaint is not abusive. Abusive complaints do not get responses.

SelfhelpMagazine *gives a wealth of information and support to visitors from more than 110 countries every month. The magazine is accessible 24 hours a day. This format is only one of many large and creative endeavors offered by mental health practitioners who are exploring how to best advance their professions and deliver information using the power and reach of the Net.*

SelfhelpMagazine is a leader in combining professionalism; a user-friendly presentation; a rich selection of well-written, peer-reviewed articles; and a wide array of active consumer forums while avoiding blatant commercialism.

Self-Administered Quizzes and Tests. The use on Web sites of self-administered psychological tests, quizzes, or other assessment instruments is hotly debated. They can draw tremendous traffic to a site. Consumers of mental health information are proving to be eager self-assessment takers. In fact, some Web sites offer dozens of such instruments.

The problem with such offerings is that consumers may base decisions about or opinions of themselves or other people on the results of instruments that have no proven validity or reliability. Internet users cannot be expected to know the amount of time and research energy required to validate measures of behavior. The methodology of constructing valid tests for the worldwide population, speaking many different languages, and representing the hundreds of different cultures served by the Internet, is complicated. Easily constructed self-tests that exist on the Net at the time of this publication typically haven't undergone the rigors of scientific research. Although they may draw much traffic, their appropriateness for professional Web sites is in question. This topic is discussed in more detail in chapters 6 and 7. For now, suffice it to say that such features are to be used cautiously and only in accordance with suggestions made by the professional mental health associations.

WEB SITE MAINTENANCE

In psychotherapy research, it is much easier (and less disappointing) to study "process" than "outcome." The same applies to evaluating Web site performance. Quality control activity (the equivalent of research on process) can monitor downtime, broken internal and external links, system response delays, compatibility with various user configurations of equipment, browser and operating system, and the "user friendliness" of the presentation formats and navigation system. Usability is best measured with frequent small tests, with a few volunteers thinking out loud as they try to accomplish an assignment, such as locating a specific item of information on the Web site (Nielsen, 2001b).

Error Management

Errors and complications dismay visitors, creating a sense of powerlessness and preventing them from forming a robust conceptual model of the Web site (Nielsen, 2001a). Every page should be spell checked. "Orphan" or "cul-de-sac" pages in a site, the former with no links into it and the latter with no links out, may cause the visitor to leave one's site instead of backtracking.

HTML TIDY (http://www.w3.org/People/Raggett/tidy) is a free service for analyzing and fixing defective HTML code. Visitors appreciate Web pages that display the date they were last updated. This service is particularly helpful when pages are referenced in research papers or professional publications. Obsolete pages should be removed, along with any links to them. If articles are relocated to another part of the site, it is wise to construct a redirect page, so visitors who may have referenced the original page can find it easily on the Web site. An alternative is to have an internal search engine placed in the site, allowing easy access to moved pages. One advantage of maintaining a site with a dedicated authoring program, such as Microsoft Front-Page, is that Web site links are automatically analyzed and broken ones are flagged for the author to repair. Other link-check programs are available from the free download Web sites, such as C\NET. The following kind of experience is not always amusing.

> A visitor clicked on the link to the "National Nurses' Society on Addictions" link in the Pulier's Personal Psychiatry Pages Web site (http://www.umdnj.edu/~ pulierml). Up came a full-bore pornography site that immediately began spawning new windows to other porn Web sites. With difficulty, the visitor deleted all the browsers from her monitor screen and e-mailed a complaint to Dr. Pulier. This incident occurred at work, so that henceforth her computer's archives would indicate that she was being naughty on company time.
>
> It turned out that more than 80 nursing Web sites linked to the same pornography page. The Society had reorganized and moved to a new Web address, leaving its old URL to be snapped up by the pornographer in question. The new International Nurses Society on Addictions (http://www.intnsa.org) had not informed Web masters of the linking sites about their new address.

Many Web sites have moved to a new host server or may have changed their domain names. In some cases, the old site persists, abandoned, for years. A visitor may have bookmarked one of the pages and will return to find unchanged information without realizing that an updated page exists at the new location. The old sites are typically stripped down to a single page, the home page, and simply display a notice about the relocation and provide a link to the new home page. A brief "redirection" script can be included that will automatically move some browsers to the proper site; however, that may not motivate visitors to update their bookmarks.

Traffic Statistics

To keep count of how many different people look at a Web site, one identifies *unique visitors*. A Web site's log files give information about the number of people visiting a site per day, week, month, or any interval of time. The files can provide a variety of useful types of information. Web site owners are encouraged to review their log files weekly to determine how best to use their Web site to meet consumer interests and demand. For more information about where to find a log file in a Web account, speak with a representative of the company selling the account. Log files ought to be a free aspect of owning a Web site.

The server can also insert a small text file called a *cookie* into a user's computer for subsequent retrieval. The cookie helps the server keep track of a user (or at least of the computer) so that it can tailor the pages it produces in light of previous interchanges with the user. The cookie does not gather personally identifiable information. Cookies are often deposited without the users' consent or knowledge and can serve as clues to users' past behavior on the Web and their responses to questions. Web browsers, such as Internet Explorer, allow users to specify whether their computers accept cookies.

A site that deposits cookies is under no legal obligation, at present, to advise its users of this practices. The evolving law and ethics of the Internet are moving toward full disclosure about the use of cookies. Certainly, a site that posts a privacy policy, as any commercial site should, ought to be candid about its use of cookies. Not only should the owner indicate the use of cookie technology where applicable, but it also could benefit by providing brief instructions on how to circumvent cookies if the visitor so prefers. Although the outcome is not easily predictable, it is likely that claims may arise against site owners' using cookie technology without advising visitors of this practice. Even if this does not occur, however, disclosure avoids misunderstandings and tends to enhance the perceived professionalism of the site.

Intermediate between process and outcome research is quantitative assessment of Web site traffic. Facilities that host Web sites usually amass log files of every request to the server for a Web page. Statistics derived from such data can reveal how many unique visitors view the home page each hour and each day of the week, which pages are most frequently used as entry points to the site, and which pages are most and least often visited. Other useful statistics involve how long a visitor stays on a particular page, where people are clicking on each page, how often a particular page feature was used, and which pages tend to result in error messages presented to the viewer. Logs can also show which sites "referred" a visitor (if he or she clicked on a link to one's Web site) and how many visitors deliberately entered one's URL on their computer keyboard.

It is possible to contract for sophisticated analysis of each visitor's path through a Web site, including determining the point where each left the site, and to determine the physical location and e-mail address of most visitors, albeit at considerable financial cost and with the disadvantages entailed in encroaching on personal privacy. There may be some risk of litigation if this behavior is discovered by a visitor who becomes unhappy about it. Before incurring this risk, give serious thought to whether the information to be obtained is of value sufficient to offset the potential consequences.

Visitor's Reactions

A Web site owner may also collect data on subscriptions requested, renewed, and dropped and on purchases made through the site. Online polls, satisfaction surveys, and feedback comments can contribute further valuable material for a market analysis. Perseus Development (http://www.perseusdevelopment.com) offers information and assistance about survey construction and interpretation. Polls and surveys can be implemented by special programs on the main host computer for the Web site. A limited number of such data collection features can be set up more easily using free services, such as Alxnet (http://www.alxnet.com), that run on a separate computer. One must be careful about privacy and security vulnerabilities when using such an outside service.

A highly productive and low-cost way of gathering information is posting checklists requesting visitors' opinions wherever possible. As Figure 4.2 illustrates, every news and feature article can collect ratings on issues that are meaningful to both visitor and Web owner: usefulness, clarity, technical level, trustworthiness, and others.

Although a text-entry box can elicit some thoughtful comments, checklists are easiest to aggregate and interpret. Much to the dismay of many beginning Web owners, open text fields to be used by the mental health community sometimes result in unsolicited requests for emergency services, such as suicide notes, homicide threats, and child abuse reports, regardless of the instructions for how to use the open text field or disclaimers surrounding the open field. Open text fields on Web sites should be kept to a minimum, so that site owners provide explicit admonitions and disclaimers about appropriate subject matter. One very effective technique is to use pull-down menus and checklists rather than allowing free-form comments.

A focus panel discussion with a few visitors may illuminate issues of Web site performance, content, and expansion. This discussion could be conducted through a telephone conference call, an Internet chat, a discussion board, or e-mail. Assessment activity that clarifies the characteristics of visitors enables the tailoring of material to particular segments of the audience, as well as suggests what new kinds of user to attract. Visitors can also be asked about what they want and how effectively the Web site is delivering distinctive value.

To collect and analyze information about outcome, the most difficult part of judging Web site performance, the site owner must return to the basic goals and specific objectives defined in the formal plan described earlier in this chapter. The plan should include explicit criteria for determining whether the Web site is succeeding or failing. Discussing results with people outside the organization may provide new perspective and surprising conclusions to apply when overhauling the Web site's overall aims and goals during the next planning cycle.

This and the previous chapter have outlined text-based telecommunication issues. We now turn to telecommunication technologies that offer more interactive information: audio and video. Telephones and videoconferencing equipment and their relevance to psychotherapy are the topic of the next chapter.

Telephonic and Videoconferencing Technologies

You see, wire telegraph is a kind of a very, very long cat. You pull his tail in New York and his head is meowing in Los Angeles. Do you understand this? And radio operates exactly the same way: You send signals here, they receive them there. The only difference is that there is no cat.

—Albert Einstein (Hamilton, 2003)

Einstein's paradox of the missing cat may refer to deep concepts of modern physics,[1] and it indirectly speaks to the realities of delivering mental health care by telephone (and other audio means) or videoconferencing. In distance treatment, the medium is shaping what can be done, attracting attention to itself, influencing patient and therapist both subtly and overtly, and always threatening to shift from being a means to being an end. The "cat" demands attention not only for its helpful and occasionally troublesome role in health care but also for its effect on what may be considered the postmodern online version of transference and countertransference (Schachter, 2002).

Einstein's cat is all over the place. Psychotechnologies are providing services in prisons, clinics, schools, and homes. The challenges, however, are to disseminate these strategies more broadly in order to improve care throughout the mental health delivery system and also to make their use normal operating procedure and part of the standard of care. In 10 years, we will be asking, "Where did that cat go?"

For practical purposes now, the real question about distance therapy is whether to rely on the telephone as the primary vehicle or to use videoconferencing technologies. The terms telephone and audio will be used interchangeably in our discussions. Telephones, which are used for many activities related to health care, nearly always play a supportive rather than a primary role. Interactive videoconferencing is the preferred technology for direct care of patients by licensed health care practitioners in all aspects of health care, including mental health. To meet standards of care that have evolved for traditional in-person diagnosis and treatment, videoconferencing is the "next best thing to being there" although simply using the telephone or email can be tempting to the unequipped practitioner. Technology increased ease of use and manageability in videoconferencing units has attracted more users (Moore, 2001). Videoconferencing

---

[1] According to relativity theory the movement of a photon carrying a radio signal from transmitter to receiver takes place instantaneously, a notion that plays havoc with our conventional ideas of space and time.

in mental health is gaining momentum for a number of specific tasks (Baer et al., 1995; Burton, 1997; Cukor et al., 1998; Sampson, Kolodinsky, & Greeno, 1997).

The model for videoconferencing that many researchers in mental health care describe involves a local practitioner's in-person evaluation of a client, followed by consultation or treatment with a remote specialist over a live interactive two-way video connection (Baer et al., 1995; Brown-Connolly, 2001a, 2001b; 2002a; Cukor et al., 1998; Glueckauf et al., 1998; Huston & Burton, 1997; Jerome, 1986, 1993; Sampson et al., 1997; Stamm, 1998; Troester, Paolo, Glalt, Hubble, & Koller, 1995). In this model, in-person contact with the local or referring professional seems to bring the experience closer to the traditional practice of being in the same room as the patient. Perhaps, paradoxically, treating a patient over the telephone, which seems a more radical departure from the traditional in-person venue, rarely involves a local practitioner. As for any telephone conference "model," practice in this modality has generally been conducted informally rather than being a central focus for training, regulatory bodies, professional associations, or the research community.

This chapter is an introduction to the benefits of and barriers to both telephone and videoconferencing technology. We look at some of the still scanty professional literature in this area and end with a call for research that, we hope, will inspire students and researchers alike.

BENEFITS OF AND BARRIERS TO THE TELEPHONIC AND VIDEOCONFERENCING TECHNOLOGIES

Notwithstanding the venerable history of telemental health (Allen & Wheeler, 1998; Benschoter, 1971; Dwyer, 1973; Greist et al., 1973) whenever the topic of electronically mediated mental health service arises in casual conversation, people tend to regard it as a novel idea. In fact, it might even be a social gaffe to suggest that the humble telephone has long been an independent, established, widely used, versatile, and important, if underappreciated, tool for scheduling and delivering mental health care[2] (Haas, Benedict, & Kobos, 1996). When more recently given specific consideration, some writers have convincingly argued against its inclusion in the telehealth toolkit (VandenBos & Williams, 2000). However, the telephone of yesteryear is not the telephone of today or of tomorrow.

Many newer telephones have already been merged with other technologies and are fast becoming a versatile tool for mental health professionals. A good example is the videophone, a small device that plugs into almost any telephone and television. The videophone is likely to be the next low-technology device that mental health professionals use. During the war in Iraq, television viewers witnessed the wonders of the videophone.

Mobile telephones are now available with videophone technology, so the average citizen can relay real-time video to anyone with a compatible mobile phone using cellular telephone technology. Anytime, anywhere: Access by mobile telephone has suddenly and without much fanfare been delivered not only to psychotherapist and

---

[2] Supposedly, the first real telephone message was Alexander Graham Bell's call for help after he spilled battery acid on his clothing: "Mr. Watson, come here. I want you." (For a fine example of how to present an exposition on the Web, see http://www.iath.virginia.edu/albell/homepage.html)

client desktops but also to their schools, jobs, trips to the in-laws, backyards, kitchens, pockets, and purses. Of course, videoconferencing through a square inch or two of LCD display on a mobile telephone has its limitations, but it also has a breadth of possibilities for psychotherapists to explore. And yes, more elaborate technologies are available for videoconferencing, as discussed later in this chapter. The next sections more specifically consider the overall benefits of and barriers to using the telephonic and videoconferencing technologies.

Benefits of the Telephone and Videoconferencing

Professionals have no difficulty accepting the use of the telephone and voice mail for initial contact and screening, scheduling and rescheduling regular and emergency sessions, and making referrals. This psychotechnology is already being applied extensively for extracting patient history from previous professionals, conducting follow-ups, refilling prescriptions, and dunning clients for payments. The client uses these devices to inform practitioners of homicidal or suicidal feelings (Liebson, 1997). In addition, as Waters and Finn (1995), state, telephones are widely used to:

> check on the status of the elderly and people with disabilities, [for] radio and television call-in lines, information lines with recorded messages on mental health issues, coverage for vacationing therapists, "warm lines" for latchkey (self-care) children, confidential lines for runaways, contact between recovering substance abusers and their sponsors, the police emergency or 911 lines, and even psychotherapy that is billed to the caller's telephone or credit card number. (p. 254)

Reflecting on the fundamental and essential mental health tasks dependent on telephone communication, one is reminded of Molière's play *Le Bourgeois Gentilhomme*, in which Jourdin is delighted to learn that he had been speaking prose for more than 40 years without even knowing it!

We might, however, mention that what is really new are the rapidly expanding telecommunication infrastructure, decreasing costs of products that have converged with telephones (such as the videophone), increasing funding, and the development of specialized telephone lines and other technology to combine video with an electronic whiteboard, high-quality audio, store-and-forward technology, and many other services. This expanding telecommunication infrastructure is delivering mental health care to a growing number of patients.

Let us begin by examining one main benefit of the telecommunications technologies—its ability to provide increased access to mental health care.

Increased Access. Of course, the need for increased access to mental health care is "nothing new under the sun" (Ecclesiates 1:9): The Old Testament has young David making home visits to assuage King Saul's depressive episodes (1 Samuel 16:14–23). Millennia later, Joseph Breuer's talking treatment in Fräulein Anna O's boudoir initiated the psychoanalytic revolution (Breuer & Freud, 1955).

Technology is overcoming the difficulties in reaching mental health services. The telephone has helped patients overcome the barrier of access to several types of mental health care. Few practitioners in the United States realize that, for example, it is legitimate to take a 2-month vacation from one's in-person practice and to deliver services via telephone with established patients. Caveats for spending this time away from the office include:

- Adequate emergency backup is supplied (another practitioner has agreed to cover during the absence).
- The consent agreement fully describes details of contact and emergency backup during travel times (sections of appendix C may be useful in drafting such an agreement, but checking with legal counsel is warranted for drafting a sound agreement).
- Third-party carriers have approved the remote contact if they are reimbursing the practitioner for the service.

Geographic Distance.   Of course, travel within one's state of licensure is potentially less problematic than travel across state lines. Nonetheless, most states do not regulate the delivery of psychotherapy or counseling by telephone to established patients while one is out of the state of licensure. Interested practitioners should check with licensing board authorities and legal counsel. A careful review of all related state statutes with one's counsel before attempting such remote telephone delivery might lead to more flexibility than imagined.

Even though videoconferencing does not enjoy the latitude given to telephone contact with established patients in geographic areas beyond one's licensure, it nonetheless promises to provide different types of access. Sophisticated video links that connect widely separated clinical facilities are rapidly advancing to bring health care modalities within the reach of more clients and to increase access to care, regardless of geographic location. For example, half of Georgia's 159 counties have no psychiatrist, but Johnson County clients who engage in video-mediated psychiatric sessions through their primary care physicians' offices claim that their telepsychiatric care is comparable to in-person encounters. The psychiatry residents providing their treatment from the Medical College of Georgia, 80 miles away, receive supervision twice a week relevant to the video-mediated psychiatric sessions. This supervision also qualifies for board certification in psychiatry (Baker, 2002). Videoconferencing may help rural hospitals in the United States deal with the nationwide scarcity of pharmacists as well (Lorden, Vorhees, & Richards, 2002). Videoconferencing truly allows care to be rendered as and when needed.

The following case demonstrates how this video technology is being used. The benefits to this client, her family, and the health care system are obvious.

Lieutenant Colonel Mary Clement, 38, had been stationed on the island of Guam for nearly 18 months with her husband and three children when a routine screening mammogram disclosed ominous microcalcifications. There was no significant past medical history, but Clement's mother had died of breast cancer. Understandably, the patient and her husband were quite anxious about the mammogram results.

Before 1993, the patient would have faced the alternatives of either relying on the limited medical resources available at her small island army base or separation from her family and evacuation to Tripler Army Medical Center in Hawaii. Now, however, the case was referred to the Internet Tumor Board (ITB) for consultation and treatment recommendations.

The ITB includes a surgeon, a pathologist, an oncologist, a radiologist, and a psychologist, and it brings in other disciplines as needed. It uses several modalities simultaneously to communicate with client centers. Voice is handled by a high-quality speakerphone. The personal computer workstation uses NetMeeting's free desktop conferencing system (http://www.microsoft.com/windows/netmeeting). *An offline film digitizer prepares pathology and radiology images for transmission from the client center to the ITB in advance of a consultation session. Thus, a relatively low transmission-line rate allows both the local team and the ITB to view the images simultaneously during the live consultation session with their respective InFocus digital projectors* (http://www.infocus.com); *they can independently enlarge details in selected areas of the images. A "markup" feature makes arrows, lines, and circles sketched on an image by one party immediately visible to the other to facilitate discussion.*

After the ITB team considered Clement's history and studied her biopsy, they offered a working diagnosis and outlined a plan for oncology care that specifically included organizing appropriate family support and addressing her anxiety, insomnia, and distress.

—Leigh W. Jerome, Ph.D.
Tripler Army Base

Bringing care to where the patient lives or works delivers more than simply access (or convenience, which is often minimized when it comes to mental health care). It is easy to see that the clinical use of telephones is within the standard of care when initial assessment and perhaps psychotherapy are in-person, backed by appropriate local emergency clinical backup. When delivered in situ rather than in an office or clinic, assessment, patient education, and skills training can be more directly applicable, immediately implemented, practiced, and therefore more effective by telephone.

Reliability and Effectiveness of Using Telephones. The telephone has been shown to be as reliable as in-person methods for specific and limited purposes, even when an entire assessment is automated rather than performed by a human interviewer for surveying and screening certain mental disorders (Aneshensel, Frerichs, Clark, & Yokopenic, 1982; Desmond, Tatemichi, & Hanzawa, 1994; Fenig, Levav, Kohn, & Yelin, 1993; Gallo & Breitner, 1995; Go et al., 1997; Gonzalez, Costello, La Tourette, Joyce, & Valenzuela, 1997; Kobak et al., 1997a; 1997b). The telephone also is reliable for rendering diagnoses (Paulsen, Crowe, Noyes, & Pfohl, 1988; Rohde, Lewinsohn, & Seeley, 1997; Wells, Burnam, Leake, & Robins, 1988). Telephones have been shown to be reliable for assessing severity of syndromes and disorders by clinical interview (Go et al., 1997; Kobak, Greist, Jefferson, Mundt, & Katzelnick, 1999; Kobak et al., 1997; Monteiro et al., 1998; Mundt et al., 1998; Potts, Daniels, Burnam, & Wells, 1990; Roccaforte, Burke, Bayer, & Wengel, 1992; Simon, Revicki, & VonKorff, 1993; Tunstall, Prince, & Mann, 1997).

Studies demonstrating that the telephone can reliably convey clinically important information do not imply that treatment by telephone is comparable to sitting in an office or may further enhance distance therapy. In practical terms, two kinds of study are needed. One involves comparing treatments delivered by telephone with video-mediated and in-person therapies and measuring their relative effectiveness. A design using control patients would be necessary to show that real effectiveness was achieved by the active treatments. A second type of study should assess relative costs. Even if treatment via telephone is less effective, cost and availability may sometimes make it the best approach.

As it happens, the telephone is increasingly considered quite effective for delivering psychotherapy and counseling with specific populations, such as with patients struggling with multiple sclerosis (Mohr et al., 2000), tobacco smokers (Orleans et al.,

1991), and clients with mild depression (Lynch, Tamburrino, & Nagel, 1997). Further evidence indicates that mental health professionals can deliver useful psychotherapy over the telephone (Reese, Conoley, & Brossart, 2002).

However, other studies have uncovered factors that may reduce the effectiveness of telephone contact. For example, people with fewer economic resources and subjectively greater distress may do less well with telephone counseling than with in-person treatment (Reese, 2001). One may further speculate that youngsters and other people who have difficulty maintaining dutiful focus may do better with a more immersive videoconference than with a telephone session. On the other hand, someone who is camera shy may feel closer and cozier conducting a tête-à-tête by phone.

Telephone-mediated contact can enhance clinical outcome even when the intervention is brief and not intensive. Emotional support and focused behavioral interventions delivered by primary care nurses in ten 6-minute telephone calls to patients beginning antidepressants in a primary care practice were associated with significantly greater improvement in depression scores and satisfaction at 6 months in one study (Hunkeler et al., 2000). Wasson et al. (1992), in a study of 470 primary care patients, found that substituting three clinician-initiated telephone calls for otherwise routinely scheduled clinic visits over a 2-year period was associated not only with fewer in-person visits but also with less medication use, fewer admissions, and shorter hospital stays, resulting in an annual saving of $828 per patient as compared with usual-care control patients.

After primary care physicians instituted antidepressant therapy for 613 patients studied by Simon, VonKoff, Rutter, and Wagner (2000), 306 of the patients were randomly chosen to received systematic telephone follow-up by care managers, with their physicians receiving treatment recommendations and practice support. Compared with the other patients, the experimental group fared much better, at a mean cost of $80 per patient. More intensive counseling delivered by a masters-level therapist over the telephone to 28 patients beginning antidepressant pharmacotherapy in a primary care setting was associated with lower depressive symptoms at 3- and 6-month follow-up at an extra cost per patient of $150, compared with 94 patients receiving usual care (Tutty, Simon, & Ludman, 2000).

There is reason to believe that telephone communication can sustain prolonged psychotherapy. Mark Leffert, a training and supervising analyst, described having continued nine courses of psychoanalysis and five of psychotherapy by telephone after moving to another state (Leffert, 2002). (It may be of interest to the U.S. reader that many state licensing boards do not prohibit telephone contact with patients across state boundaries but do prohibit videoconferenced contact.) Leffer noted that some patients seemed to experience less shame in conversing over the telephone. For patients who did not take well to the telephone, he reasoned that it was an unsatisfactory substitute, owing to a patient's intense and ambivalent transference dominated by feelings of abandonment. The technology itself quickly became "transparent" and was not much of an issue. However, the loss of the "container" represented by the therapist's office did arise as a source of difficulty for some patients but as a liberating experience for others. Leffert suggests that in-person sessions be included in analytic treatment using telephones. As for selecting patients, he suggested that the decision to use telephones may not rely exclusively on diagnosis but may include the patient's subjective opinion after a few trial telephone sessions. This particular report's sample size is by no means adequate to generalize to the mental health population, but, combined with the previously mentioned studies, these reports suggest that continued research into the use of telephones is warranted.

Reliability and Effectiveness of Videoconferencing. The reliability and effectiveness of the telephone as a medium for mental health communication between therapist and patient do not necessarily extend to videoconferencing. Video is not simply audio with an added visual component. For example, as we note earlier in this chapter, shame at being seen may interfere with treatment. Furthermore, technical problems could make video unreliable. We must therefore look to studies that have examined the reliability of specific functions using videoconferencing technologies. For instance, in a study by Ruskin et al. (1998), two interviewers assessed 30 psychiatric patients; 15 patients received an assessment from each interviewer in-person, and 15 patients received assessments from one in-person interviewer and one remote interviewer. Interrater reliability was either identical or nearly identical under both conditions for major depression, bipolar disorder, panic disorder, and alcohol dependence.

Similarly, Baer et al. (1995) found that interrater agreements in the diagnostic assessment of patients with obsessive-compulsive disorder was nearly perfect when comparing in-person and videoconferencing results. In general, in comparisons of videoconferenced to in-person evaluations, patients with schizophrenia and obsessive-compulsive disorder seem to receive the highest interrater reliability (Baer et al., 1995; Baigent et al., 1997; Ball, McLaren, Summerfield, Lipsedge, & Watson, 1995; Zarate et al., 1997). Zaylor (1999) found no significant difference in Global Assessment and Functioning (GAF) scores when comparing videoconferencing and in-person outcomes of 49 patients with major depression or schizoaffective disorder. The videoconferencing group did show higher attendance rates, and the time used for a follow-up visit was cut in half. Because various uses of videoconferencing are growing rapidly in mental health, the reader is encouraged to contact researchers in appendix A to see whether they might be conducting other studies in this area.

If we can accept videoconferencing as generally reliable, we can then ask whether it supports effective therapy. Early studies indicate that telepsychiatry using videoconferencing technology could effectively assist clients and practitioners, as well as support a therapeutic alliance (Baigent et al., 1997; Ball et al., 1995; Baur & Doering, 2000; Brown-Connolly, 2001a; 2001b; D'Souza & Hawker, 1998; Ghosh, McLaren, & Watson, 1997; Jerome, 1993; Kennedy & Yellowlees, 2003; McLaren, 2003; McLaren, Blunden, Lipsedge, & Summerfield, 1996; Montani, Billaud, Tyrrell, & Fluchaire, 1997; Simpson, 2003). A recent study in Australia using videoconferencing to deliver psychoeducation to clients and their families identified significant improvement in longitudinal outcomes for clients with serious mental illness in treatment adherence, decreased adverse medication reactions, reduced relapses and hospitalizations, high satisfaction, and improved quality of life (D'Souza, 2002). Rather than list more studies and their findings here, the reader can review appendix A for studies comparing the clinical efficacy of various psychotechnologies.

Barriers to Using the Telephone and Videoconferencing

If research has indicated that therapy mediated by telephone and videoconferencing is efficacious, why is it not more common? There are many reasons. Inertia is not an explanation—adequate telephone technology has been available (and in use) for decades. First, we should note that even though research has shown promising results, there is little of it. In particular, outcome studies clearly showing that electronically mediated therapy (or indeed any therapy) is effective for mental health problems are few and difficult to generalize. Cost is another factor. Some other barriers to using the telephone and videoconferencing include general telehealth challenges that result from:

- A clinician's preparation for managing emergencies from afar.
- Interstate and international practice and related licensure law.
- Lack of specific practice guidelines for appropriate use of various technologies.
- Privacy, security, confidentiality, and data integrity with telecommunications and the handling of electronic medical records.
- Adequate and timely staff training.
- Overall practitioner and patient acceptance.
- The reliability, affordability and compatibility of technologies.

Maheu, Whitten, and Allen (2001) have detailed each of these challenges. This section examines several barriers directly related to the delivery of mental health care via the psychotechnologies.

Nonverbal Cues. In the real world, animals regulate many of their relationships within and between species by exchanging nonverbal signals. Human language extends these functions by setting and reinforcing and by interpersonal boundaries, by unifying a group into a single speech community, and by excluding outsiders (Saville-Troike, 2003). On the Internet and through the telephone, however, nonverbal signals are poorly transmitted. In both media, language tends to be compressed, especially if it is in the form of text rather than speech.

Mental health practice depends on both verbal and nonverbal communication, for gathering data and also for providing treatment. Personal and family history, recitation of symptoms, and even observation of most signs of pathological mental status rest on words. Meanwhile, the stream of nonverbal data flowing from a client may be useful where it is discrepant, incongruous, unexpectedly absent, emotionally affecting, or apparently false. However, the verbal material usually dominates in the clinical record, the working diagnosis, the choice of therapy, the team meeting, and the supervisory session.

Surely, there are important exceptions to this. However, in psychoeducation, cognitive-behavioral therapies, and even psychoanalytically inspired approaches, verbalization appears to be primary. Implementing the psychoanalytic slogan "*Wo Es war, soll Ich werden*"[3] (Freud, 1923, p. 80) involves putting matters into words rather than into facial expressions, body postures, or other nonverbal channels. For many purposes, adequate sound quality would thus be much more important in general electronic audiovisual communication than would high-quality video (Finn, Sellen, & Wilbur, 1997); the same may hold true for clinical interventions resembling in-person psychotherapy.[4] Of course, if (or when) "irrational," nonverbal factors or insight are much more crucial for clinical diagnosis or as with those diagnoses that require the clinician to identify visual symptoms, as per the *Diagnostic and Statistical Manual* (DSM-IV) of the American Psychiatric Association (2000a), our rationalization of the relative importance of words fails. Early research in communication has shown evidence that video supports the importance of social cues and information about affect.

---

[3] "Where id was, ego shall be."
[4] Note that we are careful to say "resembling" rather than "substituting for."

Thus, it follows that a serious barrier with the use of telephones in consultation is that it deprives the participants of essential nonverbal cues (Haas et al., 1996). This disadvantage is remedied only partially by whatever quality of video service might be substituted for, or added to, the telephone (Cukor et al., 1998). Reactions such as a smile or a sympathetic look are lost in telephone, e-mail, and chat room interactions (Anderson, Newlands, & Mullin, 1996). This does not necessarily impede the use of these technologies, but the clinician needs to be aware of the missing information and to recognize the situations in which using each of these technologies might be appropriate.

Let us remember that many adolescents conduct intense relationships and convey strong feelings during hours spent on the telephone. To be sure, the lack of nonverbal cues does not automatically prevent a professional from conducting therapy. Visually impaired trainees are regularly accepted into psychotherapy programs and go on to practice quite successfully. Tone of voice, inflection, speech rhythm, alterations in word pronunciation, sighs and giggles, and the poetry involved in word choice all convey nonverbal material quite effectively (Tausig & Freeman, 1988). Telephones carry such information successfully.

Popular as telephone sex may be, easy access over the Internet to visible depictions of sexual material has been an even greater industry boon. The auditory is powerful, but the visual is yet more compelling, at least for the majority of such users (Carnes, 2001).

Providing mental health assistance to a distant client is supported by an informal but natural test under the extreme parameters that characterize crisis telephone hot lines. The fact that Befrienders International (http://www.befrienders.org) has organized 357 telephone support centers in 41 countries attests to the viability of their activity. The Befrienders Web site (an example of supplementing POTS, Plain Old Telephone Service, with another psychotechnology) can quickly put a visitor in touch with trained volunteers speaking Arabic, Chinese, Danish, German, English, Spanish, French, Magyar, Dutch, Portuguese, Russian, and/or Suomi. At their telephone support centers, volunteers commonly form a temporary working relationship with desperate and sometimes anonymous strangers who call from a distance, often about a life-threatening situation. The volunteers do not ask for the caller's name or location and have no access to relatives, clinical records, or professionals who have treated the caller. Nonetheless, the volunteers manage to get a sufficient grasp of the caller's immediate problem, provide assistance, and usually avert catastrophe.

Extrapolation—no, actually, interpolation—from this extreme to more favorable circumstance usually exists in a professional practice. Experienced licensed clinicians have managed, for the most part, to be reasonably safe when conducting something akin to psychotherapy by telephone with well-known clients in the context of ongoing therapy, particularly when it is conducted predominantly in-person and is supplemented by traditional collateral meetings with family members and contact with other professionals. Of course, a statement that service delivery seems "reasonably safe" does not satisfy ethical requirements, and mental health organizations remain wary about defining ethical standards or even guidelines for psychotherapy at a distance.

The next question becomes, "Does the addition of video to the telephone offer telemental health comparable enhancements?" Research in communication has shown evidence that video supports social cues and information about affect and attitude. For example, nonverbal cues to a stranger's altruism might be recognizable over video. These cues may involve contraction of the *orbicularis oculi* and other involuntary muscles that distinguish a genuine from a fake smile (Brown, Palameta, & Moore, 2003).

Whitaker and O'Conaill (1997) state the following:

> Adding video information to the speech channel changes the outcome and character of communication that require access to affect or emotional factors. Example tasks here include negotiation, bargaining and conflict resolution. Participants focus more on the motives of others when they have access to visual information, and video/audio conversations are more personalized, less argumentative, more polite, and broader in focus. They are also less likely to end in deadlock than speech-only communications. (p. 38)

Research must decide the actual relevance to satisfaction and clinical outcome of missing nonverbal material. Rice (1993) conducted a study comparing social presence in written memo, in-person, video, and audio contact. For such criteria as decision making, problem solving, conflict resolution, and generating new ideas, in-person communication was consistently superior, followed by video, audio, and, finally, written memo. Social presence was found to be dependent on the communication context and on the full range of verbal and nonverbal cues, not solely on the words involved in the communication. For people who want to roll up their sleeves and get started, other studies comparing audio, video, and in-person groups are emerging (Glueckauf et al., 2002; Pelletier, 2002; Schneider, 1999).

Acceptance. Studies of client and professional acceptance of telephones for particular mental health applications are increasing; for instance, according to a survey of 121 psychologists (Richards, 2001), 74% had conducted therapy by telephone. Clearly, more studies with large samples are needed.

As for general health services delivered through videoconferencing , research has shown that clients and clinicians are generally satisfied (Brown-Connolly, 2002a; Gustke, Balch, West, & Rogers, 2000; Hartley, Bird, & Dempsey, 1999; McLaren, Ahlbom, Riley, Mohammedali, & Denis, 2002), but much of this research has been conducted with general patient populations, not with mental health patients. Another study has indicated that services accessed via video are as satisfactory to patients as is in-person consultation (usual care); in transfer of knowledge for educational purposes, such video services were rated as better than usual care (Brown-Connolly, 2002a). The latter study included mental health services, but the report describes combined results drawn from a sample of patients across medical specialties.

When video is used in conjunction with telephone or other high-quality audio channels for psychiatric purposes, the technology is apparently acceptable (Baer, Cukor, & Coyle, 1997). In Texas, telepsychiatry was compared to in-person appointments and found to have satisfactory levels of client satisfaction and clinical outcome (Rohland, 2001). Conversely, Dongier, Tempier, Lalinoc-Michaud, and Meunier (1986) asked participants to compare a videoconferenced psychiatric interview with previously experienced in-person psychiatric interviews. Most patients gave the videoconferencing session an above-average rating, but the consultants disagreed; they rated global assessment, diagnosis, and written consultation by videoconferencing as slightly inferior.

Cost-Effectiveness. The factors most germane to decisions about treatment by telephone or videoconferencing are not merely cost-effectiveness but also who bears the cost and who receives the benefit. Reducing a patient's travel expenditure does not affect reimbursement of the clinician or directly benefit a third-party payer. If a practitioner can charge for time spent with a patient on the telephone, this modality is likely to be used more often. Before investing in the special equipment and communication service needed for videoconferencing, a practice or a clinic will tend to weigh its own financial advantage against any financial or clinical benefit to its patients. Currently, in the United States, payment for remote mental health treatment is usually confined to videoconferencing conducted under defined circumstances (as discussed in chapter 13), unless arrangements are made with the patient to pay out of pocket. Ideally, the health care system will evolve to reward using electronic communication vehicles whenever it is in the best interest of patients.

Several studies have shown that delivery of health care service over the telephone can result in considerable financial savings overall. This chapter has described some reports showing minimal cost involved in some effective telephone interventions. Although the cost savings of using telephones for psychotherapy were established in the 1980s and 1990s, the marketplace did not sustain businesses based on such technology at the time.

This trend may be changing, with new models surfacing from managed care organizations as they combine telephonic with Web-based services and information. As we discuss in chapter 1, feasibility studies have shown a renewed interest in telephone counseling now that it is accessed anonymously through private employer Web sites (Masi & Freeman, 1999). Research and the market will help decide the cost-effectiveness of using videoconferencing to deliver mental health services. In a preliminary study, Doze, Simpson, Hailey, and Jacobs (1999) assessed a telepsychiatry pilot project using questionnaires concerning ease of use, cost-effectiveness, and quality of care. The results came back positive for all three criteria and suggested that telepsychiatry was a viable and cost-effective option for an integrated, community-based mental health service. In another study, videoconferencing was found economically advantageous compared with in-person medical consultation for patients at some distance from services, indicating a cost saving to patients on an average of $83 for one-way travel alone in California (Brown-Connolly, 2002a). Furthermore, in North Carolina, 71 consultations were held over a 2-year period, mostly for dementia or depression.

Researchers reported the benefits of using videoconferencing as including timely consultation and a reduced need for travel for nursing home residents (Johnston & Jones, 2001). Finally, the National Institute on Disability and Rehabilitation Research's Videocounseling for Rural Teens with Seizures Project seeks to assess the cost-effectiveness, impact on family relationships, and improvement of specific problems for home-based video, speakerphones, and office-based counseling (Center for Research on Telehealth and Healthcare Communications, 2002).

Full video capability is not yet common to most mental health professionals, but the cost is dropping for both the high-speed connection service it requires and for the equipment. Some communities are finding that sharing their videoconferencing facilities with other communities can make the initial cost of installation and ongoing cost of maintenance and use well worth the investment. Duffy Soto, executive director of technology and innovation at Lake City Community College in northern Florida, tells of his attempt to make videoconferencing more affordable:

Even though prices for equipment have been steadily coming down over the past few years—and will continue to decline—the real cost of operating a network is in the recurring monthly circuit costs paid to the service providers. Costs vary, depending on the complexity of the infrastructure, as well as on what transport modality you settle on. Other factors that ultimately determine your recurring costs include the location of your network in relationship to provider LATA (local access and transport area) boundaries and even how individual states' public service commissions might regulate pricing and access. Simply, it's difficult to predict what you might pay in your specific area without consulting a service provider. One thing, however, remains consistent regardless of what state or states your network encompasses: The service providers must recover their pretty hefty investment in digital connectivity, so the term recurring costs *will be quite relative, depending on your area of desired coverage.*

Lake City Community College's televideo network is spread over rural central north Florida. At first, we couldn't even get digital connectivity. When we finally could, we were afraid we couldn't afford it. But surprisingly, our costs came out to be less than they would have been if we were located in a much larger metropolitan area. Lake City's annual fee for connectivity averages about $5,000 per month for up to seven sites that cover roughly 2,000 square miles. Although five "big ones" a month may sound expensive, it's really a bargain when you consider that we can operate the system 24 hours a day, 7 days a week for this cost. At that rate, our costs come out to about one dollar per hour per site. Now, that's cost-effective! Of course, it becomes incumbent on management to make sure that the system is booked for as many hours a day as possible, in order to keep the system cost-effective as well as to generate revenue for operation.

Not long after we completed our own system, we needed to expand. Students in other areas needed access to our distance learning programs. The more sites we could access, the more people we could reach (or conference with) and the more courses we could deliver. However, the $100,000 per site cost (plus recurring costs) would severely limit our growth rate to less than one per year, which was much less than our plan called for. We needed a plan that would enable us to acquire more sites without going into debt and that would also allow us to grow at a more rapid rate. Thus, the idea of the "e-community" was born.

The e-community concept is simple: Seek out an area in which we would like to have a presence, then recruit partners whose businesses would benefit from televideo. Our plan was to convince them to build the site, using their resources. The college would provide the partner with a multitude of "up-front" services, such as planning and design. After the site was completed, the new partners would then allow the college to access the site on an "as-available" basis at reduced cost. Essentially, their site would become our site, but we didn't have the expense associated with building and operation. In exchange, the college would help the partner with such tasks as helping choose a vendor, overseeing project construction (if needed), training the users, providing tech support and help-desk maintenance, and, finally, granting the partner access to our existing sites on an as-available basis as well. Thus, our sites now become their sites.

The e-community partnership concept makes sense to Lake City Community College in two ways. First, we get a new site (or sites) designed to be compatible with our other sites at no direct expense to the college; second, we can perpetuate the expansion of a "common" network infrastructure to include still more e-community partners down the road. In essence—and theoretically—we're building our own interactive network across the state with little or no third-party intervention. The concept provides that each e-community partner bear the cost for construction and operation of its site (or sites) while giving other partners access to those sites at reduced or no cost in exchange for the same consideration. In other words, each partner pays all the expenses associated with its own site or sites buts lets e-community partners use the site as needed and on as available at reduced or no cost. The goal is to keep all sites as active for as many hours as possible to be cost-effective.

The e-community concept can be compared somewhat to the system of railroads owned by different rail companies. Trains owned by all companies are free to use the tracks, yet each company is responsible for the repair and upkeep of its own system of track. We use interactive televideo sites, not rails, but the principle is loosely the same.

I envision that great telemedicine networks can be built quickly and with greater prominence using the e-community concept. If so, then many rural health care givers would have access to a myriad of otherwise unavailable services via the e-community network.

As with any idea, naysayers think that a large e-community network would be unmanageable and expensive to maintain and therefore is impractical—especially as an H320 standard. Internet, or IP, they say, is the standard that offers the best solution for long-distance video. Sounds good. Unfortunately, IP video as a source for high-quality and viable interactive conferencing—especially as a telemedicine platform—isn't ready and likely won't be for a while. I agree that when looking at IP from the top, it shows an extreme amount of potential. However, keeping it back is the lack of sufficient bandwidth available with some modicum of QoS (quality of service) to support many interactive users. High-quality interactive video simply isn't practical using the World Wide Web yet, and it is practical only when used within an enclosed or private H323 network. However, you are then homebound, with little hope of linking at will to other sites off that network.

Can a low-cost alternative to H320 provide quality and security as well? Possibly, as more wireless broadband becomes available, but even that is several years away. Broadband offers good bandwidth, but its range is limited. As well, vendors can make more money selling high-speed data and Internet access to the masses, so bandwidth availability for quality video even with wireless broadband will still likely come at a premium. So if you're waiting to see what might be coming over the top of the hill, you could be losing a lot of time. Your best bet for setting up a cost-effective televideo system, quickly and with the least amount of investment, may lie in developing of your own e-communities.

—**Duffy Soto**
Executive Director of Technology and Innovation
Lake City Community College

As Duffy Soto describes, we can expect distance technology to be more cost-effective as well as convenient over the next decade or so. With the U.S. government promising to promote expansion of broadband communications nationwide, and with improved security in Internet transmissions, a video hookup in a mental health practitioner's office is likely to become routine within the decade. For now, high-quality videoconferencing for mental health is found mainly where there is no good alternative access, for demonstration or research projects, and in e-communities.

Videoconferencing is attracting substantial mainstream attention and funding. Revenue from videoconferencing equipment is expected to increase from $780 million in 2001 to $1.1 billion by 2005 (Moore, 2001). The September 11, 2001, terrorist attacks, coupled with a slumping economy, have led many companies to cut their travel budgets and look for new solutions for conducting business (Moore, 2001). Expanding office locations, technical advances, air travel security concerns, travel costs, and stretched schedules may all result in the cost of videoconferencing technology falling and may hasten its social acceptability. Moore (2001) also reported that one company saved between $150,000 and $200,000 per month in travel expenses with its new videoconferencing unit.

Need for More Research.   Empirical data on behavioral telehealth care are just beginning to emerge (Rabasca, 2000). Appendix A mentions several recently published articles. Of course, more extensive research is clearly needed, with larger samples, longer trials, and different clinical populations. A review commissioned by the U.S. Agency for Healthcare Research and Quality (AHRQ at http://www.ahcpr.gov) identified 13 mental health store-and-forward programs and 66 mental health clinician interactive programs (Agency for Healthcare Research and Quality, 2001). The AHRQ recommended randomized controlled trials to assess the benefit of telepsychiatry. The need for these research studies is acute, especially as the social fabric advances parity for mental health care.

More specifically, research is needed to determine how to recognize situations and clients for whom two-way audio would be adequate, where low-quality or high-quality video should be used instead (Zarate et al., 1997), or where a mental health professional must have in-person contact with a client to provide service that meets professional standards (Zarr, 1984). The fact is, we are still gathering data about how various videoconferencing methods are either helpful or detrimental to mental health practice. For example, on the Internet, some practitioners are already offering video-enhanced personal computer–based mental health services using the World Wide Web.

One of the largest and most recognized systems online is offered by eGetgoing (http://www.egetgoing.com), an Internet-based company affiliated with CRC Health Corp., one of the nation's largest traditional drug and alcohol treatment systems. The Web site uses audio, visual, and text-based Internet environments to provide online treatment for chemical dependency. Clients use video links to talk with the professionals and other group members. Reportedly, eGetgoing use cognitive behavioral techniques that teach the clients in its group sessions solutions to problems related to chemical dependency. Psychoeducational modules are also available to improve the clients understanding of themselves and their drug and alcohol abuse. Other services include video vignettes of simulated treatment interactions, slide shows, and a personal home page. Clients can use the personal home page before and after each counseling session to record personal progress, write e-mails to group members or professionals, and/or enter a professionally mediated chat room. All eGetgoing programs are encrypted to meet HIPAA security regulations for patient–clinician contact through the Internet.

An interesting aspect of this program is that clients can see the professional but not each other. The professional also cannot see the client. Some critics might claim that one-way videoconferencing, with the camera focusing on the therapist rather than on the client, is a serious impediment to mental health care, particularly with chemically dependent patients. However, patients report an enhanced group experience with the ability to see their counselor. They also report that the anonymity reduces anxiety, increasing their willingness to self-disclose. Similarly, patients with concurrent social anxiety disorder appreciate the benefit of anonymity, which permits them to participate without the paralyzing anxiety they normally experience in such programs (P. Rosenberg, personal communication, October 20, 2002).

Research is being conducted at eGetgoing and other Web sites. Although programs such as eGetgoing are creatively using technologies as they become available through the Internet to access clients who otherwise might not be serviced, the professional community at large has yet to determine issues related to the clinical appropriateness of the psychotechnologies used over the Internet. The research outcomes will tell which model(s) are great, good, or just plain bad ideas. Ethics and legal case law will establish appropriate limits and standards.

Notably, eGetgoing was the first online treatment organization approved by the Joint Commission on Accreditation of Healthcare Organizations (JCAHO), having measured up to the same standards applied to traditional programs (Joint Commission on Accreditation of Healthcare Organizations, 2002). The eGetgoing Web site has met with good response and plans to expand, having already produced an extension for adolescents, called teen Getgoing (https://www.teengetgoing.com). We await the research results and the professional community's reaction to this intervention model. The bottom line: Tha'r's gold in them tha'r hills, as well as the possibility of accreditation. The next section discusses other audio and video technologies and their contributions to mental health care.

TELEPHONIC PRACTICE ENHANCERS

Basic telephones have expanded into other audio technologies. Attempts to clarify a utility bill, purchase airline or movie tickets, and/or report a stolen credit card by phone usually lead automated response systems. These systems are improving rapidly, ideally to reduce the frustration often experienced while punching numbers and waiting "on hold." Advances in technology are likely to enable enhancement of electronic audio communication in mental health care as well. The following section discusses examples of newer audio technologies for the professional to consider for clinical practice. Meanwhile the following cartoon demonstrates a more unlikely possibility.

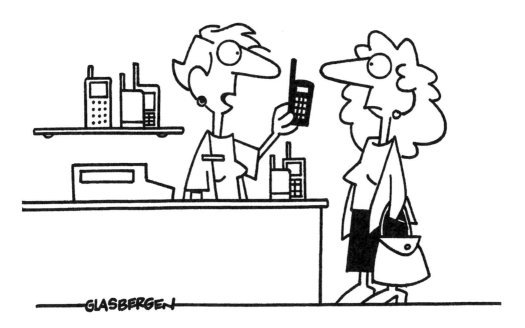

"This phone has a special filter that makes calls from your mother 20% less stressful."

Wireless Telephone Technologies Combined with Text Messaging

Many mobile phones can now send and receive text messages. Until recently, low cost and high accessibility of voice service have impeded the growth of mobile text messaging in the United States, but text is very popular in Europe, particularly among adolescents, who have developed an efficient jargon that is delightfully incomprehensible to adults. One can sneak a peek at a message or send one during meetings without alerting family, friends, teachers, or peers. This practice offers reasonable de facto privacy, although technical security of current implementations of text messaging is low.

Telephone texting can be very effective in enhancing patient compliance. Couching messages in a form congruent with the interests and communication pattern of young people in Scotland, researchers found that "reminders about treatment and useful tips on education may be a medium to allow people with chronic health problems to make their disease comply with their lifestyle and not the other way around" (Neville, Greene, McLeod, Tracy, & Surie, 2002, p. 600). A colleague from Australia tells about the newest combined applications he has reviewed for psychotherapists:

I recently upgraded my mobile phone. I had no plans to purchase it, but I couldn't resist after I saw it had Triband capacity, which allows the phone to be used on all populated continents. Most phones in Australia are tuned for dual-band systems, allowing the phones to be used in Asia and Europe but not North America.

When I was away in August, I had my service provider install its Surepage service, which meant that all calls to my phone were answered by a live operator, who then typed my messages into my phone by virtue of its built-in SMS, or Short Message Service.[5] In the UK alone, where the system has been maturing for a number of years, some 1.4 billion (yes, billion) SMS messages were sent in February 2002, according to one estimate.

Mobile phones also allow "always-on" contact with the Internet for Web surfing and e-mail exchange. The best search engine, Google, even has a mobile text-only search location specifically set up for mobile phones. Some phones even allow photographs to be taken and sent phone-to-phone while you are also holding a regular phone call. Companies such as Sony (http://www.sonyericsson.com) and Nokia (http://nokia.com) are continually inventing new and exciting ways to improve mobile telephone features.

Can mobile phones and SMS be incorporated into our practices in useful ways? At their most basic, mobile phones can supply us with a lifetime telephone number. Many businesspeople now give out their mobile numbers and list them in phone directories. The mobile number has become their primary telephone number, allowing contact almost anywhere in the world.

SMS messages can also be used to communicate with clients for appointment keeping. I now routinely ask my clients for their mobile numbers (8 in 10 bring a phone into their sessions, and 5 in 10 forget to turn them off at least once during our contact). I now also ask whether clients send and receive SMS messages; if yes, I also suggest that clients may use the system to alter their appointments. Naturally, I ask whether they would like me to contact them via SMS should I need to make changes, and most say yes. The traditional method of contacting clients by telephone might involve leaving a message through an unreliable receptionist, family member, or roommate. With messages going directly to the client's mobile phone, immediate access is more likely. One can also leave

---

[5] SMS (Short Message Service) is a wireless sysem for sending messages of up to approximately 160 characters (224 characters if using a 5-bit mode) to mobile phones using the Global System for Mobile communication (GSM). SMS is somewhat akin to *paging*, except that SMS messages are captured by mobile phones even if the phone is turned off and out of range. Messages are held for a number of days until the phone is active and within range. SMS messages can also be sent to digital phones from a Web site equipped with PC Link or from one digital phone to another. SMS and GSM services have gained their greatest popularity in Europe.

a voice message or a text message that can be stored in the phone's memory. If the client and I agree to use SMS, we also agree that a confirmation SMS is sent to be sure that the message has been received and understood. I have found that young people in particular are very savvy in this area and think it cool that their psychotherapist is up with their preferred technologies.

Software also allows automation to schedule appointments; iCal (http://www.apple.com/ical) is a free calendar software application that enables you to keep track of your appointments and manage your contacts. But iCal offers a new twist. Users of iCal can publish their calendars on the Internet, allowing others to both see them and enter their own data. If you are part of a collaborative team, you can share one calendar and thus synchronize meeting times; or, each individual can post his or her calendar, allowing for easier organization of meetings.

Professionals can also place their calendars on the Web, which enables existing and new clients to select their own appointment times. Some professionals may choose to make this service available only to existing clients, having explained how the system works. The site is then password protected so only select clients can access at.

Using iCal, conference organizers can place the conference program on the Web and allow workshop-goers to enter their names on preattendance sheets. Friends and colleagues can see who else is attending the same workshop. Organizers can quickly rearrange oversubscribed workshops. Interest groups and hobbyists can place their monthly activities on the Web for all to see and then download into the PCs, PDAs, or mobile phones—yes, mobile phones also come with built-in calendar software.

There is one more spin to how iCal can be used, which is why I acknowledge the program when other programs exist. The iCal diary allows each appointment to have numerous details recorded in a central address book. When an individual rings your mobile phone, linked to your computer either via a physical connection or wireless (up to 10 meters away), an Address Book application pops up and recognizes the phone number (as long as it is not blocked) and automatically pulls up the individual's details, including an area to make notes during the call. For new callers, a blank Address contact area opens, allowing details to be recorded as the call continues. To see this operation in action, see http://www.apple.com/macosx/jaguar/addressbook.html. Going in the other direction, one can type messages in the address book's contact area, which can be sent via SMS or e-mail to the client.

Here is the fun kicker: One can set the iCal diary to automatically send a message by SMS at a predetermined time. So, by agreement, a client can receive an SMS the night or morning before the appointment with a reminder of any homework or materials to bring.

The psychotherapist and the client can work out the message to be sent at the conclusion of the current session and also agree on its timing. For some clients, this small feat of technology may enhance therapeutic alliance as well as compliance with treatment. By automation, the software takes care of both the sending of the message and keeping a record in the contact manager of the address book.

Of course, there is no need to restrict oneself to mere appointment reminding. The psychotherapist for example, could remind the client of between-session activities, such as breathing or relaxation exercises and recording of thoughts or anxiety levels, or could simply send encouraging messages, perhaps reinforcing a particular cognitive or behavioral intervention. Or perhaps the client could report to therapist when these activities have been completed.

Dozens of similar calendar programs are available, including the free Palm Desktop. By the way, in the Windows world, Microsoft Outlook XP allows calendar sharing too, albeit a tad more complicated (http://www.uwec.edu/help/outlookXP/CAL-PERMISSIONS.HTM). *Eroom.com and Yahoo! each has its own way to allow work groups to work together, sharing calendars and resources.*

When more people have new mobile phones that accept the next iteration of SMS, known as MMS, or multimedia message system (as do the Sony Ericsson and Nokia phones, mentioned earlier), psychotherapists as well as clients can send sounds, pictures, and videos from their PCs or mobile phones. This ability will open a new window into the world of the client, allowing the psychotherapist to see and hear daily interactions that the client has chosen.

—**Les Posen, Ph.D.**
Psychologist
St. Kilda South, Australia

Once mobile phones and SMS systems are introduced into a patient's treatment, such innovations may be difficult to remove. Before inviting all one's patients to use any of these new technologies, it may be wise to consider the added cost to the patient and the patient's diagnosis (especially personality disorders), as well as how using the technology will fit into the treatment plan. Impact on the clinician should also be considered. Much as it has added convenience and access to patients seeking immediate contact with their psychotherapist, the telephone has also imposed on the clinician responsibility for being available by telephone or beeper. Using a psychotechnology with even one patient may become a problem in communities in which information about a professional's innovative toolbox can spread quickly and may have other patients wondering why they have been excluded from the extra service.

Furthermore, until cellular, mobile, and other wireless communication devices improve to the point of being more secure in the United States, wireless telephone calls intercepted and the client's confidentiality compromised. Many people would be surprised to learn the range of eavesdropping activities considered legal the United States. See http://www.MonitoringTimes.com for more information.

Nonetheless, some clinicians use mobile phones after securing consent agreements from their patients. Consider how Tim Hodgens has applied the mobile phone creatively:

Concerning innovative use of cell phones, I have worked with fearful fliers and make good use of their cell phones. I have them call me from the airport, before and/or after they go through the security gate, and also inside the plane before they take off if they need an extra boost. They usually like to call after they land so they can share their exuberance with someone right away. I was able to help one person through a particularly nasty anxiety surge associated with a feeling of falling apart by identifying hypoglycemia as a contributing factor. She was told to eat something the first time this happened and then before all future exposure trials and also to carry food in case her blood sugar dropped again at any time.

On a slightly different note, I sent one woman off to drive across an especially troubling bridge (bridge phobia) and had her check in a few times on her cell phone. Just before she went across the bridge (before the last exit) she pulled over and called me. Prior to the start of our discussion, a state trooper pulled over to see whether she needed assistance. She said, "No, I'm just calling my therapist because I'm afraid of bridges." I could hear him saying, "Oh, this isn't all that bad," and he left. She said that she would call me later. A few minutes later, she pulled over and called again. She ecstatically told me that she

*had done it! I asked her to take the long way home, to immediately build on her success,
and go across two more bridges.*

*Of course, I have all my patients sign a consent agreement stipulating that they
understand the risks to confidentiality posed by the use of cellular telephones.*

—Tim Hodgens, Ph.D.
Psychologist
Westborough, Massachusetts

Voice over Internet Protocol

In larger corporations, it has become commonplace to replace the traditional point-
to-point telephone service with Voice over Internet Protocol.[6] (VoIP). Using VoIP, the
corporate computer network carries transmissions between what look like ordinary
telephone devices. VoIP offers considerable cost savings and enables such extra features as speech recognition, text-to-speech technology, and interactive voice response.

Extending VoIP beyond the corporate network to the Internet, however, opens the
door to serious security vulnerabilities (Molitor, 2001). In contrast to having a dedicated wire connection between the users' telephones, VoIP has data skipping between
a series of server computers until assembled at its destination, exposing the data and
the system to many attack strategies. Furthermore, although tapping a telephone is
typically accomplished one connection at a time, software can alert an eavesdropper
to the occurrence of keywords in any of thousands of Internet transmissions scanned
simultaneously.

Nonetheless, progress is being made toward developing sufficient security measures to make VoIP safe enough for mental health care delivery. A VoIP service that allows customers to make telephone calls from personal computers using the Microsoft
Windows XP operating system is available in the United Kingdom (Rhode, 2002).
Whether it meets security requirements in other countries needs be ascertained by
professionals using such technologies, however.

VIDEOCONFERENCING PRACTICE ENHANCERS

As with any other type of device, video equipment comes in diverse configurations
and qualities, each useful for different purposes. Videoconferencing can be accomplished through videophone over ordinary telephone lines, through high-speed point-
to-point leased lines, and by Internet. With high-capacity connections, a videoconference can involve more than two locations with several cameras operating at each. But
we should begin our discussion with types of connections (channels), because they
determine the type of equipment to be used (devices).

Transmission Channels

Chapter 2, carefully distinguishes between telecommunication transmission channels
and telecommunication devices. Decisions about devices are based on the type of

---

[6] VoIP (voice delivered through an internet Protocol) generally refers to sending digitized voice information
in discrete packets through the Internet rather than through the public switched telephone network. An
advantage if VoIP is that it avoids fees charged by traditional telephone services.

transmission channel to be used. Smoke signals, beacons, carrier pigeons, and other envoys are fine for some types of communication, but they won't do for remote mental health services! It's all about bandwidth.

Bandwidth limitations in low-speed transmission channels make it difficult to transmit audio and visual signals at a quality that adequately approximates in-person communications (Fussell & Benimoff, 1995). If POTS is the only available transmission channel, then only audioconferencing and crude videoconferencing devices are possible. For the video portion, adequate bandwidth is essential to convey motion smoothly and to capture brief events, such as an eye blink or other subtle nonverbal behavior (Zarate et al., 1997). Impact of video quality on treatment outcome, however, has yet to be determined.

Quality of Video. Research has not yet clarified when high-quality video is necessary and when low-quality video suffices for assessment, psychotherapy, psychoeducation, or other mental health services (Day & Schneider, 2000; Kaplan, 1997). Zarate's study (1997) suggested that high bandwidth is better for assessing negative signs of schizophrenia. A good-quality image may even boost the effectiveness of psychotechnology beyond what is ordinarily achieved with standard in-person encounters. The touchstone for video adequacy is the opinion of the clinician referring or treating the patient. If the clinical question posed cannot be answered or the service request fulfilled with the existing technology or video quality, then the use of that particular system or piece of technology is probably inappropriate.

In the United States, psychopharmacologic practice has been reduced in many clinics to a series of "med checks." A med check allots a psychiatrist 15 minutes to review a client's record, take an interim history, perform an examination, prescribe, and make a record, sometimes of a client who is usually tracked by a different psychiatrist. Often, the med check session is curtailed by scheduling problems, telephone calls, crises, and other distractions. It is not difficult to envision doing better than this "standard practice" with even a relatively low-quality videoconferencing system.

Additionally, the zoom feature on some videoconferencing units can be useful for closer scrutiny when monitoring a client's reactions to psychotropic medications (Smith & Allison, 2000). Comparing digitized and bookmarked video records from previous sessions could enable a remote practitioner to detect extrapyramidal impairments, early tardive dyskinesia, alleviation of overactivation, and other changes. If the video system is a component of a comprehensive secure online workspace (Gonsalves, 2002) with access to the clinical record and decision support features, then the clinician could be quite effective within a narrow time span.

Broadband Connections. Developers of telecommunication channels for videoconferencing are envisioning broadband Internet connections to desktops at home, at school, and at work. As broadband Internet connections become more available, high-quality video and multimedia services will become more practical for general mental health care, using low-cost off-the-shelf equipment. Just as televisions have become ubiquitous in the past 50 years, so video services are being developed with the same goal in mind—and only for videoconferencing.

Already, broadband carrier services, such as DSL (Digital Subscriber Lines) and digital cable, are shifting our emphasis from pure videoconferencing toward techniques that integrate streaming video with other ways of collaborating, such as whiteboards (described later in this chapter). Also, slides and sessions are beginning to shift from special institutions to the patient's home and the professional's office. Of some interest to psychotherapists, Internet2[7] will offer greater transmission speeds (Barrett, 2002), and enable broader use of videoconferencing devices in primarily academic and quasi-military settings. If Internet2 or its equivalent is opened up for health care, the quality of videoconsultation images will rival that of digital television.

For professionals who must be at the head of the curve, having an ISDN (Integrated Services Digital Network) connection (or funding for ISDN) puts one into a very different realm than does using POTS. Today's high-end videoconferencing systems typically connect to a personal computer and run through ISDN lines (Gale, 1992). ISDN is the preferred carrier service for telemedicine and accounts for approximately 85% of all such videoconferencing. As a point-to-point delivery channel, ISDN has an important security advantage over Internet connectivity, potentially allowing any number of points to connect to a psychotherapy session. Despite its popularity, ISDN may be overshadowed in a few years by the more cost-effective Internet protocol (IP)–based videoconferencing (Lindemann, 2001), once the security issues are addressed.

An example of creative applications of video-based communication supported by three ISDN lines is the work of University of Rochester psychologist Robert Pollard (Pollard, 2003). Strong Connections (http://www.urmc.rochester.edu/strongconnections), a not-for-profit service of the University of Rochester Medical Center, provides an interpreter service via a high-bandwidth videoconferencing connection for deaf patients and medical professionals when the parties cannot wait for a local interpreter to arrive. The service is available 24 hours a day, 7 days a week. Deaf patients are reportedly happy with the service; they say that the medically experienced sign language interpreters provide better quality interpretation than do less medically experienced interpreters and that service is comparable to on-site interpreters. The program's Web site home page explains that using video is helpful: "The cumbersome, error-prone communication methods of note-writing and lipreading are avoided (University of Rochester Medical Center, 2003)." Although some work with the deaf community is conducted with low-bandwidth POTS connections when resources are limited, higher bandwidth effectively reduces the possibility of error in communication.

A high-speed DSL, trunk, or cable connection to the Internet elevates frame rate and resolution to much more acceptable standards than does POTS, but the image remains grainy and jerky. Bottom line—Internet delivery mechanisms involve packets. Rather than streaming video information continuously, as does ISDN, Internet-based communication involves sending a message piecemeal, then accumulating the pieces and delivering the message only after it can be reassembled at the other end. Although this process may be adequate for e-mail, it complicates interactive video by interfering with smooth two-way transmission of motion and synchronizing it with sound.

The time delay in sending and receiving packets of audio or video information can be a serious impediment to evaluating neurological signs. The time delay also is detrimental to assessing quality of eye contact, hesitancy, and a host of other nonverbal cues. Lack of continuity in showing a client's movement obviates much of the advantage of video over the telephone. A possible cure for this deficit would be a protocol for prioritizing packets involved in streaming video communication. Although this works for store-and-forward technology, it is unlikely that mental health professionals

---

[7] The Internet2 is a collaboration of many universities to develop advanced networking applications for learning and research.

will be able to wrest priority from the giant multinational corporations taking advantage of the limited priority opportunities available on the Internet.

ISDN is potentially available even where DSL and cable are not (as discussed in chapter 2). Nonetheless, experience in California has shown that not all local telephone companies are ready to handle the demand for ISDN installation or us (Brown-Connolly, 2002a). It is wise to inform the telephone company that one's ISDN lines are intended for delivering medical care so they won't be "borrowed" without notice and sessions won't be interrupted without notice.

For sufficient bandwidth to pass nonverbal communication in amounts necessary to detect signs of schizophrenia, one may have to install equipment to bridge at least two ISDN lines (Zarate et al., 1997). Going to three or more lines yoked together for even better quality entails much higher costs not only for line charges but also for the equipment needed on both ends to distribute the signals into the lines and later recombine them. Although rates vary geographically, it is useful to compare costs (installation and operational) for ISDN. Note that some European companies report ISDN connections running up to $500 per hour (Lindemann, 2001).

Secure options other than ISDN are available. They often involve VPNs (Virtual Private Networks), which use Internet Protocol (IP) to communicate over wide area networks (WANs) and local area networks (LANs). One example is the Federal Bureau of Prisons in the United States, which is moving to a WAN using Internet Protocol in its large telemedicine system.

Videoconferencing Devices and Programs

Not all videoconferencing devices are the same. Wise investors will consider their needs, the options, and the applications of such technologies by other clinicians before purchasing equipment. The next sections discuss information that might influence the purchase of videoconferencing devices. Whether the connection uses low-end videoconferencing programs (such as the Internet-based NetMeeting program), a videophone, or a more expensive videoconferencing unit, all parties must have compatible equipment. Compatibility extends to the software installed on a personal computer, connecting the computer with others on a network, and matching the computer with the transmission carrier type to be used (Puskin, Mintzer, & Wasem, 1997). A high-speed videoconferencing system is unsuitable for a target group that is connected using a POTS line.

The quality of videoconferencing technology depends on *resolution, color depth, frame size,* and *frame rate*. Essentially, resolution is the number of *pixels* (picture elements) displayed. Resolution may be specified as 640 × 480, which means that there are 640 columns and 480 rows of pixels, for a total of 307,200 pixels. Obviously, in depicting the same scene, more pixels could convey more detail. If pixels can be only black or white, color depth is minimal. If a pixel can be any of 256 colors, more information is conveyed; in television-quality pictures, millions of colors are available for any pixel.

Merely making a video picture larger does not make it more detailed or clearer (except for the visually impaired). It is nice to have a larger screen (frame size), but the magnification can make the individual pixels seem blocky and the image grainy. This occurs because each pixel is shown larger on a big screen (the size of a pixel on a monitor is expressed as its *pitch*).

To create a sensation of motion, a videoconferencing system redraws an image repeatedly, each time with a small modification. The frame rate is the number of times per second that the image changes. If this rate is too slow, movement seems jerky. Frame rates for movies and television are typically 24 to 36 per second. Telecommunications carrier limitations may bring frame rate down far below this (Whatis.com, 2001a). For a computer to display a smooth *full frame* (a reasonably large picture), the hardware must be fairly fast; thus, most of last generation's personal computers may not be suitable for video work.

Videophones. A *videophone* is a small, easily installed unit that attaches to a telephone and some type of monitor. Depending on the videophone model, the image can be shown on a computer monitor or a television, although some devices have their own small built-in monitor. The videophone unit includes a camera to allow the remote party to see the message sender in real time (i.e., synchronously). These units also sport a telephonelike apparatus with excellent voice quality.

Videophones support low-resolution videoconferencing with anyone using similar equipment. The resolution of a videophone image may be only as high as 176 dots across by 144 down. This is comparable to the resolution of a crude, ineptly drawn tattoo. The videophone usually supports a frame rate below 15 to 20 frames per second (fps), which yields jerky motion. Some newer videophones claim to have better frame rates, and further improvement is likely over time. Specialized assessment and treatment protocols may not run adequately through videophones and may require more sophisticated technology (Squibb, 1999).

Videophone vendors include Connectix, Intel, InnoMedia, Leadtek, Microsoft, Philips, Smith Micro, Tandberg, and Video Con. Interactive technology, such as the CareStation126 videophone from Motion Media Technology, permits simultaneous two-way transmission of voice, video, and data over regular telephone lines. These videophones also include integrated electronic plug-ins for peripheral medical measurement devices, such as pulse oximetry, stethoscope, and thermometer, and they support output to external devices (a VCR, television, etc.).

The two-way videophone is finding its way into regular use in many telemental health programs. In delivering contact to family members, it is easiest to use a videophone with a built-in monitor at the home site; the unit can be plugged into the phone jack and serve as both a telephone and a monitor. These units can also be a great source of comfort to homebound adults and children who cannot obtain easy access to a hospitalized family member. Children have been particularly uninhibited in using videophones to communicate with their hospitalized parents. Children readily put their hands, noses, or lips up to the cameras and ask their loved ones to do the same. Children draw pictures and show them to each other. In fact, videophones are so adaptive that they could conceivably be used in a variety of settings to connect patients to their distant family and loved ones for daily psychosocial support. These psychotherapeutic applications may make do with low-quality video transmission.

Other Videoconferencing Technology. Several companies have products that allow two-way video communication to occur as simply as dialing the telephone number on a push-button telephone (see http://www.Motion-Media.com or http://www.8x8.com). Accordant Health Services provides an example of an integrated multimodality system offering visitors real-time conversations with nurses (http://www.accordant.net).

Aethra (http://www.aethra.com) is another company that offers devices for practitioners who want to start using advanced telecommunication. This company delivers audio- and videoconferencing and videostreaming services to a global telecommunications market. The company's products range from high-performance video systems for large conference rooms to highly mobile compact video systems for personal use. The Voyager, a videoconferencing system contained in a single briefcase, can transmit simultaneous audio and video signals at 30 frames per second over an ISDN transmission channel. In addition to selling a range of products, Aethra.net delivers video streaming, videoconferencing, and audio conferencing services through the Internet; the company also rents videoconferencing facilities throughout the world. The company reports that all products are compliant with key international standards.

Other technologies have become much more commonplace than videophones. For example, the Internet's reach is expanding dramatically, and several companies have been offering videoconferencing software to be used over the Internet. In fact, because the Internet can carry synchronous two-way voice communications supplemented by text and other modalities, it is poised to replace a standard telephone network for many purposes, including videoconferencing.

It is possible that as the Internet develops, videophones will give way to high-speed *webcams*. Designed for the Internet, webcams are digital cameras that allow for videostreaming. Pornography has driven much of the webcam technology on the Internet and will continue to encourage improvement in clarity and increased functionality. Although webcams do not allow for synchronous video transmission, they can supplement synchronous text-based communication with one-way video.

NetMeeting and CU-SeeMe offer free video transmission over the Internet. A basic webcam used in such applications retails for about $50. Resolution and frame rates may be comparable to poorer videophones. Frame rates via a POTS modem are sometimes up to 10 frames per second, but the video signal can interfere with audio transmission. Motion is jerky, and sound is often impaired, making these connections impractical for traditional psychotherapy or counseling. Their performance could be improved by advances in technology; it will not be surprising to find webcams competing with videophones in quality within a decade.

Other videoconferencing services are available. Some are marketed through a variety of online videoconferencing companies tailoring their services to a variety of industries, including, fortunately, mental and behavioral health care entities. Some services claim to offer added value and to have wide experience with employee assistance programs but do not give out their client lists as references. Other services are more reputable—they claim such experience, and can substantiate their claims with the names of satisfied customers who have offered to answer questions from other mental health professionals. Interested readers can investigate such companies as BeBetterNetworks, located in Atlanta, Georgia (http://bebetter.net).

A neat trick is to use a telephone for secure, reliable, and fair-quality audio communication while simultaneously using a webcam for a bit of video. This is not a bad solution for people with two telephone lines available, but most patients will not be able to participate in such an arrangement, and for practitioners in the United States, such video practices fail under federal security regulations and are not allowed without encryption of the video connection.

Whiteboards. In addition to audio and video, one can communicate synchronously by drawing pictures and lines. A *whiteboard* serves the same function as the a schoolroom's chalkboard, except that it's white. This system allows a user to put various marks (or to post pictures) on a screen and have the same material show up on the screens of others participating in a conference. Whiteboarding is thus a useful tool for distance education. Whiteboards are most commonly used in connection with a videoconference, where the whiteboard occupies part of the monitor screen alongside a video "window" with, perhaps, a third area devoted to showing text messages. A whiteboard can show text, a graph, a clinical picture, X-ray, or testing summary; one or more conference participants can then move a pointer or draw lines and arrows or words on top of it.

The whiteboard, once found only in the fanciest corporate dedicated videoconferencing systems, is now becoming available at a reasonable cost for Internet-mediated conferences between two or even many personal computer users. Simple whiteboarding is available on some of the common free instant messaging systems on the Internet, along with audio, but not video, interchange.

The following fictionalized vignette illustrates how a number of modalities are combined in an enhanced videoconferencing system:

Dr. Garcia was having trouble communicating to his client about the idea of choice points during her child's temper tantrum. Rhonda was unable to change the behavior of both her child and herself during these tantrums. Dr. Garcia had been intermittently providing therapy through a secured (encrypted) videoconferencing connection located in a rural clinic close to Rhonda's home. He was located 300 miles away, in an urban hospital setting.

Dr. Garcia felt that he needed to take a different approach to clarify the choice points. He asked Rhonda to videotape an episode between her and her child to bring in to the next videoconferencing session. The following week, Rhonda played the tape for Dr. Garcia, using a VCR connected to the videoconferencing unit. To make the videotape visible to them both, they switched their respective videoconference unit options to subdivide the screen on both their monitors, creating a checkerboard "Brady Bunch" effect. The top two windows displayed both Dr. Garcia and Rhonda. The bottom left window began showing the videotape. The bottom right window displayed a whiteboard that could be used by either party as they reviewed the videotape of the child's tantrum in front of his mother during dinner. In reviewing the tape together, Dr. Garcia and his client were able to identify several key points at which Rhonda could have made different decisions.

Dr. Garcia also asked Rhonda to make a list for herself on the whiteboard of these key points and of how she might react differently. She wrote "Remain calm" on her whiteboard, and these words appeared on the shared whiteboard they were both viewing on their monitors. Dr. Garcia congratulated her on using the technology efficiently, and they proceeded through the rest of the videotape. Rhonda was then able to print the notes she had made on her whiteboard, so she could take them home. Rhonda felt proud not only that she learned how she might interact with her child more effectively but also that she was interacting with Dr. Garcia efficiently. Dr. Garcia commented, "You seem to have gotten the idea. All it took was a little guided learning. I think you'll do fine next time this situation arises." He closed the window displaying the tape and opened an article that he believed would help Rhonda. The two reviewed the article together and concluded the session. "Thank you so much," Rhonda smiled and announced, "I think I learned a lot today!"

The gambit of technologies and techniques suggested in the previous vignette should prompt conversation about this fascinating topic. This depiction of how family psychotherapy can be conducted when only a mother is available and she is located in a remote facility illustrates technologies and techniques that have been available for almost a decade.

Purchasing Videoconferencing Equipment. The price of desktop videoconferencing units ranges from $400 to $5,000, and quality varies accordingly. A full-fledged room-based videoconferencing system can start at about $100,000 (Orubeondo, 2001). Such an installation may be necessary for certain medical specialties, but it is likely that maximum effectiveness for most mental health purposes can be achieved at a much lower cost. As we discuss later in this chapter, good audio function (clarity, ability to pick up quiet sounds, close synchronization, minimal delay, and near absence of noise) is the most important attribute of a videoconferencing system.

Allotting money to a high-quality lens is prudent, as it makes quite a difference in picture quality. The bells and whistles, such as connections for physiological monitors, that are available on the more expensive videoconferencing products are not necessary for most mental health practice, yet they may be worth considering.

Purchasing decisions should take into account the speed of transmission required for the chosen clinical application (text can be transmitted over POTS, whereas live video needs at least 384 kbps), scalability (for future expansion), initial and long-term maintenance and upgrading issues, availability of technical support, and level of expertise needed for use (Orubeondo, 2001). Check out vendors with other customers, particularly to see whether repairs, servicing, and technical assistance are completed promptly. Add to the contract language committing the company to its service promises. A trial run for all equipment is a must. If the system is having problems, get them fixed before signing off on the order.

Not all brands of videophones are compatible with one another, even if specifications are similar. When considering purchase of additional computer systems or videophones to work with existing units, be sure to have the vendor physically demonstrate the ability of the new model to connect to the old model and system. Such demonstrations are particularly important if one unit will be located within a corporate office, where telephone systems and networks are complex and often involve firewalls that make connection more difficult. Just because something looks like an ordinary telephone doesn't mean it acts like one. Special in-house telephone networks (a private branch exchange, or PBX) may present voltages that will fry a computer's modem and may use transmission protocols that are incompatible with a newly purchased computer system or videophone. Some so-called telephones are really little computers built for voice over Internet Protocol (VoIP). Ordinary videophones will not work if simply substituted for such a telephone and may be damaged. It is important to find the right information technology expert and ask the right questions or to have the salesperson demonstrate the model by putting a demonstration unit at risk.

Videoconferencing Practicalities

The successful use of videoconferencing technology in mental health depends on a number of factors (Barker & Alessi, 2001), including telepresence, technical audio and video considerations, and cleaving to videoconferencing etiquette. These factors in turn are limited by the kind of videoconferencing software and equipment used, as previously discussed. As the sophistication of technology increases, common problems and general social and business etiquette for conferencing will be worked out. The professional is advised to watch for special options improving the audio and video on newer units, such as upgraded sound and video cards, HIPAA-compliant software, and compatibilities among software in multiple sites. One source for updates on the state of videoconferencing is the Video Development Initiative Web site (http://www.vide.gatech.edu/cookbook2.0). Add-ons to the main videoconferencing unit, such as a whiteboard, document camera, or DVD player, may also enhance video-conferencing sessions (Video Development Initiative, 2000).

Telepresence. When thinking about the clinical environment, mental health professionals need to be aware of the remote site as part of their clinical milieu. All the considerations required for an in-person visit also apply to the remote location:

- Who is in the room? Only persons known to all parties and announced should be in the room. If other people enter during a consultation, they need to announce their presence.
- Does the client have privacy during a therapy session? Unwittingly, clients may compromise their own privacy. For example, an overly enthusiastic client at work in an office cubicle may be overheard by coworkers.
- Are the rooms in both locations sufficiently soundproof?
- Is on-site support staff available?
- Backup services for client support should be identified before routine remote consultation is started.
- Emergent support services should be available for client protections.

Telepresence, or the social presence created by a video connection (Anderson, Newlands, & Mullin, 1996; Cukor et al., 1998; Prussog, Mühlbach, & Böcker, 1994; Sellen, 1995), helps both parties feel more comfortable discussing emotional issues. Participants experience a stronger sense of "social presence" when using a "rich" communications medium, such as high-quality videoconferencing. Clients and professionals can feel more connected and may therefore pay better attention. This conclusion, of course, still needs to be proven through empirical research. Research has found that facial expression can give both parties a level of mutual understanding (Whittaker & O'Conaill, 1997). Thus, the parties must see each other clearly.

Because of the potential of videoconferencing to create telepresence and to support transaction of mental health treatment, we are careful to use the term *in-person* when patient and therapist are in the same room, so that *face to face* includes videoconferencing as well. However, face to face is not necessarily eye to eye. So-called eye contact has strong emotional impact on social beings (e.g., one should avoid eye contact with potentially hostile animals and even with a police officer who is considering issuing a traffic ticket—it implies challenge). Furtive glances, avoidance of the other's gaze, and staring deep into the eyes of another person carry clues to people's attitude and state of mind and can communicate sincerity, evasion, or submission, for example. It follows that participants in psychotherapeutic videoconferencing should be able to see each other's eyes.

One disadvantage of most videoconferencing equipment is that a person cannot simultaneously look into the camera lens and watch the other party in the monitor. The continually averted gaze that results creates a sense of alienation. Television newspeople make it a point to look directly at the camera as much as they can. A good primer for the neophyte in using videoconferencing for clinical care is *Telemedicine: Practicing in the Information Age* (Dunn & Viegas, 1998).

Room lighting can have a profound effect on telepresence, as we discuss in detail in the following sections. The camera's ability to capture the room used for videoconferencing is related to telepresence. Human figures appear more clearly through a camera lens when they are placed against a light blue or eggshell background. Aesthetically, books or an organization's logo can be strategically placed to create a professional ambiance. Solicit input from people at the remote site regarding how the decor comes across in their view. The resulting suggestions can be eye-openers.

Audio and video transmission should be clear. Transmission speeds required to create telepresence are minimal by today's standards and can be achieved with low-cost videophones that use POTS (Croweroft, 1997). More important than image quality is reliability, which is better with POTS and ISDN than with Internet-mediated videoconferencing (as discussed previously in this chapter). Occasional freezing or loss of video, particularly common with Internet transmission, is tolerable, but audio clarity and continuity are essential to maintain a sense of presence. However, if video signals are too frequently interrupted, therapy sessions will become more frustrating than therapeutic. Likewise, delayed video images can be disruptive and possibly cause confusion, particularly if facial expressions are displayed after the speaker has switched to another topic (Whittaker, 1995) or the speaker's lips are not synchronized with the voice.

Audio Matters. The audio channel is the most important component of the videoconferencing system. Delays in audio response can be annoying (Hapgood, 1998), and disruptions in the turn-taking process of communication can occur if audio quality is sacrificed for the sake of boosting video images (Tang & Isaacs, 1993). Check to make sure that any system you buy has a high-end sound card as part of its hardware package, or upgrade the sound card before delivery so it can be installed professionally.

Type, quantity, and location of the microphones and speakers strongly affect audio quality (Video Development Initiative, 2000). Speakerphones or headsets transmit audio information and leave one's hands free (Fussell & Benimoff, 1995). If speakers are used, it is important for the equipment to include echo and feedback cancellation features. It is disconcerting to hear one's voice repeating a split second after speaking (Video Development Initiative, 2000). A small high-quality microphone that is part of a headset may give excellent results. Microphones placed right in front of the mouth tend to produce pronounced popping sounds when a person pronounces a word beginning with the letter *p* or hissing sounds with the letter *s*. Sometimes, entertainers wave their handheld mike around as a prop and occasionally look as if they are about to swallow it. Those microphones either have special pop-block features or are fakes. A microphone clipped to clothing may pick up rustling noises. Good microphones don't and are probably the best solution for videoconferencing. Little two-headed lapel mikes are now standard for interviewees seen on broadcast television.

Any extraneous noise that is captured disturbs telepresence. Consider soundproofing the videoconferencing rooms at both locations. In small rural communities, privacy and confidentiality are particularly important. A lack of attention to thin walls and the potential for eavesdropping can create potentially embarrassing situations for the client and can inhibit persons from seeking or continuing care. If treatment occurs at home or in a school environment, the clinician needs to be assured that the area is private. Many mental health consultation rooms are far from soundproof, but people in adjacent rooms are usually so absorbed in their activities that they do not notice what they can hear from next door. Someone on the remote end of a videoconference will be much more aware of concurrent activity in the therapist's environment and thus may lose confidence in the therapist's dedication to confidentiality. We should point out that the usual solution therapists adopt—operating a noise machine in their office—makes them less able to overhear conversations in other offices, but this machine does not block sound leaking out of their own consultation room. Such a noise machine or music might be needed in the waiting room but not in a videoconferencing room.

The videoconferencing room should be located where there is minimal background noise from both inside and outside the room. Humming air conditioners, air purifiers, busy stairs, vacuum cleaners, adjoining snack or kitchenette areas, ringing telephones, fax machines, noisy streets, airplanes, and even trains might be accommodated in-person. Through a videoconferencing technology, however, such sounds produce inescapable disruptions and probably annoyances to a psychotherapeutic conversation. Similarly, professionals also should avoid making small but noisy personal movements, such as tapping fingers or chewing a pen. Plush couches, pillows, drapes, and carpeting absorb noise and reduce the reverberation that otherwise make a room sound like an echo chamber to the person at the other end, even when the effect is not noticeable locally. A white noise machine should not be used during a videoconference. Each party can keep the audio channel clear by muting his or her microphone when not talking, but automating this practice may cause undesirable delays, depending on the audio components being used (Video Development Initiative, 2000). Testing the audio channel before every videoconferencing session is highly recommended.

A final audio consideration is audio delays. Generally, the sound transmission ends as soon as a telephone is hung up. However, when using a computer to transmit audio, clicking on the End Call button may not stop voice transmission for a few seconds. During this delay, both parties may not see each other, but they may still be heard. As related by author Nancy Brown-Connolly, the following true story is related in staff training at new telehealth sites to increase awareness and sensitivity to audio issues:

> A psychiatric nurse had clicked on the button ending the videoconference meeting with a medical group. She remarked about the tie one remote physician was wearing, saying it was "a particularly awful color and pattern." The next regularly scheduled videoconference included that same physician, who opened the meeting by asking the nurse if she preferred the tie he was wearing that day, as it had been picked especially for him. This proved to be an embarrassing but useful lesson for both parties, who then joked about how videoconferencing can create different types of exchanges between communicators.

Imagine how many times remarks are made following a telephone call. Avoiding such comments is particularly important when using video technology, especially when video involves direct care with a client.

Visual Basics. It is important that both the client and the professional see each other clearly when using videoconferencing technologies. The quality of the camera and speed of the transmission channel will markedly affect how each party is viewed (Video Development Initiative, 2000). Lighting, personal appearance, background, and the position of the camera will also affect the experience of the parties when using video. Table 5.1 outlines several audio and visual considerations for optimal communication transmission.

Frontal lighting sufficient to illuminate the face is necessary for proper viewing. A consultation with a photographer can be of some assistance, or a little experimentation may suffice. A face in shadows (or a person wearing sunglasses) perturbs a viewer's

TABLE 5.1
Audio and Visual Considerations

Audio

Ensure Privacy and Confidentiality
Soundproof room	Ask whether anyone is in remote room
Prevent eavesdropping	Close all doors

Optimize Audio Clarity and Continuity
Select microphone to match needs	Microphone placement
Location of speakers	Speakerphones or headsets
Echo cancellation	Equipment quality

Minimize background noise
• Busy streets	• Children
• Telephones and fax machines	• Stairs
• Public kitchens	• Delivery people
• Trains and airplanes	• Janitorial services

Reduce reverberation
• Carpeting	• Plush couches
• Drapes	• Pillows

Avoid
Audible bodily functions (and leather)	Sniffling
Scratching	Rustling papers
Tapping fingers	Pen chewing

Video

Optimize Video Clarity and Continuity
Transmission channel speed	Camera quality
Camera positioning	Test reliability of technology

Consider lighting
• Natural vs. artificial light	• Gel filters
• Shadows	• Facial illumination
• 60/40 split frontal top and bottom	• Hot spots

Use makeup (powder)
• Chin	• Forehead
• Balding spots	• Nose

Enhance room functionality
• Books and diplomas	• Plants
• Nameplate with city of origin	• Clock

Avoid visual distractions
• Loud clothing	• White clothing
• Checkered clothing	• Striped clothing
• Sharply contrasting colors	• Reflective jewelry
• Pictures	• Eyeglasses
• Other glossy surfaces	• Excessive gesturing
• Rocking or side-to-side movements	

Avoid
Nose scratching	Sneezing
Pants unzipped	Odd facial expressions

sense of trust. Backlighting can create on the viewer's monitor a *hot spot* that dazzles out a person's visage and reduces him or her to a silhouette. Lighting sources above, below, or to the side of the speaker can create undesirable shadows and a campfire atmosphere. Shadows can obliterate the face, and, as we know, trust in part depends on seeing the "whites" of the other parties' eyes.[8]

A 60/40 split between frontal top and frontal bottom lighting can control shadows nicely (Video Development Initiative, 2000). Avoid sharp reflections from eyeglasses by diffusing light sources positioned directly in front of a person. Excessive natural and artificial lighting can cause squinting and a look of pain on the speaker's face. Video cameras are quite sensitive and do not require high illumination. *Gel filters* on the light source (a colored translucent film available at video and lighting stores) can soften the speaker's appearance. The filter color can be matched to the speaker's complexion and clothing. Of course, a red gel filter can imply danger, a green filter can make a professional look sick, and a blue filter can make a professional look like a cartoon character.

Even careful lighting is likely to create glare on a person's face. Makeup (at least face powder) should be applied to areas, such as the nose, chin, forehead, and balding spots, that otherwise will create an annoying shine. Vanity aside, makeup can compensate for the tendency of video cameras to exaggerate skin roughness and blemishes. Ideally, the professional will come across on video much the same as in person.

The appearance of the room, as seen through the camera lens, may affect telepresence. A logo or a few well-placed books, plants, and diplomas not only create a professional appearance but also warm up the scene. Pictures, eyeglasses, and other glossy surfaces can create undesirable glare or distracting mirror effects that reflect parts of the room. Diplomas displayed under glass could produce a glare spot on the other participant's screen. Proper placement of light sources could avoid this, but it is necessary to inspect the scene using a monitor screen before going on the air.

Video cameras, especially combined with low-bandwidth transmission channels, can create psychedelic illusions from checkered, striped, or brightly colored clothing or from sharply contrasting adjacent colors. Pastel hues are easier on a camera than is white clothing. Experts say that Richard Nixon may have lost the 1960 election in part because he wore a white shirt during the televised debate, whereas John Kennedy wore blue. Close-up shots of Nixon showed him clearly sweating, while Kennedy appeared cool and dry. Conservative, nonreflective jewelry is also recommended. Large, dangling earrings or necklaces may be appropriate for in-person interactions, but they may be distracting on the viewing monitor. Quick side-to-side movements can cause blurring, as can excessive gesturing when speaking.

The location of the transmitting camera can also affect the speaker's appearance. A camera placed high on a viewing monitor can make the speaker seem to be looking upward or to be gazing at something other than the audience. It is recommended that the camera be placed just to the side of the viewing monitor to give to the appearance of an eye-to-eye conversation. Looking slightly to the right or left can be difficult to distinguish from looking straight ahead, which is why on many television shows, cue cards are placed by the camera. When speaking, one usually should look directly into the camera to emulate making eye contact. Then again, in some cultures, looking

---

[8] Actually, during the American Revolutionary War, seeing the whites of the enemies' eyes was a signal to shoot them.

directly at another person is considered offensive. Knowing or asking about the cultural sensitivities of one's patient is important when making these decisions.

Some videoconferencing units allow the observing party to adjust the picture, pan the room, zoom in or out, and freeze a frame. These functions may capture unintended images. Scratching one's nose, sneezing, or accidentally leaving one's pants unzipped may result in an unflattering or damaging appearance. Where possible, preparation for a videoconference should include having someone check out the professional's on-screen appearance. Videoconferencing units may also feature a picture-in-picture function, which allows the speaker to see how he or she appears to the other party.

Videoconferencing does not convey the depth dimension well. The proximity of parties in an in-person interaction plays a role in the comfort of the interaction. This topic deserves research (Jerome & Zaylor, 2000). Violation of one's personal space can trigger strong primitive reactions. Objects closer to the camera will appear bigger, and the combination of a large screen and a head shot could make the speaker appear to be a "close talker." Leaning forward to adjust the monitor or camera during a conversation can unleash the *giant palm monster* (Video Development Initiative, 2000). Conversely, a camera placed too far from a professional, combined with a client's small monitor, could produce a feeling of emotional distance.

The professional's side of the videoconference may be arranged to create as good an impression as is practical. The client's side, however, is more likely to involve inferior video equipment, poorly arranged lighting, echoes, and external noise. Just as it is important to be aware not only of transference but also of one's own countertransference reactions, the professional must compensate for the way a patient may seem hostile, tired, or ill simply as an artifact of the communication setup. Because "seeing is believing," it may be difficult to imagine that audio without video will have distinct clinical advantages when subjected to empirical comparison. Research is undoubtedly needed in this area and, more specifically, research with specific diagnostic groups.

The importance of testing the communication setup is crucial. Jiggle all the connections to make sure they are secure. Don't run wires where people might trip over them in their enthusiasm about particularly insightful therapeutic intervention. If possible, act out a bit of a session into a recording device, then see how it looks and sounds on playback. Alternatively, feed the video into a monitor to assess the image for lighting, background, decor, and other factors. Try out the videoconferencing setup well enough in advance of each session to allow enough time to take care of glitches.[9] Test the system again just before the session. Then, as the session begins, part of the initial "handshaking" should involve an inquiry about transmission quality. Patients may notice problems the professional overlooked or cannot see. Conversely, an experienced professional may readily solve minor technical problems on the client's end: "If you try closing your Venetian blinds, you may see the screen better."

VIDEOCONFERENCING APPLICATIONS IN THE REAL WORLD

As we've discussed, videoconferencing is the primary modality for online consultation. Whether videoconferencing is used in a given case is typically determined by the patient's venue or circumstances rather than by the diagnosis or treatment

---

[9] A glitch is an equipment (hardware) dysfunction; a bug is a programming (software) problem.

method. Most likely, this is because the costs of videoconferencing are easiest to justify where difficult access makes no other care or limited care available. Frontrunners in the development of videoconference-based mental health programs are found in several arenas, including rural communities, military venues, correctional facilities, and schools. The use of videoconferencing in each of these settings is discussed next.

Rural Area Programs

Contrary to common belief, rural areas exist in all states. In fact, depending on the definition of *rural*, nearly one in four (Murray & Keller, 1991) or one in five Americans live in rural areas (Mohatt & Kirwan, 1995; Office of Technology Assessment, 1990). In most rural areas, distance, weather, and difficult terrain hinder clients from visiting clinics. Furthermore, the population base is too small or too poor to support a behavioral health practice, or the limited career opportunities and the limited opportunities for collegial collaboration discourage professionals from setting up practices. As a result, health care specialists in particular are thinly distributed (First Consult Group, 2002). A rural community mental health center catchment area may cover 60,000 square miles. Thus, as previously discussed in this chapter and also in chapter, one main goal for technology in rural health care is to improve and expand access to medical and mental health experts (Ax, Fagan, & Holton, 2003; Cornish et al., 2003; Fahey, Day, & Gelber, 2003; Farrell & McKinnon, 2003; Mistretta, 2002; Rohland, Saleh, Rohrer, & Romitti, 2000; Sheahan, 2002). The difficulties of providing access are compounded by state licensing issues. (See chapter 9 for a discussion of licensing across state and national borders.) It is usually fairly easy to obtain licensure in a state abutting one's own, but the procedural hurdles can be discouraging.

Often, residents receive mental health services from the de facto mental health system composed of family members, friends, religious leaders, and self-help groups (Fox, Merwin, & Blank, 1995). People in rural areas are less likely to seek mental health treatment, because of various factors, including the stigma attached to mental illness (First Consult Group, 2002), lack of understanding about mental health services, lack of knowledge about how to obtain services, and inability to pay for services (Mulder et al., 2001). Rural residents seeking mental health services must often travel long distances, only to receive treatment from a professional with less training than urban professionals (Wagenfield, Murray, Mohatt, & DeBruyn, 1994). Collaboration between local and remote professionals within telehealth projects has been shown to have a positive impact on knowledge about treatment for clients and practitioners alike (Brown-Connolly, 2001b).

A rural program can encompass a broad array of medical and mental health services, including videoconferencing technology. Several countries have developed large-scale programs. The University Hospital of Tromsø, Norway (http://www.telemed.no), and Australia's Center for Online Health at the University of Queensland (http://www.coh.uq.edu.au) have been pioneers in rural applications, including online mental health services. Finland, with its vast, sparsely populated territory, provides telepsychiatry consultation and began mobile telemedicine and social services in 1998 (http://www.sonera.fi). China, Japan, Korea, and Sri Lanka have set up rural programs to provide consultation to specialty centers, alleviating long-distance travel and associated costs. Indeed, it is difficult to find a country that either has not participated in rural telehealth or is not planning to launch a telehealth program.

In the United States, the Department of Psychiatry at Cedars-Sinai Medical Center in Los Angeles has an online program to provide services to clinics more than 8 hours distant for child developmental psychiatry via videoconferencing and other technologies, a subspecialty that has traditionally been available only in large urban centers. The following vignette describes the medical center's developmental psychiatry program:

Cedars-Sinai Medical Center, Department of Psychiatry, began its first telepsychiatry clinic in 1997. Since that time, the department has expanded to three regular weekly clinics. All the clinics are devoted to patients with both developmental disabilities and mental illness. The telepsychiatry program presents an opportunity for the child psychiatry department to share our expertise with distant families and practitioners. The clinics are staffed by child psychiatrists because their expertise is essential to understanding the population we are serving, whether children or adults. Besides assisting with therapy, the clinics have been used to train medical students, residents in child psychiatry and in family practice, fellows in child psychiatry, social workers, psychologists, and early-childhood experts. The clinics serve remote locations that include inpatient developmental centers, regional centers, and outpatient and group homes for children and adults.

Each satellite clinic has a coordinator who schedules patients, as in any other clinic. Many people are invited to join for the sessions: parents, teachers, a pharmacist, a psychologist, a therapist, a day program professional, siblings, and other people who want to be present. If some people aren't available, we call them and talk on a speakerphone. The consultation is very collaborative and interactive. The patient is involved as much as possible, and most of our clients enjoy the idea of being "on TV."

It took a while for many caretakers to be comfortable with a "dial-in-the-doctor" clinic, especially because they live in rural areas and were used to ongoing relationships with doctors whom they knew. However, the families and caretakers have accepted our physicians because of their special expertise, which is not available anywhere near them. Over the years, this consultation practice has educated local doctors so that they can provide better care using psychotropic medications. It has also influenced physicians in training to be more comfortable and interested in working with the developmentally disabled.

—**Roxy Szeftel, M.D.**
Director of Child Psychiatry and Child Psychiatric Training
Department of Psychiatry at Cedars-Sinai Medical Center

Potential clinical applications for rural programs span the full spectrum of diagnostic, treatment, management, and forensic practice. Whether used as adjunctive therapy or as the only encounter with a mental health professional, the clinical interview is frequently supported by other communication technologies, such as faxing and electronic medical records (see chapter 8 for a discussion of record keeping).

Videoconferencing technology also can provide for a timely and critical intervention in situations in which qualified personnel are unavailable. Remote professionals occasionally face behavioral or emotional emergencies for which they have had little or no training. Clinics with videoconferencing equipment might decide to use it to access mental health experts in emergencies. In summary, programs that incorporate videoconferencing technology have proved that they can help meet the needs of local communities regardless of their location.

Military Programs

Historically, the military services have been in the forefront of research on and development of telehealth care applications (Edwards, 1997). The U.S. Telehealth and Advanced Telemedicine Research Center (TATRC) (http://www.tatrc.org) develops technologies capable of providing services around the world in places where the environment is hostile or needed resources are far away. Mental health services via videoconferencing and other technologies have been offered to troops at the front lines in crisis situations in the Middle East, Kosovo, and Somalia, among others.

Behavioral telehealth is an integral part of the military health care system's day-to-day activities. On January 3, 2001, the Center of Excellence for Remote and Medically Under-Served Areas (CERMUSA) inaugurated its telepsychiatry prototype. This service allowed a psychiatrist in Bethesda, Maryland, to videoconference with clients in Willow Grove, Pennsylvania, saving up to 6 total hours of travel time. This prototype program is designed to explore the feasibility of telepsychiatric unit deployment.

The following pilot project, initiated in March 1998, has become a formalized consultation clinic for children and adolescents, using live video teleconferencing:

> *Several years ago, using teleconferencing, we at Walter Reed Army Medical Center began obtaining appropriate consultations on pediatric psychiatry cases from a pediatrician at Carlisle Barracks, Pennsyvania (about 2 hours away from us). Traditionally, the patients there would come down to our clinic and spend the better part of the day traveling and being seen in the clinic. This was not an effective use of time; furthermore, it was felt that families preferred to see providers in their communities rather than make the trek. Because of the scarcity of child and adolescent psychiatry resources, however, they were unable to access appropriate care in their communities, and we knew that many were not getting the care they needed.*
>
> *But with the use of teleconferencing, I have seen more than 70 children in that clinic over the past several years and have provided expert consultations to a pediatrician and to parents. Often, I have stayed involved in cases by meeting occasionally. The purpose has usually been to provide continued psychiatric oversight of treatment plans as well as ongoing medication management consultation to the pediatrician. We are collecting data on this; we have generally found it to be an extremely effective method of seeing children and adolescents and of providing appropriate consultation to remote sites that have no resources available to them. If I had extra time to dedicate (e.g., more than one half day each week), I suspect that I could manage all the care from a distance. So the limitations have more to do with personnel resources than with the technology. We are developing a more extensive business model that will allow expanding this service to many remote sites in the northeast United States to better serve dependent children.*
>
> **—Lieutenant Colonel Stephen J. Cozza, M.D.**
> **Walter Reed Army Medical Center**

The military also has adult telepsychiatry, automated patient records, distance learning, and colleague consultation and supervision programs and initiatives.

Correctional Facility Programs

The U.S. Constitution forbids "cruel and unusual punishment." U.S. prisons are therefore obliged to provide health care. Prison facilities experience a microcosm of the problems plaguing the health care system at large. Prisons are required to provide access to standard health services to large numbers of relatively powerless people under exceptionally challenging circumstances while keeping down costs and protecting the health care professional. Therefore, the correctional system has found videoconferencing technologies to be excellent tools for addressing the spectrum of mental heath disorders and services (Winchell & Wilbright, 2003; Zaylor, Spaulding, & Cook, 2003). The patient base has a great need for diagnostic services, acute intervention, and ongoing management of mental disorders.

More specifically, an estimated 16% of inmates in U.S. prisons suffer from a mental illness, and about 16% of probationers have mental conditions or have been treated in a mental institution (Ditton, 1999). Regier et al. (1990) reported that 82% of prison inmates abused alcohol and drugs and/or had mental disorders. Chemically abusive mentally ill prisoners were especially likely to be imprisoned for violent crimes, the majority of which were committed under the influence of drugs and/or alcohol (Ditton, 1999).

The societal benefits of providing videoconferencing services in a controlled environment without the risks incurred by having prisoners leave the facility is apparent to correctional officers and psychiatric professionals alike. The inmates' need for protection of private information is also addressed by using a secure link for communication with professionals outside the correctional environment.

Research conducted by Abt Associates for the National Institute of Justice identified psychiatry as highly effective when videoconferencing technology was used to treat patients in place of in-person visits, as occurred in the participating prisons (McDonald, 1999). Improved medication management was also noted to decrease inmate transfers for social and emotional problems and reduced the rate of violent episodes. The overall improvement in clinical services and the decrease in transfers resulted in substantial cost savings to the system.

According to the Association of Telehealth Service Providers (1999), 20% of telemedicine activity reported for 1998 was in prisons. The U.S. Federal Bureau of Prisons (http://www.bop.gov) initiated an aggressive telemedicine program for more than 90 of its facilities in 2000. Mental health professionals now have opportunities to interface with correctional facilities by contracting for services through local and federal health service offices.

Zaylor, Whitten, and Kingsley (1999) conducted a telepsychiatry project that connected inmates at the Lyon County Jail in Kansas to the Kansas University Medical Center, using videoconferencing technology. Two hundred and sixty-four consultations were conducted during the pilot project—70 initial visits and 194 follow-up visits. The demand for telepsychiatric services was five times higher than first predicted. The authors found that telepsychiatric consultations were effective for the treatment of moderate to severe psychiatric illnesses.

School Programs

It should be no surprise that public school budgets for health services are often inadequate. This is especially true in school systems in which a high percentage of children have special needs and are mainstreamed into the regular classroom. The school nurse may visit a school once every few weeks, but a child's need for medical care can occur at any time. Undiagnosed problems can lead to distractions in the classroom, erupting violence, and underachievement.

Teachers find themselves having to take on the nurse's role with inadequate training and experience. Where school nurse services are inadequate or nonexistent, a videoconferencing system can fill in ("Integrated School-Based Mental Health...," 2000).

In addition, videoconferencing consultations can help ensure that a "visit" to a professional takes place while minimizing the disruption of learning and time away from school. The TeleKidcare program (http://www2.kumc.edu/telemedicine/programs/telekidcare.htm) links the University of Kansas Medical Center with Kansas City schools via videoconferencing technology. Initially the program involved 4 schools, and because of its success, it has expanded to 12. In this program, appropriate health professionals provide cost-effective services. Behavioral health consultation accounted for 27% of TeleKidcare referrals in 2000–2001.

BEYOND MIMICRY OF TRADITIONAL CARE

Expanding the vision of online consultation beyond direct psychotherapy suggests many other useful goals, even for POTS, the answering machine, and the fax. Areas in which audio and video distance communication may be applied include screening and case acquisition, assessment, diagnosis, collaborative treatment planning, informed consent, therapeutic interventions and motivation enhancement, crisis response, client and family education, case management, medication support, consultation, case supervision, training, and continuing professional education.

The impact of the electronic medium on outcome and process is evolving; we can only speculate about its future. Certainly, the psychometric properties of many clinical assessment instruments will be altered by administering tests and questionnaires remotely, and conclusions based on them should not be trusted until the instruments have been recalibrated. Similarly, the professional's ability to discern risks and benefits or to measure success or failure of a service may be different (perhaps superior, perhaps not) when psychotechnologies are incorporated to mediate therapeutic relationships. Circumstances strongly influence cognitive processing, as reflected in the language style and jargon that characterize various communication media—how people speak on ham radios versus citizens' band radio or how they write in e-mail versus snail mail, for example. This change in language use may have a profound, but currently uncertain, impact on electronically mediated treatment (Murphy & Pardeck, 1988).

In general, studies to date have not shown significant degradation in outcome when mental health service is delivered over two-way audio or video systems instead of in-person (Day & Schneider, 2000; Glueckauf et al., 1998, 2002). Absence of proof is not proof of absence. It is simply too early in the use of technology in psychotherapy for research to have provided the answers many clinicians would like to have before working with high-risk and potentially suicidal or homicidal patients.

A convincing study would include a placebo control arm that, by incidentally demonstrating effectiveness of the standard treatment, shows that the measuring instrument is working (Klein, 1995). Even then, correlating dosage with effectiveness and uncovering reasons that treatment failed in specific instances would be needed to bolster the claim that telemental health is just as good as in-person treatment. Even if one can get past the ethical quandary (Klein, 1995; Rothman & Michels, 1994) and the technical difficulty of providing a placebo service as part of a study, it may be a long time before adequate samples of in-person versus distance-mediated services will receive funding and be implemented and replicated.

Furthermore, as we keep reiterating, what professionals need to see is not whether behavioral telehealth (or telemental health) is just as good but whether it is good enough or, more accurately, just how good it is so that they can make informed choices that balance clinical considerations with questions of cost, availability, and acceptability. To this end, evidence-based decisions on using distance communication in treatment ideally should rest in part on quantitative utility analysis, which is a long way off (Diener, O'Brien, & Gafni, 1998) and on cost studies that take into account not only immediate transactional expenses but also the impact on emergency department visits, use of all health care, medication expenses, hospitalizations of all kinds, vocational function, family burden, quality of life, and other factors. Meanwhile, behavioral telehealth should not stand still. Its use will have to be guided by professional judgment, general experience, qualitative studies, insightful case reports, and proper attention to Einstein's elusive cat.

Now that we have examined use of the various telecommunication technologies in the mental health professions, the next chapter shifts our focus to computer-assisted technologies that augment assessment.

6

Computer-Aided Assessment

Computer-aided assessment is an innovation whose time has come. This chapter looks at benefits of and barriers to adoption of such assessments, types of assessments and clinical interviews now available, a few of the Web applications and the development of guidelines for their use, electronic diaries, and interactive voice response systems. Finally, we outline developments in the increasingly important area of decision-support software. We begin by familiarizing the reader with some benefits of and barriers to computer-aided assessment.

ADOPTION OF COMPUTER-AIDED ASSESSMENT

The earliest computer programs for assessment and therapeutic support through self-help involved a single large mainframe computer serving one client at a time. The Internet now has the capability of distributing such services anywhere, anytime, and to anyone with access to a computer and modem, expanding use and encouraging development of increasingly sophisticated psychotechnologies. Old-style programs merely processed a set of data and emitted a report. New programs are interactive, responding to what a user does, awaiting further input, and responding flexibly. Both types of programs have spread to Web sites that offer analysis of personal health risk factors, self-diagnostic questionnaires, and self-care training. The Internet has developed rapidly, and enthusiasm for mental health information has surged. Furthermore, as discussed in chapter 1, the employee assistance market has been rewarded by financial profit and has grown rapidly. The mental health professional may need to be familiar with such services, their underlying concepts, and how they can influence and supplement patient treatment.

Benefits

Practice today is being driven by the increasing complexity of mental health treatments, advances in research and technology, requirements for documentation of services, and demands for greater cost-effectiveness and efficiency. Figure 6.1 illustrates the pressures these factors cause and the resulting development of behavioral health care technology.

Computerization is seen as a possible and viable solution to (as well as a possible cause of) these increasing demands. Beyond self-help, technology is improving direct care by mental health practitioners. The increasing requirements for documentation

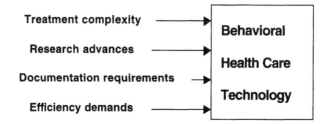

FIG. 6.1. Factors driving the development of behavioral health care technology.

of services and the demands for greater cost-effectiveness and efficiency will soon make computers an inescapable necessity for mental health professionals. Because they excel at repetitive and rule-based tasks and have virtually unlimited recall capacity, computers can alleviate the workload by administering and scoring diagnostic questionnaires, structured interviews, and remote biofeedback and by dramatically expanding psychophysiological and ambulatory monitoring for treatment.

Assessment software packages that have passed empirical testing can be a notable asset to the average clinician (Kobak et al., 1997a; Newman, Kenardy, Herman, & Taylor, 1996). As always, whether computer based or in-person, assessement strategies must involve a thorough clinical interview to provide contextual information about the individual being assessed. Nonetheless, it is reasonable to look at computerization of certain specific elements of the psychotherapy assessment, while highlighting the importance of clinician oversight and professional judgment.

Some practitioners may be tempted by services that have adapted traditional paper-and-pencil assessments to the Internet, but simply adapting existing assessment tools to the computer is questionable. Unexpected problems may arise when developing or adapting existing assessment instruments to the computer. For instance, the psychometric properties of an otherwise reliable assessment instrument may be thrown off if items are presented in a "branching" manner to avoid seemingly inefficient redundancy. In branching logic, a negative answer to a general question (e.g., about hallucinations) bypasses a series of questions that would probe details. Indeed, adequate statistical study of a branching questionnaire faces formidable scientific obstacles. Practitioners should therefore carefully examine the structure of online and computerized use of familiar and otherwise well-established instruments and techniques. On the other hand, if tests are initially constructed and normed with branching logic, this format may be a considerable improvement to traditional test administration. This determination, however, must rely on sound empirical research and not left to professionals who would circumvent the time-consuming and costly effort of developing tests specifically for self-administration over the Internet.

Barriers

Controlled clinical trials support evaluating the effectiveness of computerized assessment, treatment, and practice-management computer applications. Nonetheless, there is a significant lag in practitioner interest in these areas. We now hypothesize why this lag exists in mental health when other health care disciplines have forged ahead with wide-scale adoption of technology (Maheu, Whitten, & Allen, 2001); we hope researchers will examine this lag with appropriate scientific scrutiny.

A barrier to adopting computer-aided assessment may be a lack of outside encouragement or coercion, as would be found within a hospital. General health care enterprises began introducing mandatory adoption of computerization and concomitant training programs during the past 2 decades. Employees of such general health care organizations had to learn to use in-house communication systems. Most of those employees were exposed to completing forms (data entry), in-house messaging (e-mail), and, more recently, the World Wide Web to complete routine tasks. Mental health practitioners, on the other hand, have not felt such pressures. Many mental health practitioners work alone or in small groups of non-computerized offices.

The benefits of computerization for assessment, treatment, and practice management may not have been made as salient for mental health practitioners as for general health care professionals. Being self-selected soloists, many mental health practitioners do not work with assistants, such as nurses, who also interact with patients on a daily basis. Similarly, the advantages of sharing assessment results, progress notes, or in-house communication with other staff members may not be as apparent to practitioners working independently when compared with colleagues in hospital or private clinic settings.

Another explanation for delayed computer adoption by mental health workers might be a reluctance to invest time and energy in computers and software that could lead to unexpected and unwanted legal or ethical problems. Many practitioners were not trained in graduate settings in which computerization was modeled for any aspect of mental health care. Computer skills may be helpful for surviving graduate school, but they traditionally have not been in the repertoire of skill sets required for practice. Workshops offered at many state and national convention programs in using computers often confuse more than clarify issues for the beginner, and presentations related to computer and Internet security and confidentiality can be more frightening than inspiring.

Difficulties securing funding to investigate computer-based forms of intervention might also contribute to the relative delay in computer adoption by mental health care practitioners. At best, most empirically based evaluations are at the stage of showing the feasibility of implementing a new approach, demonstrating acceptability to clients, or suggesting effectiveness in limited samples. Without empirical validation, many computer-based assessment approaches may not meet current practice standards.

Last, being a special reimbursement "carve out" might add to the lack of marketing focused on the financially struggling and relatively indigent mental health sector. Compounding this problem, practitioners and researchers have little experience with commercializing their own products and many of their innovations receive little publicity or encouragement.

DEVELOPMENT AND USE OF COMPUTER-AIDED ASSESSMENT

Despite these barriers, computer-aided assessments are slowly but steadily gaining acceptance in the therapeutic community, both nationally and internationally. They are being developed primarily to accompany psychiatric consultation or psychotherapy. Current applications of computer-aided assessment include personality and clinical assessment by questionnaires, diagnostic interviewing, electronic diaries, interactive voice response systems, and clinical decision-support systems. Each of these topics is discussed in the remainder of this chapter.

Computer-Based Questionnaires

A specialized form of a computer-aided assessment scale is the questionnaire. Computer administration of clinical interviews and questionnaires spares professionals from filling out lengthy forms and thus can be more economical (for an early review, see Fowler, 1985). Some of the earliest mainframe computers installed in universities evaluated large databases of questionnaire items during the 1950s. The first clinical application of computers coped with the heavy influx of patients at the Mayo Clinic in Rochester, Minnesota (Swenson, Rome, Pearson, & Brannick, 1965). Patients marked their responses to Minnesota Multiphasic Personality Inventory (MMPI) on special data cards for scanning into a computer. A program then scored 14 MMPI scales, converted them into standard scores, and printed a series of descriptive statements. Although simple by today's standards, the Mayo system provided a practical means of screening large numbers of medical patients who otherwise might have received no psychological or psychiatric assessment.

Questionnaires have long elicited additional information on specific mental health issues—the Beck Depression Inventory (Beck, Ward, Mendelson, Mock, & Erbaugh, 1961) and the Mobility Inventory (Chambless, Caputo, Hasin, Gracely, & Williams, 1985). Another example is the the **A**lgorithms for **E**ffective **R**eporting and **T**reatment (ALERT[SM]) system, which analyzes self-reported, practitioner-reported, and other assessment information, using clinical algorithms (step-by-step procedures). Data gathered from the client during an initial telephone assessment are compared with those from a second telephone interview 6 months into treatment. If the observed improvement in clinical status falls significantly short of the initially calculated expected change, the treating professional receives an advisory letter such as the following:

> *Patient: B.G.*
>
> *Thank you for your recent submission of the Life Status Questionnaire (LSQ) for B.G. The purpose of this alert is to draw attention to one or more risk factors identified by the ALERT[SM] clinical information system.*
>
> *The primary reason we are contacting you is that this patient responded to substance abuse items on the LSQ in a manner suggesting that he or she may have a problem with abusing drugs or alcohol. You answered "No" to the question regarding your assessment of the presense of a substance abuse problem. We wanted to be sure that you had fully addressed the substance abuse problem. We would support your intensifying treatment with a focus on substance abuse if you feel it would benefit your patient. Please let us know if you need additional services certified at this time.*
>
> *Your patient also began treatment with an LSQ intake score of 77. This patient is expected to improve to a score of 64 or less. The ALERT system makes this determination by comparing information from your patient to a large normative sample, which enables us to determine how much change similar patients typically experience over the course of a treatment episode and to identify risk factors.*
>
> *On the following page is a summary of the clinical data for this patient. Please feel free to contact us if you have questions or wish to discuss this case further. Thank you for the time and attention to this patient.*
>
> —Edward R. Jones, Ph.D.
> Corporate Clinical Director
> PacifiCare Behavioral Health

Practitioners using the ALERT system should anticipate that, in event of litigation, the notice from ALERT is probably discoverable, and adversaries will attempt to use it as a guideline for treatment. Therefore, a clinician who disagrees with the ALERT system's recommendation should probably document carefully the basis for that disagreement and the reasons for rejecting ALERT's recommendation.

Advantages of Computer-Based Questionnaires. Questionnaires are a quick way to gather and structure clinical information and are particularly useful in large-scale psychopharmacological clinical trials. Computer administration of such assessment instruments can be more economical, standardized, personalized, straightforward, and time efficient, as well as less biased and even less intimidating (Sampson, 1990). User acceptance of computer-based questionnaires is surprisingly high (e.g., Lucas, Mullin, Luna, & McInroy, 1977; Moore, Summer, & Bloor, 1984). Several studies even demonstrated that most respondents preferred computer administration to the paper-and-pencil format (e.g., Lukin, Dowd, Plake, & Kraft, 1985), and one study found computer-based assessment to be more time efficient and also more conducive to honest responses (Hart & Goldstein, 1985).

Although the user-computer interface can distract a client and distort test results, a computer can use audiovisual effects to enhance the presentation of questions and tests. These effects may increase client comprehension, motivation, and compliance with instructions, as well as overcome barriers created by a client's visual or hearing disabilities. Such effects may even help overcome some clients' cognitive difficulties. Face-valid, systematic research is needed to support these claims.

Disadvantages of Computer-Based Questionnaires. Current programming languages make it easy to write a computer program that collects data from questionnaires. Using an appealing graphical user interface enables one to generate a detailed report of test results and their probable interpretation. However, constructing a useful automated clinical instrument is not simple. Furthermore, the mode of test administration can markedly influence its psychometric properties, so that instructions, methods, and interpretive norms standardized for structured interviews and questionnaires may require modification when data gathering is automated.

It is reassuring that the few studies conducted suggest that the mode of test administration may not be a major factor influencing test scores (French & Beaumont, 1989; Lukin et al., 1985; Waller & Reise, 1989; Wilson, Genco, & Yager, 1985). However, the current guidelines for computerizing an established paper-and-pencil questionnaire call for reestablishing item construction and selection, internal consistency, test–retest reliability, and internal and external validity (American Psychological Association, 1999a).

Ease of Use Invites Misuse. The impression of objectivity and accuracy elicited by computerized reports through their professional-sounding language may mislead both clients and unwary professionals (Groth-Marnat & Schumaker, 1989). Interpreting questionnaire and psychological test data entails much more than scoring and selecting statements from a cookbook. Professionals must integrate information from multiple sources, including direct examination, and must take into account patterns and discrepancies among subscales (Fowler, 1985). Doubts have been raised in the professional literature as to whether mental health professionals can ever rely on automated condensation of questionnaire information (e.g., Burke & Normand, 1987).

In fact, computerized test interpretations have been sharply criticized for decades (Matarazzo, 1986).

Ease of Use Invites Enhanced Use.   On the other hand, questionnaires and tests could generate an individually tailored framework for an initial evaluation report, treatment plan, or a progress note that a professional could then adjust and flesh out. Because computers are unlike most of us, a computer need not simply fill in for a live professional when communicating directly with a client. The computer can approach a case from a unique angle and pick up different information than might the human eye, ear, or mind. In fact, if the test is properly developed, the computer can be used as a more precise measurement tool than can a human examiner, and as a tool, it might have the capacity to detect more subtle differences in the respondee's behavior, including movement and verbalizations.

We can also envision that future computer testing systems will be able to process a respondee's wide range of behavior and compare it all to norms established with other test takers. To the extent that a computer's analysis of test results can be deemed a separate source of expertise, programmers should anticipate that creative lawyers will attempt to bring them in as defendants if something goes wrong or if there is a need for additional evidence.

Computer-Based Tests

A wide range of human psychological responses are shaped by processes of which a person is unaware. Beyond what a person is able to report, the implicit measurement of moods, attitudes, and personality variables is increasingly recognized as important for understanding human behavior (Kihlstrom, 1987; LeDoux, 2002; Tallis, 2002). Explicit questionnaires assess introspectively accessible self-descriptions and self-evaluations; implicit tests tap introspectively unidentified traces of past experiences that influence current behavior (Greenwald et al., 2002). To some degree, such tests can also detect a client's conscious efforts to conceal or fabricate material.

With the exception of the lie detector, or polygraph (Board on Behavioral, Cognitive, and Sensory Sciences and Education, & Committee on National Statistics, 2003), implicit tests are applied predominantly in research settings. The efficacy for individual testing needs to be established before practitioners can find widespread application for them. Implicit, but not explicit, self-esteem has been associated with apparent anxiety during a self-revealing interview (Spalding & Hardin, 1999). Implicit racial prejudice exhibited by Caucasian participants correlated with MRI-assessed amygdala activation and eye-blink startle responses when participants were shown black compared to white faces (Phelps et al., 2000). Taken together, implicit measures seem especially promising for predicting behaviors not normally subject to conscious control, such as nonverbal behavior and physiological responses.

Dot-Probe Task.   A computer program that measures implicit anxiety is the attentional dot-probe task (MacLeod, Mathews, & Tata, 1986), which can be implemented using Micro Experimental Laboratory software (Schneider, 1988). The software assesses automatic attention allocation to threatening stimuli by presenting pairs of threatening and neutral words simultaneously on different areas of a computer screen. Attention is measured by a secondary task that involves the detection of a dot, which appears in the spatial location of either word immediately after the display of that word was terminated. By examining the differential impact of threat versus neutral words on the speed of dot detection, the researcher can compute an index of attention allocation toward or away from threat—independent from general vigilance.

This kind of testing has demonstrated that clinically anxious clients focus on threatening stimuli in their environment more than do normal controls (Mineka & Sutton, 1992). Furthermore, the dot-probe test predicted cardiovascular reactivity to an evaluated speaking task, whereas an explicit anxiety measure did not (Egloff, Wilhelm, Neubauer, Mauss, & Gross, 2002). The dot-probe test and other implicit tests have been used to examine the role that biases in attention and memory may play in the etiology of depression, in recovery from this disorder, and in relapse of depression (for a review, see Gotlib & Neubauer, 2000).

Response Latency Tests. Response time to a test item may be determined largely by such factors as a person's age or fluency in the questionnaire language (Slack, Leviton, Bennett, Fleischmann, & Lawrence, 1988). Differences in response time to various items presented by a computer can provide information that is difficult to obtain manually about an individual. Fekken found an association between response latency and changes in response on retest a useful indicator of falsified responding (Fekken & Holden, 1992; Fekken & Jackson, 1988). Questions about emotional health produced greater latency than did questions about general medical or lifestyle issues (George & Skinner, 1990). Abnormally short response latencies, particularly toward the end of a questionnaire, may also suggest that clients are responding haphazardly.

Clinical Interviews

Attempts began by the late 1960s to computerize clinical interviews (Kleinmuntz & McLean, 1968; Stillman, Roth, Colby, & Rosenbaum, 1969). Many studies have shown that reliability and validity of computer-based structured clinical interviews are comparable to clinician-administered interviews (for reviews, see Newman, Consoli, & Taylor, 1997; Plutchik & Karasu, 1991). For example, in a comparison of three versions of the Diagnostic Interview Schedule of the National Institute of Mental Health (Robins & Helzer, 1985)—conventional interviewer administered, interviewer prompted by computer, and fully computerized administered—pairwise diagnostic agreement was good for the various psychiatric diagnoses (Erdman, Klein, Greist, & Skare, 1992). Reading level did not bias the results in the fully computer-based administration, and acceptance was high; indeed, responding to the computer was considered least embarrassing.

More Empirical Support. Computer-administered versions of clinical scales are available for the assessment of depression, anxiety, obsessive-compulsive disorder, and social phobia (Kobak, Greist, Jefferson, & Katzelnick, 1996). Studies support the reliability, validity, and equivalence of these scales. More specifically, computer administration and scoring of mental disorders are available through such programs as IShell, a general-purpose interview tool developed at the World Health Organization (WHO). When downloaded from its Web site (http://www3.who.int/cidi/index.htm), Ishell automatically installs under Windows operating systems. The program includes the CIDI2.1 interview (Lifetime version) in English, Spanish, or French; help files; and a data export module that allows interfacing with SPSS, Inc. (http://www.spss.com), statistical software. Compatible SPSS scoring programs are available from the Web site.

The CIDI (Composite International Diagnostic Interview), developed by WHO, is a comprehensive, standardized instrument for assessment of mental disorders according to the definitions and criteria of ICD-10 (World Health Organization, 1990) and the *Diagnostic and Statistical Manual of Mental Disorders* (4th ed.) (American Psychiatric Association, 1994). The CIDI is validated for use in epidemiological and cross-cultural studies, as well as for clinical and research purposes (Wittchen, 1994).

Several studies have evaluated the computer-based version (Peters & Andrews, 1995; Peters, Clark, & Carroll, 1998; Rosenman, Korten, & Levings, 1997; Rosenman, Levings, & Korten, 1997), including administration over the Internet (Carlbring et al., 2002). These studies concluded that the self-administered computer-based CIDI is an acceptable substitute for the clinician-administered CIDI for selected populations—for example, for patients presenting at an anxiety disorders clinic. However, although patient acceptance was high, it had unsatisfactory validity measured against psychiatrist diagnosis for hospitalized patients of acute psychiatric services.

Over the years, clinicians and researchers have speculated about the use of computer-based clinical interviews. Many clinicians considered (and might still consider) their use as taboo in mental health care, much in keeping with this early 20th century warning:

> A man burdened with a secret should especially avoid the intimacy of his physician. If the latter possess native sagacity, and a nameless something more, let us call it intuition; if he show no intrusive egotism, nor disagreeably prominent characteristics of his own; if he have the power, which must be born with him, to bring his mind into such affinity with his patient's that this last shall unawares have spoken what he imagines himself only to have thought; if such revelations be received without tumult, and acknowledged not so often by an uttered sympathy, as by silence, an inarticulate breath, and here and there a word, to indicate that all is understood; if, to these qualifications of a confidant be joined the advantages afforded by his recognised character as a physician; then, at some inevitable moment, will the soul of the sufferer be dissolved and flow forth in a dark, but transparent stream, bringing all its mysteries into the daylight.
>
> —(Hawthorne, 1906, p. 151)

Therapeutic Alliance. Despite the power of a therapeutic relationship to uncover long-held secrets, clinicians seeking a more scientific approach to optimizing efficiency are finding that structured interviews are successful with patients in a number of clinical settings. For instance, the Structured Clinical Interview for the DSM-IV (SCID-IV) (First, Spitzer, Gibbon, & Williams, 1995) has become the widely accepted research standard for diagnostic assessment of mental disorders. In fact, it has proved more reliable and valid for diagnostic purposes than are other modalities of assessment, such as unstructured interviews or questionnaires (Segal & Falk, 1998). In clinical practice, structured interviews are used much less frequently, perhaps because of some combination of lack of practitioner training, pressure to accomplish more than simply make a diagnosis in the limited time available with the patient, and/or concern about establishing an adequate therapeutic relationship.

Nonetheless, there are many possibilities for using structured interviews while helping to develop a therapeutic alliance. For example, the computer could be used to conduct a preliminary structured interview that could serve as a guide for a clinician's subsequent, more flexible diagnostic interview. Alternatively, a computer-based diagnostic interview as a follow-up to the clinician's initial evaluation could be more extended and comprehensive, filling in areas on which the clinician did not focus, perhaps uncovering important information and diagnostic possibilities the clinician did not consider, or perhaps adding information to support the clinician's impression and enhance confidence in the clinician's working diagnosis.

Computers can serve effectively as an initial interviewer by following a branching algorithm. However, when they learn that positive answers to screening questions can lead to several follow-up questions, clients may tend to avoid giving positive responses. This cause of underreporting of symptoms can be skirted by asking all the screening questions first and only then returning to a close examination of promising leads. More sophisticated methods may revisit denied topics using different phraseology and may probe for specifics if a contradictory response is received.

Advantages of Internet-Based Clinical Interviews. Used in accordance with established ethical guidelines and in appropriately selected cases, Internet administration of computer-based assessments promises inexpensive, accessible, and time-efficient means of assessing or monitoring stress levels, self-care behaviors, compliance with medication, and mental disorders. At this time, however, more research is needed to evaluate reliability and validity (compared to in-person interviewing) of computer-based interviews, particularly those delivered through the Internet. Computer-based assessment can clarify a diagnostic impression, but clinicians might want to avoid using such assessments with clients who are difficult to diagnose, such as those with comorbid diagnoses, language difficulties, personality disorders, or acute psychiatric episodes.

Professionals need to consider several issues before encouraging clients to locate psychological, personality, and/or behavioral monitoring sites on the Web without assistance. Professionals referring clients to Web sites for testing or monitoring their behavior may want review such services to determine whether they were developed and validated in accordance with the established guidelines for computerization of tests. Norman Hoffman gives the reader added insight into the advantages and disadvantages of computer-based assessment on the Web:

> Clinicians, as well as consumers of behavioral health services, should be cautious about unconditionally accepting computer outputs from psychological assessments, whether from freestanding computers or Internet sites. The old adage of GIGO (garbage in—garbage out) has been supplanted in the minds of some Internet users by GIDO (garbage in—deification out). These individuals tend to confer greater credence or validity on output from a computer than from other sources. Just because a result has been produced by a computer or a Web site does not in itself confer on it any greater validity than that for paper tests or clinician-administered tools or procedures. Yet Internet consumers may not know the difference between validated and nonvalidated tests and may alter their lives in accord with a home-brewed test they took on a mental health professional's Web site.
>
> This situation suggests that clinicians exercise caution in selecting and using software, whether on an office computer, provided through a service, or from an Internet site. The appropriate function of such programs is to provide the best information and integration of data for the clinician to evaluate, along with whatever other information might be available. Programs can produce a result at variance with the judgment of the clinician, who may have access to additional information. In this case, the clinician's expert judgment based on the broader scope of information is best integrated with computer-generated output. As always, clinicians and not computers should be making diagnostic determinations for clients and patients, even if the programs are new and seemingly sophisticated.
>
> Use of the Internet carries a need for additional caution. Reputable developers and distributors of assessment tools not only adhere to established principles in how the tools

are developed and in the claims for their tools but also provide contact information for questions related to test development, administration, and interpretation. Internet sites can be relatively anonymous in terms of where the site is located or who is responsible for its development and maintenance. Because the Internet is worldwide, a Web site could be on the far side of the planet—next door. When Web site users cross international boundaries, issues of accountability, and security, as well as multilingual and multicultural factors influencing test interpretation, can be compromised.

Despite the limitations and prudent cautions, automated systems and Internet-based assessments hold a great deal of promise. Internet systems can provide updates in a way that is seamless and even imperceptible to the user. Such systems also have the capacity to capture large quantities of information that can be of great value to advancing scientific knowledge and providing enhanced clinical services. As with any technology Trained professionals, must offer Internet-based assessments with prudence and objective clinical judgment.

—**Norman G. Hoffmann, Ph.D.**
President
Evince Clinical Assessments

Computer-based diagnostic assessments have these specific advantages:

- They are administered anytime, anywhere, and in a manner that precludes the introduction of differences owing to administrator differences and associated personal biases.
- They are highly acceptable to many clients, or in some instances even preferred, because clients feel freer to take their time with answers (e.g., Greist, Klein, Erdman, & Bires, 1987).
- Clients may tend to reveal more sensitive information (e.g., substance abuse, sexual disorders, and/or suicide attempts) because they feel less embarrassed providing this information to a computer (e.g., Erdman, 1987, Lucas, Mullian, Luna & McInroy, 1977; Millstein, 1987).
- Computer-based interviews can be translated into different languages and can facilitate access to mental health services for minorities. Performing these translations can present a problem, as will be discussed in the following section on disadvantages.

Disadvantages of Internet-Based Clinical Interviews. As for disadvantages, many of the plethora of tests already available on the Internet are poorly validated or inappropriate for a given client. A mental health professional should consider relevance, relationship issues, ethics, and standards for necessary professional training in interpreting results before recommending particular tests to a particular client. The professional needs to decide which results should be returned directly to the client (American Psychological Association, 2002a). Other, specific disadvantages to computer-based assessment may include the following:

- Standardization of administration can be compromised if the client is interrupted by a telephone call, a child, a pet, or a ringing doorbell.
- The computer cannot gather and evaluate nonverbal behaviors that convey many cues to emotional states that are relevant to successful therapeutic intervention.

- Professionals often have insight that is based on years of experience with a client. The degree to which insight is influenced by nonverbal behavior between professional and client is unknown.
- Computers are not programmed to adapt their language to the needs of individuals, as when some people cannot comprehend certain words.
- The effectiveness of computers with clients depends on the client's reading ability. The validity and reliablity of programs with reading abilities that vary from one client to another are still to be improved.
- Automatic branching algorithms may miss important problems if a more general screening question is negated. (However, this is also true for highly structured clinician-administered interviews.)
- Computer interviews are economical only if they are used often enough to offset initial costs for installation and training.
- Posting psychological assessments on the Internet can compromise test security. That is, public dissemination can seriously compromise and render ineffective secured tests whose psychometric integrity depends on the test taker's not having prior access to test materials (American Psychological Association, 1999b).
- Web sites may ask patients for personal information and may log all mouse clicks and keystrokes, without the knowledge of a referring practitioner. This practice can expose a client to violations of privacy, especially when highly sensitive data are involved. Furthermore, moving a test result from a Web site to a client's clinical chart adds an extra opportunity for inadvertent privacy violation. Owners of such sites need to be cognizant of federal and state laws applicable to privacy issues and should strongly consider adopting, posting, and abiding by a privacy policy that takes such authorities into account. Practitioners may want to obtain HIPAA-compliant business agreements with such vendors.

While this fast moving area is still fraught with uncertainty we will discuss a few potential problems of computerized test construction and administration. We encourage the interested reader to regularly consult with test development specialists for updates. There is the risk of administering a test via psychotechnologies for a population for which research findings have not been determined. For example, it might seem easy to translate a test's words into a client's native language but languages change. Also, current subtleties may be lost to a foreign speaker who learned a language several decades ago. Furthermore, idiom, dialect, and colloquism make translation difficult even with widely spoken languages, such as Spanish and French. Spanish and French colonization of diverse geographic areas has resulted in local expressions that have evolved into a rich blend of region-specific dialects. Take, for example, the differences in French as spoken in France, Haiti, Québec, and New Orleans. A native speaker in any of the cities or countries may be able to decipher the gist of a spoken message delivered by a native speaker from another region, but specific words or phrases might be misunderstood or lost entirely. Translate these four dialects of the French language from the spoken to the written word, and inevitable time delays in reading will ensue.

Constructing a test to be administered to a worldwide audience is a significant challenge: It will require much more than taking an existing paper-and-pencil test, coding it for a Web site, and inviting the Internet audience to respond. The task of developing psychological tests for use on the Internet is best left to trained diagnosticians who know the guidelines for test construction and standardization and also the limits of interpretation.

Few structured interviews have been studied in other than controlled settings, where interviewer characteristics include being especially motivated, trained, and monitored. In practice, clinicians tend to merely skim through or skip the basic manual, to omit items, and to drift in their interpretation of the items rather than to remain anchored to the text. A hurried clinician who has a rich array of instruments readily available may not treat each one with much respect in its administration yet may, paradoxically, harbor unrealistic beliefs of its accuracy. False attribution of accuracy may tend to snowball as the result of a supposed objective assessment technique. The sentiment can then make its way from one clinician to the next. As the distance from raw observation increases, from the interviewer or tester, the professional may tend to put more faith into test results than into the original clinician's supposedly more subjective opinions and writings. These fundamental factors and their related hazards will only become more pressing with the widespread availability and use of computer-aided clinical instruments.

Nonetheless, where adequately skilled professionals are not available but a diagnosis is needed in a crisis, a computer will undoubtedly be used as a stopgap diagnostician until proper consultation can be obtained. The use of such applications is suggested very cautiously; as due consideration is needed when replacing a sensitive and insightful clinician with a mechanical device. The danger, of course, is that practitioners motivated by profit rather than patient-centered care will eventually seek to replace time-intensive psychodiagnostic processes with an increasing number of computer-based interviews and assessments. Furthermore, given the time and expense of developing valid and reliable assessment tools, existing assessments could be used on professional Web sites without regard to the vagaries of nonstandardized testing situations. Test administration could be interrupted by telephone calls, visits from the neighbor, sick children, or angry mates.

Home-brewed assessments can and are offered to the world at large without considering the traditional rigors imposed on the development of psychodiagnostic measures. Throwing together a series of questions and posting them on a Web site without regard to the seriousness imparted to psychodiagnostic measures by the average person is unconscionable. Tests that lead users to conclude that they are "stupid, selfish, greedy, needy, dependent, or narcissistic" can be outdone only by people who would use Web-based tests that lead a user to decide that "this employee must be a thief," or "the baby-sitter is a child molester." At the opposite end of the continuum, empirical evidence shows that computers can be of remarkable assistance to patients, practitioners, and yes, third parties. However, scientific rigor and clinical judgment must bridge the gap.

Use of language is another serious and complicated issue. Without specific referral by a knowledgeable clinician, then, sending clients to unverified Web sites offering psychological assessment or self-monitoring could lead to a host of unwarranted problems. Without appropriate referral and interpretation of results, clients could find themselves categorized as mentally disordered without receiving any further information on the limitations of such remote and automatic assessment, without understanding the implications of a diagnosis (if the test is valid), or without being given emotional support, if needed. Should any people so categorized come to harm as a result, the chances are good that some of them claim will be asserted against the individuals or companies responsible for operating the program. Providing a warning to the public on the self-test might not provide a complete defense, but it is better to err on the side of posting a well-drafted disclaimer. This area of the law is very new and rapidly evolving; practitioners should watch it closely and to adapt as it changes.

To avoid some limitations of computer-based assessment and yet to preserve their advantages, some professionals prefer to conduct diagnostic interviews themselves, using the computer program to prompt them as they complete the multiple-choice questions. The professionals use the automatic branching capabilities of the computer and get scores immediately.

Electronic Diaries

Paper-and-pencil diaries have long been used in clinical studies to track a client's state in his or her natural environment. The prospective assessment achieved with immediate report of moods, symptoms, cognitions, and behaviors can bypass problems of clients' retrospective assessments and their biases in judging what constitutes the reply "often" or "rarely." Arthur Stone coined the term ecological momentary assessment to describe the collection of data about client experience in an ecologically valid setting at the moment it occurs (Stone & Shiffman, 1994). This term has helped demonstrate, for example, that retrospective reports of panic attacks are exaggerated (Margraf, Taylor, Ehlers, Roth, & Agras, 1987) and that smokers actually underestimate their smoking behavior. Such diaries have been implemented on palmtop computers (also known as personal digital assistants [PDAs]) (Fahrenberg & Myrtek, 1996; Kenardy, Evans, & Oei, 1988; Newman et al., 1996; Shiffman, 1993; Taylor, Fried, & Kenardy, 1990) and are now commercially available. Examples can be found at http://www.invivodata.com, a clinical trials service provider; and at http://www.pendragonsoftware.com, a software manufacturer that generates electronic surveys, field databases, and diaries for PDAs.

With improvements in hardware and software and a growing number of published studies on the use of electronic patient diaries, more and more pharmaceutical companies are adopting electronic patient diary technology for clinical trials. A major reason for the marked increase in the use of this technology is the consensus among researchers and the Federal Drug Administration that paper diaries do not yield accurate data. More advanced versions even collect physiological data concurrently (see, e.g., http://www.vivometrics.com).

Electronic diaries can expose precursors of transient clinical episodes, as in eating disorders, anxiety disorders, and addictive disorders (Kenardy, Fried, Kraemer, & Taylor, 1992). Clinically important antecedents are often unreported by the retrospective narratives of clients but can become quite clear when information is systematically elicited within problematic situations. Electronic diaries can be more accurate, complete, and accessible than their paper-and-pencil counterpart in the following ways:

- Electronic diaries may be filled out immediately and not after the fact, thus bypassing retrospective memory biases.
- Entries are automatically time-stamped and are not subject to retrospective alteration ("cheating"), thus providing a detailed record of compliance.
- Respondents' input can be checked for completeness and reasonableness interactively during data entry. For example, missing or contradictory entries and ratings outside of the scale's range can be queried again.
- Queries and their frequency can be programmed to adjust to response patterns. For example, when monitoring panic attacks, it might be useful to increase the

frequency of queries during periods of elevated anxiety in order to better capture the time course of the attack. An anxiety level that exceeds a threshold may trigger evaluation of specific bodily symptoms.

- An electronic diary may (or may not) be more private than a paper-and-pencil one. Privacy and confidentiality are functions of the security precautions to protect any document on the Internet.
- Data can be quickly and accurately downloaded to the professional's computer for immediate graphing and analysis.

The efficiency in data handling compared to the paper-and-pencil method makes electronic diaries especially useful in larger clinical trials. A client's daily experience can be sampled at regular intervals (e.g., hourly with an "alarm clock" feature to remind the client). Such biopsies can also be triggered by a quasi-random signal to obtain a representative sample of a client's momentary states, because the client cannot anticipate the timing of the signal. Alternatively, clients can be instructed to make entries immediately after a defined clinical event (e.g., a panic attack, nail biting, or an intense worry episode).

The electronic diary method has its disadvantages as well:

- It may be more costly than the paper-and-pencil approach if equipment and setup expenses cannot be amortized across many clients.
- Programming an electronic diary for a specific diagnosis may be difficult and thus may be best suited for research studies of many clients with the same diagnosis. Although they offer useful and otherwise lost information, diaries present problems that are not easily remedied by computerization. Specifically, electronic diaries produce a large amount of data and require special logistical and interpretive skills from professionals. Such diaries also typically demand effort, honesty, and cooperation from clients.
- Certain clinical groups may have difficulty with electronic diary assessment (e.g., audible prompts may be overheard at work, and screen contents may be illegible to elderly or visually impaired clients).
- Clients may be reluctant to use technology or find it intrusive. Some clients may resist using an electronic device in public or may be unable to operate it.

A digital voice recorder can be added to a PDA to collect complex annotations and remarks that would be difficult to capture by structured input menus or by writing on a touch-screen (see, e.g., http://www.admobis.com). Data collection similar to electronic diaries can be achieved by using cellular or mobile telephones. A computer can dial a telephone at regular intervals to collect information from patients through an automated voice response system (as discussed in the next section of this chapter). Patients can also be asked to call in at regular intervals. One advantage of having the computer call a mobile telephone is that professionals can assume that it is the patient who is responding; no elaborate password-mediated sign-in procedure is required. However, automation of this sort still has problems, particularly when the call is intermittently severed as the user is moving in and out of an area with adequate signal strength. Researchers have struggled with the convenience of such systems versus the participant's objections to being asked to respond to a mobile phone that terminates the call and then rings again to resume the sequence of questions from the beginning rather than at the point of interruption.

When initiated by a therapist instead of a computer, on-the-spot phone assessment can be easily integrated into remote psychotherapy, as, for example, when supervising self-exposure trials as part of homework assignments in the treatment of phobias.

Interactive Voice Response Systems

Clinical rating scales and structured interviews can be delivered via interactive voice response (IVR) systems to allow computer-based assessment of clients' mood and symptoms via regular telephone lines. IVR technology, which is commonly used with voice-mail systems, has been expanded to conduct clinical telephone interviewing by computer. IVR interview systems can be installed on a centralized computer that users can dial toll-free anytime and, with a mobile phones, from any location.

This technology extends the reach of practitioners and can facilitate longitudinal monitoring of patients without requiring office visits to collect data. IVR applications increase the accessibility of information to the clinician and thus may improve the quality of patient care through more informed decision making.

IVR typically presents preprogrammed questions using digitized human speech. The system waits for clients to respond by keypad to indicate yes (1), no (0), or to type in a number—for example, the number of clinical episodes or the severity of a symptom. Many systems do not require touch-tone phones; they can recognize the voice input. These systems can also record entire sentences for later retrieval by practitioners. IVR interviews can be programmed to skip and branch depending on the input, to provide immediate feedback to clients, to accumulate data and prepare computer reports, and/or even to alert a clinician by beeper if necessary (Greist, Jefferson, & Wenzel et al., 1997).

An IVR interview has been successfully applied to monitor symptom severity in patients with obsessive-compulsive disorder (OCD; Baer, Brown-Beasley, Sorce, & Henriques, 1993). Scores derived with this system agree well with scores from human administration of the assessment scales by telephone and paper-and-pencil scales returned by mail. Results indicate that this approach provides reliable, low-cost, and instantaneous data acquisition. IVR has been used in conjunction with a self-exposure treatment program for OCD to monitor patient progress at their homes (Marks, Shaw, & Parkin, 1998). Of the 63 participants who used the program, 84% completed the self-assessment module. Participants initiated most calls outside usual office hours. Completion of the self-assessment predicted later improvement with self-exposure treatment.

IVR reporting proved superior to the usual retrospective query method for monitoring binge eating. In a study of 43 subjects, significantly more binge episodes were described using an IVR system than were mentioned in a subsequent Timeline Follow-Back interview covering the same 12-week period (Bardone, Krahn, Goodman, & Searles, 2000). IVR technology has also shown promise in general clinical screening for mental disorders. A computer-assisted telephone-administered version of the Primary Care Evaluation of Mental Disorders (IVR-PRIME-MD) was compared with clinician administration, and both were compared to a clinician-administered Structured Clinical Interview for DSM-IV (SCID) (Kobak et al., 1997b) in 200 outpatients. The authors concluded that the high agreement between methods supports the IVR-PRIME-MD as a valid instrument for making treatment decisions with primary care patients. An IVR interview for screening for mental disorders uses a 26-item scale that takes only about 5 minutes to administer and has shown high agreement with the written version (Leon et al., 1999).

One technology leader in this arena is Healthcare Technology Systems, founded by pioneers in the exploration of its use in clinical studies (http://www.healthtechsys.com).

Advances in speech recognition technologies are making possible significant improvement in the management of chronic diseases, medication use, and monitoring for adverse events. For instance, Gerene Schmidt, founder of (SB&E), conducted a study in 1997 at the Spokane Heart Institute to gather clinical data from 1,515 patients with congestive heart failure to explore the accuracy and user acceptability of an automated telephone monitoring system. Accuracy averaged nearly 95%, and two thirds of the users said that they would welcome regular use of the system.

Schmidt believes that telephone monitoring of mental health status can contribute to preventing acute episodic illness by adapting clinical protocols to an automated telephone dialogue. We are working on the development of other chronic disease systems that will allow patients to be closely monitored by telephone or any digital communication device, such as pagers, instant messaging, e-mail, or PDAs. Physicians will receive alerts when their patients' monitoring levels or symptoms are out of an acceptable range. We are also developing programs to integrate digital output of monitoring devices into the patient record as part of the monitoring process.

—**Mark Lediard**
Consultant
Science Business and Education, Inc.

The COPE program is a fully self-administered self-care program using cognitive-behavioral interventions for the treatment of mild to moderate depression. In its current implementation, it is not Internet based. Rather, it uses a computer-aided IVR system that can be accessed via regular telephone lines. We focus on this program here because it contains several groundbreaking ideas on how IVR can bridge assessment and treatment. The fact that this program can be implemented on an Internet Web site illustrates how the distinction between regular telephone calls and Internet use will become fluid as the information superhighway infrastructure expands (Gates, Myhrvold, & Rinearson, 1995).

The COPE program was developed by an international team of researchers, including Deborah Osgood-Hynes, Lee Baer, and Isaac Marks in association with John Greist of Healthcare Technology Systems, LLC, in Madison, Wisconsin, to provide fully automated treatment to depressed patients. The program has IVR technology and the Parameter Driven Interview Driver™ software at its core, installed on a centralized computer that can be dialed toll-free at any time, and by cell phones, from any location. The software presents information and questions to clients by playing prerecorded voice files over the telephone (selected from a set of more than 700 text segments). Clients answer questions by pressing the numbers on the telephone keypad; the computer responds with prerecorded voice messages that depend on the specific answer.

Here is an example of how COPE works:

During a call, clients may be prompted to select a statement from a list of negative thoughts they say to themselves. The list includes such statements as "I am worthless," "Making mistakes is terrible," "I have made a mess of my life," or "I can never control my emotions." After clients select a statement by keypad, the computer asks them to come up with constructive thoughts. Then COPE provides constructive thoughts and asks clients to compare these to their own. If "I can never control my emotions" was selected, COPE provides the following constructive thoughts: "At times, my feelings can seem out of control, but I've learned some skills I can use to help me feel more in control of my emotions and more in control of what I choose to do. No one can control all their thoughts all the time, but I can practice ways to change my thinking from negative to constructive, and this will help me feel more in control. And is it really true that I can never control my emotions? No. I can think about the times when I do have better control over my emotions."

The efficacy and acceptability of the COPE self-help system were evaluated in 41 depressed patients from the United States and England during a 12-week treatment (Osgood-Hynes et al., 1998). The efficacy and acceptability of the telephone-based COPE were comparable to other established therapies. Expectation of effectiveness and time spent making COPE calls correlated positively with improvement over 12 weeks. As a safety measure, suicidal patients were excluded. The version of COPE commercially available through the Internet (http://www.healthtechsys.com/products/edcare_cope.html), lets clients choose a male or female voice.

Clinical Decision Support

Of particular interest to mental health professionals is the emerging area of clinical decision support, in which computerized assessment, treatment planning, and practitioner selection all come together in new and very exciting ways (Health Informatics, 2004). Although such support is not available to the solo practitioner, knowledge of this burgeoning area may help practitioners who work for managed care organizations. These and other large organizations will undoubtedly be using such software in the near future, if they already do not.

Decision-support software in mental health brings together information about optimal treatment assessment, planning, and practitioner selection, it also fits into the U.S. government's overall goal of developing computerized patient records (CPRs) to meet the needs of all health care practitioners. True, CPRs for mental health are not yet widely used. Although some practice management software companies identified in chapter 8 are touting inclusion of electronic patient records in their software, the full functionality to be delivered by computerized patient records is still on the horizon. Nonetheless, significant progress is being made on one aspect of the CPR as defined by the Institute of Medicine (Institute of Medicine, 1997).

For now, let's look at an area that is gaining increasing attention—clinical decision support. Several researchers from around the world are creating a tidal wave in mental health treatment research. The next section discusses how this research has evolved and, more important, what it means for practitioners in the immediate future.

Mental health practitioners daily make decisions about treatment planning, treatment modification, or treatment termination and referral. Protocols for empirically based treatment are surfacing from various specialty associations and organizations, workshop presenters, and conferences. When shopping for therapists, patients are requesting more information about the treatments being offered. Patients want to know more about the choices they have, particularly when treatment has not gone well with another therapist, is not going well in the current therapy, or when they are overtly dissatisfied and considering termination of their own accord. Patients may soon be able to access Web sites that assist with these types of decisions (Majeski, 2003).

Decisions related to treatment assignment, modification of treatment plans, and optimal termination and referral are issues that sometimes plague practitioners as well. Errors in decision making can have negative consequences for the patient, as well as for the practitioner. These important issues have not traditionally been well addressed by the research community despite valiant attempts with both efficacy research (Kendall, 1998; Lambert & Bergin, 1994; Lipsey & Wilson, 1993; Smith, Glass, & Miller, 1980) and effectiveness research (Mintz, Drake, & Crits-Christoph, 1996).

More recently, patient-focused research is being considered as a possible bridge between mental health treatment research and practice (Chambless & Ollendick, 2001; Lambert, Hansen, & Finch, 2001). Decision-support technology is an outgrowth of patient-focused research, with emphasis on monitoring the progress of individual patients. The patient-focused research approach asks individuals to complete standardized tests, from which the expected outcome can be established for each individual. Progress over time is analyzed for each patient, using statistical regression techniques in the context of normative data for groups of individuals with the same diagnosis and healthy comparison groups. Compared to the improvement rates of similar groups of clients, recovery curves can be calculated at any time during treatment. Clinicians can then interpret any deviation from expected progress. Some patients may be ahead of their expected recovery rates; others may be behind. Early recovery may suggest the opportunity for early termination or the time to begin treatment for a secondary problem. If a patient's progress is slower than expected, there may be a need for a change in treatment strategy or an outside referral to a specialist. Research advances have allowed researchers to define clinically meaningful change judging whether treatment has led to satisfactory progress in treatment (Kendall, Marrs-Garcia, Nath, & Sheldrick, 1999; Tingey, Lambert, Burlingame, & Hansen, 1996).

Although several research groups are working on decision-support programs, five research programs are worth mentioning in this context. References and brief descriptions are provided for the interested reader:

- Since 1990, a project started by the late Ken Howard is ongoing at Northwestern University and affiliated institutions. His colleagues and successors have continued his work on this, the oldest and best established, patient-focused research program. It is a patient-tracking system used mostly outside the United States. Eli Lilly and Company offered it free to primary care practitioners as a screening tool. It has been researched widely across other countries as well (Lueger et al., 2001).

- Michael J. Lambert, of Brigham Young University, has developed a symptom- and problem-orientated measure that, taken at various times, tracks and measures change and gives feedback to the clinician about treatment efficacy (Lambert et al., 2001).

- In Stuttgart, Germany, practitioners are creating computer software to identify patients in need of additional treatment, thus helping clinicians focus more directly on case conceptualization. This software uses established measures so a clinician can pick any one of a variety of measures (Kordy, Hannover, & Richard, 2001).

- Michael Barkham, from the United Kingdom, does not create a projection of change but measures symptoms at a specific time. He presents his work within the British health care system (Barkham et al., 2001).

- Larry E. Beutler's systematic treatment selection (STS) system grew from the seminal work of Beutler and Clarkin (Beutler & Clarkin, 1990). Their measure of assessment seeks to match specific treatment modalities with individual patients before monitoring the effects of treatment. They developed their program based on specific algorithms.

Because Beutler's system is the most complex and has benefited from extensive computerization, it is detailed here. As a computer-interactive, clinician-based measure of behavior, the STS is designed to both track patient progress and help clinicians develop effective treatment plans. The STS is based on the conclusion that patient factors interact with type of treatment. In other words, the STS is based on the premise that patients respond differently to different kinds of treatment as a function of their own response and coping styles.

The researchers demonstrate their premise by citing the example of treating 100 randomly selected moderately depressed people with similar socioeconomic status characteristics, all with Beck Depression Inventory (BDI) scores of 20 to 25, given by 10 experienced clinicians with the same experience and education level. If the patients were randomly assigned to clinicians so that each had 10 clients and all patients were given the same treatment, there would be significant improvement over time in the mean of the BDI across weeks. However, a look at each patient individually reveals considerable variation across those 20 weeks. Why is that? Could the patients all be considered to have had the same type of depression if considerable variation existed across 20 weeks?

Beutler and his associate, Oliver Williams, examined this situation further and concluded that successful outcome can be better predicted by matching a therapist and patient to a specific manualized treatment, based on patient characteristics and not diagnosis characteristics. These patient characteristics include:

- The individual's distress (motivational distress) at any given time.
- The patient's complexity (one who experiences depression as a situational event, such as bereavement or separation or recent relationship demise versus someone who is chronically depressed with many types of issues). In one case, we have a situational, acute problem; in other cases, we have someone who is complex.
- The individual's resistance or reactance. Reactance is a constellation of parameters that define patient autonomy, need to control, opposition, passive-aggressiveness, antiauthoritarianism, and competition. These types of continua more or less determine how directive or nondirective the therapist can be. Therapists tend to be constant once they start with an approach.
- The individual's coping style, internalizing to externalizing. For example, some people cope with anxiety by externalizing, acting out, using aggressive behavior, blaming, projecting, or developing somatic complaints. Other people cope by internalizing; they may ruminate, control, compartmentalize, or worry. The more externalizing someone is, the more he or she may benefit from a therapy approach that is behaviorally oriented; someone who is more internalizing is often a better fit with a therapy approach that is more insight oriented.

Along these four dimensions, the STS identifies the principles of change that best fit each patient's style. That is, the STS fits classes of interventions to patient qualities, on the assumption that the greatest power is at the level of what the therapist does, not the particular model to which he or she subscribes. This is at a more specific level than are treatment manuals, but it also is more general in the sense that the STS treatment planning is based on a set of optimized principles of change that cut across manuals and models.

Translated, this means that the STS goes beyond merely suggesting that Aaron Beck's cognitive treatment (CT) is the most appropriate. The STS isolates which aspects of that approach are responsible for the particular fit. For example, among externalizing patients, any set of procedures that tend to be symptom focused and skill focused seems more advantageous than procedures that focus on insight or awareness. Thus, behavior therapy procedures and interpersonal therapy (IPT) procedures, as well as CT procedures, may be effective. For internalizers, procedures that foster awareness, self-understanding, and insight seem to work best. Thus, Beutler talks about classes or families of interventions. A manual for how to implement these interventions is incorporated into the STS system (Beutler & Harwood, 2000).

For more information, see Beutler and Clarkin (1990); Beutler and Williams (1995); and Fisher, Beutler, and Williams (1999). For guidelines related to the treatment of depressed patients, see Beutler, Clarkin, and Bongar (2000). For a recent paper on personality assessment, see Beutler and Groth-Marnat (2003).

The elements that Beutler's system tracks require time-intensive analysis. Researchers of decision support, then, have turned to computerization to help improve clinical treatment. Computerization of patient-focused research in large health care settings has been developed and empirically validated. Clinical decision-support computer systems are now available for practitioners in a variety of settings. When it makes a projection, the STS doesn't simply do it on the average outpatient, but rather on the basis of the patients most similar to this patient. This comparison can be done on the clinic level, regional level, or national or international level; it can also be done through the Web (http://test6.graphxink.com), where all data available are entered into a database and the computer extracts the patients most similar to a particular patient, based on dimensions more relevant than diagnosis. These other dimensions might include gender, severity of the problem, personality characteristics, the complexity and chronicity of problems, level of social support, and age.

When using the Web, patients calls their health management organization (HMO), which connects them to the computer STS. It asks questions through an aural (vocal) component, and the patients answer yes or no by voice or keypad. The entire process takes 10 to 15 minutes. A complete treatment plan is written and goes into a database, which searches to find the most appropriate therapist for that particular patient. The even draws a graph over time, stating that if the patient is matched with a particular therapist, the patient can expect a 42% improvement rate over 10 weeks, for example. If the program cannot find a match within 5 to 10 miles of the patient's residence, then video teleconferencing to an optimally matched therapist would be appropriate.

The patient visits the doctor, who has received the treatment plan from the HMO. The treatment plan suggests the issues to focus on, the length of treatment to be expected, whether to use medication, and whether hospitalization might be needed. If the doctor wants to claim payment, he or she logs on to the Web site, provides the authorization number for the patient, and completes an update for that session. The secured Internet connection does not exchange names at any time.

The STS is being used in San Juan, Argentina; Barcelona, Spain; Las Vegas, Nevada; Santa Barbara, California, and several other locations to track patient change over time. In these settings, the STS provides a description of treatment, including an example of treatment, and a projection of change for such problems as depression, anxiety, chemical abuse, general psychiatry, relationship, work, and retirement issues.

Although first evaluations justify the use of computerized assessment methods, much more research is needed to establish the specific benefits of and barriers to the various modalities. Furthermore, as with conventional assessment methods, computer-generated information needs to be placed within the context of the client's overall life situation. It is the practitioner's responsibility to be aware of a test's validity, to understand the methods by which computer-based interpretations are derived, and to determine the applicability of the test within a specific context. Until clear guidelines are established, practitioners need to be cautious when using computer-assisted assessments in their practice. The following chapter describes the next logical step in computerizing a clinical practice: using computers to support therapeutic services to clients.

7

Computer-Aided Psychotherapy

The controversy and derision associated with computerized forms of psychotherapy are almost as old as George Orwell's (1949) classic book *1984*, and the two are often compared. The 1980s have come and gone, making Orwell's projections of dystopia seem a bit naive yet still somehow relevant. The same might be said of many early conceptualizations of computerized psychotherapy. To the relief of many clinicians whose livelihoods depend on the practice of psychotherapy, the state of the art with respect to psychotherapy is computer-aided and not computer-replaced treatment.

BENEFITS OF COMPUTER-AIDED PSYCHOTHERAPY

Known as "therapy-support programs," or more popularly, "therapy extenders," most computer-aided psychotherapy programs are still in the developmental stage. Some have been launched and reported in the scientific literature, but few have yet been thoroughly evaluated. Preliminary indications are that outcomes with computer-based interventions may be comparable to in-person therapy (Jacobs et al., 2001). This chapter discusses many of these new applications. Most computerized therapy programs on the open marketplace are stand-alone applications running on individual personal computers. Some of the programs available in the marketplace are discussed in chapter 13, as part of our detailing of the Online Clinical Practice Management model.

Most of this technology developed as stand-alone applications probably will be available within the next 5 to 10 years through the Internet. In fact, distributors will most likely rely at least partially on the Internet for sales, as this is the best worldwide distribution channel. The global distribution of computer-aided psychotherapy programs raises a number of multicultural and multilingual challenges, however. Web consumers may not always be in the best position to determine how to interact with materials developed for specific cultural or linguistic groups. Nonetheless, practitioners are also likely to depend increasingly on the Internet for various functions related to the delivery of services to mental health patients, including the upgrading of programs, knowledge supplementation, record storage, sophisticated data analysis, and direct delivery of services.

Ken Weingardt is a clinical psychologist investigating how the field of instructional design and technology can be used to transform empirically validated treatment manuals into interactive, media-rich Web applications. After several years working in the online learning industry, he shares his view of this emerging field:

Although a Web application for guided self-change is no substitute for a traditional, in-person psychotherapeutic relationship, I believe that this type of resource has tremendous potential to serve as an effective and engaging adjunct to therapy. Even though much of the psychological literature over the past 2 decades has empirically validated the use of cognitive-behavioral therapy (CBT) and skills-based interventions, much of this work doesn't find its way into day-to-day clinical practice. One reason for this may be that practicing therapists don't have time to learn about these new therapies. Another reason may be that more pressing emotional issues often surface during the therapy sessions, pushing the CBT work to the back burner. And finally, let's be honest, running through the same structured exercises over and over isn't the most interesting way to spend clinical time.

Using the processes and tools of instructional design and technology, psychologists can create instructionally sound online interventions that efficiently teach clients the knowledge and skills that they need, leaving us with more time to concentrate on the myriad of other tasks that psychotherapy involves.

— Ken Weingardt, Ph.D.
Center for Health Care Evaluation
Veteran's Administration Palo Alto Health Care System
Stanford University School of Medicine

Although many of Weingardt's applications are available through the Web, they are not yet accessible to the general public. Therefore, to help readers understand the benefits of referring their patients to self-instructional programs on the Internet, he has contributed this fictionalized account of a client's potential experience with a self-guided Web-based program:

Mark P. was referred to my private practice by his managed care company immediately following the loss of his job. He is a 46-year-old married Asian American engineer who lives and works in Santa Clara, California, and he had been employed for the past 23 years by the same Silicon Valley technology company. Throughout the 1980s and 1990s, he gradually worked his way up through the ranks from manufacturing engineer to managing a design team working on the next generation of computer processors.

During our initial session, Mark shared his initial reaction to being laid off last week: "When they came around and told me I had to clear out of my cube by noon, I just completely fell apart." It took several days for the initial shock to wear off, after which he found himself getting extremely angry. In his words, "My entire life revolved around that company, and then one day, poof! It's all gone. What gives them the right to do that to someone?"

I spent the first three sessions with Mark establishing rapport, doing my standard intake, some short-term crisis management, and giving him the space he needed to vent his feelings of anger and loss. It didn't take very long to see that he was a highly intelligent, well-adjusted individual with no preexisting psychopathology. His long and profitable career had just been abruptly derailed, and he was in the process of experiencing some predictable, though extremely unpleasant, emotions as he negotiated this major life adjustment.

Toward the end of our fourth session, I let Mark know about a Web application that I had helped develop. We designed it for people who were in similar situations to his own—folks going through a major life transition. "It's normal to have trouble adjusting to a major change," I began. "Whether its a negative change, such as getting laid off, or a positive change, such as getting married or buying a new home, you need a similar set of interpersonal and self-management skills to make the most of your situation. These skills are things like learning how to be an effective communicator, how to be resilient and bounce back from setbacks, how to become more flexible—that sort of thing."

Mark seemed receptive to the idea of using this application, so I brought it up on my office computer and gave him a quick overview: "For each skill, there are three or four interactive exercises you can complete. Some exercises involve watching a video role-play and answering questions about it; others ask you to identify a challenge that you've really been wrestling with and lead you through the process of breaking it down into concrete, specific goals that you can accomplish in a limited amount of time. So—does this sound like something you're interested in checking out?" With a less than enthusiastic "I guess it can't hurt," Mark went home with a URL, user ID, and password.

Mark appeared for our next session with a sheaf of papers in his hand. He had printed out some of the online change management exercises from the program. "Ken, this Web thing is really interesting, but it brought up some serious questions for me. Can we talk about them now?"

"Absolutely!" I said with a smile, thinking that this was exactly how I hoped he would react to the experience. We could now use the session to work through some of the emotions and thoughts that the exercises had stirred up and decide how best to use both our time together and the online resources to help Mark get his career (and his mental health) back on track.

— Ken Weingardt, Ph.D.
Center for Health Care Evaluation
Veteran's Administration Palo Alto Health Care System
Stanford University School of Medicine

Dr. Weingardt has illustrated how a program can take on specifically selected elements of the therapeutic process. Cognitive behavior therapy in particular is one approach replete with linear processes that a computer could teach, such as relaxation training, systematic desensitization, developing thought records, and challenging negative thoughts. The vignette shows how ongoing contact with a clinician is essential to making best use of the computerized program. Such adjunctive programs are discussed in more detail later in this chapter.

BARRIERS TO COMPUTER-AIDED PSYCHOTHERAPY

A common criticism of computer-assisted therapy is that it may alienate clients. Research (e.g., Cavanagh, Zack, & Shapiro, 2003; Ghosh, Mclaren, & Watson, 1997; Yellowlees, 2003) indicates the opposite: the accessibility and privacy of computerized interventions can enhance client comfort and receptivity. A comparison of standard in-person therapies with computerized therapies also shows that dropout rates do not differ (e.g., Carr, Ghosh, & Marks, 1988; Newman, Kenardy, Herman, & Taylor, 1997).

There are serious cautions regarding the use of computer-aided assessment (discussed in the previous chapter) and computer-aided treatment. At this early stage of exploration, practitioners might optimistically assume that empirical validation of treatments justifies using computerized versions of them in clinical practice as long as the procedures are inexpensive, easy to disseminate, and do not cause harm when in a supplemental role. However, this view assumes that a computer implementation of a successful in-person treatment modality will not degrade outcome. For all we know, however, much of the effectiveness of mental health treatment may be a nonspecific result of interpersonal exchanges that are not addressed by formal descriptions of treatment and that are not even mentioned, let alone captured, in the protocols of manualized treatment approaches. Furthermore, professionals are highly adaptive to the specific needs and personalities of clients, whereas computer programs are typically more rigid. This inflexibility can lead to poor compliance or premature treatment termination in some cases.

Computerizing aspects of psychotherapy raises other problems. In the event of a lawsuit, all data collected by desktop, laptop, or handheld computer or Internet-based programs are likely to be discoverable. That is, the plaintiff may be able to learn about these data and obtain printed copies of them. The presence of these data may legally oblige the practitioner to be aware of them all and to have considered all the information in making a decision. To strain a metaphor, discovery of the material can result in a field day for Monday-morning quarterbacks.[1] Apart from cost-effectiveness issues discoverable information, raises the question of how technology might place new burdens on practitioners, thereby creating the health care equivalent of an unfunded mandate.

Similarly, the issue of informed consent may also arise. Before exposing the patient to a computerized therapy, did the clinician ensure that the patient understood the risks and benefits of such therapy? In the United States, the practitioner's obligation to disclose information is governed by case law. In some states, the practitioner has a duty to reveal whatever the patient subjectively might want to know. In these states, it is easy for dissatisfied patient–plaintiffs to claim that whatever they were told was not a sufficient response to their questions. In some states, the practitioner is obliged to reveal what reasonable patients in similar circumstances would want or need to know even if they had not explicitly asked. The best approach, from a practitioner's perspective, is to reveal to a patient whatever reasonably prudent practitioners in the same geographic on local community would reveal under similar circumstances.

As is true with other theories of tort liability, a plaintiff alleging lack of informed consent must prove that lack of consent caused actual harm. In some states, the test of causation is whether the particular patients (plaintiffs) would have declined the proposed intervention had they known of the risk allegedly not revealed. Like the subjective test of disclosure previously described, this test is subject to manipulation; plaintiffs can always claim that had they known of Risk X, they never would have agreed to the procedure. Again, there is a more rational, objective approach to the causation question: Would a reasonable patient, advised of the risk allegedly not disclosed, have nevertheless agreed to the procedure? Legal systems around the world have yet to answer these and similar questions.

With any unbounded excitement somewhat abated by the realities of the challenges to computer-aided psychotherapy, we now discuss some of the most notable developments in computer-aided psychotherapy—guidance and psychoeducation as applied to psychiatric problems, habit disorders, and health promotion. Before delving into modern computer-aided psychotechnologies, however, we look at the predecessors

---

[1] Ready access to extensive raw detail can encourage critics to second-guess the therapist.

of many modern-day technologies—ELIZA, PLATO-DCS, psychoeducational programs, therapeutic computer games, and the Therapeutic Learning Program.

HISTORICAL ROOTS

In the 1970s and 1980s, society moved from the industrial age to the information age with the invention and widespread adoption of inexpensive microcomputers to perform both routine and specialized tasks. Researchers and mental health therapists began seeking ways to increase efficiency by using these microcomputers. The first applications included unstructured therapeutic interventions, personality testing, and career guidance (Alpert, Pulvino, & Lee, 1985). ELIZA was the first use of computers for therapeutic purposes, although it was not intended as such. Joseph Weizenbaum, ELIZA's developer, was not a clinician; nor was he attempting to develop a treatment protocol. Rather, he was trying to show that computers cannot conduct psychotherapy. He was surprised to learn that his secretary was using ELIZA during her lunch hour for personal treatment sessions. We begin our discussion with ELIZA.

ELIZA

In 1966, Joseph Weizenbaum, a researcher at the Massachusetts Institute of Technology, introduced ELIZA, the first and perhaps the most famous computerized therapy program (Weizenbaum, 1966). His objective was to develop software that would respond to natural written language and simulate client-centered therapy (Cabaniss, 2001). The program simplistically emulated therapy by merely forming questions from words used by "patients," with special twists on words that matched those in its internal dictionary. Even today, the concept of a machine "comprehending" anything remains philosophically undefined and a matter of dispute. Weizenbaum knew better than to aim for ELIZA's understanding of anything. Rather, he attempted to get the machine to parse natural language accurately and to recognize key terms. He did not work on assessment of context or recognition of recurrent themes, as newer versions of ELIZA are able to do. Surprisingly, early users of this program seemed to respond well (Weizenbaum, 1976). Internet users can still consult with ELIZA at http://www-ai.ijs.si/eliza/eliza.html.

A typical ELIZA dialogue could go something like this:

ELIZA: How do you do. Please state your problem.
PATIENT: Men are all alike.
ELIZA: Would you like it if they were not all alike?
PATIENT: No, I guess not. But my husband is a real nerd.
ELIZA: Your husband is a real nerd?
PATIENT: Yes, he's constantly sitting at his computer and doesn't seem to care about me anymore.
ELIZA: Do computers worry you?
PATIENT: No, but my husband should pay more attention to me.
ELIZA: Your husband should pay more attention to you?
PATIENT: Well, I'd like to go out with him more.
ELIZA: Please go on.
PATIENT: At the time we married, we were always doing a lot of great stuff together, and now things have changed.

ELIZA: Can you think of a specific example?
PATIENT: For example, we used to go hiking together almost every weekend.
ELIZA: What does that suggest to you?
PATIENT: Maybe my husband doesn't love me anymore.
ELIZA: You don't seem quite certain.
PATIENT: Well, he sometimes tells me he loves me, but I think he's lying.
ELIZA: Please go on.

Early attempts by Weizenbaum and others ultimately led to a consensus that computers could not replace a nondirective therapist (Colby, Watt, & Gilbert, 1966). Computer systems could not deal with the ambiguity, complexity, idiosyncrasy, emotional connotation, and social context of natural language occurring in the psychotherapeutic process (Murphy & Pardeck, 1988). For instance, such expressions as "A cat's got my tongue" were often taken literally by the program. Weizenbaum (1976) also voiced pragmatic and ethical concerns about what he called the illusion of understanding.

Despite these misgivings, software is being developed to parse natural language accurately into parts of speech in order to facilitate entry of handwritten and spoken data into automated systems (Markoff, 2002).

PLATO–DCS

More than a decade after ELIZA's debut, Programmed Logic for Automatic Teaching Operations–Dilemma Counseling System (PLATO–DCS) was introduced as an interactive computer program to teach problem-solving skills to clients (Wagman & Kerber, 1980). PLATO–DCS is based on the assumption that most problems can be considered dilemmas in which one must choose between two undesirable alternatives.

This computer counseling was as effective as standard counseling for dilemma type problems with a large sample of students (Wagman, 1982). Of course, failure to find a difference is not proof of effectiveness. In any case, many students preferred working with the computer to seeing a counselor. Unfortunately, study of this program was not systematically expanded beyond student samples in order to identify characteristics of clinical populations that would benefit. For an in-depth description and discussion of PLATO–DCS, see Wagman (1988).

The progress in the dialogue of ELIZA depended on the user, with the program reacting in an essentially passive manner by issuing prompts for the user to continue. PLATO–DCS brought into the discussion between computer–therapist and client a structure intended to organize the target problem in a way that could lead to a solution. In part, this approach to computerizing therapy was selected because of conceptual difficulties in operationalizing therapeutic techniques (Selmi, Klein, Greist, Sorrell, & Erdman, 1990). Developments in cognitive-behavioral therapy for depression suggested ways that computers could more actively bring informational content, in addition to structuring exchanges, into the therapeutic dialogue. In particular, demonstrating the efficacy of cognitive-behavioral protocols (Miller & Berman, 1983) encouraged controlled experimental comparison of computer-aided therapy, with a trained professional delivering treatment.

Psychoeducational Programs

The late 1980s saw the first computer-assisted psychoeducational programs for preventing dysfunctional health-related behaviors or promoting positive health behaviors. Such programs often use guided-learning principles established in educational psychology (Kulik & Kulik, 1991). Examples include computer-assisted programs for drug and alcohol abuse prevention (Moncher, Parms, Orlandi, & Schinke, 1989), promotion of responsible sexual behavior (Kann, 1987), and enhancement of self-esteem (Robertson, Ladewig, Strickland, & Boschung, 1987). A comprehensive educational computer program covering five health areas (alcohol and other drugs, human sexuality, smoking prevention and cessation, stress management, and diet and exercise) was effective in a large sample of adolescents in providing confidential, nonjudgmental health information, behavioral change strategies, and sources of referral (Hawkins, Gustafson, Chewning, & Bosworth, 1987).

Computer Games

At about the time that psychoeducational and other programs appeared, computer games became available. Their potential as therapeutic tools inspired a series of empirical studies. Ultima, one of the first therapeutic graphical fantasy games, was designed to stimulate persistence and to decrease impulsivity in children with behavioral problems (Allen, 1984). The child selected a character to be challenged with obstacles and dangers along the path to a castle containing a princess perpetually in need of rescue. The game rewarded functional behaviors and discouraged dysfunctional behaviors. As in conventional play therapy, children developed coping strategies that the therapist then related to real-life situations.

Clarke and Schoech (1983, 1994) describe a similar game for impulse control in adolescents. The player took the role of commander of a small force on a quest to recover a lost crown, necessitating facing dragons and other obstacles. Problem-solving skills, such as goal orientation and careful planning, were rewarded. No controlled studies were published on Ultima, but this and similar programs led to the development of many other programs for children, teens, and adults.

Therapeutic Learning Program

The Therapeutic Learning Program (TLP), developed by Colby, Gould, and Aronson (1989), adds computer interaction to direct contact with a therapist in a group setting. The TLP is a structured, 10-session computer-based treatment designed to help clients counter self-doubts that interfere with personal development (Gould, 1990, 1996a).

The TLP applies Gould's theory of adult development (Gould, 1978) to unearth "hot spots," whereby what first appears to be an adaptive need in fact arises from a developmental issue that arouses, or threatens to arouse, emotionality. Intervention aims not at simple support or exploration of historical meaning but at clarifying the current meaning of key actions a person fears to undertake and encouraging the patient to go ahead, do what works, and thus unblock natural psychological developmental processes (R. Gould, personal communication, May 29, 2001).

Of a large sample of patients in a managed care setting, two thirds reported general reduction in distress with the TLP, and nearly all acknowledged improvement in their ability to handle the identified problem (Colby et al., 1989). Recently, the TLP achieved gains similar to those of traditional individual psychotherapy in a controlled experimental study of 90 clients with a variety of problems (Jacobs et al., 2001). The TLP has pioneered the path for other effective programs. The next section samples some of these interactive programs and points to their clinical utility.

APPLICATIONS OF COMPUTER-AIDED PSYCHOTHERAPY

Early experiments with computers helped set the stage for currently available software. To help the reader understand both the hardware and the software aspects of this material, the remainder of this section organizes clinically relevant programs first at the level of hardware (desktop, handheld, or wearable computerized devices) and then, within each category, the clinical problems addressed by samples of the software programs shown effective through clinical trials.

The boundaries have become fluid. Software programs are typically developed for desktop computers, and then special applications are often developed for handheld computer devices, the Internet, or both. Most programs developed today will soon migrate to the larger audience made available by the Internet. The next section of this chapter acquaints the reader with several desktop computer software programs.

Desktop Computers

Social stigma, geographical distance, financial limitations, inconvenient timing, lack of child care, and physical or emotional disability, such as agoraphobia, are some obstacles preventing people from seeking professional help. In response, manuals, videos, and self-help workbooks have been created (Rosen, 1987); self-help has become the largest section in general-purpose bookstores. A review of self-help workbooks by L'Abate (2002b) is a first step in helping professionals identify potential areas that can be adapted to the Web.

An interactive self-help computer program can improve on books by adapting guided learning to the client's input. A meta-analysis found such computer-assisted instruction effective (Kulik & Kulik, 1991). Most such programs aim to help people modify specific behaviors, such as phobic avoidance and smoking, or to control dysfunctional cognitions associated with depression or other maladaptive thought patterns.

Bibliotherapy and video training have become well-accepted therapeutic modalities. Professionals can use the similar but potentially more powerful and flexible therapeutic supplements that computers deliver to augment their practice. Advantages include the client's ability to access the supplements privately in an atmosphere of comfort and safety, the supplements' affordability for single or multiple use, the ease of distribution to multiple locations, and the minimization of scheduling problems for both client and professional. Compared with the "one-size-fits-all" limitation inherent in books and videos, computer programs can query a client for comprehension and repeat misunderstood information in varied ways and with inexhaustible patience.

Although the literature is still relatively recent, a few controlled studies indicate that computer-aided interventions can be effective in treating depression (Selmi et al., 1990) and anxiety disorders (Newman et al., 1997), for general psychiatric disorders (Jacobs et al., 2001), in helping with weight regulation (Taylor, Agras, Losch, & Plante, 1991), and in treating a variety of other medical problems (Lewis, 1999; Noell & Glasgow, 1999). Many researchers have conducted pilot studies of Internet-based educational programs (e.g., DeGuzman & Ross, 1999; Helwig, Lovelle, Guse, & Gottlieb, 1999; Stroem, 2000; Winzelberg et al., 2000) and have reviewed the role of distance writing in computer-assisted interventions (L'Abate, 2001, 2002a). A host of software packages have also passed empirical testing and can be a notable asset to the average clinician's toolkit (Hester & Delaney, 1997; Kobak et al., 1997a).

Psychotherapy Extenders. Recent developments of instructional design and technology (IDT) have led to the creation of self-instructional programs that can be used adjunctively with psychotherapy. This area shows the greatest immediate potential for psychotherapeutic applications of the Internet, pending the arrival of HIPAA-compliant, two-way videoconferencing on the Web.

Stress. Psychiatrist Roger Gould created a commercial Web site (http://www.masteringstress.com) based on the demonstrated success of his Therapeutic Learning Program. The core of the site is a set of interactive modules for PCs, called Solution Sessions; each session takes 20 minutes of a user's time to develop personalized suggestions for dealing with problems the user raises:

> USER: I'm angry when people start going on about their grandchildren.
> COMPUTER: So tell them.
> USER: I can't do that. That's rude.
> COMPUTER: Find a way that's not rude.
> USER: I just can't confront people. Never have.
> COMPUTER: That's the real issue to work on.
> —(R. Gould, personal communication, May 29, 2001)

The Solution Sessions modules were created, revised, and tested in several studies involving more than 20,000 research participants, establishing their scientific validity. On the Mastering Stress Web site, paid subscribers can receive online therapy that includes the modules and consultation sessions with Roger Gould by e-mail. He does not take responsibility for patient care on his Web site and does not keep medical records or collect contact information. The Web site restricts itself to helping people think clearly about the conduct of their lives and recommends "professional therapy and/or counseling" or contacting a physician if necessary.

Mastering Stress is an example of using existing technology to deliver a mental health approach that is solidly grounded on sophisticated theory and research. Thus program does not try to recreate a traditional treatment technique in cyberspace or substitute for professional treatment, yet the edges are a bit blurred, suggesting that Mastering Stress presages the redefinitions of therapy and the roles of therapist and patient.

As will be discussed in chapters 9 and 10, health care professionals risk sanctions by state boards and ethics authorities if they provide treatment where they are not licensed and without some in-person contact with the patient. We also describe professional liability issues raised when a practitioner does not have good contact information and local backup for a patient who develops an unexpected crisis. Merely, making this statement does not eliminate responsibility through the disclaimer that one is not doing "treatment" or "therapy" or functioning as a physician, psychologist, or other practitioner. Ideally, Mastering Stress will not become a test case with regard to these concerns. As for technology, Mastering Stress combines stand-alone computer programs, e-mail, static Web pages, and Web-mediated testing with automated scoring and interpretation (Gould, 1996b, 2001).

Anxiety. Exposure to an irrationally feared object or situation is an effective pathway to ameliorating a phobia (Barlow, 1988). FearFighter was developed through collaboration with Isaac Marks, long a leader in clinical anxiety research (Marks, 1978, 1995) and the ST Solutions Ltd. (STS) company. This program provides in vivo self-exposure exercises for the treatment of phobic disorders and presents psycho-educational material related to the causes and symptoms of anxiety.

FearFighter is now an ordinary fixture in West London's Stress Self Care Clinic, and it is freely available without a physician's prior authorization. In a recent randomized controlled study, the outcome of self-exposure guided mainly by FearFighter was as effective as with self-exposure guided entirely by a professional and significantly better than the outcome by using self-relaxation. FearFighter saved three fourths of professional time without impairing client outcome or satisfaction (I. Marks, personal communication, July 22, 2001). One can meet and greet FearFighter at http://www.fearfighter.com. As discussed in chapter 4, similar features will soon be playing at a Web site near you.

By the early 1990s, enthusiasm for integrating computers into psychotherapy had ebbed because of software unavailability, high cost, and lack of experienced professionals. Low-cost personal computers and the widespread use of the Internet have rekindled interest in the potential of computerized therapy aids. With such aids, a specialist can open a door for clients who otherwise would not seek mental or behavioral health care.

Professional literature by health care practitioners on the use of computer software to deliver psychotherapy and psychoeducational interventions is expanding rapidly. Recent computerized therapy tends to involve a highly structured and very specific approach for a restricted type of clinical problem, such as major depression, generalized anxiety disorder, or alcohol abuse. Systematic and well-delineated therapy methods, such as cognitive behavior therapy, are particularly suited for translation into computer programs (Newman, Consoli, & Taylor, 1997).

Alcohol. To avoid problems with computer inflexibility, the professional may be better off restricting work with a computer to selected, highly specialized parts of the treatment. An example is the Behavioral Self-Control Program offered by Behavior Therapy Associates (http://www.behaviortherapy.com). This program is designed to augment rather than replace a professional's intervention. Presented as appropriate for heavy drinkers but not alcoholics, the program implements a therapy approach previously shown to reduce drinking behavior (Hester, 1995). Alcoholic behavior is identified by the user's initial completion of two self-administered tests, including the Michigan Alcoholism Screening Test (MAST). Behavioral self-control training uses behavioral techniques and the learning of alternative coping skills to pursue a goal of either abstinence or moderate and nonproblematic drinking. The program teaches skills for moderation of drinking behavior. In a pilot evaluation, the Behavioral Self-Control Program was shown to be more effective than was a wait-list control group at posttreatment and follow-up (Hester & Delaney, 1997).

The program is being adapted for the Windows CE operating system for palmtops and personal digital assistants (PDAs). The reader may also find it illuminating to scan a description of plans for research on a computerized implementation of another tool by the same researchers—the Drinker's Checkup. Information on this program is available at the Behavior Therapy Associates Web site. Additionally, the following are some of the other alcohol programs found on the Web:

- Alcohol 101 Plus (http://www.alcohol101plus.org).
- Alcohol Edu (http://www.alcoholedu.com).
- e-CHUG (http://www.e-chug.com).
- MyStudentBody (http://mystudentbody.com).

General Health. In addition to psychoeducational applications, software is available to supplement the treatment of medical patients, mainly in the area of chronic disease (for reviews, see Lewis, 1999; Noell & Glasgow, 1999). Gustafson and colleages were quick to recognize that it is difficult to grasp the full potential of computer-based promotion of health behavior (Gustafson, Bosworth, Chewning, & Hawkins, 1987). Nonetheless, in his development of the CHESS Program in Madison, Wisconsin (Gustafson, Bosworth, Hawkins, Boberg, & Bricker, 1992), David Gustafson has shown the effectiveness of computerized educational and telecommunications programs for a variety of mental health issues, including those related to breast cancer (Gustafson et al., 1993), HIV and AIDS (Gustafson, Hawkins, Boberg, Bricker et al., 1994), and several other areas (Gustafson, Hawkins, Boberg, Pingree et al., 1999).

Dental Fears. Among people treated for specific dental phobia, fear of dental injections and drills was the most frequent (Roy-Byrne, Milgrom, Khoon-Mei, & Weinstein, 1994). Dental fear is a significant barrier to regular care for 5% to 10% of the population, even when financial and access barriers are eliminated (Kaakko et al., 1998). Dentists can handle moderate fear, but they usually refer patients with severe phobia for specialized psychological treatment. However, a widely disseminated and inexpensive computer-aided treatment may be a viable alternative. This vignette is an example of how such treatment might be delivered:

> *Sandy, a 34-year-old horticulturalist, has been phobic for both medical and dental injections since childhood. She avoided situations that might involve needles and found it difficult to make dental or medical appointments. She often became angry and embarrassed for what she termed "acting like a baby."*
>
> *Through a newspaper advertisement, Sandy learned of the computer-assisted relaxation learning (CARL) program study to reduce the fear of needles. After months of delay and deliberation, Sandy finally called for an interview appointment. At the screening interview, the study protocol was discussed, and she was introduced to the CARL program.*
>
> *Sandy spent 1 visit per week working with the self-paced hierarchical program. After 14 sessions, she felt confident enough to proceed with an injection. Later that week, Sandy sat waiting for her first injection in years. A wave of anxiety rushed through her body in the waiting room. Before the anxiety took control, Sandy began to practice the relaxation skills she had learned through the CARL program. When the time came, Sandy calmly allowed the doctor to administer the shot. On finishing, Sandy cried tears of joy and relief, and shouted, "I did it! I did it! I didn't like it, but I did it!!!" Six weeks after Sandy completed the study, we received a card. She wrote, "Thank you. Thank you. And my physician thanks you! I was able to have my blood drawn at my annual exam. I shall never forget all of you."*

— Sue Coldwell, Ph.D.
— Agnes T. Spadafora, RDH, BSDH
Dental Fears Research Clinic
University of Washington, Seattle

The Dental Fears Research Clinic at the University of Washington in Seattle investigated combining antianxiety drugs with the CARL program to treat fear of needles and injections (Coldwell et al., 1998). The controlled exposure therapy paradigm commonly applied to simple phobia gradually presents increasingly anxiety-provoking situations, each to the limit of tolerance, while the client is induced to interfere with the anxiety by using relaxation techniques. The CARL program conducts such exposure therapy in two modes: in vitro, by presenting a digitized, videotaped exposure hierarchy on the computer screen; and in vivo, with scripts for a dentist or hygienist to use while working with a client.

The in vitro mode of the CARL program seats a client in a dental chair and plays an interactive video that begins with muscle relaxation, paced breathing, and cognitive coping strategies for the client to use during the procedure. In each of the seven video segments, the hygienist informs the client about a particular aspect of the dental injection procedure and explains common misconceptions about the procedure. Periodically, the video queries the client about his or her understanding of the procedures and anxiety levels and replays the segment if the anxiety is too high.

The in vivo mode presents to the hygienist or dentist conducting the therapy scripts that mimic the video segments. The client continues these processes until able to tolerate dental injection. The course of treatment usually requires several 1-hour sessions (typically 5 to 10).

Preliminary evaluation (Coldwell et al., 1998) indicated that the CARL program was successful. That is, a majority of the dental patients were able to receive two dental injections at the end of therapy, and all reduced their general dental fear. An expanded trial (unpublished data, P. Milgrom, personal communication, May 21, 2001) indicated that CARL was very effective, even when operating solely in the in vitro mode. Plans are under way to test a new version of the CARL program in rural dental offices in preparation for disseminating the program to underserved areas of the United States.

An Internet-based CARL program is expected to be available within 5 years (S. Coldwell, personal communication, June 18, 2002). Ultimately, the CARL program and many other therapeutic programs will likely be adapted to the smaller screens of portable handheld computers to further enhance dissemination and to make the programs directly available to clients in their problematic situations. The following section describes how these compact but powerful devices can be used to support therapy.

Depression. Offered "for informational purposes only," the MoodGym (http://moodgym.anu.edu.au) developed by Australia's Centre for Mental Health Research at Australian National University (http://www.anu.edu.au/cmhr) introduces visitors to a combined cognitive-behavior therapy and interpersonal therapy approach and advises "individuals who feel stressed or depressed" to "talk to a health professional." Although it is unclear whether going through the program will in fact help visitors, MoodGym uses some clever strategies, including interactive games, that designers of other psychotherapy extenders should study.

Therapeutic Computer Games. By taking advantage of the natural attraction of play and exploration, psychotherapists working with children and adolescents have been able to foster expression of emotional distress in clients who otherwise are difficult to engage in therapeutic exchanges. Playing games with children and teens focuses their attention and helps them tell their stories. Playing games has been shown to promote socialization, encourage development of identity and self-esteem, and help master anxiety (Schaefer & Reid, 2001). Computer games can also be programmed to deliver health information to clients in an entertaining way. Correct answers or desirable behaviors can be rewarded by moving the plot of a game along, by adding points to a player's score, or by advancing the player to the next challenge level. As an imaginative extension of computer games, the Virtual Reality Medical Center (http://www.vrphobia.com) uses robots as an adjunct to traditional child therapy.

Schizophrenia. A particularly promising area of research is the use of computer games with patients suffering from severe and persistent mental illness, particularly schizophrenic-spectrum disorders. Various games have been used in rehabilitative treatment for such cognitive deficits as impairment in attention, pattern recognition, memory, and executive function, which are commonly associated with schizophrenia. A limitation of these initial proof-of-concept-type studies is that they generally enrolled only a small number of participants.

In an empirical evaluation of the complex Cognitive Remediation Program, which included a game component, several cognitive deficits were alleviated on posttreatment assessment (Cassidy, Easton, Capelli, Singer, & Bilodeau, 1996). The positive reaction in a majority of a group of patients with chronic schizophrenia suggested that computer games could be useful for evaluation of attitudes and motivations or as reward (Samoilovich, Riccitelli, Schiel, & Siedi, 1992). A series of studies with inpatients, showed that computer games could be used to attract the attention of patients who were socially intractable (Matthews, de Santi, Callahan, & Koblenz-Sulcov, 1987).

Traumatic Brain Injury. Computer games can also be an efficient therapeutic tool in treating patients with traumatic brain injury. One computer game designed to help with rehabilitation of sensorimotor functional deficits asked patients to make certain finger movements in response to visual displays (Taylor & Berry, 1998). The patients were able to improve speed and accuracy of movements during therapy. Another computer game was shown to assist older adults in improving memory function (Ryan, 1994). An intensive 12-hour computer game training program significantly improved scanning and tracking abilities in patients with severe attention difficulties with or without cerebral dysfunctions (Larose, Gagnon, Ferland, & Pepin, 1989).

Safer Sex. In a study with adolescents, an interactive computer game helped to increase skills and self-efficacy regarding the negotiation of safer sex practices (Thomas, Cahill, & Santilli, 1997). The program used a time-travel adventure format to provide information and nonthreatening skill practice. Users recorded and played back their responses as they negotiated with their virtual chosen partners. The participants achieved significant gains in their health attitudes.

Computer action games are very popular. Modern commercial computer games use three-dimensional simulations with realistic graphics and sounds. Many Internet users participate in elaborate multiuser games that involve forming alliances with other players, making independent decisions, sensing impending betrayal by an erstwhile partner, and other intensive social behaviors.

However, the development of therapeutic computer games has not kept pace with the computer industry, which is intensively promoting elaborate games to play over the Internet. Most existing therapeutic programs, which were developed several years ago, operate with older, slower graphical interfaces that resemble games from the early 1990s. Funding for such applications is also lagging. Nonetheless, the potential for this therapeutic approach has just begun to be tapped.

A growing concern with computer-game use among adolescents in particular is that the amount of time spent engaging with these games can be so significant as to interfere with social skill development at a time when peer interaction is considered crucial. Parents and clinicians are advised to stay informed about how children and teens are spending their time with various forms of technology, including computer games on and off the Internet, as well as with cellular telephones. Used as an adjunct and kept in perspective with a patient's future other needs computer games could be an engaging part of treatment programing.

Therapy Assisted by Handheld Computers

Programs developed for handheld portable devices promise significant advantages over desktop or laptop computer-based programs. Such devices include the Casio PB-1000 or Hewlett Packard 200LX and, more recently, PDAs, such as the Palm Pilot or Handspring Visor. These devices can accompany the client and professional all day and night, extending treatment beyond the therapy hour and into the client's home and work environments and, most important, making treatment available within problematic situations. The devices can continuously and unobtrusively collect and process data related to treatment adherence and the subjective, behavioral, and psychophysiologic impact of therapy.

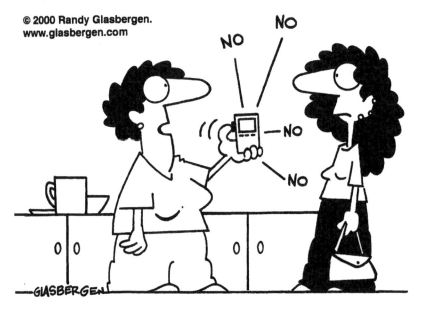

"I REMEMBER HOW HARD IT CAN BE TO SAY NO TO BOYS, NO TO DRUGS, NO TO ALCOHOL, NO TO CIGARETTES... SO I MADE A TAPE YOU CAN PLAY IN AN EMERGENCY."

The following example illustrates how handheld computers can help the professional as well. Practitioners who carry pocket PCs and mobile phones feel safer in rundown neighborhoods. The handheld computer can also greatly enhance coordination of services and provide access to records and support in the field:

> "Experience taught me to carry a small multiple-purpose tool in my belt (near the pocket PC and cell phone) when making home visits. When people lock themselves in rooms, you need tools to break in without damaging the door."
> —(P. Negro, personal communication, September 3, 2002)

Dr. Negro's remark is rich with implication. It illustrates how today's mental health professional may practice in various environments, with a broad range of technical needs. The array of skills and instruments needed may range from a screw-driver to the latest personal digital assistant (PDA). Although this example suggests, rather graphically, that not every patient can be treated at a distance, the peripatetic Dr. Negro clearly keeps his antenna tuned to technology.

Psychotherapy Homework Compliance. Lack of compliance with psychothera-peutic homework is one of the biggest barriers to success of cognitive-behavior ther-apy. Handheld devices that accompany clients can motivate compliance with home-work assignments and issue reminders on a preprogrammed schedule. The devices can provide structure by prompting practice of techniques step by step the moment a problem resurfaces. With anxiety or mood disorders, such practice opportunities occur many times a day, making handheld computers particularly appropriate for anxious or depressed clients. In general, a computer can also monitor the clients' mo-mentary response to intervention techniques, providing guidance to the professional in making clinical decisions.

Anxiety Disorders. C. Barr Taylor and Michelle Newman have been major in-novators in developing handheld computer programs for professionals conducting cognitive-behavior treatment. In a series of studies conducted in the Laboratory for Behavioral Medicine at Stanford University, they explored the utility of handheld devices as an adjunct to standard treatments for a variety of anxiety disorders.

An initial case description demonstrated a module for restructuring of catastrophic cognitions occurring during intense anxiety in patients with panic disorder (Newman, Kenardy, Herman, & Taylor, 1996). For example, the cognition "I'm feeling weak and dizzy and may pass out" may be challenged and can then be replaced by the client with the more likely cognition "I feel weak now, but I've never passed out when I was anxious. I will feel better soon." The program also incorporated instructions for breathing training.

A controlled clinical trial of 18 participants (Newman et al., 1997) used this ap-proach to reduce the standard 12 weekly sessions of in-person cognitive-behavioral treatment (Barlow, Craske, Cerny, & Klosko, 1989) to 4 sessions with a professional. Clients carried the computer at all times during these 4 weeks and continued to use it for 8 weeks after termination of the in-person therapy. Both treatments reduced panic attacks and other symptoms significantly after the 12 weeks and at follow-up. The computer-assisted therapy proved more cost-effective than the 12-week treatment.

Another version of the software incorporates additional therapeutic techniques to emulate the current standard therapy for generalized anxiety disorder (Borkovec & Costello, 1993). Generalized anxiety disorder is characterized by persistent anxiety and excessive worry, unrealistic worry, or both. The program includes cognitive re-structuring, imagined exposure to feared situations, breathing training, relaxation, pleasant imagery, and continuous self-monitoring of moods and symptoms. Clients can initiate therapy whenever they feel anxious or want to practice the techniques. Detailed flowcharts of the software are provided in Newman, Consoli, and Taylor (1999).

Social Phobia. A handheld computer program developed by Gruber, Moran, Roth, and Taylor (2001) was also successfully used as an adjunct to cognitive-behavioral group treatment (CBT) for social phobia. CBT for social phobia typically consists of 12 weekly, 2½-hour group sessions with exposure to simulated phobic events, cogni-tive restructuring, and homework assignments (Heimberg, Hope, Dodge, & Becker,

1990). The handheld computer was used primarily to facilitate homework assignments, including self-exposure to a variety of social situations and cognitive restructuring. Adding the computer eliminated the need for 4 group sessions with a professional without reducing program effectiveness. Similarly, handheld computer-assisted therapy for the treatment of obesity was found equally effective with or without group therapy (Agras, Taylor, Feldman, & Losch, 1990).

Although the cost of handheld computers can be up to $500 per unit, more than one client can use each computer. (As discussed in chapter 10, security protections so that confidentiality is protected need to be in place for Client 2 to not gain access to data recorded from Client 1.) Handheld devices can be helpful to adults, and computer games are showing much promise for working with adolescents. For further information, the Arizona Health Services Library has compiled an extensive bibliography on the use of handheld computers in health care (http://educ.ahsl.arizona.edu/pda/art. htm).

Virtual Reality–Assisted Therapy

Virtual reality (VR) creates a "sense of place and being which exists in cyberspace.... Virtual reality commonly implies full-immersion technologies using goggles and similar devices.... The objects in the virtual world are modeled using 3D modeling techniques.... The [VR] system provides random interactivity" (CyberEdge Information Systems, n.d.). VR projects real-time computer graphics onto special devices, such as head-mounted visual displays, and plays accompanying sounds through headphones. At the minimum, VR reacts to horizontal head movements by changing the projected graphics in accordance. Sometimes, body tracking and other sensors are integrated to create a computer-generated *virtual environment* (VE). Virtual environments are a three-dimensional data set describing an environment based on real-world or abstract objects and data. Typically, the terms *virtual environment* and *virtual reality* are used synonymously, but some authors reserve VE for an artificial environment the patient uses (Blade & Padgett, 2002; Roessler, Mueller-Spahn, Baehrer, & Bullinger, 2000).

More specifically, a VE is a three-dimensional computer simulation that incorporates audio, visual, vestibular, olfactory, and vibratory stimuli to produce a realistic situation (Wiederhold & Wiederhold, 2002). Rizzo, Wiederhold, and Buckwalter (1998, p. 2) define VR as it relates to psychology as "an advanced form of computer interface that allows the user to 'interact' with and become 'immersed' within a computer generated environment." One main application of this technology is game playing, particularly with a peer group, but the potential assessment or treatment applications are immense. A person with a fear of spiders may, for example, be exposed to realistic, three-dimensional depictions of large spiders in the distance and be asked to approach or even handle the animals in VR to overcome the phobic response. In many clinical studies, patients require approximately 8 to 12 VR sessions to overcome a phobia (Wiederhold & Wiederhold, 2002).

Circumventing imagination and almost directly evoking a feeling of immersion in an artificial world, virtual reality takes a major step beyond standard audiovisual presentation. Ordinarily, questionnaire items may be so abstract that clients' responses misrepresent their real life-reactions. The immersive context, in contrast, can provide specific situational cues in at least two modalities (picture and sound), which enable clients to access relevant emotional memories more easily. For example, presenting lifelike images of spiders, heights, or other phobic stimuli before requesting fearfulness ratings may make these stimuli more representative of real-life phobic encounters. The professional may even accompany the client into the synthesized world to guide the assessment and observe behavioral reactions to various stimuli (L. Hodges, personal communication, August 2002). We discuss already existing computerized versions of clinical interviews in the following section.

VR treatment research and technology have advanced significantly in the past decade. The average professional can now afford VR. A typical equipment package from Virtually Better, Inc. includes a computer, tracking device, headset, and treatment manuals providing a session-by-session outline of specific treatment approaches for various disorders. Cost for the program, including the nonrecurrent initial fee to buy computer, head-mounted display, and a tracking system, is $5,000; the monthly fee for a 24-month use and update contract is $400. Companies in Spain, Italy, and Korea are developing other systems. The initial body of research demonstrates that use of the virtual world can help people in the real world.

Although most research involves small, uncontrolled studies (Schuemie, van der Straaten, Krijin, & van der Mast, 2001), the results are encouraging; VR is emerging as a viable tool for psychotherapy and other mental health applications (e.g., Glantz, Durlach, Barnett, & Aviles, 1996). Among apparently successful areas of application are eating disorders or body image disturbances (Riva, 1998; Riva et al., 2001; Riva, Bacchetta, Baruffi, Rinaldi, & Molinari, 1999; Riva & Melis, 1997), developmental disabilities and autism (Brown & Wilson, 1995; Cromby, Standen, & Brown, 1996; Strickland, Mesibov, & Hogan, 1996), and phobias (Anderson, Rothbaum, & Hodges, 2000; Kirkby, 1996; Rothbaum, Hodges, & Kooper, 1997).

Body Image. In addition to assessment and treatment of phobias, the assessment of body image shows promise for the use of virtual reality technology (Riva, 1998). The three-dimensional graphical interface of the VR reality program allows respondents to select figures that reflect their current and ideal body size. The discrepancy reflects the level of body dissatisfaction.

VR has also found success in assessing executive cognitive functions (Pugnetti et al., 1998), memory (Attree et al., 1996), and attention (Wann, Rushton, Smyth, & Jones, 1997). The application of VR technology to clinical assessment is at an early stage (Rizzo, Buckwalter et al., 2001; Rizzo, Buckwalter, & van der Zaag, 2002), and imaginative applications are likely to emerge in the next few years (Rizzo, Neumann, Pintaric, & Norden, 2001). Even clinical interviews performed over the Internet within a VR therapeutic room are now technically feasible.

Anxiety. Phobic disorders successfully treated with VR technology include panic disorder with agoraphobia (North, North, & Coble, 1995), fear of flying (North, North, & Coble, 1997), and fear of heights (Rothbaum, Hodges, Kooper, & Opdyke, 1995). Clients with anxiety disorders can experience and learn to decrease their anxiety by facing its source despite knowing that they are only in a virtual world. The reduction in the maladaptive anxiety response transfers well to the real world. One important advantage of VR exposure over imaginal exposure is that VR does not depend on how vividly clients can imagine anxiety-provoking scenes.

Furthermore, VR exposure does not put the client at risk in difficult situations. For example, VR exposure was used as an alternative to typical imaginal exposure treatment for Vietnam combat veterans with posttraumatic stress disorder (PTSD). Combat-related PTSD can be quite difficult to treat. One study describes a 50-year-old male Vietnam combat veteran who was exposed to two virtual environments—a virtual Huey helicopter flying over a virtual Vietnam and a clearing surrounded by jungle. The patient experienced a 34% decrease on clinician-rated PTSD symptoms on completing treatment; this gain was maintained at 6-month follow-up (Rothbaum et al., 1999).

Barbara Rothbaum, of the Emory School of Medicine, and Larry Hodges, of the Georgia Technology College of Computing, pioneers in this field, formed a company in 1996 to develop and test VR environments for treating anxiety disorders, assisting in behavioral medicine, and making this equipment commercially available to psychotherapists. Their Atlanta, Georgia, company, Virtually Better, Inc. (http://www.virtuallybetter.com), has developed the previous applications as well as an engaging VR situated in a gorilla-inhabited jungle that help pediatric oncology patients cope with anxiety and distress when undergoing painful medical procedures. Page Anderson, director of clinical services, explained, "The level of immersion created by VR can be used not only to help people face their fears in the real world, but also as a distracter from the real world" (personal communication, May 10, 2001).

The Virtual Reality Medical Center (VRMC, http://www.vrphobia.com), founded by Brenda and Mark Wiederhold, applies the Virtually Better and other technologies (including real-time physiological monitoring) to treat a variety of anxiety and eating disorders following cognitive-behavioral protocols. In addition, their multimedia physiological systems are used to treat physiological disorders and stress-related disorders, such as headache, hypertension, chronic pain, Raynaud's disease, TMJ disorder, and attention deficit–hyperactivity disorder. VRMC offers training to graduate students in a variety of disciplines, including psychology and biomedical engineering. VRMC began using interactive technologies to treat fear of flying in 1997. In addition to therapeutic applications, VRMC is funded by government agencies, including the Centers for Disease Control, to use VR as a training tool for high school students and also for the Pentagon to train military personnel.

Many of VRMC's research studies are conducted under its nonprofit affiliate, the Interactive Media Institute (IMI). The company maintains offices in San Diego, West Los Angeles, and Palo Alto, California.

Pain Reduction and Distraction. Hoffman (Hoffman, Patterson, & Carrougher, 2000; Hoffman, Patterson, Carrougher, & Nakamura, 2001) demonstrated empirically that VR distraction is helpful in pain reduction for burn patients. For example, time spent thinking about pain during physical therapy as reported on a 100-mm Likert visual analogue scale dropped from 60 to 14 mm. Results provide preliminary evidence that VR can function as a strong nonpharmacologic pain-reduction technique. Of course, as with any other evolving technology, risks may not yet be identified. As it stands now, the future of VR-based therapy is very promising.

Clients drawn to VR-based interventions often include people who might otherwise avoid psychotherapy. Using technology legitimizes psychotherapy in the eyes of people who see themselves as needing not therapy but rather a new skill set for dealing with anxiety-arousing stimuli. Therapy may be more convenient and more efficient when conducted in VR because it gives professionals the opportunity to conduct effective exposure in the confidential and controlled office setting.

The challenge for professionals is to find appropriate off-the-shelf virtual reality programs that meet client needs. Scientific literature discussing gender issues, as well as ethical issues related to VR, can help guide such selection (Larson et al., 1999; Rizzo, Schultheis, & Rothbaum, 2002).

As with all innovative therapies, VR will have to be studied and continually reevaluated as experience with it grows. Many new therapies fail to live up to their initial promise on long-term follow-up. Others entail hidden risks that become apparent only after the passage of considerable time. An excellent example is the DES tragedy, in which a popular drug prescribed to many pregnant women between the 1940s and 1970s later resulted in severe side effects, such as cancer. Although at present there is no reason to predict any such analogous risk in using VR, practitioners are cautioned that early adopters, those who generate the early literature, tend to be the enthusiasts.

The following sections describe new avenues for adding physiological measurement to enhance clinical practice.

Biofeedback Devices

Psychophysiology explores the interactions between a person's psychological and physiological states. For example, thinking about a traumatic event can raise one's heart rate, listening to soft music can increase peripheral temperature, and ruminating about a problem can delay sleep onset. Psychophysiological research has been occupied largely with basic questions, such as identifying pathways in the brain and peripheral nervous system involved in specific emotional responses. Although this research has greatly enhanced our understanding of mind–body connections, the impact of the field on clinical practice has been small except in the assessments of sleep disturbance and pain management (Roth, 1998). The increasing availability of inexpensive yet sophisticated noninvasive measurement devices has led mental health professionals to recognize the clinical potential of psychophysiological technologies. Thus, *biofeedback* is positioned at the forefront of clinical applications.

Biofeedback involves electronically measuring a physiological value and immediately communicating any change to a client's reward apparatus to train the client to function better. Subtle body changes can be amplified and presented to the client to alter cognitive, emotional, and/or physiological behavior. Biofeedback often uses heart rate to capture the most basic of emotion-relevant factors—calm versus aroused. The so-called fight-or-flight response of acutely anxious or stressed individuals is more complex, characterized by sympathetic hyperarousal increases in heart rate, blood pressure and breathing rate, and vasoconstriction. People are not ordinarily aware of subtle bodily changes, but through biofeedback-mediated training, they can learn to reduce physiological overreaction, which also diminishes the cognitive and affective experience of anxiety.

Other bodily systems that biofeedback commonly monitors include respiration (breathing rate, depth, and pattern reflect a wide variety of emotional changes), skin conductance (sweating is a sign of stress and anxiety), muscular activity (muscular tension is a concomitant of stress), and finger temperature (cold hands are commonly a sign of sustained stress or distress) (Schwartz, 1995). Progress in microelectronics and interfaces with personal computers have filled the marketplace with devices that are simple to operate, compact, and affordable.

Biofeedback methods were researched heavily in the 1980s for treating such disorders as hypertension, headaches, and incontinence, temporomandibular syndrome, irritable bowel syndrome, and functional cardiac disorder (Lawrence, 1986). Particularly for treatment of psychophysiological disorders and pain, biofeedback has been shown to be a cost-effective option as a component of an integrated behavioral medicine treatment program (Schneider, 1987). Although the results were quite positive, the cost, size, and intricacy of the equipment and the shortage of trained professionals kept biofeedback from widespread adoption. Relatively inexpensive devices and efficient biofeedback protocols are now available (http://www.aapb.org).

Mental health care professionals often treat clients with incapacitating physical symptoms. Such clients search for alternative treatment when they do not find relief from traditional medicine. An influential article in the *Journal of the American Medical Association* reported an astounding 629 million total visits to alternative medicine professionals in 1997, a 47% increase from 1990 (Eisenberg et al., 1998). Alternative therapies were used most frequently for chronic conditions, including headaches, insomnia, anxiety, and depression. Biofeedback, which clearly has specific indications for many of these disorders, was used rarely (1%), although it had better insurance coverage than did most other alternative treatments (30% of visits were fully covered, and 44% were partially covered).

Biofeedback is also highly compatible with standard cognitive-behavioral treatment, which emphasizes self-regulation and focuses on behavior change. This compatibility suggests that biofeedback may be helpful as a secondary modality in treating psychiatric disorders (Futterman & Shapiro, 1986). Biofeedback has some important stand-alone or adjunctive applications for individuals with emotional, behavioral, or psychosomatic problems (see Table 7.1).

Remote Biofeedback. In an innovative program based in Hawaii's Tripler Army Base, Ray Folen, Mark Verschell, and colleagues are conducting research on using telecommunication technology to deliver biofeedback services to active duty military, their families, and dependents. With a catchment area that is 52% of the earth's surface, their program is a pioneering attempt for psychologists to provide tertiary care services to the more remote bases in such locations as Japan, Korea, and the South Pacific. Using real-time connectivity, they connect biofeedback equipment at the remote site to their practitioners, stationed in Hawaii. Using Norton's PCanywhere software (http://www.symantec.com/pcanywhere/Consumer) and J&J Engineering biofeedback equipment (http://www.jjengineering.com), their system allows remote control of a biofeedback computer (monitoring heart rate, breathing, skin conductance, and skin temperature) attached to the patient at the remote site. The system uses three telephone lines. One phone line is engaged for biofeedback, another uses a videophone (Teleye) with a H.324 protocol, and the third line maintains connectivity with a professional at the remote site.

The presence and connectivity of a professional are required to enhance the safety of the procedure and to provide emergency backup if needed. The professional may or

TABLE 7.1
Biofeedback Applications for Mental Health

Type of Application	Reference
EMG biofeedback-assisted progressive relaxation	Lehrer, Carr, Sargunaraj, & Woolfolk, 1994; Lichstein, 1988
Biofeedback of specific symptomatic organ systems	Schwartz, 1995
CO_2 biofeedback training for hyperventilation	Meuret, Wilhelm, & Roth, 2001; Wilhelm, Alpers, Meuret, & Roth, 2001; Wilhelm, Gevirtz, & Roth, 2001
Heart rate variability biofeedback training	Lehrer et al., 1997; Lehrer, Smetankin, & Potapova, 2000; Lehrer, Vaschillo, & Vaschillo, 2000
Frontal EEG asymmetry biofeedback training to enhance mood	Allen, Harmon-Jones, & Cavender, 2001; Davidson, 1993

may not be trained in mental health care and may occasionally be credentialed emergency room personnel. Professionals working with patients at the remote site are credentialed according to JCAHO requirements by completing a credentials packet and mailing it to the Hawaii-based program directors. The credentialing process is "fairly rigorous and thorough, so the Tripler service is credentialed at each of these sites." Procedures for obtaining referrals are the same as those of the in-person referral systems. Hawaii-based practitioners speak by telephone to the referral source to determine the appropriateness of the referral. A telephone contact is then made with the patient but only after the patient has been screened and consent forms have been reviewed both verbally and in writing. Copies of files are sent via secured fax (point-to-point telephone line), or data can be printed from the remote site through the remote computer. All patient data are uploaded to the data in the central Hawaii computer (R. Folen, personal communication, April 4, 2001).

Biofeedback Vendors. We are happy to provide Readers with information about some vendors with which we are familiar. Readers are encouraged to contact any of the following biofeedback and ambulatory monitoring vendors at their own discretion:

- Ambulatory Monitoring, Inc. (http://www.ambulatory-monitoring.com).
- BCI, Inc. (http://www.smiths-bci.com).
- Bio Research Institute (http://www.7hz.com).
- Bio-Medical (http://www.bio-medical.com).
- CRF Box, Ltd. (http://www.crfbox.com).
- HeartMath, LLC. (http://www.heartmath.com).
- Intelligent Clothing (http://www.intelligentclothing.com).
- Invivodata, Inc. (http://www.invivodata.com).
- J&J Engineering (http://www.jjengineering.com).
- Mini Mitter Co., Inc. (http://www.minimitter.com).
- Polar (http://www.polar-usa.com).
- Thought Technology Ltd. (http://www.thoughttechnology.com).

Ambulatory Monitoring. Regular monitoring of psychophysiological functions, such as heart rate, blood pressure, breathing rate, and/or skin temperature, while clients are away from the consulting room can help the professional determine the severity of a disorder and the best course of treatment. Professionals keeping in touch with clients by providing remote therapy can follow events by such monitoring even when unable to directly perceive nonverbal clues of stress and distress that are a natural part of in-person therapy, such as sweaty or cold hands (which can be diagnostically helpful when noticed during a handshake) or irregular breathing.

The pharmaceutical industry is starting to recognize the potential of ambulatory monitoring technology for enhancing clinical testing of new medications. IBM Business Consulting Services published projections of current trends and recommendations: "Promising new drugs will first be tested in [people] during late-stage discovery, to prove their safety and efficacy. They will then be launched on the market and subjected to additional 'in-life testing,' using a variety of remote monitoring devices. Collectively, these changes will blur the boundaries between discovery, development and the marketplace" (Arlington, Barnett, Hughes, & Palo, n.d.).

A simple and inexpensive wristband motion sensor (actigraph) can help tailor interventions for sleep disturbances associated with anxiety or depression and can obtain objective data about improvement with therapy (Jean-Louis, Zizi, Von Gizycki, & Hauri, 1999). Actigraphy is more accurate than a sleep diary in estimating sleep efficiency and sleep onset latency (Eissa, Poffenbarger, & Portman, 2001).

Panic disorder is associated with hyperventilation (Papp, Klein, & Gorman, 1993), slow recovery (Wilhelm, Gerlach, & Roth, 2001), tidal volume instability and sighing (Wilhelm, Trabert, & Roth, 2001a, 2001b), and frequent microapneas during sleep (Stein, Millar, Larsen, & Kryger, 1995). Respiratory abnormalities are found in patients with situational phobias during acute anxiety (Alpers, Wilhelm, & Roth, 1999; Wilhelm & Roth, 1998). Other conditions that involve respiratory dysregulation are functional cardiac disorder, chronic pain, and asthma (Wilhelm, Gevirtz, & Roth, 2001).

Unfortunately, current mental health practice often entirely neglects physiological measurement, even though many defining symptoms of the most common disorders are likely of physiological origin (Wilhelm & Roth, 2001). In contrast, most other health care specialties rely on both symptom self-report and systematic biomedical measurements (e.g., the glucose tolerance test for diabetes) to confirm a diagnosis and to follow progress.

This situation may change with the advent of the LifeShirt™ by VivoMetrics, Inc. (http://www.vivometrics.com). This adaptable and washable technological solution is an advanced *multichannel system* for detailed ambulatory measurement of EKG, heart rate and heart rate variability, respiratory sinus arrhythmia, respiratory minute volume and rate, tidal volume variability, central and obstructive sleep apnea, sighing, and coughing. Clients can type information about their specific symptoms and moods at any time into a touch-sensitive customized display, which serves as an electronic diary of clients' subjective experiences. Other peripheral diagnostic devices may be plugged into the LifeShirt system intermittently for special purposes. These devices include a pulse oximeter, blood pressure recorder, capnometer, oral thermometer, or digital weighing scale.

The LifeShirt system can be used for ambulatory monitoring of physiologic parameters during wake, sleep, and activity states. In addition, patient experience data can be gathered automatically and reliably, overcoming the limitations of retrospective reports or paper-and-pencil diaries. Intervals when patients report specific symptoms can receive special attention in the inspection of physiologic parameters. The LifeShirt also records actigraphic and posture information about the patients' gross motor behavior. This information provides the clinician with more situational information for the interpretation of physiological changes. In other words, the LifeShirt records all three emotional response systems—language, physiology, and motor behavior.

LifeShirt technology vastly expands the scope of self-report and physiological measurement. Because emotions can profoundly affect respiration, clinicians' understanding of a wide spectrum of mental disorders associated with emotional disturbance could benefit from a detailed monitoring of respiratory function. Physiological recording is particularly relevant as an interface between psychiatry and general medicine. For example, because many symptoms of panic disorder mimic those of coronary heart disease, differentiating these disorders and learning how they may influence each other are imperatives for clinical practice. Complaints of palpitations are common in both disorders, suggesting that monitoring cardiac parameters could be beneficial. Undetected breathing disturbance during sleep may contribute to the symptomatology of these and many other psychiatric and psychosomatic disorders.

The following experience of a fictionalized practitioner can give the reader insight into how such a shirt might be used in clinical practice:

Having attended a conference featuring new technologies in behavioral health care, Dr. Boivin was the first to introduce advanced technologies to the practice of psychotherapy in her metropolitan area. As a psychologist in Québec City, she had specialized in anxiety disorders for more than 20 years. Despite general success, Dr. Boivin had difficulty treating certain patients with multiple disorders that seemed stress related, as their symptoms lacked clear organic causes. Without information about the patients' physiological state, Dr. Boivin could not make accurate diagnoses or treatment recommendations. Impressed with a LifeShirt demonstration at a conference, Dr. Boivin purchased the system for her practice.

Dr. Boivin was eager to explain the new wearable LifeShirt to Mr. Lavoie, who had been suffering from a sleep disorder, unexplained neck pain, and intermittent panic attacks for more than 16 years. During his previous 2 months of treatment with Dr. Boivin, she had introduced him to the cognitive-behavioral techniques of thought tracking and relaxation training. Dr. Boivin now explained to Mr. Lavoie that the LifeShirt was to be worn as a T-shirt, under his everyday clothes, for a few days to track breathing and heart activity and to provide her with a profile of his autonomic nervous system functioning.

Sensors woven into the garment or attached directly to the skin transmit signals to a PDA worn on the belt. Mr. Lavoie would keep track of daily stressors, activities, moods, symptoms, and cognitions on the PDA computer diary customized to his particular issues. At his weekly sessions, the data would be uploaded to Dr. Boivin's computer for display. The doctor and client would then discuss connections between events and the values recorded by the LifeShirt and which cognitive techniques Mr. Lavoie had tried for each event.

Overnight recordings confirmed frequent sleep interruption, but there was no evidence of such respiratory abnormalities as obstructive or central apneas. During the course of treatment, sleep problems abated, and Mr. Lavoie was able to avert nearly all his panic attacks. His general stress level and neck pain decreased.

Such day-in and day-out monitoring can provide an unprecedented view of symptoms. A patient's complaints and diagnostic "snapshots" taken during routine exams can now be augmented with an entire "movie" of a patient's experience and physiologic function in daily life. This monitoring can also increase rapport with difficult symptom-centered clients who resist the idea of a psychological deficiency. Psychophysiological measurements and biofeedback tools can complement psychotherapy, in the office or through distance using telecommunication technology.

Other Web-Based Programs. Population-based mental health interventions using the Internet are also now appearing. C. Barr Taylor's research program at Stanford University tests the feasibility and effectiveness of bringing online clinical practice to schools, for example, to prevent eating disorders by teaching college students about healthy lifestyle choices and by using cognitive interventions to counteract media-driven weight concerns (Taylor, Winzelberg, & Celio, 2001).

Another large Web strategy targets suicide. Among U.S. college students, the suicide rate is 8.5 per 100,000, making it the second leading cause of death for this population (National Mental Health Association & The Jed Foundation, 2002). The Jed Foundation, Emory University, and the American Foundation for Suicide Prevention have mounted a Web service (http://www.ulifeline.org) that assesses students for suicide risk and steers them to proper in-person professional evaluation and support. Of 1,250 Emory University freshmen in the class of 2005, about 230 completed the survey (Ellen, 2002), a proportion that reflects both the students' discomfort with their death wishes and their comfort with using the Web for highly personal matters.

Many computerized therapeutic programs, games, virtual reality, biofeedback, ambulatory monitors, and specialized Web sites are available to the psychotherapist. These psychotechnologies enhance therapy with focused and time-limited tools developed for specific and measurable goals. This use of technology requires a shift in perspective for some psychotherapists, but it can lead to increasingly specialized practice. For instance, such technologies as virtual reality, the LifeShirt, or advanced biofeedback can prove to be effective adjuncts to everyday practice in treating a variety of anxiety disorders. Objective data on therapeutic progress are especially important when therapy is performed over distance and when the professional needs additional sources of information to compensate for the lack of in-person contact. These tools can be just what the doctor ordered to confirm a diagnosis, increase psychotherapeutic efficacy, obtain authorization for continued treatment, and establish treatment efficacy in terms of outcome. Caution is in order, however.

The next two chapters examine the legal, regulatory, and ethical ramifications of many issues discussed in chapters 1 and 3–6. Chapters 11, 12, and 13 will look at how these topics can come together in an integrated model for delivering service to mental health patients while managing risk to the practitioner.

8

Electronic Practice Management and the Computer-Based Patient Record

8

Practitioners can now rely on computers to handle the more mundane tasks associated with clinical practice. Chances are, most offices have a reasonably up-to-date computer, printer, and modem to connect to the Internet. They probably also have a facsimile (fax) machine or a fax program integrated into a computer. Of course, telephones are standard, but depending on the size of the office, the telephone system might include a messaging service that connects several people, such as an office manager, a billing specialist, and/or other practitioners, throughout the office system. An office might also have a copy machine, or at least a fax machine that can make copies. Although we will not give recommendations about any of this hardware, we do recognize that these elements are considered basic equipment for a modern mental health office.

We assume that the reader either has a desktop or laptop computer or is considering such a purchase. Software packages are designed to operate on almost any kind of computer, but some packages are specifically developed for either a Macintosh or a PC only. Be sure to thoroughly investigate the software package's requirements if you have not yet purchased a computer.

This chapter looks more closely at the various practice management systems that the everyday clinician uses. The first half of the chapter focuses on how practice management software can help centralize and streamline administrative and back-office operations. The second half covers the new and important topic of the *computer-based patient record* (CPR).

PRACTICE MANAGEMENT SYSTEMS

A number of stand-alone computer programs developed in the past several decades are available for the mental health practitioner. New developments are most often advertised in the classified and display sections of the American Psychological Association's *Monitor, Psychiatric News, Psychiatric Times, NASW Newsletter, National Psychologist, Counseling Today,* and similar newsletters, bulletins, and publications for other mental health disciplines. Booths of product displays appear at most national conferences. Experienced conference attendees know, however, that such booths are rarely crowded with practitioners sampling programs.

Despite this seeming lack of enthusiasm, practice management systems can accelerate communications, transactions, and document agreements, and also can decrease

delays, error rates, uncertainty, and cost. Third-party carriers are increasingly requesting electronic billing submissions and practitioner requests for authorizations. Such
requests will likely continue, with credentialing being automated, as are payment and
explanation of benefits.

Various software packages help with many routine office tasks. Let's examine specific features of some of these programs. Once we consider the available options, we
can discuss what it might mean for a clinician to adopt the strategies needed to integrate computers into an office and perhaps even into sessions with patients. The
following sections give more information about personal factors to consider when
choosing which psychotechnologies to introduce into a professional practice.

Practice Management Program Features

Practice management software features can range from basic billing (or claims management) functionality to the following impressive (and only partial) list offered by the
DELPHI/PBS practice management system,[1] which includes upgrades and lifetime
support:

- Accounting.
- Adjustments.
- Aging reports (who owes you money and since when).
- Assessment and intake evaluations.
- Authorization number.
- Batch payments.
- Benefit limits tracking.
- Built-in backup.
- Client statements.
- Codes.
- Copayments.
- Customer support diagnostic.
- Discounts/write-offs/hold harmless.
- Easy-to-use electronic billing.
- Error trapping.
- Expense register.
- Export data.
- Flexible fee schedules.
- General ledger interface.
- Group practices, clinics, and billing companies.
- Interest/service/finance charges.
- Labels.
- Mail merge.
- Managed care warning limits.
- Multiple providers network compat-ible.
- Online help.
- Password protection.
- Payroll calculator for providers.
- Place of service.
- Procedure codes progress/clinical notes.
- Referral source tracking.
- Refunds.
- Reports.
- Responsible-party billing.
- Risk pool deductions.
- Scheduling.

Most other programs do not have as many features and do not offer lifetime support
and upgrades—but they are not as expensive, either. Nonetheless, other programs
might have specialty features that some practices can use. A medical practice management system, topsBill (http://www.e-mds.com/emds/rodserv/tops_bill.html?ov),

---

[1] Reprinted with permission of Will Pardy for DELPHI/PBS on 10/29/2002, located at (http://www.
delphipbs.com/features.htm).

has fraud- and abuse-prevention measures that comply with the Health Insurance Portability and Accountability Act (HIPAA) and a built-in patent-pending embezzlement safeguard to help ensure collection of all copays and other monies owed (Winn & Angelocci, 2002). Other medically oriented programs tout reduced risk of malpractice, courtesy of a medical dictionary that screens entries for medication dosages and body weight and cross-checks within the record for medication contraindications.

Being able to print a report of all outstanding accounts can help a busy practitioner collect insurance deductibles. Similarly, a printout of all referral sources, divided by physicians and other sources, can also help the professional attempting to build a practice. A mail-merge feature allows the professional to write a letter to each of these groups to request payment of the deductible, thank the referral source for trusting in one's professionalism, or offer information of new services being developed. Having immediate access to financial histories, benefits warning messages, and flexible fee schedules allows a practitioner to keep track of the kinds of nuisance details that can make the clinician feel disorganized and also appear so to patients. Having a single desktop practice management program that does many, if not all, of these functions with a minimum of extra effort can be worth the time and energy involved in learning the program. Digitizing one's practice is also considered to be one of the more significant ways to offset decreasing fees being paid by third-party payers.

With easy installation and user-friendly menus, a practitioner can use software to update a patient's record, schedule appointments, and do much more with the few minutes available between sessions. With an additional few hours a week, the average practitioner or office assistant, equipped with a high-end, reliable practice management package, can accomplish all the routine tasks required to deal with managed care. Of course, the practitioner will need to do some things, such as call the managed care case worker and legitimize additional sessions. Tomorrow's competitive marketplace will require efficient technology management to keep up with other practices and organizations. Although practice management software's biggest competitor is paper- and- pencil accounting, scheduling, and note taking, the ease of use and time savings of established software packages are rendering obsolete this slower, hand-powered method.

Before we discuss the practicalities of choosing a software package, let's consider what such a change might involve for a clinician.

Changing Professional Relationships

With practices growing busier, with less time to complete and collect appropriate intake and assessment forms, obtain appropriate release forms, contact primary care practitioners, consult by telephone with case managers about problematic cases, complete outpatient treatment reports, attend to billing and claims management, as well as the day-to-day grind of taking case notes, tracking medications and dosages taken or modified, scheduling and its last-minute changes, the time may have come for automation. But is the practitioner ready?

First, the practitioner's personality must be considered. Some practitioners are comfortable introducing new elements to their office management routine; others are not. Some are comfortable introducing new approaches and related equipment with their patients; others are not. For a thorough discussion of the issues related to technology adoption, see Rosen and Weil (1997).

Introducing novel mental health practice ideas that might impinge on the professional relationship is a highly controversial topic. Nonetheless, technology moves steadily forward, and so shall we, albeit too quickly for some and too slowly for others.

Let's recall chapter 1—Dr. Dale Giolas's enthusiastic description of his current psychiatric practices. We can also mention that other practitioners are reporting similar experiments with their practices when the topic arises at our training seminars. These practitioners report having their laptops or desktops turned on during medication consult or psychotherapy sessions. When patients ask what they are doing, they explore the reasoning behind the question, of course, and then often show them the various functions the software performs. Most practitioners who publish their experiments tend to report that the patients are usually delighted to see their doctors changing with the times.

Not all patients or practitioners, however, consider such innovation to be an improvement. Patients respond according to their particular personalities. Some clinicians who occasionally choose not to use their computers with some patients base their choice on factors particular to the patient(s) rather than or an overall rejection of the idea with all patients. (We have not conducted a study of psychotherapists using innovative psychotechnologies with patients; this clinical topic seems ripe for scientific investigation for readers looking for research topics.)

Note Taking. A change now occuring in routine clinical operations is the use of computers for note taking. The old-style 50-minute hour left 10 minutes between sessions for process notes and contemplation. In some localities, an hour now takes only 45 minutes, and 15-minute medication consults are squeezed into 10. The 5 minutes thus saved can be used to make calls to managed care companies, to write notes, to do billing, or even to rest. One justification for trimmed sessions is that patients are indirectly compensated by receiving benefits from their managed care system, which can easily require the average practitioner to spend 15 to 20 minutes to achieve telephonic access.

Some practitioners maintain the traditional time allotments for meeting with patients but opt for note taking within a session. Other practitioners routinely complete request-for-authorization (outpatient treatment report, or OTR) forms during their time with patients. These professionals see this time as well spent, explaining that the patient should be involved in the authorization and record-keeping process and that this time is the most reliable source of recent information about progress, goals, medications taken, other practitioners visited, and auxiliary support groups attended. It is apparent that note taking practices are indeed changing; adding yet more considerations.

The first issues to consider when developing notes or records during the psychotherapy session are whether to introduce automation and which technology to introduce. For example, during a session, some practitioners dictate into cassette recorders for later entry into the patient record. Other practitioners, who consider this practice a serious disruption of patient contact, would not consider computer note taking to be any more disruptive than using a pencil and notepad. These practitioners might explain that they no longer have time to gather this information during the session, only to transfer it to paper or computer between sessions.

Other clinicians say they would be uncomfortable simultaneously juggling the patient relationship and the unfamiliar computer technology. It could be disconcerting to have the patient looking over one's shoulder and asking questions about the computer and program, or suggesting how to use the word processor. If the computer configuration allows the patient a view of the screen, the therapist should consider whether such visibility poses any threat to the patient, and, if so, how that threat can be avoided.

Other Patient Acceptance of Note Taking Changes. The most interesting source of information about change comes from what patients report to their psychotherapists. One author of this book describes two novel approaches described by patients seen in cotreating clinicians weekly practice:

> One patient reported a "high-tech" approach to couple's counseling taken by a colleague. He and his partner went to their usual couple's session, only to find that the therapist's office was rearranged to make space for a computer and printer. The therapist sat by the laptop and entered case notes while they were conversing. She needed to update their outpatient treatment report, so she went to the CIGNA Web site, pulled up the form, and asked them the questions needed to complete the request. The patient reported that "it took all of 5 minutes and I knew what she was saying about us to the insurance company. That made me feel a lot better than I had before, when I didn't know what was being said about me. The therapist asked us about our families of origin, and, after our discussion, used her computer again to print a blank genogram along with a sample of a completed genogram. After she explained how to complete the genogram, she sent us home with two copies, one for each of us to complete as homework. She's cool."
>
> Another patient reported being surprised when he last met with his psychiatrist. Apparently, the psychiatrist was experimenting with a new interviewing procedure. A nurse interviewed the patient first and asked the patient many behavior- and medication-related questions. They were then joined by the psychiatrist (whom I've known to treat patients traditionally for at least a decade), and the nurse reported the patient's information. He promptly made a few suggestions and decisions to change medications, discussed the change and rationale with the patient, made some notes in the patient chart, and left the room.
>
> The nurse sat with the patient and answered his questions about the medication. Although the patient found this approach to be different, he didn't consider it unacceptable. He commented, "This was my third visit, and now I've seen how things are run in that office. I guess it's gotten to be like visiting my primary care doc. I got what I needed, and that's what counts. The nurse also said I could call her anytime, which I did the next day. She was great and gave me all the information I wanted right away."

Although having a psychiatric nurse gather information before the a psychiatrist comes into a treatment session seems novel enough to appear here in the context of electronic systems, this format was pioneered a generation ago, in the late 1960s, by the renowned psychopharmacologist Nathan M. Kline. Observation of his practice by one of this book's authors showed that patients readily accepted this highly efficient system. It delivered high-quality treatment with more personal attention and also with much more of a psychotherapy component than is usual in the med check sessions so common now. Kline claimed that his arrangement presaged the practice of the future, but it has been slower to arrive than he anticipated. Clearly, patient acceptance of change in note taking is another area in need of empirical research.

Changes Implemented by Health Care Insurance Companies. A previous vignette referred to CIGNA's Web site. Let's take a few minutes to discuss what is happening with such third-party carriers, which hold large sums of money and therefore will undoubtedly shape practice in the years to come. Many of the larger managed care companies have developed Web sites for practitioners to use for automated outpatient treatment reports and requests for further authorizations. These Web sites will soon include other features. The acronym RACERB, which summarizes the goal of many of these Web sites, refers to integrated electronic handling of referrals, authorizations, certification, eligibility, reporting, and billing. Beyond these third-party payer-oriented functions, a RACERB Web site could eventually support off-site data backup, personnel management, accounting, and even clinical data processing, thus handling the bulk of health care information technology. Although a facility that performs all these functions automatically for a large insurance company might seem ambitious or, perhaps, dangerous if done primarily over the Web, a degree of centralization makes practical sense, is manageable, and can be done.

In fact, it is already being done for several companies at once, using one Web site. MedUnite's Web site (http://www.medunite.com) standardized paperwork for medical entities. It connected physicians with pharmacies, labs, hospitals, ancillary practitioners, health plans, and medical groups. MedUnite's participants included Aetna, Anthem, CIGNA, Health Net, Oxford, PacifiCare, and WellPoint, as well as tens of thousands of physicians. MedUnite's financial difficulties (Chin, 2001) led to its acquisition by ProxyMed and subsequent profitability (see http://proxymed.com).

As yet, there are no similar multipayer, inclusive Web sites for mental health entities and carve-out enterprises. Nearly all major mental and behavioral health insurance organizations have individual Web sites in the works. Some companies have operational Web services for practitioners, making requests for authorization of patient sessions by filing outpatient treatment reports as easy as entering the practitioner's name, password, identifying patients, completing fields, and checking boxes. The entire procedure can take as little as 5 minutes, complete with the printed paper copy to place in the patient's file or to give to the patient.

Organizations with such Web sites include CIGNA Behavioral Health and Value-Options. The following two statements from CIGNA and ValueOptions representatives give a better sense of the rationales and goals these companies indentify:

CIGNA Behavioral Health has established a provider Web site and new online tools for providers, aimed at improving the benefit management process. The system can support a number of different functions, including the filing of claims electronically, submission of payment authorization requests, comprehensive review of open cases for continued benefit management, closing of cases, and exchange of other clinical data. The company hopes to transform provider transactions and reduce administrative burdens.

CIGNA Behavioral Health reports that about 70% of its contracted providers have Internet access either at home or at the office and can use the system at their convenience, 24 hours a day. There are no fees for using the service, and the system will likely prove cost-effective by lowering the costs for stamps, long-distance fax transmissions, and long-distance telephone calls. The system may also prove to be time effective by reducing errors in claim submission and the time taken to fill out initial review submissions and follow-up requests.

The Secure Sockets Layer (SSL) protocol, the same protocol Web sites use for electronic banking and credit card purchases, allows secure data transmission to and from the user's computer. SSL connections can be verified by a closed padlock icon at the bottom of most Web browsers. In addition, the Web server sits behind a firewall at CIGNA Behavioral Health, protecting it from hackers and unauthorized users. Technical assistance is available to providers via a toll-free number or via e-mail. In the future, the company plans to expand the site for use with Employee Assistance Program products, to upgrade the Web claims submission capabilities, and to add the capability for electronic fund transfer. For more information, visit www.cignabehavioral.com.

— Jodi Aronson, Ph.D.
Vice President of Clinical Operations
CIGNA Behavioral Health

Several other companies offer similar services. Michael Bollini explains another aspect of the current service and rationale at ValueOptions:

Nearly all the providers contracted with ValueOptions (91%) report having access to the Internet, with more than half (56%) indicating that they have such access at work. With that in mind, ValueOptions has been exploring ways to increase the use of the Internet to ease the multiple provider-related administrative tasks.

A key element of the ValueOptions approach has been in addressing important confidentiality concerns that surround patient privacy and the Internet. The ValueOptions firewall and other technical safeguards have been established to deter unauthorized access to patient data. In addition, security measures have been implemented to simplify verification of data a billing agent submits on behalf of a provider. Such security processes continue to be strengthened as new federal privacy rules come into effect.

— Michael Bollini, Ph.D.
Executive Vice-President, Provider Relations
ValueOptions

Passwords is another important issue when considering the use of insurance Web sites. Mental health professionals associated with more than one insurance company need to access multiple Web sites to visit to fill out RACERB forms. Professionals are advised to store the log-in pages for each Web site in the Favorites or Bookmark folder of their Web browsers. Passwords (or passphrases) must be routinely changed and otherwise protected. They should be nonsensical strings of letters and numbers and not some compound of dictionary words, such as "accessVO" or "accessCBH." Passwords for various sites should not resemble one another, as they do in the example just given. When working with employees, password policy and the date of each password change can be documented for proof of security precautions.

This brief discussion of managed care Web sites can demonstrates how quickly authorizations can be obtained with a computer, and thus might inspire the reader to consider alternative ways of practicing—perhaps even introducing a computer into sessions with patients. Managed care companies are focused on developing a host of Web services specifically intended to aid practitioner in-session or out of session, whichever that the practitioner prefers.

Although they do not currently have the convenience offered to the medical community through such Web sites as MedUnite, mental health practitioners will be able to benefit from insurance companies' offering RACERB services through individual company Web sites. Supporters of such automation claim that the more comfortable professionals are with computers, Web sites developed by insurance companies, and practice management software, the more time will be available to comfortably sit with patients and do the work of providing mental health care. With any luck, mental health practitioners also will be able to improve services with such innovation.

Practical Considerations

Now that we've discussed the personal and professional issues related to using practice management software, we can discuss the practical issues. Wholesale automation of office functions carries great advantages to large-scale multisite research and exciting opportunities for quality control and cost savings by giant provider networks and payer enterprises. Such benefits might not be realistic for small or medium-size clinics or even for most university-based mental health care operations. Most clinicians are not statisticians; they are interested primarily in treating patients and getting paid. Most practices will never use all that comes as standard equipment with the more sophisticated practice management systems. What makes more sense is to introduce information technology step by step, based on priorities determined by a cost–benefit analysis.

Pinpointing Need. Practice automation is best initiated into three areas. The first is where there is repetitive paperwork. For example, registering a new patient into an electronic database is a straightforward matter with immediate benefits because a one-time demographic entry can reduce the time necessary to complete all future tasks related to that patient. The computer can automatically pull up any part of the data as needed for other functions, such as note taking or checking accounts due, often with only a couple keystrokes, such as the patient's initials. Second, look for trouble spots where fixing the problem could make a difference. For example, telling a mental health patient, "I'll call you back after I get a chance to pull up your chart" could be improved if the clinician could access crucial clinical data even while away from the office.

The third key target area for quick return on investment is inefficient charge capture. Patients may tend to feel that bills need not be paid if they were not sent promptly enough. Failure to collect copayments from patients may be a contract violation; the government may even allege fraud and abuse. Managed care refuses to pay if paperwork or preauthorizations are not done correctly. Medicaid and Medicare get picky about codes for diagnoses and fees for procedures. Plugging these leaks is money in the bank—metaphorically, of course.

Because the places that most need automation are similar in every practice, solutions are likely to be readily available. Such solutions are inexpensive, easy to use, and will disrupt the existing manual system only minimally. Many practitioners have started out with home-grown systems, perhaps consisting of only a word processor. It takes little technical know-how to put together some useful practice aids. As practitioners become more familiar with automation, they appreciate being able to add further functionalities and to evaluate commercially developed systems or to work with a consultant or developer in building a customized system.

Of course, a nice ready-made system offered for free or at a deep discount may be worth considering. It is in the best interest of third-party payers to help their providers automate.

Hardware. Minimal requirements for a laptop or desktop computer system (easily met by today's home models) include 128 megabytes (MB) of random access memory (RAM), a 1-gigahertz (GHz) processor, 10 gigabytes (GB) of hard disk space, and a 56-kilobyte (KB) modem. Newer technologies combine previously separate devices, such as telephones, PDAs (personal digital assistants), digital cameras, mobile Internet surfers (e-mail capable), webcams, and Web browsers, into one handheld product.

Some devices include a miniature color monitor, keypads, and voice-activated systems (Hao, 2002). Wireless tablet computers, which are intermediate between PDAs and laptops, are quite powerful and can store and display scanned documents and large data entry forms.

Decisions about hardware should be based on lifestyle and practice management preferences. Some discussion here of the options can help a clinician make a good choice. The pros and cons of using such devices must also be considered. Such a discussion is not within the purview of this book, however, but the reader can find an extensive Web site with articles and a well-considered discussion by informed mental health practitioners on mental health software and hardware led by Martin Briscoe from the United Kingdom (http://groups.yahoo.com/group/CIMH2000).

Software. The place to begin looking for practice management software products is through a Web search for "mental health" AND "practice management" AND "software." With this search, a good Web search engine, such as Google or Yahoo, may offer more than 15,000 options to explore. When running such a search, note that there are two ways to run software programs: stand alone and through an application service provider (ASP).

Typically, software can be purchased and sent to the purchaser through regular surface mail. Software programs can also be downloaded from a Web site. Payment is usually made by credit card through the software company's Web site, although a toll-free telephone number may be available for people who do not want to submit a credit card number through the Internet. Software obtained through surface mail and software downloaded through a Web site both function as *stand-alone* programs. That is, they do not require connection to the Internet to perform their functions. All operations occur on the computer running the software.

The second type of software format works with the help of the Internet. ASPs are third-party entities that manage and distribute software-based services from a central data center to customers across a wide area network. Web-based vendors supply practice management services to clinicians and clinical organizations for a subscription fee plus nominal transaction fees. These ASPs free clinicians and clinical organizations from purchasing software for their individual desktops. The advantages ASPs offer are the following:

- The subscriber does not have substantial up-front investment in software, because it is downloaded per transaction from the Internet.
- The subscriber does not have substantial upgrade fees, because each upgrade is handled through the main server and not on each clinician's computer.
- The subscriber has lower hardware costs, because only a very basic computer is necessary.

Despite these advantages, the challenges are significant and include the following:

- Protecting data privacy in transmission and storage of confidential patient information.
- Defining who owns the data.
- Providing quick access and transmission power over the Internet for user-friendly transactions.

- Waiting for third-party carriers to be Web-enabled to accept information from such ASPs.
- Depending on the ASP to survive in a difficult economic climate.

Viability of a Software Company. An important topic to consider when purchasing software is the health of the software company itself. In addition to the software's functionality, decisions about purchasing software should include an analysis of the viability of the vendor and manufacturer and the prognosis for their product lines. Choose software based on a company's reputation and experience in serving the mental health community. Psychologist Tom Trabin states:

> *Software is plentiful for individual psychotherapists and small-group practices. However, at least at the present time, this is a difficult, low-end market that requires considerable market share or deep pockets for a vendor to stay viable. Although it is difficult to find vendors that have been in the marketplace long enough to have developed customer confidence, at least two well-known vendors have successfully created and marketed practice management software. (Others may exist.) These vendors are VantageMed (Therapist Helper) and a partnership between Creative SocioMedics and the publisher John Wiley and Sons (TheraScribe). Both companies offer software to assist in some aspects of clinical decision making and management of the day-to-day computer functions of private practice.*
>
> *On the other hand, quite a few excellent practice management products have proved themselves for midsize to larger provider organizations. Most of these products are made by companies that are members of the Software and Technology Vendors' Association. Members are reflected on that trade association's Web site (http://www.satva.org). Look for the "Links to Vendors" page. These vendors typically offer software and training that provide clinical, financial, billing, and administrative functionality for such provider organizations as residential programs, mental health centers, social services agencies, and hospitals. Some vendors offer comprehensive applications for managed care organizations needing member services, provider referrals, provider relations, claims adjudication, call centers, and care management.*
>
> **— Tom Trabin, Ph.D., MSM**
> **Executive Director, Software and Technology Vendors' Association**
> **Co-Chair and Co-Founder, BHIT Conference**

How long has the software's development company been in business? What do other users of its products say when specifically asked? What do colleagues recommend? Practitioners who spend the time and energy to set up software and transfer information can be disappointed if the company supporting the software goes out of business. Other questions to ask such vendors are found in Maheu, Whitten, and Allen (2001).

Specific Practice Management Software. This list of specific practice management software is a start, and we encourage a more detailed search for software that is specific to each clinician's needs. Many of these programs are available as either stand-alone or ASP versions:

- Askesis Development Group, Inc. (http://www.psychconsult.org).
- CMHC Systems (http://www.cmhcmis.com).
- DuicDoc (http://www.quicdoc.com).

- Geneva Software Company (http://www.genevasoftware.com).
- Harmony Information Systems, Inc. (http://www.harmonyis.com).
- New Therapist (http://www.newtherapist.com).
- Orion Healthcare Technology (http://www.orionhealthcare.com).
- Point of View Survey Systems (http://www.povss.com).
- Secure Health, Inc. (http://www.securehealth.cc).
- Sequest Technologies, Inc. (http://www.sequest.net).
- ShrinkRapt (http://www.shrinkrapt.com).
- Synergistic Office Solutions (http://www.sosoft.com).
- Teleotech Systems (http://www.teleotech.com).
- TheraManager (http://www.theramanager.com).
- TherapistHelper (http://www.helper.com).
- UNI/CARE Systems, Inc. (http://www.unicaresys.com).

Some companies cater to all parts of the spectrum: from the individual practitioner to the clinic, hospital, or insurance company enterprise. For special applications, the reader is encouraged to investigate some of these companies as well:

- Anasazi Software, Inc. (http://www.anasazisoftware.com).
- CompuCare Management Solutions (http://www.compu-care.net).
- Creative Socio-Medics Corporation (http://www.csmcorp.com).
- InfoMC (http://www.infomc.com).

Demonstration Programs. Once the programs on our list have been reviewed and choices narrowed to about five, follow these suggestions, proposed by Larry Rosen: "First, go to the five Web sites and get a feel for the product through lists of features and other options. Select a maximum of two Web sites and download the demos or call the company who will mail a CD-ROM demo. Load one demo at a time and enter 5 to 10 of your patients. Now, bill for a month of sessions and see how the program 'feels'" (Rosen, 2000). On request, most companies will permit free downloads from their Web sites or will send free or low-cost demonstration disks through surface mail to enable interested practitioners to sample their products.

Look and Feel. The next important considerations when buying software if the so-called look and feel of a program, which is a subjective judgment. If the practitioner is going to be the primary program user then the practitioner should choose a program that feels right. If, on the other hand, the software is to be used primarily by office staff or shared with colleagues, the best approach is to get a demonstration copy for them to try and then ask their opinion. Their feedback can help decide which program to buy and can also indicate how much resistance to expect when streamlining the mental health practice with other technical time-savers. Allowing staff to help select their tools is good office management. Involving the staff will improve their degree of buy-in and may also improve office morale.

Support and Upgrades. After need and cost, availability of support and upgrades is the most essential factor to consider. Are support and upgrades of the management software included in the initial price, or will additional expenses be incurred yearly? Does the software company offer support through a toll-free line? A free phone call, however, may provide scant solace if the number is usually busy or if the caller is put on hold for a geologic era or two while being subjected to canned music.

If the software salesperson downplays or ignores these questions, take it as a bad sign and look elsewhere. Inadequate support can bring any office to a grinding halt. The lack of support and upgrades has driven many software owners to trash their expensive purchases and reach for the pen and pad.

A good way to learn about the availability of support staff is to call the software manufacturer's support line before purchasing the software. Count the number of minutes it takes to reach a live operator. This experiment can be a good, although not foolproof, test of a support staff's responsiveness. Speaking with other customers about their experiences with support is another important step. Most software companies are happy to give the names of satisfied customers who have informed them of their availability for such inquiries. If a company says, "We protect our customers' confidentiality and never give out names," don't trust it. Salespeople know they need satisfied customers, and if the company doesn't have enough of a sales force to have recruited happy and willing customers, then keep looking for a bigger and more established company. Another option, of course, is to discuss a particular software package and its support through the previously mentioned Martin Briscoe discussion forum, accessible at (http://health.groups.yahoo.com/CIMH2000).

Speech Recognition Technology. A specialty software program of particular interest and value to clinicians is speech recognition.[2] Dictate through a microphone, and computer-related carpal tunnel syndrome may become nonexistent! A speech recognition program attempts to recognize spoken sounds as corresponding to one or more words contained in its library. For some programs, a clinician can purchase an add-on health care vocabulary. The programs require time to match the user's speech to words in the software's vocabulary. Some programs can handle more than one user; each person's voice and pronunciation patterns are stored separately.

Room noise must be minimal, and a good microphone is essential for accuracy. Note that an error rate is fair if the program gets 98 words out of 100 correct (which is an expected performance level). Speech recognition programs are improving steadily and already are good enough to enhance the lot of many mental health professionals.

Some speech recognition programs coordinate with the most popular e-mail programs and word processors. Filling out computer-based paperwork is another possible use for this technology, although some programs may not be compatible. Mental health professionals can also use this technology to take notes during or after a session, rather than using a tape recorder.

The major manufacturers of speech recognition software are:

- ScanSoft (http://www.scansoft.com).
- IBM ViaVoice (http://www-3.ibm.com/software/speech).
- Nuance Communications (http://www.nuance.com).
- SpeechWorks (http://www.speechworks.com).

These software programs may have a range of editions, from the standard package to the professional edition, and may cost anywhere from about $60 to $300. Professional packages, by definition, are more likely to meet the needs of practitioners. Scrimping on voice recognition software purchases for notetaking or other forms of

---

[2] We prefer to reserve the term *voice recognition* for system that confirm a person's identity by his or her voice quality, an alternative to using fingerprints, irises, retinas, and scent.

professional record keeping may not be advisable, particularly when medical records are involved. Errors that such programs make usually involve spelling errors, which could prove embarrassing or worse at a later date.

COMPUTER-BASED PATIENT RECORDS

Even though most practice management software for mental health has not been made compatible with the larger-scale computer-based patient record (CPR), this is likely to happen. Learning about the CPR and what it entails can give the clinician a peek into what is around the corner for mental health practice. Therefore, the rest of this chapter discusses the overall plan for the CPR.

Computerized health information systems have existed for more than 3 decades. The first systems were designed primarily to support administrative tasks, such as billing and insurance. One early large-scale system that went beyond a head count and captured clinical data was the Multi-State Information System (MSIS), linking state psychiatric hospitals; this system was eventually implemented in several countries (Laska, 1975). Using computers for handling online medical information, telehealth communication networks, and electronic patient files has enabled improved health care decisions, prevented dangerous oversights, increased access to care, and reduced costs for patients, practitioners, and insurance companies (Lindberg & Humphreys, 1998).

This book uses the term *computer-based patient record* comprehensively to include all database systems capable of electronically storing information about an individual. Again, we face the problem of overlapping terminology. The scientific literature refers to the terms *electronic medical record* (EMR), and *computer-based* (or *computerized) patient record*, and many clinicians do not understand the difference. An important distinction between the EMR and CPR is explained as follows:

> As a staff member of the American Health Information Management Association, a 43,000-member association of health information managers, I and my colleagues have looked into the difference between all the electronic records and the computer-based patient record.
>
> The EMR (or electronic patient record, or electronic health record, or any derivative of electronics) is what most people have now. This is a record system based primarily on scanned images of paper records or stored files of transcribed documents. These types of EMRs have very limited functionality. The EMR has copies of files, such as the X-ray report and the dictated discharge note. It can normally be searched by document, such as Operative Report, History, or Physical, but not down to the individual word level. It can't pull information out of the report. It can't find all the elevated hemoglobin values for the last 24 hours, for example. However, the EMR is still better than the paper-and-pencil record because it allows clinicians to copy, encrypt, password protect, and transmit records that can be shared from one location to another. But it doesn't use the true capacity of the computer.
>
> The CPR is the "Big League." It is the goal. It is best defined by the Institute of Medicine's landmark book, The Computer-Based Patient Record: An Essential Technology of Health Care. CPRs make full use of features made possible by computerization.

— **Harry Rhodes, MBA, RHIA**
Director of Health Information Management Products and Services
American Health Information Management Association

An optimum CPR, as defined by the Institute of Medicine (IOM) (1997), is "an electronic patient record that resides in a system designed to support users through availability of complete and accurate data, practitioner reminders and alerts, clinical decision support systems, links to bodies of medical knowledge, and other aids" (p. 55). As described in chapter 6, clinical decision support is part of computer-based assessment. The remaining issues are discussed in the next sections.

The Institute of Medicine (1997) further defines the computer-based patient record system as "the set of components that form the mechanism by which patient records are created, used, stored, and retrieved . . . [including] people, data, rules and procedures, processing and storage devices, and communication and support facilities. Future patient records should support patient care and improve its quality, enhance productivity and reduce administrative costs, support clinical and health services research, accommodate future developments, and ensure patient data confidentiality" (p. 56). The Institute of Medicine identifies five specific characteristics of the CPR:

1. *Integrated view of patient data*—allows the clinician to see all requested data, searched by keyword, independent of where the information was created. For example, the clinician might ask for all Beck Depression Scores over the past 6 months, the presence of any physical disorder that might contribute to anxiety, or any medication that might have depression as a side effect. Better yet, recent systems can produce a graph of chosen values for the clinician to review before making clinical decisions. Constrained by a format that has not substantively differed in more than a century, the paper record does not meet the rigorous information requirements of modern-day clinical practice.

2. *Access to knowledge resources*—gives access to some of the world's largest electronic dictionaries and medical resources. For example, the clinician reading the CPR see the term *ovarian cancer*. Clicking on the term brings up most recent or most complete body of knowledge on this topic, which is then available when completing the progress note or making treatment decisions.

3. *Physician order entry and clinician data entry*—directly links treatment or medication orders to all parts of the record, so the practitioner can be alerted with an immediate pop-up window of information related to any contraindications for orders being entered. It also might pull on other knowledge resources, such as those giving the clinician a pop-up menu to access any new information about the medication or treatment being ordered.

4. *Integrated communications support*—links the patient record to e-mail and other telecommunication services. This enables and facilitates consultation or progress note entries from various geographical sites, such as home, multiple clinics or offices, or on the road.

5. *Clinician decision support*—in general health care, this term refers to such information as drug-interaction checking and changing laboratory-test result alerts. Passive data resources could match patient context and diagnosis to research-based treatment protocols or to best-practice suggestions published by specialty associations.

This description of the CPR is the ideal rather than what is currently available for mental and behavioral health practitioners. Overly eager practitioners might be fooled by crafty salespeople offering CPRs that are only repositories of information and front ends to computer workstations. For now, "Buyer beware" is a worthwhile dictum. Without a full complement of the CPR characteristics listed, many existing CPR systems are not as comprehensive as the IOM's vision (American Health Information Management System, n.d.).

Constructing the CPR record depends on using an internationally accepted nomenclature consisting of comprehensive, multiaxial, controlled terminology created for indexing data in the medical record. SNOMED International, a division of the College of American Pathologists, oversees the direction and maintenance of such a system, known as the Systematized Nomenclature of Medicine, or SNOMED®. This agreed-on nomenclature is embedded in a technology now used in more than 40 countries. The system allows for consistent gathering of detailed clinical information, enabling providers of various specialties, researchers, and patients to share a common understanding of health care sites and computer systems. More information about their contributions to the CPR can be found at http://www.snomed.org.

Because few CPR software products have been developed for mental or behavioral health care specialists, the reader may want to understand the horizon without purchasing these expensive products until they've been refined.

Benefits of the Computer-Based Patient Record

Timely provision of client information for clinical encounters provided in other clinics or locales is needed for accurate treatment decisions. The following vignette illustrates this point:

> *I consult with a psychiatrist 3 hours distant as a routine part of my day. Supervision for cases, as well as discussion to identify the best course of therapy for my patients, occurs without my leaving the local clinic. Once I have completed the consultation, a record of the encounter and a summary of treatment are dictated and available as an electronic medical record (EMR) within 3 hours of the consultation.*
>
> *This procedure was especially important in one situation in which a patient presented in an agitated and confused state, seeking additional services at another clinic many hours away. In making treatment decisions, a professional at that clinic had the benefit of a reliable, up-to-date record accessed through a private telephone connection. Medication given that morning had caused side effects in the patient, who would have received additional doses of the same medication without a record of prior treatment and presenting condition. Once the record was reviewed at the second clinic, a video connection was made with me, and I was able to confirm the patient's condition prior to initial treatment. In this situation, a medical error was avoided through access to information via an integrated technology.*
>
> **— Marybeth Goulet-Connolly, APRN, CS**
> **Acadia Healthcare, Maine**

Computer-based records will be a part of future health care and mental health care practices. With shortages of mental health in today's public health arena, CPRs offer another tool to increase the quality and integrity of the mental health services. Errors have been shown to decline when a clinician uses a computer-based systems. Financial savings can be realized through more accurate documentation as well.

Some overlap with practice management software can be seen in how CPRs are developing. For instance, both types of programs have functions that check for drug interactions and weight-based medication dosages. The fully computerized physician's order entry system in use at the Ohio State University is an example of the great advantage of just one component of an overall CPR (Hagland, 2003). Features of this system include allergy checking, drug interaction and duplication alerts, drug route restrictions, weight-based dosing, general order duplication, corollary checking, and bidirectional interfacing with ancillary systems, such as the laboratory information system. Physicians key in 80% of the orders, with nurses entering physicians' verbal orders. The extra time it takes to get to a terminal and do the typing rather than to find the chart or order book and scribble in a note is amply repaid by time saved phoning to check on orders, especially as medication, lab, imaging, and other orders are acted on much more quickly. Errors have reportedly plummeted.

One major time saver is the system's library of 450 evidence-based order sets for various diagnoses and conditions. Even though a suite of orders, plans, or to-do items is more difficult to standarize in the mental health field than in medical practice, the potential is obvious. The time necessary to enter orders can be shaved by presenting menus that can be checked off. For patient authorization, a CPR facilitates access, for legitimate users, to health data stored in multiple, dispersed locations (Computer-Based Patient Record Institute, 1999). Networks will have better access to up-to-date patient treatment and medication regimes when a patient uses a distant clinic or other network site during off-hours. Such access to information facilitates continuity of health care and contributes to research and trend recognition using longitudinal health data and public health reporting.

In addition, well-designed computer-based patient records provide documentation that is more easily accessible, manageable, and transmittable. Much like smaller and less comprehensive practice management software discussed earlier in this chapter, the CPR gives better access to information and track a patient's or member's activity over time within an organization and across various types of health care settings (Fernandes et al., 1997).

As CPRs become more common in general health care, mental health care can expect similar tools to become available. In medical practices, precious time is often wasted searching for necessary patient records even when patients are in the practitioners' offices. Several studies have reported that during patient visits, practitioners could not find necessary or desired information up to 30% of the time (U.S. General Accounting Office, 1991). To a greater extent, health care professionals simply don't bother to gather and review all the information that could be helpful during a visit.

Existing practice management software and the CPR already overlap in this area. CPRs also allow patient data to be shared remotely. They allow orders, payments, and laboratory data or referral letters to be exchanged or e-mailed (Dick, Steen, & Detmer, 1997). Electronic Network Systems (http://www.enshealth.com) offers a number of products for CPRs, claims, and communication. TeleVox® (http://www.TeleVox.com) has developed a Windows-based system that integrates telephone messaging with various administrative functions of receiving medical care, such as notification of laboratory results, appointment reminders, scheduling and medication reminders, and a number of other functions. CPR systems unify various clinical data, helping reduce the cost of filing and storing paper records, and, theoretically, eliminating such problems as illegible notes, lost charts, and illegible prescription orders. More specifically, the risk of serious medication errors or adverse drug interactions can be substantially decreased when drugs and dosages can be selected from menus on an electronic entry form and then cross-checked against the patient's current diagnosis, current medications, and history of drug reactions and allergies. Clinicians may be able to immediately access all patient medical files and quickly review whether a particular medication or dosage will adversely trigger a patient's other medical condition(s).

Several companies offer handheld PDAs that interface with the CPR for clinicians on the go. One such company is Advanced Clinical Solutions (http://www.officechart.com).

Barriers to the Adoption of Computer-Based Patient Records

A number of barriers must fall before CPRs become standard clinical tools. The cost of purchasing new systems and migrating from manual methods or from existing CPR systems to keep up with the rapidly changing technology are discouraging many clinics and individual practitioners. In addition, the CPR must be better designed to fit workflow needs, be easier to learn and use, and be more reliably maintained. Many current solutions are fragmented among vendors. Issues related to ownership must be clarified (American Health Information Management System, n.d.).

Typical CPRs work with checklists or numeric entries. If narrative responses are accepted, they sit in the record, unprocessed, albeit more legible than typical professional scrawl. The essential information involved in mental health care may not lend itself to a yes–no or "how many times per week" format. Furthermore, the CPR requirements to fill in the little boxes might seriously distort clinical practice. Progress in automatic interpretation of "natural language" offers hope that a CPR may eventually welcome narrative. The CPR could then fill in missing information and clarify ambiguities by asking pointed questions of the clinician, such as "Did that first panic attack occur before or after the patient began drinking more heavily? Select: BEFORE/AFTER/UNKNOWN/ASK ME LATER."

Patient's and Professional's Attitudes. From the patient's perspective, many Americans fear that their personal health data might be used to limit insurance coverage or job opportunities. Until people worry less about health information being shared or sold without their consent, they may remain suspicious of many types of e-health tools, such as electronic health records (Eng, 2001).

Professional qualms about using new technology are another problem. Many mental health professionals react with dismay when encountering techie-engineered computer programs that purport to save time and simplify practice. In reality, many of these programs fail to deliver, owing to either design issues or lack of training to the professional user. Relief may be forthcoming if companies follow the example of MicroFour (http://www.micro4.com); this company demonstrated its user-friendly touch screen and voice-integrated CPR to enthusiastic clinicians at the October 2002 meeting of the American Academy of Family Physicians in San Diego, California.

Security of Computer-Based Patient Record Systems. When practicing in coordination with several offices, the health information network must be designed to maximize benefits yet be secure, confidential, and user friendly for the practitioner. Unfortunately, in practice, security problems remain unresolved. In California, the primary perceived threat to CPR confidentiality is computer hackers (California Healthcare Foundation, 1999). Most people surveyed have responded that they do not want outside sources—such as drug companies—to have access to their medical records, except in cases of medical research or if they were being offered a new job. These concerns come with good reason. The 2000 Computer Security Institute/FBI annual review of more than 680 large businesses' and organizations' computer systems revealed that more than 90% had security breaches in the year before the survey, with losses totaling more than $265 million. This figure does not include lawsuit settlements still pending against the organizations (Brittin, 2001).

Computer security has serious implications for mental health professionals who computerize patient contact or information. Computer hacking can be learned online, and hacking tools can be downloaded online for free. Every few months, the media relate a story of how business or government Web sites and databases are hacked. As we discuss in the next chapter, HIPAA has established guidelines for security requirements, but much is still left to the individual practitioner to understand and implement regarding the treatment of mental health patients and their records.

It is unlikely that individual practitioners or clinics will ever be able to adequately secure a CPR on their own. Even large commercial enterprises have severe continuing security problems (Hulme, 2003). Microsoft quite often issues new patches to seal leaks in its operating system and software products. Many employees play background music on their computers after installing something like RealPlayer, but this practice can expose the entire system to hacker intrusion (TechWeb News, 2002).

Security Leaks with Paper Records.   Theoretically, computer-based patient record systems can provide greater protection of confidentiality and data integrity than can paper records. In contrast to paper health care records, an electronic system can encrypt both the data and their existence, make material available only to designated people, maintain backup copies in remote locations, and maintain an audit trail of all attempts at access and all additions and alterations to the original data. Information moved between locations can be encrypted and transmitted via secure electronic pipes rather than transported by truck, such as the paper records in the following examples. The basic technology for all this is simple, mature, well tested, readily available, and inexpensive. The U.S. Department of Health and Human Services (2000) reported:

> The health insurance claims forms of thousands of patients blew out of a truck on its way to a recycling center in East Hartford, Connecticut. (*The Hartford Courant*, May 14, 1999)
>
> A patient in a Boston-area hospital discovered that her medical record had been read by more than 200 of the hospital's employees. (*The Boston Globe*, August 1, 2000)
>
> A speculator bid $4,000 for the patient records of a family practice in South Carolina. Among the businessman's uses of the purchased records was selling them back to the former patients. (*The New York Times*, August 14, 1991)

Security Leaks with Electronic Records.   With paper records, a minor security leak in the system is usually inconsequential. Most of the 200 hospital employees who read portions of the patient's record in the previous example probably did not care about what they saw. A minor leak in an electronic system has much more potential to harm a patient because much more information is exposed, it is much easier to search for damaging data, and the number of snoops who can gain access is several orders of magnitude greater.

But minor leaks are not the issue. In larger organizations, CPR systems tend to have many serious points of vulnerability. This is true because of questions about the entire system; technology alone is only part of the problem. The system includes people; who constitute perhaps the greatest risk. People print out portions of a record, copy it to nonsecure media, paste portions into other records, select weak passwords, leave papers on desks and cabinets unlocked, tinker with programs, gossip, and blab. Worse yet are the disgruntled employees who sabotage database systems, copy them from the workplace, and use the name and contact information for other, often illicit purposes. At least on par for disruptiveness are logic bombs[3] that an insider can use to sabotage a computer system (Hulme, 2002). These vulnerabilities call for setting up, monitoring, and enforcing appropriate workplace policies.

As mentioned previously, a core system's need for maintenance and updates means the presence of outside technicians and services. More difficulty arises because the core CPR system is part of a larger, immensely complex, ever-changing, and ill-defined multiagency system. Both for clinical expediency and to meet regulatory demands, the local system must be flexibly constructed to communicate, conform, and comply into the indefinite future. Routine software upgrades and security-enhancing patches sent by software manufacturers may contain vulnerabilities, either inadvertant or deliberately planted (Yager, 2002). This possibility means that users, as well as designers, are obliged to keep up with developments and requirements, maintain vigilance, and live with considerable risk and uncertainty.

The latest industry trend is to employ an information security czar, on the level of the chief financial officer, chief operating officer, and chief technical officer, who is responsible for internal political, personnel, and policy aspects; business repercussions; physical security; and technical protection (Pope, 2002). In smaller health care organizations, this person could probably double as the chief privacy officer, required by the federal privacy regulations under HIPAA.

Any practitioner or other entity acting as the custodian of health information must engage specific security features to physically secure locations for data system components, identify authorized users, control and permit authorized local and remote user access to internal and external sources of data, control input and amendment of data by users, control outbound data transmission, protect data integrity, promote information and process completeness, manage database backup and recovery, and foster data system availability and reliability.

Backup measures are almost always inadequate. The key issue is how much data a practitioner can afford to lose. Being unable to bill for a few sessions is a problem, but not having a record of key clinical transactions can affect treatment outcome and hobble a practitioner's defense against malpractice allegations. In fact, it is not difficult to imagine a claim on two counts: one for alleged malpractice and a second for the loss of data. Practitioners should collect and record essential information in a way that permits this information to be reentered into the automated system in the event of a crash. Files should be backed up frequently enough so that the gaps left after getting a system going again following a major disruption are tolerable. Perhaps the best way to do this is to have backup performed automatically and almost continuously, rather than only at the end of a working day.

As the key issues of confidentiality and security are resolved, CPRs will take their place at the center of the information stream that supplies the entire health care enterprise. The adoption of such technology may be pushed by legislation, as in California, which has mandated that:

> this plan shall include technology implementation, such as, but not limited to, computerized physician order entry or other technology that, based upon independent, expert scientific advice and data, has been shown effective in eliminating or substantially reducing medication-related errors.
>
> —(SB 1875, 2000)

---

[3] A logic bomb or "slag code" is a time-delayed computer virus.

The Web site of the nonprofit Medical Records Institute (http://www.medrecinst.com) tracks developments in this area. Despite the issues of compatibility, security, and resource allocation, the lower costs of using advanced technology will likely be the main force driving decisions in the increasingly competitive health care field.

Legislation, Standards, and Guidelines

Although the differences between legislation, standards and guidelines can tend to blur for some readers, we will focus primarily on the topic of records here, and dissect the legal and regulatory language in chapter 9. Let us begin by first discussing legislation related to records.

Legislation. Legislation governing patients' health care records vary somewhat between jurisdictions. The paper record, of course, is most commonly used now. Various jurisdictions have established legal requirements of varying degrees of clarity on what information is to be recorded, how long information is to be retained, and what its content should be. The rules, formulated for paper records, are undergoing modification and extension to adjust to the new opportunities, cost considerations, and risks introduced by the digitization of the medical record. Nonetheless, online practice does not diminish patient protections; at least until the law becomes clearer, all applicable laws should be applied to electronic records:

> Although it is true that new laws and regulations that address the computerized record are being introduced, readers should not believe that just because a current law/regulation does not have the word *electronic* in it, they should ignore it. We often run into that problem with people who call the American Health Information Management Association (AHIMA) for advice. Many laws/regulations simply refer to the medical record or patient information and do not distinguish between paper or electronic. These laws/regulations apply to health information media; readers should believe that a health information law/regulation does not apply to them because the law is old and that they need to wait for the version that refers specifically to electronic records.
> —(H. Rhodes, personal communication, October 25, 2002)

Regulation is changing because of the rapid development of electronic commerce in health care practice, and this trend will continue for the foreseeable future. An example of such changing regulation is the broad ruling signed into law by President George W. Bush. Since the September 11, 2001, terrorism attacks, Section 215 of the USA Patriot Act of 2001 (HR 3163) allows FBI agents to apply to a judge for permission to access medical records, including psychiatric and psychotherapeutic notes, to aid in protecting the country against terrorist activities. These subpoena powers could be used in response to various threats, including medical epidemics (Mulligan, 2002a).

As most practitioners know, releasing medical information generally requires patient consent, and the release of medical information related to mental health requires additional releases. The mental health professional should check local, state, and federal requirements for details. Practitioners must follow HIPAA guidelines for security and confidentiality in the transmission of medical information where appropriate (see chapter 9). As for now, release of medical records from a treatment program to a professional is subject to limitations on further dissemination to other entities without additional release(s) from the patient. For example, a professional release of medical record information for federal programs offering treatment for alcohol and substance abuse must be accompanied by the following statement and must have the client's written consent over and above general consent for every requested release (Schanz & Cepelewicz, 2001):

> This information has been disclosed to you from records protected by Federal confidentiality rules (42 CFR, Part 2). The Federal rules prohibit professionals from making any further disclosure of this information unless further disclosure is expressly permitted by written consent of the person to whom it pertains or as otherwise permitted by 42 CFR, Part 2. A general authorization for the release of medical or other information is NOT sufficient for this purpose. The Federal rules restrict any use of the information to criminally investigate or prosecute any alcohol or drug abuse patient.
> —(National Archives and Records Administration, 2001, § 2.32)

Policies, Standards and Guidelines. The American Medical Association has promulgated a number of policies with regard to electronic communication and patient records. Practitioners can access the following policies by searching the AMA Web site (http://www.ama-assn.org):

- E-5.07 Confidentiality: Computers.
- H-315.989 Confidentiality of Computerized Patient Records.
- H-315.990 Confidentiality of Computerized Patient Records.
- H-315.993 Evolving Electronic Health Care Record Systems.
- H-478.997 Guidelines for Patient–Physician Electronic Mail.
- H-480.971 The Computer-Based Patient Record.

The American Nurses Association (ANA) (1995) issued a position paper on computer-based patient record standards in accord with the Computer-Based Patient Record Institute and the Health Information and Management Systems Society (HIMSS, http://www.himss.org). These two organizations merged to create a definitive information resource on CPR issues for the health care professions. The ANA position is also in accord with the aforementioned policies of the American Medical Association.

Psychiatric nurse practitioners and support staff should read the various position papers and standards before implementing any CPR in their offices or institutions. To protect an investment, the practitioner should comply with these standards and incorporate appropriate legal language into a contract with any vendor. The vendor's system should support current professional and applicable legal standards, including HIPAA. The system should be upgraded and tested against those standards as they evolve.

The organization formed by the merger between the CPRI-HOST and HIMSS organizations will likely issue standards and guidelines on CPR issues. The National Committee on Vital and Health Statistics workgroup is the public advisory body to the Secretary of Health and Human Services. In its statement to the committee regarding computer-based patient records, the AMA stated:

> [The AMA believes that] a patient's health record should include sufficient information for [another] health care professional to assess previous treatment, to ensure continuity of care, and to avoid unnecessary or inappropriate tests or therapy.
> —(American Medical Association, 1998)

Whether keeping a record of services delivered online, on paper, or in electronic format, mental health professionals may want to document the expanded dimensions of the online situation. For example, an online consultation between a patient and a psychiatric nurse practitioner at a primary care site and a psychiatrist via live interactive video needs to document the additional dimensions required by online service. Professional's may need to consult state regulations for specific requirements. Such regulations might include:

- Informed consent for online clinical practice.
- Time of transmission.
- Names of all involved parties.
- Primary (and secondary) practitioner identification by name, professional designation, location, and specialty.
- Signature of primary practitioner.
- Documentation of a specialist's recommendations in the medical record.
- Type of computer-based patient record used.
- The type of technology and the software systems used.
- Any known limitations for e-mail, live video, store-and-forward, or asynchronous technologies used for the online consultation.

The American Psychiatric Association (1998a) approved a resource document for telepsychiatry via videoconferencing. Regarding medical records, the document states:

> Medical records of telepsychiatric interventions are to be maintained as with psychiatric interventions in general. If the quality of a transmission was poor, this should be documented in the patient record. Telepsychiatric care is subject to Quality Assurance monitoring as with other forms of medical care; procedures should be systematically monitored and evaluated as part of overall quality improvement of a facility.
>
> The progress note for an interview by videoconference may include the following information:
>
> - The location of the clinician providing the service (this may be different from the clinician's office);
> - The location of the patient (town, facility where seen);
> - Type of equipment used and any malfunction that may affect clinical care;
> - Who was present during the office visit, and what their role was.

Choosing a Computer-Based Patient Record System

The reader will note that this section is similar to the considerations listed for practice management software purchases. The various similiarities between practice management software and the CPR are evidence that the two types of software will eventually converge. For this same reason, the forward-looking practitioner should be aware of both types of software and should seek vendors that are planning for the merger.

Making the transition to a computer-based patient record may occur in stages and will depend on the practice type, size, and location. The bottom line for many organizations is resource allocation. The initial financial outlay for a system may significantly affect the fiscal year's budget. In any practice situation, the time to implement, train, and operationalize a system can create time delays that have associated costs. It is necessary to plan carefully and to consider transitioning over time as new and continuing patients come into the practice. Top people in the practice or clinic, including senior clinicians, will have to devote time to planning, training and tweaking, and to cleaning up mistakes. It is thus necessary to plan carefully and to be ready to fall back on hand processing when the system misfires, while providing adequate service for new and continuing patients.

As with nearly every subject in this book, the decision about going digital is not whether but how, when, and how much. Increasingly, practitioners submitting claims for third-party reimbursement will benefit from moving to electronic billing services. From this point, adding clinical records bit by bit will be straightforward and rewarding both clinically and financially.

Mental health practitioners need to determine whether a CPR makes sense in their particular settings, both financially and clinically. Ancillary benefits may include lower malpractice risk and protection from embezzlement. In choosing the CPR that is best for one's practice, the practitioner should:

- Identify the functions needed in a system and not purchase functionality that will not be used very soon. Identify specific technical specifications needed in the practice environment.
- Tabulate the return on investment that can realistically be expected. It is usually best to be conservative in estimating cost savings and to exaggerate costs and implementation timing.
- Identify any hidden costs related to technical components—software upgrades, hardware, telephone lines, internal wiring, and routers, for example. Insist that the vendor include all these costs in the overall plan.
- Clearly identify technical-support requirements and resources with the vendor in areas of training and service, and specify them in the written contract along with performance penalties. If the vendor cannot provide the technical backup and training required to be successful, find another vendor.
- Check on the vendor's financial position. One difficulty in the fast-paced technology market is the merger, acquisition, or bankruptcy of the vendor or the vendor's suppliers. Contractual safeguards can limit the resulting damage, through indemnification clauses, for example.
- Identify the availability of regular clinical updates and their cost. If these are not provided, find another vendor.
- Check the vendor's experience in the relevant clinical specialty and with similar practices, and converse with some of the vendor's other customers.
- Get the vendor to ensure technical compatibility with existing systems.
- Negotiate the contract with the help of an attorney knowledgeable about the relevant issues to protect a practice or organization when things go wrong.

A stable and prosperous vendor will be eager for continuing business and strong recommendations. Signs of vendor strength include a substantial list of happy customers; a sharp focus on a core product or mission rather than a scattered array of innovations and ideals; a relatively large, well-trained, experienced, and highly organized sales force led by a head of sales who has an exceptional resume; and plenty of cash reserves (Marhula, 2003). A consultant may be able to ferret out and interpret information on acompany's reliability and financial health.

Advocacy

Another issue of importance here is the difference between the storage of notes pertinent to general health care versus those specific to mental health care. Most often, both terms refer to a patient's longitudinal health data, compiled across a lifetime. Although current systems contain information for a limited amount of time, the goals of many CPR and EMR developers are to develop and disseminate systems capable of storing a patient's lifelong history of health status and health care.

This trend offers both advantages and disadvantages to the patient, particularly to the mental health patient. For reasons ranging from error to poor memory, the desire to avoid stigmatization, and the prevention of embarrassment for unfair employment or firing practices at work, patients have had good reasons to seek protection of medical, especially mental health, privacy. Of course, some patients may wish to dupe third-party health care companies.

Nonetheless, decision makers are moving toward widespread adoption of lifelong records, typically stored on a computer chip, such as on a smart card carried by the patient, or kept in a centralized data warehouse. As we discuss in chapter 9, HIPAA makes provisions for exemptions related to psychotherapy notes. How these provisions will reflect the needs of mental health patients and their CPRs is yet to be seen. Concerned professionals are encouraged to communicate with their professional associations to determine the extent to which the associations are involved in defining the parameters of CPRs for mental health patients. The next chapter also examines legal, regulatory, and reimbursement issues that will affirm the need for increased familiariety with computerization in the practice of mental health care, as discussed in this chapter.

Legal and Regulatory Issues

By collapsing distances, crossing borders, and creating new definitions of care and new ways to deliver it, the psychotechnologies raise a confusing array of national and international legal, regulatory, and reimbursement issues. This chapter is restricted to aspects of privacy and confidentiality, security of information, regulation of health care devices, electonic signatures, licensure, and reimbursement. These are the issues of most immediate relevance to clinical practice.

Our intention is to prepare professionals to examine specific details with their local licensing bodies and regulatory agencies in order to determine how to organize their electronic practices. Professionals are advised to keep up with relevant statements published by professional societies about evolving standards and practice norms and to be aware of the latest official material published by their national government on telehealth. Such information is conveniently available in searchable format in the Code of Federal Regulations and the Federal Register (http://www.access. gpo.gov/nara/cfr). The Civic Research Institute (http://www.civicresearchinstitute. com) has issued a helpful compendium, *Telemedicine Law and Practice for the United States*, and offers additional information on its Web site (Schanz & Cepelewicz, 2001). Consultation with an attorney who has special expertise in telehealth law is also advisable for certain purposes.

PRIVACY PROTECTIONS

Privacy and confidentiality are central concerns about the use of technology in mental health services, especially psychotechnologies related to telecommunication. Approximately 6.3 million Internet users decline to access online health information because they worry about security and confidentiality (Cyber Dialogue, 2000). The Electronic Privacy Information Center (EPIC; http://www.epic.org) offers extensive information about health-related and other privacy issues.

Many professionals eagerly turn to e-mail to discuss difficult cases or to seek referrals for patients. The following two messages (edited to protect the patients) appeared on a large e-mail forum for mental health professionals. As of this writing, both messages remain available in the online archive:

1) Looking for a referral in the [MIDSIZE TOWN] [STATE] area, for a [AGE] year-old retired [DIFFERENT STATE] [UNUSUAL VOCATION], Vietnam Vet, with mild to moderate dysphoria and some (largely suppressed) PTSD. Stable, cooperative, no history of drugs or violence needs basic psychopharm and intermittent support.

2) A [AGE] yo ["RACE" & SEX] I have presented here before is moving to [CITY].
[HE/SHE] has had severe, and very difficult to control Bipolar I disorder, and also has had
innumerable psychotherapeutic issues with [HIS/HER] abusive family. ***[HE/SHE]
has been disabled for a number of years, but has made miraculous strides in [HIS/HER]
personal and professional life, and now has a job in [HIS/HER] field of [LICENSED
HELPING PROFESSION]—the first in about 7 years! [Signed by professional in named
midsized city.]

If the redacted information were restored, the patient in the first example would immediately be recognized by an acquaintance because of the very specific description. The clinician in the second example, who is in a position of great trust, is dealing with relatively powerless clients. A public-spirited citizen of the city mentioned might feel obliged to track down this recent arrival and alert the authorities or the press, especially because the original e-mail detailed the patient's psychotherapeutic issues.

Two regulatory acts dominate current practice with regard to privacy and the electronic transmission of health care information: the U.S. Health Insurance Portability and Accountability Act (HIPAA) and the EU Directive. The movement toward electronic commerce in health care is further supported by electronic signatures (discussed later in this chapter). International developments are reviewed in the annual "Privacy and Human Rights" survey (Electronic Privacy Information Center, 2002). Historical information is available in the Civic Research Institute compendium (http://www.civicresearchinstitute.com).

Professionals should be aware of the implications of the wide range of privacy issues that involve health care information and electronic commerce, so that they can respond adequately to their patients' concerns and needs.

A Brief History

A short chronology of legal authorities pertinent to privacy in psychotechnology within the United States begins with the Privacy Act of 1974. This act mandated that U.S. federal information systems protect the confidentiality of *individually identifiable health information*. Federal systems are obliged to establish appropriate administrative, technical, and physical safeguards to ensure the security and confidentiality of records and to protect against any anticipated threats or hazards to their security or integrity that could result in substantial harm, embarrassment, inconvenience, or unfairness to any individual on whom information is maintained (Health Care Financing Administration, 1998).

The Privacy Act was followed by the Right to Financial Privacy Act (1974), the Privacy Protection Act (1980), the Electronic Communications Privacy Act (1986), the Video Privacy Protection Act (1988), and, more recently, the Telephone Consumer Protection Act (1991), the Telecommunications Act (1996), the Health Insurance Portability and Accountability Act, commonly called "HIPPA" (Center for Medicare and Medicaid Services, 1996), and the Children's Online Privacy Protection Act (1998). A sizable and prospering industry has sprung up to explain HIPAA privacy regulations to administrators, information system planners, and clinicians.

A 1997 report to the U.S. President from the Advisory Commission on Consumer Protection and Quality in the Health Care Industry recognized the need for consumer protections. In 1997, the U.S. Congress passed the Balanced Budget Act (Public Law 105-34), which added language to the Social Security Act (18 U.S.C. 1852) for the protection of individually identifiable health information under HIPAA (45 C.F.R., Parts 160–164).

A global perspective on privacy concerns, both in the United States and abroad, was published jointly by the Electronic Privacy Information Center (EPIC) and Privacy International (Banisar, 2002). This study strongly suggests that neither govenmental regulations nor technological advances hold promise of strong guarantees that either professionals or patients can completely control electronic records or communications of personal health information. Privacy is always a matter of degree. Data may be released for national security purposes without consent and yet may otherwise be kept reasonably secret. Data from many patients may be aggregated for administrative or research purposes.

Attitudes to privacy differ among cultures. Many dictatorships evince little regard for human rights. In European countries, people tend to accept the advantages of governments' acquiring personal details about individuals and resent such information coming into the hands of commercial enterprises; in the United States, however, there is more resistance to the notion of governmental intrusion into private lives and relatively less concern about private-sector exploitation of personal information (Varney, 1996).

Working Definitions

A fair amount of confusion abounds about the terms *privacy*, *confidentiality*, and *data protections*. The next section outlines the key distinctions.

Privacy. According to the U.S. General Accounting Office (1999), privacy is "the specific right of an individual to control the collection, use, and disclosure of personal information" (p. 4). Consumers may not be sufficiently aware of what they should protect from whom, and why. Before involving a client in personal therapy using psychotechnologies, a professional should obtain informed consent that covers privacy and confidentiality.

Confidentiality. "Confidentiality is the right of an individual to not have personally identifiable medical or other information disclosed to others without that individual's express informed consent" (Winker et al., n.d.). Confidentiality can be seen as the tool for protecting privacy (National Telecommunications and Information Administration, 1997). A client's informed consent can authorize relaxation of confidentiality for specific information. HIPPA has many provisions under which information of various degrees of sensitivity may or must be released even without the patient's consent.

Data Protections. The professional's obligation to protect privacy also entails the need to ensure adequate security provisions of one's Internet service provider, Web site host, Web site developer, local network, and personal computer. *Data integrity* is the assurance that information is not entered incorrectly because of program coding inadequacies or does not inadvertently change, deteriorate, or get lost. New programs are notorious for having "bugs"—tendencies to misread or otherwise alter information. Some program fields are interpreted by some users to mean one thing and by other users to mean another.

Software must be field tested with a specific population (e.g., accountants, dentists, nurses, psychotherapists) in order to remove predictable errors in data entry based on specific knowledge held by a group of professionals. Once errors have been removed, policies and procedures, such as written archiving and data retrieval procedures, can be put in place to protect data integrity on a computer (Maheu, Whitten, & Allen, 2001).

The Association for Information and Image Management, an accredited organization of the American National Standards Institute, has recommend practices on a number of issues related to data integrity (http://www.aiim.org/documents/standards/AIIM_ARP1_2002.pdf).

Security. A separate but related concept is security. Security refers to techniques or methods (e.g., password protections), policies, and practices for controlling information access and data integrity. Only approved persons can become aware of, find, retrieve, and interpret secured information. We refer to security issues throughout this chapter and then discuss security issues more extensively in chapter 10.

Trust versus Trustworthiness

Health care (including veterinary medicine) depends on eliciting and deserving trust. People are often suspicious of material presented on the Internet, and they worry about privacy (Poensgen & Larsson, 2001). An analysis of the privacy practices of 21 popular e-health sites revealed that although they had clearly stated policies, the Web sites did not adhere to them, and most did not even follow minimum fair information practices (Goldman, Hudson, & Smith, 2000). If proven, these deviations could result in action by the Federal Trade Commission, by state regulatory boards, or by citizens pursuing private rights of action. From a risk management perspective, it would be better to post no privacy policy than to violate the one posted.

The sad truth is that some Web sites use privacy policy statements merely to make the consumer feel more comfortable. Meanwhile, behind the facade of a home page, those sites are careless with the information they gather from visitors. Enforced standards delineating allowable use of a person's identifiable health information can help preserve trust in the health care system and in the individuals and institutions that comprise it (U.S. Department of Health and Human Services, 2001).

A psychologist who runs an online service for consumers reported this example of the importance of trust:

> *Joanne, a 34-year-old accountant, was upset that her husband, Scott, was paying less and less attention to her and their two children. When Joanne asked Scott about his extra hours at the office and late nights on the home computer, Scott insisted that his workload had increased. Joanne accepted the answer until she caught Scott masturbating at the computer late one night. After a long talk, Scott promised to stop his online sexual activity and spend more time with his family. Unfortunately, it became apparent throughout the next month that Scott was unable to keep his promise. Joanne desperately sought the help of a psychologist. Dr. Lane met with Joanne weekly and suggested that between sessions, Joanne visit OnlineSexAddict.org for education and support.*
>
> *The OnlineSexAddict.org bulletin board service allowed Joanne to read stories of people such as herself and the struggles of men and women who felt they were sexually addicted. This helped Joanne better understand her husband's problem and gave her questions to bring to therapy. Eventually, Joanne decided to share her own experiences on the Web site, but preferred to remain anonymous because of her concerns about the confidentiality of her personal information. Joanne read the confidentiality statement and reviewed the membership benefits and guidelines. She was pleased to learn that none of her information would be shared by the Web site or its members and decided to pay a small fee to become an OnlineSexAddict.org member.*

In the member's area, Joanne chatted with several women with similar experiences; this activity provided the support and understanding she needed. The testimonials of her online friends also convinced Joanne to take a course offered through the OnlineSexAddict.org Web site. The course educated Joanne about the development of sexual problems on the Internet and taught her some treatment approaches that allowed her to communicate with Scott more effectively. The new skills helped Joanne convince Scott to enter marital therapy and resolve the problems that had damaged their relationship.

— **Dana Putnam, Ph.D.**
Owner and Founder
OnlineSexAddict.org

The security of the technology used to deliver services directly limits confidentiality. System breakdown or unauthorized users accessing data or backups of data could compromise patient confidentiality (Australian Psychological Society, 1999). Before information is digitized and entered into easily accessible and cross-referenced databases, each professional and organization needs to analyze exactly who should have access to the data and for what purpose.

When hackers gain access to confidential medical records stored in computers, there is wholesale loss of privacy. For example, a hacker infiltrated the University of Washington Medical Center medical records database and stole confidential information on more than 5,000 patients (Chin, 2001). There are many examples of medical records being maliciously published or inadvertently revealed, often because a respected corporation or medical center failed to use adequate safeguards. Certain computer viruses e-mail copies of random files stored on a victim's hard drive; unprotected patient information can thus be widely disseminated. Other viruses that harvest names from a computer's address book could determine that Person X may be a mental health patient of Professional Y. Each organization providing services must decide the appropriate amount of money to allocate to protect the confidentiality of data (Ziglin, 1995). HIPAA sets out minimum requirements, which can be quite expensive.

Health Insurance Portability and Accountability Act

As you may know, federal regulations have been promulgated by the United States Dept. of Health and Human Services to guarantee to patients new rights and protections against the misuse of disclosure of their health records by health care providers who transmit health information in electronic form in connection with specified health claim transactions.... Traditionally, privacy and confidentiality laws have been a matter of state law. Now, under federal law and regulation, the federal rule will preempt state law in some respects and state law will apply in other respects. New rights are accorded to patients and significant obligations are imposed on providers who are covered by the regulations.

—(Leslie, 2002, p. 1)

In the United States, HIPAA regulates privacy of most medical records. Its protections are the national standard for administrative and financial electronic data transactions. The U.S. Congress sought to facilitate efficiencies and cost savings through the increasing use of electronic information exchange for financial and administrative transactions while recognizing the privacy challenges engendered by the electronic interface. When Congress failed to enact standards by August 1999, the Secretary of

Health and Human Services was required to issue standards to protect the security and privacy of individually identifiable health information transmitted over the Internet (U.S. Department of Health and Human Services, 2003).

HIPAA has three rule sets; they address transactions, security, and privacy, respectively. A brief mention here of the transaction and security rules suffices, at least now, for most mental health practitioners. We then focus on privacy rules because they have the most impact on mental health professionals. A full discussion of HIPAA and the regulations promulgated pursuant to it is beyond the scope of this text; indeed, this topic could supply the material for a separate book. We touch on it briefly here because no discussion of the psychotechnologies can ignore this statute and the intricate regulatory framework to which it has given rise. For more specific information, mental health professionals are advised to review all HIPAA rules (available at http://aspe.hhs.gov/admnsimp). Another useful Web site is produced by the Workgroup for Electronic Data Interchange (http://www.wedi.org/snip).

HIPAA Transaction and Security Rules. In what is often referred to by professionals as the Transaction Rule, HIPAA requires standard formatting for certain financial and administrative electronic transactions. In practical terms, the Transaction Rule means that if using electronic media for billing, the practitioner has to be ready and able to put electronic claims data into standardized HIPAA format (Nickelson, 2002).

The security rule addresses such issues as access to computers and electronic files. This rule is not very detailed, and compliance with it will probably not be exceptionally difficult. Given the extraordinary rate at which new technologies can become obsolete, the Department of Health and Human Services (HHS) avoided specifying what measures ought to be taken and instead requires covered entities[1] to abide by a reasonableness standard. April 2005 is the compliance date for the Security Rule.

Of particular importance to mental health professionals is the requirement that any e-mail be encrypted and digitally signed.

HIPAA Privacy Rule. The deadline for most covered entities to comply was April 14, 2003 (http://telehealth.hrsa.gov/pubs/hipaatxt.htm); small health plans had until April 14, 2004, to comply. Mental health professionals are advised to check the government Web site (http://aspe.hhs.gov/admnsimp) for up-to-date information.

Penalties and Compliance. Who needs to know about HIPAA? Who is legally bound by HIPAA rules? How will HIPAA affect mental health professionals? Answers to these questions are important because noncompliance can result in significant penalties, with fines in the most egregious cases of up to $250,000 and 10 years imprisonment. However, most mental health professionals sanctioned under the regulations would have to pay much lower fines, from about $100 per violation and not to exceed $25,000 per year.

To avoid these penalties, a covered entity must take "reasonable" steps, according to its size and functions, to meet the requirements. In other words, the administrative requirements of the Privacy Rule are on a scale. The administrative burden on a

---

[1] Any health care professional who files claims electronically instantly becomes a "covered entity," subject to the full requirements and stiff fines imposed under HIPAA.

hospital is much greater than that on a solo practitioner. A hospital may be required to create a full-time staff position to serve as a privacy officer, whereas a solo practitioner may designate himself or herself as privacy officer.

HIPAA privacy regulations acknowledge that incidental disclosure may occur from time to time and is not a violation of the rule as long as reasonable safeguards and minimum security requirements have been met to protect patient information. The Department of Health and Human Services, Office for Civil Rights (OCR), will enforce HIPAA regulations and will help practitioners, health plans, and health care clearing-houses meet its requirements (see http://www.hhs.gov/ocr/hipaa). Theoretically, a practitioner can obtain assistance with HIPAA by telephone; the toll- free number is 1-866-627-7748. The TTY number is 1-866-788-4989. Readers interested in more specific information are encouraged to start with these Web sites.

- Covered Entity Decision Tools (how to tell whether you are a covered entity) (http://www.cms.hhs.gov/hipaa/hipaa2/support/tools/decisionsupport/default. asp).
- A Path to HIPAA Compliance by Paul Litwak (http://www.hipaacomplianceguide. com).
- American Psychological Association Practice Directorate (http://www. APApractice.org).

Many professional organizations, such as the National Association of College and University Attorneys (http://www.nacua.org), offer seminars on HIPAA. Of course, for application of HIPAA rules to specific situations, and in particular for help in coping with applicable state law and its interaction with federal law, consult knowledgeable counsel.

Protected Health Information. HIPAA privacy rules apply only to specifically defined health information. The final rules define *protected health information* (PHI) to include individually identifiable health information that is transmitted or maintained in any electronic form or medium. It is important for all health care professionals to realize, however, that once the HIPAA privacy regulations have been triggered, the regulations affect all patient or client information, not just information contained in electronic records. Not all providers are covered entities; only those that engage in covered transactions are covered and hence obliged to follow the privacy rules. Once a provider executes any of the specified transactions electronically (see list on page 229), that provider becomes a covered entity. HIPAA privacy regulations then pertain to individually identifiable health information any form—electronic, paper, or verbal—whether or not that particular bit of information has been transmitted or maintained electronically.

Individually identifiable health information refers to health information defined as information that health care professionals or entities create or use to diagnose or treat patients or to facilitate payment for services. Such information has components that could be used to identify the client. Individually identifiable health information includes any health or demographic information about an individual that is created or received by a covered entity; that relates to an individual's past, present, or future physical or mental health condition; that relates to the provision of an individual's health care; or that relates to the past, present, or future payment for the provision of an individual's health care. Examples of data elements that make information individually identifiable are the following:

- An individual's, relative's, or employer's name, address, phone and fax numbers, and/or e-mail address.
- Date of birth or of hospitalization.
- Photographs, video recordings.
- Social Security Number, medical record numbers, and membership, automobile license, or account numbers.

Who Is a "Covered Entity"? HIPAA Privacy Rule does not apply to everyone. For example, HIPAA does not apply in educational settings where the Federal Education and Privacy Act (FERPA) applies. Similarly, HIPAA does not apply to professionals, such as some forensic or industrial/organizational psychologists, whose services are not related to health care.

The only providers who are not covered entities are those who do not engage in covered transactions. Health plans, health care clearinghouses, and most health care practitioners are all *covered entities* and are required to comply with HIPAA requirements. As third-party payers increasingly insist on doing business by electronic transactions, the already small percentage of providers that are not covered entities will get even smaller.

Many practitioners decided to bring themselves into compliance by the April 14, 2003, deadline for two specific reasons. First, many circumstances out of a practitioner's control can trigger the rule. Suppose that a client submits a professional's bill to a health plan, which transmits it electronically to corporate headquarters with the professional's name on it. Presto—the professional has been transformed into a covered entity, responsible for complying with the rules. As soon as the law is triggered, practitioners are expected to be compliant. There is no grace period for practitioners to become compliant after they realize that they have triggered the law. Furthermore, becoming a covered entity can involve as little as one transmission, and this coverage is permanent.

The second reason for U.S. practitioners to bring themselves into compliance as soon as possible is that unless one is contemplating full and permanent retirement in the immediate future, the need to be compliant is practically inevitable. Even though many U.S. practitioners may not yet be transmitting electronic patient information, they probably will in the near future. Medicare billing is quickly changing to electronic transmission requirements, and other insurance companies are following suit because such transmission is less costly and more efficient. For years, paper record keeping has been associated with delayed payment. Soon, paper record keeping will be associated with no payment from third-party carriers.

Definitions of all entities and exceptions are available in the Federal Register (45 C.F.R., Parts 160–164) and on the Web site (http://telehealth.hrsa.gov/pubs/hipaatxt. htm). A number of foundations and nonprofit groups have developed information and reference materials of varying quality and detail for practitioners who are covered entities. One example is the *HIPAA Administrative Simplification: Tool Kit for Small Group and Safety-Net Providers*, offered by the Pacific Health Policy Group (2002). As mental health professionals prepare their respective practices to include online clinical practice services, a good rule is to search out these tools and incorporate their information. It would be wise, however, to get professional legal advice before going online, rather than to rely exclusively on generic resources, especially if one is in a special circumstance.

The privacy rules apply to the mental health professional's entire practice (including information that was not transmitted electronically) once electronic transactions are executed covering these areas:

- Health care claims.
- Health care payment and remittance advice.
- Coordination of benefits.
- Health care claim status.
- Enrollment or disenrollment in a health plan.
- Eligibility for a health plan.
- Health plan premium payments.
- Referral certification and authorization.
- First report of injury.
- Health claims attachments (American Psychological Association, 2002b, p. 3).

These operations apply to the business associates of a mental health professional as well. A business associate who handles protected health information electronically triggers HIPAA privacy rules for the mental health practitioner. (For a discussion of covered transactions, see 1173(a)(1) of the Act). Technically, the business associates of covered entities are not under the jurisdiction of the U.S. Department of Health and Human Services and are not obliged by law to comply. Covered entities, however, entering into contracts with such business associates must have them sign a business associate contract that vouches for their compliance. Covered entities, then, impose by contract substantially (though not exactly) the same requirements on the business associates as are imposed by law on the covered entities. Examples of business associates are billing, bookkeeping, accounting, and other professional support services that have or receive knowledge of specific patient health information.

Nearly all mental health professionals should consider themselves a covered entity and should behave accordingly. Before continuing, let us also say that mental health care practitioners do not need to make dramatic changes from current practice that relies on good clinical judgment and is in compliance with state law. Most mental health clinicians have essentially been in conformity with HIPAA privacy principles throughout their practices. However, now there is a requirement for extra documentation and detail. The Privacy Rule does require formal written policies and procedures for how records are handled in the office, as well as for how professionals document training and agreements with business associates and coworkers who may have access to records. For example, most practitioners have discussed confidentiality with their office staff, such as receptionists, office managers, and billing specialists. These staff members now must be trained about the Privacy Rule, and that training must be documented.

It is a good idea for all professionals, including those working outside the United States, to take a short course (perhaps online) or to read expositions of do's and don'ts (see, for example, the frequently asked questions resource at http://www.hhs.gov/ocr/hipaa/assist.html). This research can remind the clinician about many privacy issues, such as calling out the name of a patient in the waiting room or leaving a message on a patient's answering machine. Such actions may be permissible under HIPAA but may call for special discretion with mental health patients. Note also that the Privacy Rule gives patients the right to inspect and copy their records and to amend certain information, to have an accounting of what use has been made of their records, and to restrict their future use to some extent.

Psychotherapy Notes. HIPAA gives psychotherapists the option of keeping psychotherapy notes separate from the remainder of a clinical file. Psychotherapy notes have been given special protection under HIPAA because they contain sensitive information that is never intended to be shared with other parties. It is understood that patients receiving mental health treatment may have greater privacy needs than do people receiving general health care. Many of these needs result from the societal stigmatization of mental disorders. Also, many patients fear that disclosure of their psychotherapy records could cause irreparable harm to their relationships with family, friends, business associates, and/or acquaintances. Practitioners have long been trained to restrict access to patient's intimate thoughts, words, and emotions.

A number of court decisions, including the U.S. Supreme Court *Jaffee v. Redmond*, 518 U.S. 1 (1996), have set forth legal protections of the content of psychotherapy sessions. In this decision, the Supreme Court emphasized the importance of protecting the privacy integral to the patient and psychotherapist by contrasting physical health care with psychotherapeutic care:

> Treatment by a physician for physical ailments can often proceed successfully on the basis of a physical examination, objective information supplied by the patient, and the results of diagnostic tests. Effective psychotherapy, by contrast, depends upon an atmosphere of confidence and trust in which the patient is willing to make a frank and complete disclosure of facts, emotions, memories, and fears. Because of the sensitive nature of the problems for which individuals consult psychotherapists, disclosure of confidential communications made during counseling sessions may cause embarrassment or disgrace. For this reason, the mere possibility of disclosure may impede development of the confidential relationship necessary for successful treatment.

Traditionally, mental health professionals took notes after psychotherapy or counseling sessions. Managed care began demanding increased documentation, requiring preauthorization of further sessions, and lowering reimbursement rates. Practitioners responded by shortening sessions and by taking notes (often during sessions) that served several purposes simultaneously. Many third-party payers have asserted the right to audit these notes in an effort to curb billing misrepresentation. In addition, requests for authorization of future sessions often required detailed accounts of the patient's status with respect to suicide or homicide and also emotional, cognitive, and physical states, such as tearfulness, hopelessness, irritability, hostility, lability, paranoia, delusions, level of participation in treatment, weight changes, physical illnesses, medication taken, types of problems experienced (such as with family, friends, or coworkers), days of work missed owing to mental health, and many other related issues. Answers to these mandatory questions were archived, sometimes handled quite casually and sometimes entered into electronic databases.

HIPAA Privacy Rule does not compel, but does permit, the creation of separate psychotherapy notes so that some sensitive information can now be exempted from most requirements to produce records. The term psychotherapy notes means

> notes recorded (in any medium) by a health care provider who is a mental health professional documenting or analyzing the content of conversations during the private

counseling session or a group, joint, or family counseling session and that are separated from the rest of the individual's medical record. Psychotherapy notes exclude medication, prescription and monitoring, counseling sessions, start and stop times, the modalities and frequencies of treatment furnished, results of clinical tests, and any summary of the following items: diagnosis, functional status, treatment plan, symptoms, prognosis and progress to date. (45 C.F.R. § 164.501)

Under the Privacy Rule, patients have relatively free access to their own records. Under 45 C.F.R. 164.524, however, individuals have no automatic right to inspect or obtain a copy of protected health information about themselves where that information is recorded in psychotherapy notes. A patient's access to such notes may be restricted under specific circumstances.

Disclosing information from psychotherapy notes to people other than the patient is also subject to special HIPAA privacy protections. The professional maintaining psychotherapy notes, then, can record highly sensitive information and keep it away from most peering eyes. To benefit from this protection, the practitioner must carefully segregate psychotherapy notes from other medical records. Clearly, maintaining separate psychotherapy notes may be useful if patients, on seeing them, might be inclined to harm themselves or others. Segregating the notes can also mean that other people will have greater difficulty gaining access to them, which would tend to preclude any claim of an HIPAA violation, any claim of invasion of privacy or breach of confidentiality under applicable state tort law, or liability on any other theory.

The downside, obviously, is that maintaining a separate record, and the complexities and disadvantages of taking notes at all, are compounded by the need to take two sets of notes. The practitioner must take special care to ensure that the psychotherapy notes are not intermingled with other notes, lest their special protected status be diminished or destroyed. No additional reimbursement, of course, is available to compensate professionals maintaining separate psychotherapy notes as defined in the Privacy Rule. There is an extra burden to exercise special care in handling psychotherapy notes (keeping them out of sight when they are not in use, locking them in a special area inaccessible to other staff members, or having special provisions for electronic psychotherapy notes, retrieving them in addition to the rest of the clinical record, etc.) Of course, a clinician might ask whether this practice should not be done routinely even if HIPAA did not exist. For a discussion of these topics from the American Psychiatric Association, see http://www.psych.org/archives/200201.pdf.

The Privacy Rule protection is not absolute. Under 45 C.F.R. 164.512(j), protected health information, including that contained in psychotherapy notes, can be used or disclosed to avert a serious threat to health or safety. Such disclosures and uses presuppose that the covered entity has formed a good-faith belief that the notes are "necessary to prevent or lessen a serious and imminent threat to the health or safety of a person or the public." Permitted uses and disclosures may be made only to "a person or persons reasonably able to prevent or lessen the threat, including the target of the threat." The Privacy Rule creates a presumption of good faith "if the belief is based upon the covered entity's actual knowledge or in reliance on a credible representation by a person with apparent knowledge or authority."

Note, however, that under HIPAA preemption rules, covered entities might have less freedom to disclose such information if they are practicing in a state that imposes a more narrow definition of the circumstances under which uses or disclosures may be made to avert harm or for other purposes defined in 45 C.F.R. 160.203(b). In Virginia, for example, according to Va. Code Ann. s. 32.1-127.1:03(f), such a disclosure may be made only when there is a threat to the health or well-being of the patient; this is a more narrowly defined circumstance than the federal Privacy Rule provides.

If notes on mental health issues are contained in a larger record concerned with other health matters, such as a psychiatry consultation report in the inpatient chart of a pneumonia patient, those notes cannot be defined as psychotherapy notes, because they are not segregated from the rest of the record. A similar situation results under the laws of a number of states, which, like HIPAA Privacy Rule, seem to emphasize separating psychotherapy notes from all other health records.

Covered entities are obliged under the Privacy Rule to disclose only the minimum necessary information to comply with a valid request (45 C.F.R. § 164.502 [b][1]). Compliance with many such requests might not require disclosure of the psychiatric consult. Moreover, under the HIPAA approach to preemption issues, a clinician practicing in a state that provides more stringent protection for mental health records than HIPAA does is to be bound by the requirements of state law, not federal. (See 45 C.F.R. § 160.203 [b].)

The special protection for psychotherapy notes states that no insurer can require disclosure of these notes as a condition of enrollment (45 C.F.R. § 164.508[b] [4][ii][B]). In addition, the provision does not require that the professional share psychotherapy notes with a patient even if the patient demands the records, as the patient is generally permitted to do under the Privacy Rule.

Although the issue is not free of doubt, it is probably wisest to assume that most other information that a mental health professional obtains and records about a patient—information that cannot be characterized as psychotherapy notes—would be treated no differently from information that, say, an internist gets when evaluating chest pain.

Ordinarily, a covered entity is permitted to disclose protected health information (PHI) to its subject, the patient (45 C.F.R. § 164.502 [a][1][i]). Psychotherapy notes are an exception (45 C.F.R. §§ 164.502 [a][1][iii]; 164.524 [a][1][i]). Release of such notes requires specific authorization from a client (45 C.F.R. § 164.508 [a][2]; see the following section for guidelines on patient authorization beyond general consent). An authorization for a use or disclosure of psychotherapy notes may not be combined with any other document except another authorization for a use or disclosure of psychotherapy notes (45 C.F.R. § 164.508 [b][3][ii]).

Because the new HIPAA protection significantly reduces risks that another person, will see psychotherapy notes, the professional may have more freedom to make notes "without distraction, fear, and self-censorship" (Fridhandler, 2002, p. 9). There are many guides to taking psychotherapy notes (e.g., Cameron, 2002). In discussing how the designation for psychotherapy notes came about in HIPAA, developers of HIPAA Privacy Rule noted:

> In response to commenters who opposed this proposal as a potential weakening of privacy protections or who wanted the minimum necessary requirements to apply to authorizations other than disclosures to the individual, the Department notes that nothing in the final Rule eliminates an individual's control over his or her protected health information with respect to an authorization. All authorizations must include a description of the information to be used and disclosed that identifies the information in a specific and meaningful fashion as required by [45 C.F.R.] § 164.508(c)(1)(i). If the individual does not wish to release the information requested, the individual has the right to not sign the authorization or to negotiate a narrower authorization with the requestor.
>
> Additionally, in response to those commenters who raised specific concerns with respect to authorizations which request release of psychotherapy notes, the Department clarifies that the final Rule does not require a covered entity to use and disclose protected

health information pursuant to an authorization. Rather, as with most other uses and disclosures under the Privacy Rule, this is only a permissible use or disclosure. If a covered health care provider is concerned that a request for an individual's psychotherapy notes is not warranted or is excessive, the provider may consult with the individual to determine whether or not the authorization is consistent with the individual's wishes.

Further, the Privacy Rule does not permit a health plan to condition enrollment, eligibility for benefits, or payment of a claim on obtaining the individual's authorization to use or disclose psychotherapy notes. Nor may a health care provider condition treatment on an authorization for the use or disclosure of psychotherapy notes. Thus, the Department believes that these additional protections appropriately and effectively protect an individual's privacy with respect to psychotherapy notes.... The implementation specifications describe what covered entities must do reasonably to limit uses, disclosures, and requests to the minimum necessary.

> —(U.S. Department of Health and Human Services, 2002)

We strongly advise mental health professionals to check with their respective mental health professional association or with the Federal Register itself (http://www.hhs. gov/ocr/hipaa/privruletxt.txt) to seek updates, to determine what qualifies as psychotherapy notes, and to see how the notes should be handled.[2]

Practicalities. Some psychotherapists are more focused on patients (or other things) than to keep two separate sets of notes. They simply write everything down on the same sheet of paper. Unfortunately, with the new HIPPA definitions, session notes that constitute the only record of attendance, billing, scheduling, and so forth are not separated from the rest of the record, so the entire record—session content, therapist's impressions, and doodles—is the record. There may be no special HIPAA protection for any part of it. This record would be treated as protected health information but not as psychotherapy (or process) notes, and therefore open for inspection without patient consent in numerous circumstances.

Although there is no private right of action under the Privacy Rule, do not underestimate the creativity of the plaintiffs' bar. An attorney could easily argue, for example, that compliance with HIPAA regulations, and taking the precautions they permit and encourage, have now become an integral part of the standard of care. Hence, the argument goes, there is a seemingly valid claim for malpractice against a psychiatrist, for example, whose patient comes to harm because the practitioner put all the patient's records together and failed to segregate the most sensitive data. The fact that the argument is made, of course, does not mean that it will prevail, but the practitioner should strive to prevent claims from arising and not merely gear up to defeat claims that arise. If the practitioner decides to keep separate psychotherapy notes, then he or she needs to keep these notes separate from the patient's clinical file.

Patient Rights. HIPAA privacy regulations give patients greater access to their records. Except in special circumstances, such as those in which a minor is legally authorized to consent to treatment, parents and other legal representatives of minors have the same rights as the patient. Under HIPAA, patients have the right to see a copy of their records (excluding psychotherapy notes in most cases), to request

---

[2] When looking at long, small print in government documents online, select the Adobe Acrobat version of the document, if it is available, (using the free Acrobat Reader software at http://www. adobe.com/products/acrobat/readstep2.html.) You can run searches for specific words, such as *psychotherapy notes.* Some Web browsers also allow searches for specific words on a Web page (for example, Internet Explorer→ Edit→ Find (on This Page).)

correction in some cases, and to be notified about certain information-handling processes. Practitioners and health plans are required to give patients a clear written explanation of how they use, keep, and disclose their personal health information (PHI) and also to state what rights the patient is granted under HIPAA privacy rules. Patients can request reasonable disclosure restrictions of their PHI (if the request does not compromise the practitioner's professional judgment or conclusions). Such restrictions can include limiting the individuals or institutions to which the PHI can be sent (45 C.F.R. § 164.522 [a]). The Notice of Privacy Policies required under the Privacy Rule must indicate, however, that the covered entity has the right to decline (45 C.F.R. § 164.520 [b][1][iv]); 45 C.F.R. § 164.522 [a][ii]). Patients have the right to complain to a covered professional or health plan or to the secretary of Health and Human Services if they feel that their privacy protections have been violated (45 C.F.R. § 164.520 [b][1][vi]).

In most cases, patients can request a detailed list of all disclosures of their PHI in the previous 6 years except those for treatment, payment, or health care operations (quality assurance, for example) (45 C.F.R. § 164.528). In addition to the date of transaction and name and address of the PHI recipient, the list must provide a brief description of the information disclosed and the purpose of the transaction. The need to track these disclosures started on the compliance date.

The great exception to these requirements is that for many defined business and clinical purposes, information (including sensitive personal information) has and might continue to be transferred between clinicians and health care entities without regard for a patient's consent and without disclosure to the patient. How HIPAA will influence this flow is yet to be seen. Some state laws and professional canons of ethics are more restrictive than is the HIPAA privacy rule, and some professionals would argue that information has flowed all too freely for decades.

Nonetheless, HIPAA is here, and covered entities must wrangle with its requirements. With all the emphasis on HIPAA, practitioners may forget that long before Uncle Sam weighed in, there was abundant legal authority for the proposition that confidentiality and privacy of patient records must be protected. Most of this authority originates in state law and varies in details from one jurisdiction to another.

HIPAA is not the only pertinent federal law. Consider the Children's Online Privacy Protection Act, as well as the Food and Drug Administration's regulation of telemedicine devices and electronic signatures. While making no attempt to describe U.S. state laws with specificity, we note that, in broad outline, such laws enshrine the Hippocratic principle of confidentiality. Do not underestimate their power. Under current law, the consequences for violating applicable state law may be more serious than for violations of the federal privacy rule. Although admittedly an overgeneralization, it is largely true that professionals who are guided by common sense and the ethics of their profession will usually make the right decisions. For specific technical questions, legal advice may be helpful.

Preemption is a thorny issue for U.S. practitioners living in states with stringent privacy laws. Usually, under the U.S. Constitution's Supremacy Clause, federal law overrules conflicting state law. Under HIPAA privacy regulations, however, state law controls whether state law is more protective of the patient's right to privacy. If compliance with both state and federal law is impossible or if compliance with one entails a significant obstacle to compliance with the other, then HIPAA requires that a covered entity determine which legal authority, federal or state, furnishes more stringent protection of PHI and obey it. Even for lawyers, identifying all potentially applicable state laws can be challenging. Given the differing objectives of the people who enacted the relevant statutes and regulations, making the necessary comparisons after the authorities have been identified can be difficult. As of this writing, most professionals who have attempted such an analysis within a given jurisdiction have confined themselves to comparing state and federal statutes and regulations and have largely ignored common law.

Law makers are attempting to make order of this confusion. Eventually, the uncertainty will diminish, although probably never be eliminated. By staying tuned to discussions and guidelines of professional organizations, health care professionals can keep abreast of developments in this area and thus be able to stay within the law and provide appropriate protection to their patients. The following sections give a general view of what administrators and clinicians need to study in detail.

Consent and Authorization. Patients have the right to grant or to decline consent, to treatment, and also to release of their records. Traditionally, practitioners have been restricted from using sensitive information outside of one-to-one treatment without patient consent. Under HIPPA, however, patient consent is not necessary for a health plan, practitioner, or clearinghouse to use protected health information for treatment, payment, and certain "health care operations."[3] For some but not all of these health

---

[3] *Health care operations* means any of the following activities of the covered entity to the extent that the activities are related to covered functions and any of the following activities of an organized health care arrangement in which the covered entity participates:

a. Conducting quality assessment and improvement activities, including outcomes evaluation and development of clinical guidelines, provided that obtaining the generalizable knowledge is not the primary purpose of any studies resulting from such activities; population-based activities relating to improving health or reducing health care costs, protocol development, case management and care coordination, contacting of health care providers and patients with information about treatment alternatives; and related functions that do not include treatment.

b. Reviewing the competence or qualifications of health care professionals; evaluating practitioner and provider performance, and health plan performance; conducting training programs in which health care students, trainees, or practitioners learn under supervision to practice or improve their skills as health care providers; training non-health care professionals; and accreditation, certification, licensing, or credentialing activities.

c. Underwriting, premium rating, and other activities relating to the creation, renewal or replacement of a contract of health insurance or health benefits, and ceding, securing, or placing a contract for reinsurance of risk relating to claims for health care (including stop-loss insurance and excess of loss insurance), provided that the requirements of Part 164.514(g) are met, if applicable.

d. Conducting or arranging for medical review, legal servies, and auditing functions, including fraud and abuse detection and compliance programs.

e. Business planning and development, such as conducting cost-management and planning-related analyses related to managing and operating the entity, including formulary development and administration, development or improvement of methods of payment or coverage policies.

f. Business management and general administrative activities of the entity, including, but not limited to:

   i. Management activities relating to implementation of and compliance with the requirements of this subchapter.

   ii. Customer service, including the provision of data analyses for policy holders, plan sponsors or other customers, provided that protected health information is not disclosed to such policy holder, plan sponsor, or customer.

   iii. Resolution of internal grievances.

   iv. Due diligence in connection with the sale or transfer of assets to a potential successor in interest, if the potential successor in interest is a covered entity or, following completion of the sale or transfer, will become a covered entity.

   v. Consistent with the applicable requirements of Part 164.514, creating de-identified health information, fundraising for the benefit of the covered entity, and marketing for which an individual authorization is not required as described in Part 164.514(e)(2).

care operations, personally identifying data must first be stripped from the data by the covered entity. While the remaining data may identify a particular patient in some instances, covered entities are required to make only a good-faith effort to deidentify information.

Some examples in which a patient's release of information is not mandatory (see 45 C.F.R. 164.501) are the following:

- Emergencies.
- Quality assurance activities.
- Public health concerns.
- Identification of the body of a deceased person.
- Activities related to national defense and security.

Separate patient authorization is required to release personal health information for operations above and beyond treatment, for payment, and for health care operations as defined. For example, a covered entity would need patient authorization if an employer requested personal health information.

Although HIPAA generally conforms to common sense when consent is not required, professionals should be familiar with the specific exceptions listed in the Privacy Rule. Even after practitioners are satisfied that a given disclosure is not barred by HIPAA, they should consider whether such disclosure might be barred by another authority, notably state law. Some circumstances might warrant further inquiry about disclosure.

In practical terms, a mental health clinician should obtain consent for nearly any disclosure. The processes involved in arranging for informed consent are part of treatment and can be deliberately fashioned to advance therapy.

Notice of Privacy Practices. Patients have the right to receive a paper copy of a formal Notice of Privacy Practices that is written in plain language and explains the following items:

- Uses and disclosures.
- Separate statements for certain uses or disclosures stated in the regulation.
- Individual rights.
- The covered entity's duties.
- Complaints.
- The identity and contact information of the covered entity's contact person.
- Effective date of the notice.

The heading of the notice must contain the following statement in bold type: "**This notice describes how medical information about you may be used and disclosed and how you can get access to this information. Please review it carefully.**" Such notices can be readily obtained from professional organizations and adapted to one's own practice.

Professionals practicing outside the United States should become familiar with the HIPAA Privacy Rule to enhance their awareness of patients' needs for privacy and their rights.

Children's Online Privacy Protection Act

Congress passed 15 U.S.C. §§ 6501-6506, the Children's Online Privacy Protection Act (COPPA) in 1998 (see http://www.ftc.gov/ogc/coppa1.pdf). This discussion highlights the issue for clinicians to keep in mind when working online. The Act's primary goal was to place parents in control over what information is collected from their children online. COPPA applies to operators of commercial Web sites and online services directed to children under the age of 13 that collect personal information from children and also to operators of general audience sites who know that they are collecting information from children under age 13.

These Web site operators must do the following:

- Post clear and comprehensive privacy policies on the Web site, describing their information practices for children's personal information.
- Provide notice to parents and, with limited exceptions, obtain verifiable parental consent in person before collecting personal information from children.
- Give parents the choice of whether to consent to the operator's collection and use of a child's information and to prohibit the operator from disclosing that information to third parties.
- Provide parents with access to their child's personal information in order to review it, have it deleted, or both.
- Give parents the opportunity to prevent further collection or use of the information.
- Maintain the confidentiality, security, and integrity of information they collect from children.

In addition, the Act prohibits Web site operators from conditioning a child's participation in an online activity or the child's providing more information than is reasonably necessary to participate in that activity.

The Federal Trade Commission (FTC) monitors the Internet for compliance with the Act and brings enforcement actions to deter violations. The FTC has set up a special Web page designed for children, parents, businesses, and educators (http://www.ftc. gov/bcp/conline/edcams/kidzprivacy). Professionals can obtain further information or file a complaint by calling (877) FTC-HELP. Complaints can also be submitted to the FTC through a Web site (http://www. ftc.gov).

Web site operators violating COPPA could be liable for civil penalties of up to $11,000 per violation. Penalties are based on such factors as the number of children involved, the amount and type of personal information collected, how the information was used, and whether the information was shared with any third parties (Federal Trade Commission, n.d.). When serving this population online, mental health professionals are encouraged to seek legal counsel about issues related to children and privacy within their respective jurisdictions.

International Privacy and Security Measures

Clinicians in the United States could benefit from considering how privacy issues are handled in other countries. In October 1998, the European Union (EU) issued a directive establishing a framework for regulating privacy protections for personal and electronic data in all member countries. Personal data protection is a constitutional principle in Europe, unlike in the United States. Before the directive was issued, however, differences between and among national data protection laws had created barriers to the transfer of personal data. Each member country is now instructed to enact the EU directive into law within its jurisdiction (European Union, 1998a).

The EU directive describes an obligation to collect and process personal data (including health data) only for specified, explicit, and legitimate purposes and to see that such information is relevant, accurate, and up-to-date. By fostering consumer confidence and minimizing differences between member countries' data protection rules, the directive facilitates the development of electronic commerce. The directive also establishes rules that personal data are transferred outside the EU only when the data's continued privacy is legally safeguarded, so that the directive's high standards of protection are not undermined (European Union, 1998b). Without such provisions, it was argued, by the provision's developers, one could transfer personal information to a data haven in another country and sell it to an intermediary, who could then send it back to its country of origin stripped of all protections. This requirement is roughly analogous to the business associate provisions under the HIPAA Privacy Rule.

The EU also has standard contractual clauses establishing safeguards for personal data transferred from the EU to other countries. The decision obliges member countries to recognize that companies or organizations using such standard clauses in contracts concerning personal data transfers to locations outside the EU are offering adequate protection of the data. The EU's data protection directive (95/46/EC) requires all personal data transferred to countries outside the EU to benefit from adequate protection. Use of these standard contractual clauses is voluntary, their use gives companies and organizations a straightforward means of complying with their obligation to safeguard personal data transferred to non-EU countries that the Commission has not recognized as providing adequate protection. So far, only Switzerland, Hungary, and Canada have been approved. The EU's safe harbor provisions enable individual companies to receive protected data even if laws in their country were not recognized as adequate. Internal Market Commissioner Frits Bolkestein said, "This new practical measure will make it easier for companies and organizations to comply with their obligation to ensure 'adequate protection' for personal data transferred from the Community to the rest of the world while safeguarding individuals' right to privacy," (European Commission, 2001, p. 1).

The British technical standard BS 7799, intended to protect security of e-commerce worldwide, later became the International Standards Organization ISO 17799. The standard's management includes certification programs and 10 areas of organizational control to protect the security and integrity of transmitted data. BS 7799 identifies these 10 controls for a successful information security program (Stacy, 2000):

- A documented information security policy.
- Allocation of information security responsibilities within the organization.
- Information security education and training.
- Security incident reporting and response.
- Virus detection and prevention controls.

- Business continuity planning.
- Control of proprietary software copying.
- Critical record management processes.
- Protection of personal data (privacy).
- Periodic compliance reviews.

These security measures are part of society's efforts to deserve the consumers' trust.

REGULATION

A practitioner must overcome many hurdles to practice in multiple states using tele-health technologies and licensure mobility is one of the most pressing of these hurdles (Levant, n.d.). Many states have laws requiring a practitioner to obtain full licensure in that state before conducting any type of health care service. Full licensure can often be obtained by reciprocity; that is, a practitioner licensed in state X can become so in state Y without the need to pass Y's examination. Apart from fees to pay, papers to push, and form-mongers to satiate, the task is relatively modest. In other circumstances, however, becoming licensed in another state can be difficult (DeLeon, 2000).

A number of states allow limited telephonic or in-person consultation by practitioners not fully licensed in that state. Some states permit a practitioner in an adjoining state to provide a limited number of such consultations per year; other states allow consultations by practitioners living within a certain number of miles of the state's border or in emergency circumstances. Practitioners using these exceptions are not permitted full-fledged practice in the state and could not, without becoming fully licensed, set up an office and see patients there on a regular basis.

Such laws made sense when practice was ruled by distance and discrete lines could be drawn between states and countries. Their continued viability remains to be seen in the 21st century, as remote patients and practitioners seek and demand optimal healthcare. Telecommunication technologies are bound by no borders, and their service delivery knows no distance. Interstate and international treatment are potentially available without special effort. State laws do not address the current capabilities of technology, and lawmakers are considering the passage of new laws to accommodate it. The longer this issue remains unresolved, the longer licensed professionals are constrained from expanding into cyberspace, leaving this new frontier open to exploration and exploitation by unlicensed and otherwise unregulated would-be healers and helpers. The American Psychological Association and Practice Directorate publications (e.g., Smith, 2001; Sullivan, 2000–2001) are good sources to check for the most up-to-date information on the status of mobility issues.

Allowing unlicensed practitioners to address a sizable proportion of the nation's mental health needs promises short-term budget relief for the government, insurers, employers, and other entities that otherwise would have to reimburse professionals for services rendered. To counter this trend, professional organizations should demonstrate the advantages (including overall cost savings) of maintaining high standards for behavioral e-health services.

Avoiding regulation on the Internet is presently rather easy, as demonstrated by the adult entertainment and casino industries. Companies simply buy Web hosting services in any one of numerous countries with lenient Internet laws, set up their Internet businesses, and open their doors to an international population. Similarly, so-called health care and mental health care practitioners are operating Web sites and telephone call centers from around the globe. We should note that not all health professionals providing services across international frontiers are of dubious legitimacy. Some well-trained nighthawk radiologists in south Asia and elsewhere, for example, take advantage of the time differences to provide real-time, after-hours interpretations of diagnostic images of patients in locations especially rural locations, of the West, where emergency physicians value consultations when local radiologists are asleep. On the other hand, other people offering services electronically may be less ethical and much less well trained. If regulatory bodies threaten to act, people seeking to avoid regulation may be tempted to relocate Web site operations to another Web hosting service, possibly in another country. This activity can be seamless; users are unaware of the behind-the-scenes activity.

The Telemedicine Report to Congress (U.S. Department of Commerce, 1997) reviewed alternative licensure models. A national licensure system implemented at a state level would require states to voluntarily incorporate the national standards into their laws; this step would be intended to prevent states from imposing additional standards.

One large legal issue for many states may be the ability to enforce their own laws. For example, a consumer in state A sues a practitioner who, via the Web, transmitted to the consumer state B allegedly harmful advice that traveled across states C and D (as the crow flies) and possibly also through states E, F, and G (as the Internet packets fly). Which governing body has jurisdiction? How does a successful plaintiff collect a judgment? What happens if the Web site itself was created, incorporated, and staffed outside the United States? What recourse would the consumer have if the Web site were taken down immediately but reconfigured under a different address the next day? Existing law provides few answers.

The Internet pharmacy is a practice area that illustrates both the risks and the benefits of high technology in health care. Some online pharmacies operate outside accepted pharmaceutical practice limits. A recent article in the FDA *Consumer* magazine (Henkel, 2001) argued that consumers must be wary of other online pharmacies using the Internet as an outlet for products or practices that are illegal in the offline world. These rogue sites either sell unapproved products or, if they deal in approved ones, often sidestep established procedures meant to protect consumers. For example, some sites require customers only to fill out a questionnaire before ordering prescription drugs, bypassing any in-person interaction with a health professional. One physician explains his concerns in this text:

> "This practice undermines safeguards of a direct medical supervision and physical evaluation performed by a licensed health professional," says Jeffrey Shuren, M.D., medical officer in the Food and Drug Administration's Office of Policy, Planning and Legislation. "The Internet makes it easy to bypass this safety net. Skirting the system this way sets the stage for problems that include dangerous drug interactions and harm from contaminated, counterfeit or outdated drugs. Web sites that prescribe based on a questionnaire raise additional health concerns," says Shuren. Patients risk obtaining an inappropriate medication and may sacrifice the opportunity for a correct diagnosis or the identification of a contraindication to the drug.... The FDA is investigating numerous pharmaceutical Web sites suspected of breaking the law and plans to take legal action if appropriate. The agency has made Internet surveillance an enforcement priority, targeting unapproved new drugs, health fraud, and prescription drugs sold without a valid prescription.
>
> —(Henkel, 2001)

Although abuses have occurred, many Internet pharmacies are just as responsible and valuable as conventional drugstores. Some Internet pharmacies require legitimate prescriptions from licensed physicians before they dispense drugs. Such pharmacies may facilitate delivery of needed medicines to patients in remote areas and also may decrease the cost of prescription medication for patients everywhere. For the elderly and homebound, the Internet's ability to overcome mobility problems may provide not merely convenience but even survival.

Because Medicare does not provide a drug benefit, older Americans pay the full price of their prescriptions. About 70 million Americans, including the one third on Medicare, do not have prescription drug insurance benefits. Discount plans enable patients to obtain medications through mail order or visits to local pharmacies. Internet pharmacies can serve a similar function.

According to its Web site (http://www.nabp.net), the National Association of Boards of Pharmacy (NABP) was established in 1904 to help state licensing boards develop, implement, and enforce uniform standards to protect the public health. The association includes pharmacy boards from all 50 states, the District of Columbia, three U.S. territories, several Canadian provinces, and four Australian states.

In 1999, the NABP implemented the Verified Internet Pharmacy Practice Site (VIPPS) program to provide criteria to certify Internet pharmacies. A coalition of state and federal regulatory associations, professional associations, and consumer advocacy groups developed the criteria. Pharmacies displaying the VIPPS seal must demonstrate compliance with the licensing and inspection requirements of its state and each state to which it dispenses pharmaceuticals. These pharmacies must also comply with additional VIPPS criteria, including privacy, authentication, and security, adherence to a recognized quality assurance policy, and provision of substantive consultation between patients and pharmacists.

The VIPPS hyperlink seal displayed on its Web site identifies a VIPPS pharmacy site. By clicking on the seal, a visitor can read verified information about the pharmacy as maintained by the NABP. The public is welcome to access the VIPPS Web site itself to search for a certified Internet pharmacy. The existence of this system does not mean that all problems related to Internet pharmacies have been solved. It does identify a current system that the pharmacy profession is using to govern itself for the benefit of the public. Perhaps other branches of health care could adapt its approaches to the needs of their respective professions in the same responsible manner.

Food and Drug Administration Regulation of Telemedicine Devices

In the United States jurisdiction of technology, telecommunication devices and software to deliver health care may be with the Food and Drug Administration (FDA) because of the broad definition of *device* in the Federal Food, Drug and Cosmetic Act (1997). The FDA defines *Device* as

> an instrument, apparatus, implement, machine, contrivance, implant, *in vitro* reagent or other similar or related article, including any component, part or accessory which is (1) recognized in the official national formulary, (2) intended for use in the diagnosis of disease and other conditions, or in the cure, mitigation, treatment or prevention of disease in man or animals, or (3) intended to affect the structure or any function of the body of man or other animals.

Much telehealth equipment then is regulated by the FDA.

More specifically, the FDA's Center for Radiologic Health (CDRH) defines telemedicine to include a wide range of technologies for the delivery of medical information or counseling to patients online (Center for Devices and Radiological Health, 1996).

Mental health professionals planning or engaged in telehealth activities should ask any vendor of devices (medical instruments) or clinical software whether it has FDA approval for its devices or applications. If the vendor's device or application is currently not approved and in common use, ask whether the vendor is considering submission for FDA approval or has a quality assurance process in place.

Information on whether a device is FDA regulated can be found on the FDA Web site (http://www.fda.gov/cdrh/devadvice/index.html). An informed purchaser of any application can check this site before buying equipment or signing a contract. FDA approval indicates the agency's conclusion that the device or software application meets all applicable technology standards necessary to store, transmit, and receive data. Many clinics in remote locations using telecommunication technologies have multiple-use systems for counseling and medical services. These systems are often on telephone lines (POTS or ISDN) and not the Internet. Such systems may not be subject to HIPAA guidelines, but application devices and, in specified clinical circumstances, the software may require FDA approval. Always check the FDA Web site for approval before purchasing equipment. Personnel at local FDA offices throughout the United States can assist the mental health professional identify when a device or software application requires approval.

Electronic Signatures in Global and National Commerce Act

The Electronic Signatures in Global and National Commerce Act (ESIGN) (Federal Trade Commission & Department of Commerce, 2001) is federal legislation that became effective in the United States on October 1, 2000. ESIGN notes that electronic signatures and records are legally equivalent to pen-and-ink signatures and paper records for most transactions.

The Uniform Electronic Transaction Act is a related piece of legislation developed at the state level (Schanz & Cepelewicz, 2001). Practitioners may also be interested in reading the position statement of the American Academy of Child and Adolescent Psychiatry Task Force on psychiatrist's signatures. This statement provides guidance on incorporating electronic signature function into a practice (American Academy of Child and Adolescent Psychiatry, 2000).

The task force's goal was to identify situations in which a psychiatrist's electronic signature might be needed or required. These situations include, but are not limited to, diagnoses, consent to treatment, plan of care, prescriptive signature, insurance forms, peer review and utilization documents, agency contracts, progress notes, physician orders, signatures for other physicians, forensic certification, treatment necessity, medication authorization, disability evaluation, treatment authorization requests, admission and discharge notes, and other medical-psychiatry documents (American Academy of Child and Adolescent Psychiatry, 2000).

The task force was mindful of the often erratically changing practice climate of the past several years and of the strains that these conditions place on psychiatrists' ability to practice in the best interests of patients. Previously unforeseen clinical, financial, and administrative relationships among and between psychiatrists, patients, and administrative and business entities have developed and continue to evolve in a dizzying way.

State Licensure and Liability

Licensing laws in the United States have traditionally been based on the individual states' constitutional authority to protect the health and safety of their citizens and to determine the standards and criteria necessary to manage citizen protections through an ongoing licensing system. Critics of this system argue that the rationale for "partitioning" licensing authority in this manner is rapidly eroding. Telehealth is becoming the focus of a struggle to eliminate the barriers between states.

But psychotechnology and telemedicine partisans should recognize that this is not a turf dispute among bureaucrats. The founding fathers of this country recognized that tyranny depends on power. They created a federal system, with its ingenious checks and balances and its deliberate, careful division of power between state and federal sovereigns, to "secure the blessings of liberty to ourselves and our posterity." To enlarge federal power at the expense of the states might facilitate the progress of psychotechnology, and, in our view, doing so has the potential to bring great good to many people. But if doing so wrests power from statehouses and transfers it to Washington, the price could be unacceptable. Enabling medical progress without jeopardizing liberties is the challenge we all face.

The urgency of regulating cross-border licensing issues relates to the concern that some professionals may try to use the Internet and other online technologies to circumvent existing licensing laws and to practice outside the accepted and legally defined scope of their respective specialties or to provide services for which they are ill trained or even incompetent. Some professionals present a danger to the public and could give their professions a bad reputation.

The nature of the information age and the proliferation of electronic media make it difficult for traditional oversight agencies to keep up with professionals practicing on the Internet. It is difficult for the average consumer to know whether the professional they have contacted is licensed. Online mental health consumers must be cautious and must make sure that they are dealing with credible practitioners. Professionals also need to be diligent in identifying unlicensed individuals practicing mental health and must report them to licensing bodies. Individual professionals can improve the status quo by making available to the consumer reliable evidence of their own legitimacy, licensure, and credentials. Making this standard practice by contrast can reveal the frauds and nonprofessionals.

Federation of State Medical Boards Model Act. In the fall of 1995, the board of directors of the Federation of State Medical Boards (FSMB; http://www.fsmb.org) adopted a model statute recommended by the Federation's Ad Hoc Committee on Telemedicine. The FSMB Model Act acknowledges that because of changes in the practice of medicine and technological advances, the practice of medicine often crosses state lines. The Act would require physicians to obtain a limited license to engage in the practice of medicine across state lines. Reciprocity would be granted to physicians in another state. The Act, defines the practice of medicine across state boundaries as follows:

- The rendering of a written or otherwise documented medical opinion concerning the diagnosis or treatment of a patient within this state by a physician located outside this state as a result of transmission of individual patient data by electronic or other means from within this state to such physician or his or her agent; or

- The rendering of treatment to a patient within this state by a physician located outside this state as a result of transmission of individual patient data by electronic or other means from within this state to such physician or his of her agent. (Federation of State Medical Boards of the United States, 1995)

The FSMB Model Act would establish a special license for telehealth practitioners to provide medical services across state lines. One clause in the Act includes regulations prohibiting the practitioner from physically entering another state and practicing without that state's license. Other clauses extend the limited license only to licensed practitioners who "regularly and frequently" practice interstate telehealth and require the practitioner to be readily available for investigations by the issuing state's medical board regarding any reports of misconduct. This Act pertains to practitioner-to-patient consultations only and excludes practitioner-to-practitioner and emergency consultations (Federation of State Medical Boards of the United States, 1995; Young Lawyers Division, Health Care Law Committee, 1998).

States are moving slowly to enact the FSMB Model Act. For future licensing alternatives, practitioners should watch an interim governing committee for the International Association of Medical Licensing Authorities (Schanz & Cepelewicz, 2001).

The model with the best reception to date is the Interstate Nurse Licensure Compact, which we now discuss.

Interstate Nurse Licensure Compact

Nursing is reconsidering its regulation process today in response to the many inquiries to boards of nursing about regulatory dilemmas raised by changes in the health care practice environment. Innovations in the health care delivery system have driven many of these changes. Many questions are being raised because of the increasing number of nurses providing care across state lines and in situations in which the patient is in a different state than the one in which the nurse is licensed and located.... Some might ask whether using electronic technology to provide care indeed constitutes the practice of nursing. In fact, there are those who suggest that, since electronic care does not include hands-on care and that typically telephone triage nurses use physician approved protocols for reference, this practice is not in fact nursing practice. Nurse Practice Acts in all states define nursing more broadly than "hands-on care," therefore, a consensus has been reached by boards of nursing that a nurse utilizing the knowledge, skill, assessment, judgment and decision making inherent in nursing education and licensure is indeed practicing nursing.

—(Hutcherson & Williamson, 1999)

Following the long-established precedent of states seeking to share waterways divided by state lines, the National Council of State Boards of Nursing (NCSBN) has made it easier for nurses to practice across state boundaries by promoting the Interstate Mutual Recognition Compact:

An interstate compact is an agreement between two or more states, entered into for the purpose of addressing a problem that transcends state lines. Compacts are created when two or more states enact identical statutes establishing and defining the compact and its role. The result is the creation of both state law and an enforceable contract with other states that adopt the compact.

—(Hutcherson & Williamson, 1999)

The head of the nursing licensing board administers the compact in his or her state. The compact applies to a license to registered nurses and licensed practical or vocational nurses. Under the compact arrangement, party states recognize licenses granted by the other party states. Each state, however, retains the right to sanction nurses who violate state laws or practice acts in the patient's home state (Waters, 1999).

> Notably, the interstate compact changes disciplinary action from state of practice to state of residence, an acknowledgement that a nurse may not have a license issued by the state in which she is practicing. The compact does allow states to restrict or revoke a nurse's privilege within its borders, however, regardless of the licensing state. Home states may take disciplinary action against a license based on a violation in another state.
> —(McPeck, 2001, p. 25)

Twenty or more states have entered into the compact. It may be a promising model for remote practice for other professional specialties to note. You can obtain an update on activity by visiting the NCSBN Web site (http://www.ncsbn.org). The NCSBN is also developing a compact for advance practice registered nurses. This action supports the use of technology and telepsychiatry between states and assists in making mental health care more accessible.

Association of State and Provincial Psychology Boards. The Association of State and Provincial Psychology Boards (ASPPB; http://www.asppb.org) is an alliance of state, territorial, and provincial agencies responsible for the licensure and certification of psychologists throughout the United States and Canada. Formed in 1961, the ASPPB created the Examination for Professional Practice in Psychology (EPPP), which licensing boards use to assess candidates for licensure and certification. The ASPPB also offers mobility programs to assist boards in licensure of psychologists already licensed in another state, province, or territory. Through its mobility program, the ASPPB is attempting to standardize the disparate state and provincial regulations of practice. The ASPPB offers a program for psychologists holding a license to practice in another state or province. Four ASPPB programs help facilitate professional mobility:

- The Certificate of Professional Qualification in Psychology, or CPQ (http://www.asppb.org/mobility/cpq.htm). Psychologists must meet core licensure criteria but need not document them again each time they move or practice in a new state or province.
- The ASPPB Agreement of Reciprocity (http://www.asppb.org/mobility/reciprocity.htm). Participating states and provinces bring their licensure requirements into conformity with the standards in the agreement and accept each others' licensees.
- The ASPPB Score Transfer Service (http://www.asppb.org/mobility/transfer.htm). This service gives the EPPP score to a licensing jurisdiction. This service also checks the applicant's name against the ASPPB Disciplinary Data System to determine whether disciplinary action has been taken against a license.
- The ASPPB Credentials Bank (http://www.asppb.org/mobility/cpqbank.asp). This service archives information pertaining to education, training, and experience and can verify original documentation years after the last contact with educational institutions or supervisors. (Association of State and Provincial Licensing Boards, n.d.)

Definitions of Practice

States define mental health practice differently in their statutes. All too often, these definitions are overly inclusive and might as well include the services of a hairdresser or bartender. Let's consider the "practice of psychology" as defined by California:

> [The] rendering or offering to render for a fee to individuals, groups, organizations or the public any psychological service involving the application of psychological principles, methods, and procedures of understanding, predicting, and influencing behavior, such as the principles pertaining to learning, perception, motivation, emotions, and interpersonal relationships; and the methods and procedures of interviewing, counseling, psychotherapy, behavior modification, and hypnosis; and of constructing, administering and interpreting tests of mental abilities, aptitudes, interests, attitudes, personality characteristics, emotions, and motivations. The application of such principles and methods includes, but is not restricted to: diagnosis, prevention, treatment and amelioration of psychological problems and emotional and mental disorders of individuals and groups.
> Psychotherapy within the meaning of this chapter is the use of psychological methods in a professional relationship to assist a person or persons to acquire greater human effectiveness or to modify feelings, conditions, attitudes and behavior which are emotionally, intellectually or socially ineffectual or maladjustive.
>
> —(California Business and Professions Code, § 2903)

The statute defining the practice of clinical social work in California provides this definition:

> Psychotherapy, within the meaning of this chapter, is the use of psychosocial methods within a professional relationship, to assist the person or persons to achieve a better psychosocial adaptation, to acquire greater human realization of psychosocial potential and adaptation, to modify internal and external conditions which affect individuals, groups, or communities in respect to behavior, emotions, and thinking, in respect to their intrapersonal and interpersonal processes.
>
> —(California Business and Professions Code, § 4996.9)

The practice of marriage, family, and child counseling is defined in California as:

> That service performed with individuals, couples or groups wherein interpersonal relationships are examined for the purpose of achieving more adequate, satisfying, and productive marriage and family adjustments. This practice includes relationship and premarriage counseling.
> The applications of marriage, family and child counseling principles and methods includes, but is not limited to, the use of applied psychotherapeutic techniques, to enable individuals to mature and grow within marriage and the family, and the provision of explanations and interpretations of the psychosexual and psychosocial aspects of relationships.
>
> —(California Business and Professions Code, § 4980.02)

Broad definitions raise crucial questions. Case law or legislative reform will further delineate these definitions and answer some of the related questions about the differences between the professions, as well as between non-mental-health-trained individuals. In the meantime, it appears that according to the broad definition of psychological practice in California, for example, almost any e-mail exchange with a licensed psychologist in which "feelings or attitudes have been modified" could be considered psychotherapy. Clearly, legislative reform is needed to bring legislation into line with evolving technology. Because the issues are complex, however, legislative reform may take years.

Readers are encouraged to locate the exact wording of their relevant state definitions of practice and then to consider the ramifications in a court of law. Technologically imprecise and as yet undeveloped state definitions of professional practice could make a case more difficult to defend if it involves, say, a teenage suicide or homicide. Over time, case law will undoubtedly drive the development of more distinct regulatory language for psychotherapy. Meanwhile, practitioners beware. Adhering to recognized professional limits is the best strategy for risk management.

A Department of Health and Human Services report entitled *Wired for Health and Well-Being* states:

> The extent and nature of liability associated with interactive health communication applications are unclear. Providing medical advice through these applications, including Web sites, increases the potential liability for developers, and others involved in the design and implementation of the application. Who will be liable for damages is unknown. In the absence of precedents in this area, future legal action and case law may provide some clarity on these issues.
> —(Science Panel on Interactive Communication and Health, 1999, p. 88)

One thing, however, is certain: In a lawsuit, plaintiffs will seek to name as many defendants as possible. The advantages in so doing are numerous. The more defendants there are, the better the chance that the jury will dislike at least one of them, the larger the pot of money that will be available for paying a judgment, and the better the chance that the defendants will attack one another. Too often, the disadvantage of naming multiple defendants is more theoretical than real. In most state courts, and in all federal courts, the judge can impose sanctions for frivolous claims or motions. Of course, the fact that there is more than one defendant does not prove that adding the others was frivolous. Also, courts vary widely in their willingness to impose sanctions, and plaintiffs continue to bring frivolous claims.

Precedents may be difficult to find and enforcement of existing codes even scarcer. Future laws will regulate whether a practitioner needs to disclose a licensure when professesing to offer only relationship advice through e-mail, or coaching via chat rooms, or e-therapy, for that matter. At present, it is probably wise to disclose. Regulations to enforce these decisions are likely to be the laws already in existence, such as this one from California. The California Medical Board has taken the position that any person

> who practices or attempts to practice, or who advertises or holds himself out as practicing any system or mode of treating the sick or afflicted in this state, or diagnoses, treats, operates for, or prescribes for any ailment, blemish, deformity, disease, disfigurement, disorder, injury or other physical or mental condition of any person, without having at the time of doing so a valid, unrevoked, or unsuspended certificate... is guilty of a misdemeanor (California Business & Professions Code, 2052 n.d.)

On the international front, some countries are adopting their own restrictive licensure provisions. Commentators recommend that individuals wishing to provide consultation to a foreign country through telehealth technology contact the specific country's ministry of health to ensure that they meet all applicable local licensure requirements (Waters, 1999). For example, Malaysia has a law specifically requiring local licensure to provide telehealth services there.

Several good resources for online legal issues, discussion, and updates are available at the Telemedicine Information Exchange, Telemedlaw (http://tie.telemed.org/legal/pubs.asp), and the Center for Telemedicine Law (http://www.ctl.org). Federal medical programs and states include pertinent information on their Web sites, with current contact information and identification of the department or organization with jurisdictional oversight.

SELECTING LEGAL COUNSEL

Selecting an attorney can be challenging for any legal issue. As with psychotherapists, not all attorneys are alike. Training and experience can differ widely. Telehealth is a sufficiently novel concept that the number of lawyers with relevant experience is limited. The fact that a mental health professional elects to provide care through the psychotechnologies does not, of itself, establish a need for representation. As we note in this chapter, however, the array of legal issues involved in use of psychotechnologies is wide, even dizzying. Legal advice might be helpful.

However, attorney selection may be difficult because few, if any, lawyers are experts in each areas. The defamation scholar is unlikely to be sophisticated about reimbursement questions, for example, and the labor expert may know little about copyright. Yet, depending on how the provider decides to use the psychotechnologies, all these branches of the law, and more, may be involved. A provider may need to consult with a law firm that offers expertise in each area of concern. A cost-efficient approach could be to work through a professional association to engage lawyers with appropriate credentials. All association members could benefit from counsel's advice and information, but none would have to bear the costs alone. When individual issues arise, counsel could then be separately retained to address them.

Attorney selection is especially complex and important when one is sued. In all litigation, there are commonalities, and seasoned trial lawyers should be able to apply their skills in a wide variety of contexts. The genius of the common law, after all, is its ability to apply principles originating centuries ago to fact patterns that could not have been conceived of when the principle was new. Even so, some peculiarities of telehealth may not be obvious to all attorneys. As is true in other endeavors, experience with the field is valuable.

Even if a client finds a lawyer whose background seems well suited to his or her needs, the attorney–client relationship is highly personal. A defendant may spend more time, perhaps much more time, with counsel than he or she expects at the outset. Their interactions will take place in an inherently stressful atmosphere. They will need to collaborate closely and effectively over an extended period. It is important, then, just as between psychotherapist and patient, that attorney and client develop healthy rapport. The world's best legal technician is a poor choice if the client and the attorney have personality conflicts that prevent or hinder the forging of a strong alliance.

The considerations do not stop there. The telehealth practitioner may be insured against liability arising from the conduct criticized. If so, the insurance carrier(s) potentially liable for successful claims often retain control of the choice of counsel. Carriers often maintain lists of approved counsel within a given region and will decline to engage attorneys not listed. Of course, carriers are mass consumers of legal services and can be quite sophisticated in their selections. They may be well positioned to identify the most able counsel in a given field. Many insurance defense counsel are superb trial lawyers. On the other hand, insurance carriers always strive to contain defense costs, and, as in a health care setting, they tend to shop for price. This trait is not necessarily bad, but it can mean that the insured may not be permitted choice of counsel. An important consideration in defense counsel selection is that the lawyer agreed to offer services for the lowest cost. This could mean that the lawyer appointed to defend the insured is especially efficient. It could also mean that, in forms of litigation in which fee sensitivty is less important than it is in insurance defense, counsel is not competitive.

When an insurance carrier appoints a lawyer, the insured is of course at liberty to engage personal counsel separately and at personal expense. Usually, insurance defense counsel will work with personal counsel. Two heads may be better than one, and one laywer may spot an issue the other misses. Each can bounce ideas off the other. Typically, insured practitioners are better represented than they would be if they relied on insurance counsel alone.

Hiring a personal lawyer brings the assurance of that counsel's undivided loyalty. Insurance defense counsel is loyal to both the insured and the insurer. This is permissible, as long as all parties are aware of the dual loyalty and no quarrels arise between counsel's two clients. Occasionally (although less often than one might anticipate), disputes arise between insurer and insured. An insurance carrier's counsel cannot, ethically or legally, advise either party to such disputes. Personal counsel, on the other hand, can and does advise the insured in such circumstances. The insured party pays the costs and fees of hiring a personal lawyer. However, the insured's premiums do not give him or her the right, ordinarily, to compel the carrier to pay a lawyer it does not wish to hire. In most insurance defense work, the insured avoids the cost of retaining personal counsel. In selected cases involving a professional's career and reputation, however, retaining personal counsel may be prudent, and it is a common practice.

Now that we have reviewed many legal and regulatory issues, the following chapter highlights ethical issues associated with behavioral telehealth and begins a discussion of relevant technical, clinical, and administrative standards.

10

Standards and Guidelines

> *Thus conscience dooes make cowards*
> *And thus the native hiew of resolution*
> *Is sicklied o'er with the pale cast of thought,*
> *And enterprises of great pitch and moment*
> *With this regard their currents turn awry*
> *And loose the name of action.*
>   (Shakespeare, Hamlet)
>   Act iii, Scene 1, Line 98

Mental health professionals thinking about using the psychotechnologies should review current ethical guidelines when considering practice innovations. The technological landscape is so diverse and changeable that most codes and rules are subjected to complaints, appeals, and desperate searches for loopholes by professionals and clients alike. Mental health professionals have only begun to collect data about the degree to which members believe in or comply with their professional associations' standards of conduct (e.g., Pope, Tabachnick, & Keith-Spiegel, 1987). Data are not readily available to inform either the clinical decisions of individual practitioners or the attempts of relevant professional associations to extend formal standards of practice to new areas, such as online clinical practice.

This chapter focuses on the many statements and publications of state and professional associations that address ethical issues related to online clinical practice. These documents contain essential information for mental health professionals considering practice in this area. Both the risks and the benefits of such practice are high. On one hand, enforcers and attorneys await the missteps of professionals who make uninformed decisions about online clinical practice. On the other hand, practitioners and patients look eagerly toward the possibilities inherent in new forms of service delivery.

Before we introduce relevant publications, let us remember how media can change perception. First, online clinical practice may markedly flatten the social hierarchy. Even though this result may be helpful in some circumstances, it may lower the barrier for a dissatisfied patient to initiate litigation. For example, when communicating through newspaper columns, radio, television, or stage, mental health professionals often try to reduce social unease by minimizing their status, such as by giving themselves a diminutive name—"Dr. Pat." However, the reverse is needed when using some technologies, particularly the text-based media. For instance, in communicating chiefly through e-mail, discussion forum, or chat room, the professional's image needs shoring up, not whittling down. The combination of ready accessibility, physical distance, and anonymity destabilizes (i.e., either exaggerates or reverses) the respect people hold toward one another, often causing them to "criticize, praise, attack or confront in unheard of ways" (Florey, 2001a, p. 10). During online clinical practice via text-based environments, participants may deluge a professional with pleas for help along with unrestrained expressions of adulation or condemnation.

Furthermore, in cyberspace, essential professional barriers tend to be washed away by waves of quackery, fraudulently promoted nostrums, blatantly commercial health care Web sites, floods of data from search engines, and unscientific opinions spammed by phony pundits, as well as by excellent and extensive resources maintained by dedicated, highly knowledgeable professionals and laypeople. The fads that permeate human history (Garber, 2000) can develop and collapse much more quickly on the Internet (Anderson, 1998), making paranoid group reactions quite common (Kernberg, 1993). Even professional e-mail discussion groups restricted to members with scientific training and clinical responsibilities are regularly rocked by unsubstantiated rumors of computer viruses, jury verdicts, and actions by insurance companies—stimulating a flurry of alarmed postings until someone locates the source of the deception or provides a reference to an authoritative refutation. At one time, insults tacked to a post outside a tavern could be settled by a simple duel; in cyberspace, the audience is vastly greater, and corrective communications can be disseminated much more quickly, although misinformation can never be totally wiped out.

The Internet may be shifting the power balance in health care toward clients, but commercial and government bodies are gaining overall power by avidly acquiring personal data (Hausman, 2001). Similarly, during online clinical practice through videoconferencing with severely disturbed clients, the practitioner may need to anchor his or her image with an identification card on the desktop, stating name, title, city, and facility at the remote site to avoid misperception based on diagnosis (e.g., ideas of reference, cognitive deficits resulting in disorientation, etc.).

What does professionalism bring to this sprawling bazaar? If professionals are too restrained in using the psychotechnologies and colonizing the Internet, progress will be impeded, opportunities for valuable service will be missed, and the field will be left open for exploitation by the untrained, the unskilled, and the unlicensed. This and the next three chapters deliberate on the question of professionalism related to online clinical practice in the mental health disciplines. This chapter reviews standards and guidelines from clinical, technical, and administrative perspectives.

Before we proceed, we note several other important issues. First, this book is primarily for practitioners living in developed countries, where in-person treatment is the community standard of care. In locations in which lack of availability moots the issue of standards, psychotechnologies may offer the only accessibility to mental health care. In particular, it may be difficult or even disruptive to require formal, signed confirmation of informed consent in places where illiteracy is rampant, or where women's choices are decided by their husbands, or where everyone's choices are dictated by community elders or vengeful tyrants. Obviously, there is a need for more dialogue between the developed and underdeveloped nations; the views of people in underdeveloped nations should be considered in appraising and revising statements, guidelines, and standards (Richards, 2002).

Second, readers need to be sensitive to the terms we use in discussing ethical and other professional matters, as various professionals attribute divergent meanings to these words. For example, the American Psychological Association distinguishes between practice guidelines and treatment guidelines (each defined later in this chapter). The American Psychiatric Association uses the term *practice guidelines* for guidelines related to both practice and treatment. Other associations may use the term *clinical guidelines* in the same manner.

Third, this chapter distinguishes between the use of a technological device and a new area of clinical practice. For example, just as the use of voice mail does not constitute voice mail therapy, the use of e-mail does not constitute e-mail or online therapy. A professional conducting a medication evaluation or psychotherapy via telephone, Internet, or interactive video, is practicing mental health care, and existing ethical guidelines apply. Fourth, rather than providing only answers, we raise salient questions that mental health professionals need to ponder. Finally, the chapter does not address all relevant standards and should not be taken as comprehensive.

ETHICAL FOUNDATIONS

Ethics ranges from the open-ended reflective application of ordinary human moral principles (Ladd, 1991) to explicit codes of behavior formally adopted by particular professional associations. Each professional must decide how to deal with ethical dilemmas while using the ethical code specific to the relevant professional association. As Pope and Vasquez (1998) state so succinctly:

> Ethics codes cannot do our questioning, thinking, feeling, and responding for us. Such codes can never be a substitute for the active process by which the individual therapist or counselor struggles with the sometimes bewildering, always unique constellation of questions, responsibilities, contexts, and competing demands of helping another person.... Ethics must be practical. Clinicians confront an almost unimaginable diversity of situations, each with its own shifting questions, demands, and responsibilities. Every clinician is unique in important ways. Every client is unique in important ways. Ethics that are out of touch with the practical realities of clinical work, with the diversity and constantly changing nature of the therapeutic venture, are useless. (pp. xiii–xiv)

Ethics are a level above the law; they are a higher set of rules that determine how professionals should act. Nonetheless, written professional ethical codes are legalistic and often serve as a basis for, or an influence on, legal decisions as well as public policy. For example, the APA *Statement on Services by Telephone, Teleconferencing, and the Internet* (American Psychological Association, 1997) is the sort of document that may influence public policy.

Some professional associations are developing clinical standards and guidelines for behavioral telehealth; others have put these issues on the back burner, reportedly because clinicians are not interested. Readers who belong to professional associations are encouraged to contact their associations and ask whether ethical principles, standards, and/or guidelines about behavioral telehealth have been endorsed and, if not, why not. Such inquiries could help bring about the adoption of specific behavioral telehealth standards. Until professional associations more clearly address ethical issues, professionals must ensure that the client interaction is in accordance with current practice, licensing laws, technical standards, administrative standards, and informed professional judgment.

The major advances in mental health practice may have been spurred by benevolent motives, but sometimes their creation and early elaboration overstepped then current ethical limits. Many rejected treatments strike us now as not just wrongheaded but even cruel (Zilboorg, 1967), and many treatments within current standards of care remain unproven. Some treatments eventually may be regarded as abusive mis-treatment. Similarly, ethical constructs may change with time, partly in response to the dissemination of new technologies (Hsiung, 2003; Maheu, 2001). For example, today's professional advertising would have been shocking one generation ago. Consider also how the new self-help treatments (American Psychological Association Task Force on Self-Help Therapies, 1978) have become intensively commercialized (Eng, 2001; Rosen, 1987), and consider the reengineering of the once nearly sacred right to privacy from a right to a commodity (Davies, 1997; Dyson, 1998).

As behavioral health care establishes outposts in cyberspace, some innovative concepts will undoubtedly stretch professional ethics. Mental health professionals should not disparage the adventurous clinician–hero who explores new online approaches.

Clinical practice continually requires pragmatic compromises with unconditional ethical demands and firmly held theoretical convictions. It's a matter of striking a balance. Treating a patient in cyberspace by introducing or omitting factors that crucially affect diagnosis, treatment planning, or outcome may amount to conducting an experimental procedure. Avoiding the rigors of institution-based research could be tempting to the practitioner who wants to try something new rather than to deal with academic world of human subject committees and institutional review boards. Online treatment may not always be justified, however, even if provided gratis, and it could get the practitioner into trouble if the wrong patient is involved.

Some forms of online clinical practice have been studied by mental health professionals for several decades, and many are considered less experimental because of empirical validation of their effectiveness and safety (Zarr, 1984). Appendix A's reports of controlled research into psychotherapy or counseling delivered online show several cognitive-behavioral treatment studies using various forms of online contact with subjects. Restricting telemental health to research settings and underserved communities has been put forth as another way to temporarily cleave to ethical rectitude (Baer, Elford, & Cukor, 1997). On the other hand, all health care is in some sense experimental, even a standard appendectomy. Human biology is almost infinitely variable, and a surgeon could make a case that each appendectomy is unique. Similarly, a mental health professional could make a case that every cognitive-behavioral course of treatment for depression is in some way unique.

Despite the unique aspects of clinical care, some groups have been developing guidelines for professional conduct in new practice areas related to service delivery through telehealth. The authors of the *Report of the Joint Interdisciplinary Telehealth Standards Working Group* (Milholland & Reed, 1998) anticipate changes in standards of professional conduct:

> *Standards of professional conduct are unlikely to change simply as a result of developing telehealth technology. However, the professions will likely need to develop interpretations of their standards of professional conduct as they apply to telehealth, since the application of the standards and the measurement criteria used to assess them may be different in this area. There will be a need for ongoing evaluation by professions of these issues. The most important question in professions' examination will be whether the use of telehealth technology allows professionals to meet the standards of professional conduct of their profession. Telehealth technology must be applied in a manner that does not interfere with a health care professional's ability to uphold and comply with these standards. In rare cases, evolving technology may require changes in or additions to standards of professional conduct, but standards of professional conduct should not be changed merely because they are difficult to meet with telehealth technology.*

An example of a standard of professional conduct common to all health care professionals concerns health care professionals' responsibility to protect client confidentiality. The use of telehealth technology, such as Internet-based data transmission and electronic medical records, may create serious difficulty with professionals' ability to meet standards of professional conduct in this area, and must be examined in this light.

Now, several years after the report's publication, practitioners need to reconsider their current needs. Ethical dilemmas are surfacing in multiple areas. If a former patient e-mails his or her therapist with a message that reveals sensitive information, the therapist might reply with a warning about security and a statement that he or she will not engage in such communication. But should this response be made by e-mail, telephone, or a formal letter? The most routine yet subtle problem the authors of this book experience involves how a professional who doesn't want to risk engaging with patients in e-mail should educate a colleague who thinks nothing of sending unencrypted e-mail on the open Internet to or about patients. Practitioners knowledgeable about Health Insurance Portability and Accountability Act (HIPAA) and the ethical ramifications of sending such e-mail messages are encouraged to police and correct colleagues. But what if the ethics code isn't clear about when and how to use e-mail? Practitioners vary in their attitudes toward following ethical guidelines (Pope, 1987). Engaging colleagues over an unsettled issue is likely to be burdensome, provocative, or negativistic.

Is this task to be addressed only by graduate and postgraduate training programs and professional associations, or should it also be pursued by a grass-roots effort on the part of clinicians? The next section discusses these and similar questions. The standards that apply to telehealth fall into three categories—clinical standards, administrative standards, and technical standards (Brown-Connolly, 2001b). The interplay of these standards builds a strong foundation for the delivery of quality services.

CLINICAL STANDARDS

Clinical standards cover professional conduct, practice and treatment (clinical) guidelines, standards of care, scope of practice, and other related issues. Standards and guidelines are rules promulgated by professional organizations and associations and by professional licensing boards, which in many cases are government agencies. In the United States, state licensing boards enforce legal and regulatory requirements and regulate areas of professional practice. In addition, professional associations police their own ranks. They may take action against members who do not adhere to their ethical standards by means of sanctions, expulsion, or reporting them to the appropriate state board. Because of the skepticism about health care delivered over the Internet, practitioners should be aware of the evolving law (R. Waters, personal communication, September 11, 2002).

Other concerns include malpractice coverage and liability (Office of Technology Assessment, 1990), the ramifications of practicing outside what some practitioners deem the current "standard of care," emergency backup of data files, storage of videotapes of therapy sessions, and proper documentation of services delivered (Brandt, 1996). In addition are the precautions about the treatment of minors without parental consent and regulations about patient rights (California Healthline, 1999).

Practitioners should use the word *standard* with great care. In tort law, the standards of the relevant profession provide the test of a professional's conduct. In a malpractice context, the "standard of care" depends to some extent on common law—the law that develops from a series of court decisions. What constitutes minimal acceptable care therefore differs among states. At one time, and even today in some states, standards also varied among localities, so that, for example, rural practitioners were not held to the same criteria as those near large medical centers.

Advances in communication and transportation have largely eliminated local rule in most jurisdictions to the point at which out-of-state experts are often permitted to testify about the standard of care relevant to a malpractice action. States also differ in the extent to which they recognize the pronouncements of specialty societies, professional associations, textbooks, and journal articles and the even rules and regulations of other governments as evidence of the standards of care. From a defense perspective, there is generally no advantage in expanding the number of proof sources for establishing the standards of care. After all, the more standards there are, the greater the chances that a practitioner might engage in conduct that someone is prepared to claim falls below a particular standard.

Standards of Professional Conduct

The standards of professional conduct that a health care organization sets forth define the responsibilities for which the organization holds its members accountable. In jurisdictions in which the standards of professional conduct provide the basis for licensing laws, these standards are stated in the code of ethics and policy documents for health care professionals (Milholland & Reed, 1998). These standards do not change with the integration of technology into professional practice. Rather, mental health professionals must assess their ability to adhere to these standards while working with remote sites and new technologies. For example, emergency backup services will be needed, in remote sites, and support from midlevel personnel may be desirable to foster client safety in the event of an untoward occurrence.

Standards of clinical practice include how professional practice is conducted and the quality of care delivered. The American Medical Association (AMA) policy statement identifies the need to develop practice standards and guidelines for new and developing technologies. According to the statement, the AMA:

> 1) encourages all national specialty societies to work with their state societies to develop comprehensive practice standards and guidelines to address both the clinical and technological aspects of telemedicine; 2) will assist the national specialty societies in their efforts to develop these guidelines and standards; and 3) urges national private accreditation organizations (e.g., URAC and JCAHO) to require that medical care organizations which establish ongoing arrangements for medical care delivery from remote sites require professionals at those sites to meet no less stringent credentialing standards and participate in quality review procedures that are at least equivalent to those at the site of care delivery. (American Medical Association House of Delegates, 1999, p. 3).

Ethical Principles for Online Clinical Practice. In response to the unprecedented growth of the Internet in the past decade, a number of groups have set forth ethical principles for health care delivered through the Internet (Wooton & Blignault, 2003). Such principles cover advertising, commerce, partnerships, and practice for both general and specific types of health care delivery (Eng, 2001). Organizations issuing technology-specific ethical statements include the following:

- American Accreditation Healthcare Commission (URAC) (http://www.urac.org).
- American Association of Marriage and Family Therapy (http://www.aamft.org).
- American Counseling Association (http://www.counseling.org).
- American Health Information Management Association (http://www.ahima.org).
- American Medical Association (http://www.ama-assn.org).
- American Medical Informatics Association (http://www.amia.org).
- eRisk Working Group for Healthcare (http://www.medem.com/corporate/corporate_erisk_guidelines.cfm).
- Health on the Net Foundation (http://www.hon.ch).
- Healthcare Internet Ethics (Hi-Ethics) (http://www.hiethics.org).
- Internet Healthcare Coalition (http://www.ihealthcoalition.org).
- National Board for Certified Counselors (http://www.nbcc.org).
- National Council of State Boards of Nursing (http://www.ncsbn.org).
- World Health Organization (http://www.who.int).
- Several branches of the United States government.

New groups are forming and old groups are disbanding. Some group founders and/or members may not understand psychotherapy practice or ethical principles as defined by any state or provincial licensing board. When joining a society, association, or organization issuing ethical statements for mental health professionals, readers should question the leaders about their licensure and experience with in-person practice. A group may appear credible, but a background check may reveal unlicensed leaders and/or inexperienced mental health practitioners.

Practitioners can also look into specialty behavioral health care organizations. For example, considering the proliferation of employee assistance program offerings online, it might be useful here to review the guidelines provided by one oversight organization, the Council on Accreditation (COA). An international, independent, nonprofit accrediting body, COA publishes standards for the full array of child and family services, behavioral health care services, financial management or debt counseling services, and community services. In collaboration with the Employee Assistance Society of North America (EASNA), COA has developed employee assistance program standards that cover Web-based services and the use of other technologies. These standards are published in the *Employee Assistance Program Standards and Self-Study Manual*, now in its second edition (Council on Accreditation, 2002). The COA's Web site is (http://www.coanet.org).

Without established rules governing the rapidly evolving area of distance therapy in a particular mental health discipline, practitioners must rely on basic ethical precepts. Once promulgated, online standards must undergo continued review and revision (Plaut, 1997). Professionals should take reasonable steps to protect clients, students, supervisees, research participants, and other people from harm or exploitation. When harm is foreseeable and unavoidable, professionals should take reasonable steps to minimize it. The treating professional should observe general professional principles regarding advertising, assessment, boundaries of competence, confidentiality, financial arrangements and fees, informed consent, interruption of services, and multiple relationships, just as with in-person services.

Mental health professionals should avoid, or fully disclose, any potential or perceived conflicts of interest, such as advertising a workshop on a Web site used for client transactions. Likewise, mental health professionals should not take advantage of an audio- or videoconference to urge clients to purchase their self-help book, just as physicians should not prescribe and then dispense medications for extra income.

Videoconferencing sessions, like in-person sessions, may need to be logged and described by means of session notes, but they generally do not need to be recorded. Recording may create unnecessary interpersonal, procedural, and legal complications. HIPAA and other federal and state laws will govern the use, disclosure, and storage of recorded videoconferenced sessions. Video recording may fall under the definition of "psychotherapy notes," which are given special protection under HIPAA (see chapter 9).

Although applying these concepts to actual situations is usually straightforward, a professional can be led astray by enthusiasm, overconfidence in the technology, the sense of freedom afforded by distance, and the lack of oversight in cyberspace. In fact, telecommunication technologies are now so powerful that they can require considerable extension of the traditional ethical rules for psychotherapists. Consider, for example, a practitioner's excitement over instantaneous satellite communication with a client's rural family thousands of miles away in a remote area of Canada. The technology's novel ability to shrink time and space may obscure ethical considerations in the mind of the law-abiding, ethical practitioner. The practitioner may forget that he or she is unaware of local occurrences in the family's geographic region or, if dealing with another cultural group, may not understand the ramifications for the client of contacting the family. The practitioner may not remember to obtain consent from each participating member and/or to document such consent.

Professionals are bound by ethical principles, yet extenuating circumstances presented by the psychotechnologies may obstruct compliance with these principles. For example, most psychotherapists must explain the limits of confidentiality at the onset of service provision. This initial step may be complicated for a psychotherapist who has a poor understanding of the technology and how it affects the security of information. More specifically, many practitioners cannot explain the need for encryption in e-mail, are unaware that encryption also is needed in videoconferencing through the Web, and, even if this fact were known, would not understand why encryption is not needed in videoconferencing by videophone. Being familiar with these distinctions is essential if practitioners are to abide by the ethical principle that requires explaining the limits of confidentiality.

Similarly, safeguarding professional records may become difficult when a psychotherapy session is videotaped by an employer who owns and creates backup data files for video equipment the psychotherapist uses. Suppose that the psychotherapist, having received the employer's verbal promise that videoconferencing sessions were not being backed up, learns that they were backed up as a matter of hospital policy. The employer may later explain that copies of videotaped sessions are made only when the patient is suspected of abusing a child, spouse, or elderly person, for example. What can practitioners do about the backups that were completed without their knowledge? Now that they have a therapeutic relationship with clients using the hospital's system, how should these practitioners handle that relationship if the employer will not alter its policy?

The process of service delivery can shift dramatically in other situations, such as when emergency interventions are delivered remotely. Because the current lack of knowledge and standards offers little support for providing emergency remote mental health services, the authors cannot endorse such practice. In coming years, there are likely to be many instances in which professional intervention in an emergency from a distance has succeeded and others in which it has resulted in harm to the practitioner or made matters worse for the patient.

In some cases, an emergency may develop during the course of ongoing distance therapy. As an example, in an electronic world in which distance initially seemed irrelevant, a psychologist responding to a crisis might not remember licensing or confidentiality restrictions. In delivering consultation services to a Zambian community leader struggling with the ravages of starvation, drought, and war or to an abused spouse who has fled to Tennessee, a Utah psychologist might forget local licensing limitations and not have the backup suddenly required to deal with the situation. Ideally, such experiences will allow realistic new standards to be formulated for responding to such emergencies from afar.

Perhaps a professional should be licensed in a particular state or country in order to render remote consultation in those locations. Is licensure required to provide other services via computer, such as through an interactive program delivered over the Internet or on a compact disk? Which computer-based services are acceptable (or unacceptable) without licensure in the remote location? Clearly, although general professional standards of conduct exist, many practitioners, when dealing with new contexts, might not remember the repercussions of a nonspecific ethics code.

The most recent revision of the ethical code of the American Psychological Association (2002a) offers a general approach to applying standards of professional conduct to the psychotechnologies. It states that the ethical standards apply to various named activities of psychologists across a variety of contexts, including the "Internet and other electronic transmissions[1]." It also states that a "lack of awareness or misunderstanding of an Ethical Standard is not itself a defense to a charge of unethical conduct" (p. 2).

When an activity is mentioned, such as psychotherapy via e-mail, but the specifics of the context are omitted, inexperienced practitioners might incorrectly believe that they are dutifully following all applicable ethical standards. If professionals are not intentionally given direction regarding their use of e-mail with specific patient populations, what harm can be done? Let's examine the possibilities in this fictionalized example:

A well-meaning psychotherapist establishes a professional–patient e-mail relationship with an individual who convincingly portrays herself as a single female, aged 22, struggling to overcome a social phobia. She states that she lives in a nearby city within the therapist's state of licensure. The therapist has 4 weekly online sessions with this client.

---

[1] The document reads as follows: "This Ethics Code applies only to psychologists' activities that are part of their scientific, educational, or professional roles as psychologists. Areas covered include but are not limited to the clinical, counseling, and school practice of psychology; research; teaching; supervision of trainees; public service; policy development; social intervention; development of assessment instruments; conducting assessments; educational counceling; organizational consulting; forensic activities; program design and evaluation; and administration. This Ethics Code applies to these activities across a variety of contexts, such as in person, postal, telephone, internet, and other electronic transmissions" (American Psychological Association, 2002a, p. 2).

The client promises to send the therapist a duly executed written consent form, but never does. Despite not receiving the consent form, the therapist proceeds to negotiate behavioral objectives with the patient. She fails to make much progress and decides to discontinue treatment, expressing gratitude for the therapist's attempts but moderate disappointment at her inability to overcome her shyness. A month later, the therapist is served with a summons related to the case. The plaintiffs are the girl's parents.

The patient was 15, not 22. She committed suicide after their last e-mail exchange, and her parents are outraged. The therapist hires an attorney, who appropriately responds to the summons with a request for discovery (evidence). The therapist explains to his attorney that the parents have printouts of all the therapist's e-mail exchanges with their daughter. They have credit card statements showing that they were billed for his services. Their daughter had used her mother's name and credit card. The parents also have printouts from the therapist's Web site that show his credentials. These printouts also indicate that the therapist is not licensed in their state, which is 2,000 miles away.

Who has been harmed? Who, if anyone, is responsible for the girl's suicide? How could this professional have been guided by a general ethics code? He acted in good faith. He is not a detective and, like most clinical psychologists, considers it the client's responsibility to be truthful in treatment. Will he be found to have violated any current ethical standards for his discipline? Has he violated any laws?

Patients as well as professionals are at risk. The therapist in this fictional case might be found responsible to some degree. The laws of his state and of the patient's will define the nature of his legal responsibility. The courts will decide the other issues of this case.

Do any current ethical codes indicate how the therapist could have avoided this predicament? Obviously, professionals may need to receive training to help them understand how to apply these standards to any relationship other than in-person contact with patients. Until appropriate training is available, the pilot telehealth and telemedicine projects conducted during the past few decades are good sources of information. The general model in these programs involves a professional performing a local evaluation, then referring a client to a specialist through interactive videoconferencing technology. Details of this model, the Online Clinical Practice Management (OCPM) model, are discussed in the next three chapters.

Confidentiality. Whatever the situation, whatever the technology, practitioners should always apply common sense. Make sure that cleaning staff and clients in the waiting room can't overhear messages left on the office answering machine and that fellow restaurant patrons or the movie audience cannot overhear a mobile phone conversation with or about a client. When leaving a message on a client's answering machine, remember that anyone might retrieve the message. It is best for professionals to be terse, leave off the "Dr." in their names, and supply minimal information, such as the time of day and a call-back number (Melonas, 2002).

By making massive amounts of information readily available and easy to store, retrieve, and search, the psychotechnologies have highlighted the importance of many confidentiality issues. Must video via Internet be encrypted or otherwise secured to meet HIPAA standards? (Yes.) Are chat rooms, confidential? (Not typically, despite Web owner claims.)

Many other ethical issues are involved in the collection, storage, transmission (electronic or physical), and use of confidential data and their incorporation into records. Obviously, encryption is required for data stored in electronic records to prevent the inclusion of individual identifiers. Even if practitioners meet all basic requirements, surprising dilemmas can surface. For example, if law enforcement officials suspect an impending terrorist attack, they may request electronic mental health records to screen for potential malefactors. How much access should be given, and exactly what powers should be entrusted to the law enforcement officials (Bayer & Colgrove, 2002)? Should the confidential mental health files of a parent violating a court order for child support be used by an enforcement agency to locate the delinquent parent (Ziglin, 1995)? When should a health professional balk at a demand for information and turn to the courts to overturn the demand?

Avoiding Harm. Serious potential for damage to online clients can arise from many sources. To avoid harming a client, the professional should gather pertinent information, such as the location of the client during the current transaction and the presence of third parties. Imagine, for example, the repercussions when a mental health professional sends an e-mail message alluding to the client's infidelity, unaware that the client's spouse recently entered the room. Even if the spouse did not read the message, it could remain on the client's computer or in the old e-mail file of the client's ISP. If the client's e-mail account is not password protected (and in some circumstances even if it is), a family member could eventually read the message.

It is no trivial matter when a patient receives a professional's message that was intended for someone else or when a message about the patient was inadvertently missent. A patient with a serious disorder, such as borderline personality disorder, who is involved in a cybersnafu might abruptly pull out of the therapeutic relationship and suffer undisclosed harm.

Using proper language in a written communication is essential for avoiding harm to the client. The amount of time spent writing a message may be reduced (or expanded to days) in e-mail or chat communications when compared to the time it takes to pen a note. A hastily composed note can lead to significant problems. When dashing off an e-mail message, the author may not carefully consider all phrases, and the message could be misinterpreted. Material composed on a computer may pass muster when the author reviews it on the screen and scrupulously corrects the spelling and grammatical errors, but the author may see mistakes when the file is printed. If possible, e-mail message writers should examine their output in at least two different ways (on screen and as hard copy) and should consider taking a break (preferably a night's sleep) between composing messages and sending them off to sensitive recipients.

Professionals may gain experience in composing text-based communication by joining a discussion list or chat room to learn the basic rules and norms. By doing this, professionals can discover how unintended nuances make their way into e-mail or other text-based messages. It may be wise, even in this setting, to lurk for some time before submitting a contribution.

Terminating a relationship is very easy in e-mail—one click and you're gone. If in an office, an agitated patient needs only to stand and walk out of the office. Even though this action may not involve much time, it does give a quick-thinking practitioner the time to ameliorate the situation with compassionate questions or statements to promote reality testing. Most seasoned clinicians have dealt with stressed, volatile, severe personality disordered, and/or intoxicated patients. Some of these patients might experience narcissistic wounds when no harm was intended.

How might a practitioner handle anger and distancing when working in e-mail or chat rooms? What might a professional do when the patient misinterprets an attempt to rectify an obvious empathic break? Does the professional keep sending e-mails to further attempt to rectify such a situation? What should the professional do when the patient expresses anger by failing to respond? Should the professional try calling on the telephone? If so, how many times? Leave a voice message requesting a return call? Send a snail mail letter? After how much time? If no response is received, when would a termination letter be appropriate? Should the professional decide that termination was all for the good, as the patient obviously wasn't capable of benefiting from an e-mail relationship? Is it fair for the professional to have engaged to the patient in a medium that would allow for immediate and absolute termination without having first screened the patient in-person for appropriateness based on diagnosis? Should the practitioner have discussed the possibility of such termination as part of the informed-consent activity that should be continuous throughout therapy? What repercussions will this experience have on the patient's willingness to engage with future therapists, either online or offline? These questions need to be explored through research.

On the other hand, if a socially phobic patient sustains contact with an online therapist, this contact may lead to increased connection with the outside world. It is reasonable to assume that many patients who otherwise would never approach a therapist can benefit from such treatment. The task for the professional, and the professional community, is to determine which patients are likely to benefit and which are likely to be harmed by which psychotechnology or blend of psychotechnology and in-person treatment. This issue also needs to be researched.

The ease of impersonation in e-mail transactions raises other issues. If a therapist never meets the client, how does the therapist know who is on the other end of the interaction? Males could pretend to be females, and teenagers could pretend to be adults (as in the previous fictitious example). The misleading information would contaminate any response from the psychotherapist.

In traditional treatment, coordination of care and designation of a primary mental health care provider need to be worked out when the client seeks treatment from a second or third professional. With treatment conducted over a distance, it is much easier for a patient to engage an additional mental health professional and not disclose to anyone the multiplicity of therapeutic relationships. Casually striking up a relationship with an online therapist may become so common that proper practice will require that a therapist confront this possibility at the outset of any therapy, including in-person therapy, and periodically inquire whether the patient has become involved with anyone else in this way. Physicians face a similar issue with patients who consume alternative health food nostrums that are incompatible with their prescription medications.

Boundaries of Competence. Realistically, of course, online practice not only calls for additional education and new skills but may also involve types of service that the professional was not previously providing. Psychiatrists who start doing extensive clinical work over the Internet must be careful not to administer and interpret assessment instruments in which they have not been trained. As discussed in chapters 6, using Web sites to offer psychological tests designed for in-person administration or normed with an in-person population may lead to biased results and unfounded interpretations. The general public places a high level of confidence in psychological and other health-related tests and assessments. Professionalism therefore requires that test administrators know the harm they could cause and the specific needs of the population they are serving. Similarly, remote treatment of patients from a wide geographic area may require greater cultural competence than a psychologist has attained.

As seen in the criteria delineated by the American Psychological Association, issues related to boundaries of competence are well delineated. In the 2002 revision of the 1992 APA, standards have been expanded as quoted here:

- Psychologists provide services, teach, and conduct research with populations and in areas only within the boundaries of their competence, based on their education, training, supervised experience, consultation, study, or professional experience.
- Where scientific or professional knowledge in the discipline of psychology establishes that an understanding of factors associated with age, gender, gender identity, race, ethnicity, culture, national origin, religion, sexual orientation, disability, language, or socioeconomic status is essential for effective implementation of their services or research, psychologists have or obtain the training, experience, consultation, or supervision necessary to ensure the competence of their services, or they make appropriate referrals, except as provided in Standard 2.02, Providing Services in Emergencies.
- Psychologists planning to provide services, teach, or conduct research involving populations, areas, techniques, or technologies new to them undertake relevant education, training, supervised experience, consultation, or study.
- When psychologists are asked to provide services to individuals for whom appropriate mental health services are not available and for which psychologists have not obtained the competence necessary, psychologists with closely related prior training or experience may provide such services in order to ensure that services are not denied if they make a reasonable effort to obtain the competence required by using relevant research, training, consultation, or study.
- In those emerging areas in which generally recognized standards for preparatory training do not yet exist, psychologists nevertheless take reasonable steps to ensure the competence of their work and to protect clients/patients, students, supervisees, research participants, organizational clients, and others from harm.
- When assuming forensic roles, psychologists are or become reasonably familiar with the judicial or administrative rules governing their roles. (American Psychological Association, 2002a, p. 5).

Continuing education in applying the emerging area of psychotechnologies is needed. Our vision of such training is discussed in chapter 11.

General accreditation information, such as from a page on the American Psychological Association's Web site (http://www.apa.org/ed/accreditation), can inform practitioners about accreditation standards in graduate and postgraduate psychological clinical training. Other associations have similar guidelines for the training programs they accredit. Adhering to such standards is important not only for the practitioner but also for patients who are savvy enough to ask about a professional's training. As patients become better able to determine whether they are being treated by a well-qualified clinician, attending a training program that exhibits proper credentials will become a distinct advantage for practitioners.

Structuring a Professional Relationship. The American Psychological Association's statements on ethics state that all ethical standards and guidelines apply from the moment a professional relationship begins, whether or not a fee is charged. However, determining when and whether a professional relationship has been established during e-mail contact, for instance, although crucial for professionals (and often for their lawyers), can be impossible. This is another issue in need of definition.

According to some authorities, a professional relationship may be construed to commence the moment the client feels that a professional relationship exists or entrusts treatment to the professional. Showing up for a scheduled initial appointment arranged entirely through a receptionist or central telephone access center may suffice to start the clock ticking (*Lyons v. Grether*, 1977). Definitions of professional relationships vary among jurisdictions, so practitioners are advised to refer to the relevant law defining practice.

Whether and under what circumstances the professional relationship is established is important for legal as well as ethical reasons. Malpractice is a breach of duty, and no duty exists where no therapeutic relationship exists. On the other hand, if a therapeutic relationship has been established, the law imposes on the practitioner duties that, if breached, may be actionable.

When courts have been obliged to determine whether a physician–patient or other practitioner–patient relationship existed in a particular telehealth context, they have looked to telephone cases for guidance. In these cases, courts have considered such questions as whether the practitioner (generally, a physician) spoke directly to the patient or to another physician, whether the physician knew the patient's name, whether the consultation occurred in an emergency context, whether the physician made any written record of the interaction, and whether the physician rendered a bill. It is reasonable to assume that until the law on these issues becomes clarified, many courts will continue to generalize from past telephone cases (McMenamin, 1996).

Professional associations also may have a voice in determining whether a professional relationship exists. As noted in this chapter, the American Psychiatric Association (2000b) states that an initial in-person meeting should precede telepsychiatry. If an in-person meeting is not possible, the therapist may wish to consider reasonable risks and benefits carefully before engaging in care. A meeting by video of sufficient quality probably will be considered enough of a "face-to-face" encounter to satisfy ethical criteria.

Assuming that the therapist decides to proceed, the consent agreement is the most common way to document a professional relationship. The client can endorse a preliminary agreement (an agreement to forge an agreement) almost immediately; thereafter, the informed consent can be continually modified and the modifications documented. As part of Step 4 of the Online Clinical Practice Management (OCPM) Model, mental health professionals should, as early as possible in the therapeutic relationship, expand the informed-consent agreement to describe the nature and anticipated course of therapy, the fees, the involvement of third parties, and the extent of confidentiality (Fisher, 2001).

According to the early research (outlined in appendix A), various types of media may alter the therapeutic relationship in various ways. Each type introduces its own elements into interactions with clients. E-mail and chat rooms transmit a minimum amount of information, and interactive videoconferencing delivers a maximum amount of information to both the professional and the client. Here, we first discuss text-based interactions, then videoconferencing.

The issues in text-based interactions are complicated, and the medium may alter the rules. If several queries and responses are e-mailed between a mental health practitioner and a client, when might that client legitimately assume (and later claim) that a professional relationship has been established (Kuszler, 2000)? Questions arise as to how to define a professional relationship. Vague parameters define psychotherapy, counseling, coaching (Naughton, 2002), media psychology, and online mental health (Sleek, 1995).

Vague definitions were helpful in casting a wide net over services for which practitioners could obtain reimbursement, but such vagueness now causes a problem with the psychotechnologies. For instance, practitioners often appear on talk shows in which callers question them. These interactions are assumed to be didactic, and no therapeutic relationship is established. Would the same be true for a mental health professional moderating a chat room several times a week? General advice given in a public forum to an individual is usually not considered therapy, but if general advice is given a number of times to a member of an established group online, at what point, if any, does the relationship become professional? Which types of direct e-mail discussions meet the criteria for psychotherapy? Moreover, specifically, which types of newsgroup or chat room discussions go beyond providing general information? These questions have not been answered clearly by the professional associations or by the courts.

A professional relationship brings with it, explicitly or implicitly, a responsibility for the client's care (Kane & Sands, 1998). A plaintiff's lawyer may claim that any harm arguably caused to the client by a text-based interaction when some other available communication method would have sufficed can be considered a breach of the standard of care. Having patients sign a document under which they take the responsibility for choosing a medium, such as the telephone, may be useful. The patient's counsel will argue, however, that such an agreement does not relieve the professional from responsibility, because the relationship between the parties is not equal. The patient is relying on the professional's superior knowledge about how to conduct the therapy. Stated differently, the professional's judgment is not independent. The law today on questions such as this is too limited to allow firm conclusions to be reached. Professionals therefore should draft a consent document carefully and use it conscientiously; they also should be prepared for attacks and should be ready to amend the document as needed and as the law evolves.

Often, the issue about whether a professional–client relationship exists will be clear and noncontroversial. A professional could unwittingly stumble into an implicit contract, however, that creates an opportunity for lawyer to allege a duty relationship. In one study, 41% of anaesthesiologists responding to an e-mail inquiry by an unknown client suggested a diagnosis (Oyston, 2000). Their proclivity to offer their opinions, including diagnoses, makes it crucial for professionals to realize where identifiable pitfalls lie, to use carefully drafted consent agreements, and always to err on the side of caution.

As detailed in chapter 5, choices related to the use of videoconferencing can influence social presence and therapeutic contact. Videoconferencing may have benefits not inherent in in-person encounters. It can decrease social restraints and enable clients or families and professionals to speak more freely. Critical factors in this regard might include quality of eye contact, distance from the camera, lighting so that facial features are clearly visible, size of the image, resolution, and movement as delivered through various transmission speeds. Elements of the exchange, such as facial expressions, can be relevant. Similarly, choices related to the use of e-mail or chat rooms can also influence therapeutic contact, as discussed in chapter 3.

Professional Personal Disclosure. The standards of the American Accreditation HealthCare Commission (2001) provide that the address and legal name of a health Web site owner appear on the site. The Internet Healthcare Coalition (2000) adds that Web sites should also indicate any other parties that have a significant financial interest in the Web site. Furthermore, Web site providers should post such information as credentialing and registration status (Health on the Net Foundation, 1998; Internet Healthcare Coalition, 2000) as well as licensure, if applicable (Internet Healthcare Coalition, 2000). Web sites can and should clearly distinguish advertisements and paid promotional materials from editorial and journalistic content.

The Internet allows clients to research professionals extensively and even to discover highly personal information. The reliability of the information may be uneven. Consequently, a professional is advised to be aware of the types of information available on the Internet. As an example, consider the following story, which concerns an article written by one of this book's authors:

> *In 1995, I coauthored an article in* SelfhelpMagazine *about libido. Several months later, one of my established clients came into the office, cheerfully plopped herself down in a chair, and started the session with, "So, you think a person married to someone with lupus can't expect to have sex once in a while?" I responded with a clarifying question and learned that she had read the* SelfhelpMagazine *article and wanted me to know she had learned something on the Net about my views regarding libido. Although she had misquoted my statement, she was clearly more delighted in announcing that she had learned something about me outside of our relationship than in discussing the facts of the article. She was amused that she had caught me off guard, and her provocative behavior made for a lively and productive psychotherapy session.*
>
> *Since then, other clients have reported finding information written by or about me online and have used it in various ways to elicit responses from me. To make such situations therapeutically beneficial, I have learned to expect clients to find information about me online and then to interpret their reporting style in a way that enhances our relationship. I have also learned to minimize the amount of personal information I put on my Web sites. For instance, rather than including my full curriculum vitae, I now provide only a condensed version online.*

Professionals can use various search engines to find references online to themselves and/or their practices. Professionals also should realize that any one can easily access this information. Personal information could be disadvantageous to the therapeutic relationship or harmful to the psychotherapist. Not all of the online information may be accurate. If the information is inaccurate, the professional should demand corrections.

Too often, psychotherapists using e-mail and chat rooms for contact with clients disregard norms established for in-person treatment. For example, initial contact tends to occur without any explanation of risk or the signing of a client consent agreement (Maheu & Gordon, 2000). Furthermore, the efficacy of presenting disclaimers on a Web site has not been demonstrated. Little is known about what happens when people with undiagnosed psychiatric disorders engage in e-mail—or chat room–mediated psychotherapy—or read consent agreements. Posting such agreements, however, and requiring prospective clients to click through them, is preferable to not doing so.

Attention and Distraction. The ethical standards Haas, Benedict, and Kobos (1996) describe for patient–practitioner interactions by telephone may also apply to text-based therapy via the Internet. E-mail and chat room discussions resemble telephone interactions in their absence of visual cues and the client's ability to break off communication without warning. Relevant issues include client protection and confidentiality, the ability to deliver competent service through a relatively novel medium, and informed consent.

In their review of issues related to using the telephone for psychotherapy, Haas et al. (1996) expressed particular concern about the possibility of distractions. The Internet and personal computers offer many temptations to the client and professional during text-based communication, including games, pornography, and e-mail. (It would be difficult to provide meaningful advice to a client while he or she was playing Donkey Kong at a strip club.) Distractions could undermine the therapeutic work by catering to the client's impulsivity. Both parties might also find it easy to focus attention on other happenings around the office or house or could become bored (Martin, 2000). Children, television, and/or food could distract either party, and the splitting of attention would likely reduce the benefit for the client. The focus of both parties needs to be on the task.

Even though some professionals try to make their consultation room relaxed, informal, and cozy, it remains the professional's territory, carries a certain mystique, and sets a tone designed by the professional and shared by professional and client. Videoconferencing does not involve this shared ambience. Patients at home during a remote session are on their own turf in a venue used for many activities other than therapy. This location might be less conducive to entering states of mind that are optimal for progress in psychotherapy. To some extent, similar considerations may apply to therapists practicing from home—unkempt, unwashed, and in a setting into which they would never consider having a patient enter in person. Certainly over e-mail, neither patients nor therapists are likely to feel they need to look their best.

Owing to the relative paucity or total lack of visual cues, telecommunication makes it difficult for a mental health professional to determine whether a client is fully attentive, and vice versa. Distractions may be real or imagined; in some cases, only increased access to information will help the clinician know which it is. Similarly, lapses in time during a synchronous communication may result from technological complications, unidentified social or emotional problems, poor reading comprehension, extended contemplation of an issue, limited writing ability, alcohol or drug use, or poor typing skills. Directly asking clients whether they have been distracted may not always elicit the truth. Similarly, an unusually quick reaction time may result from drug or alcohol use, mania, other sources of poor impulse control, poor reading comprehension, or limited writing ability, for example. The point is that reaction time may indicate a clinically relevant issue, but the medium makes it difficult to identify the source of the problem, because the usual contextual cues are lacking.

Problematic behaviors can arise on the clinician's side of the communication as well. Professionals may become temporarily distracted by paperwork or other tasks pursued while awaiting a client's response. Some clinicians may access e-mail while awaiting a chat room response. While reading a long-awaited e-mail, the clinician can lose track of a chat room encounter with a patient. Similarly, it is obviously rude for a professional to talk on the telephone during an in-person session (although such things happen). The important question is what the hurried clinician would do if a long-awaited telephone call arrived during a text-based exchange with a client. During such a session, a professional might be tempted to engage in potential distractions with full but false confidence that this behaviour would make no difference or that the dalliance would never be discovered. Whatever the reason, the clinician can more easily be distracted in text-based communication. The literature regarding telephone use in psychotherapy (Haas et al., 1996) discusses other ethical issues relating to attentiveness and distraction.

Providing Care to Children. According to the U.S. Surgeon General, approximately 20% of U.S. children and adolescents between 9 and 17 years of age experience a diagnosable psychiatric disorder (U.S. Public Health Service, 2000). Because children are avid consumers of electronic devices, the psychotechnologies seem particularly appropriate for pediatric mental health. However, although their use with adults has been written about extensively, little attention has been paid to their use with children, including pertinent ethical issues. One exception is an intriguing ongoing collaborative study by schools of the University of California (Henker, Whalen, Jamner, & Delfino, 2002). Ninth-grade adolescents who kept track of their moods and activities by filling in a form every 30 minutes on handheld computers showed clear correlations between their surprisingly frequent negative moods and such problem behaviors as smoking, drinking, eating, and withdrawal.

Therapists who use psychotechnologies to work with minors confront ethical issues associated with the generation gap, the rights of adolescents, the ownership of information, confidentiality, and standardized information systems. As Alessi (2001) wrote, children are dependent on other people for most health care decisions, yet children and adolescents may become better informed about health care options using psychotechnologies than are their parents or guardians. This generation gap adds confusion to the already difficult dilemmas regarding the rights of children to make their own health care decisions. In chapter 1, we discuss a recent trend in health care—the tendency of clients armed with information from the Internet and news media to present an array of health care options to their physicians instead of the other way around. Suppose that, in similar fashion, children were to present their parents with a wealth of health information obtained from the Internet. If the parents were to disregard pertinent information that could have influenced their decisions, could they be considered negligent? Currently, at age 14, adolescents are allowed to receive counseling from U.S. schools and clinics without their parents' knowledge. Depending on the state, adolescents may be deemed able to consent to confidential treatment for substance abuse or reproductive health at an even earlier age. They can readily receive support from peer groups on the Internet. If a mental health professional is participating in a discussion, what is the threshold beyond which parental permission is required? Will children seeking mental health care through the psychotechnologies be especially influenced by false or damaging information from an unreliable source, and are special methods designed for the young needed to protect them?

The Children's Online Privacy Protection Act (COPPA) requires Web site operators in the United States to obtain verifiable parental consent before collecting personally identifying information from children under age 13. A mental health professional who receives unsolicited e-mail from a child under 13 may respond once but should then delete the child's e-mail address so as not to run afoul of the law. However, it may be necessary and legitimate to retain the child's name and e-mail address to report to law enforcement authorities or to protect the Web site. Of course, this situation raises the question of how one ascertains the child's true age. At present, the law would seem to allow a professional to rely on the child's self-report if no evidence reasonably suggests that the self-report is false. Professionals who wish to engage in online therapy with a child will, of course, have to maintain records about that child. To do so lawfully, they need to obtain consent from the parents. Such consent must be obtained during an offline discussion. The identity of parents should be authenticated. Of course, consent agreements need to be documented and preserved. Note that even though taking these steps will help avoid COPPA violations, professional liability issues remain in the shadows of such practices, and professional liability can still be found on other grounds, perhaps unrelated to COPPA requirements.

Some Web sites allow visitors to set up a personal account and then to maintain a diary or journal that they may keep private or share openly or with selected guests. Some uses of these Web sites may cross over into the mental health area, such as for tracking recovery from an eating or chemical abuse disorder. Some sites provide relatively unstructured file space. There is no practical way to prevent children from opening accounts at many of these Web sites or to monitor the material deposited. Even though these sites may technically not run afoul of COPPA or be considered as holding personally identifiable medical information, they can effectively undercut the law's intent in many respects. LiveJournal (http://www.livejournal.com) now posts a notice that it will no longer accommodate children under age 13, although it is unclear how the site could enforce this policy. Another example of readily available general-purpose online file space is Yahoo!Briefcase (http://briefcase.yahoo.com).

A related issue involves electronic medical records and the ownership of information. Adolescents may wish to access their electronic medical records when seeking mental health services independently of their parents. Problems arise when the electronic medical records are controlled solely by their parents. If children are allowed to make decisions about their mental health care, should they not also be allowed to control, or at least read, their own medical records? Does this control apply to the entire record, or can a child gain partial control? An adult client's rights include the power to annotate or amend information or to remove incorrect information. Can children do this too? Can they take such action after they reach a certain age? What is the harm in allowing children to add their own comments to the record? (This is not a rhetorical question; adding comments may indeed pose a risk to the children.) Note that records of juvenile legal problems are often sealed and unavailable for review even if they include health care information. To get an idea of how quickly these issues can snowball, consider the variation in state laws regarding parental consent for an abortion performed on a minor or the variation in the ability of minors to make life decisions.

Managing Crises and Emergencies. Crises and emergencies lead to heightened (but not novel) risks. It's all a matter of degree. There is no standard definition of an emergency or a crisis. In practice, labeling a situation an emergency is a mechanism for justifying a course of action selected on the basis of numerous considerations, many of which may be subject to dispute or difficult to describe. Unless the concept of what constitutes an emergency situation is widely misused, society prefers to avert its gaze and rely on the responsible judgment of the people on the front lines. Of course, there are occasional gross misjudgments or people who exploit the looseness of the definition or cases of negligence or simply unfortunate results; any of these occurrences can lead to a lawsuit and an adverse outcome for the defendant. Thus, practitioners are forced to weigh the benefits of professional freedom (which speaks to their strengths) against the benefits of constrictive standards (which may protect against their weaknesses).

Our stance throughout this book is to recommend full prohibition of e-mail clinical practice in emergencies. To be, sure, some online programs have been effective at helping suicidal patients. But the truth is that a suicide or a homicide threat online might be a hoax or a desperate last-minute attempt to reach out for help. Practitioners might not be able to tell, especially if their response does not elicit an immediate client reply. How many average practitioners can handle not only an unknown patient at such times but also their own sleepless nights that are likely to follow?

When receiving an unexpected e-mail message describing suicidal or homicidal intent, a practitioner may not be able to thoroughly assess the patient. The truth is that a solo professional operating online may be less able to gather crucial information or to act with sufficient speed than someone who can actually go to the emergency scene. Furthermore, a remote professional may tend to overestimate the immediate effectiveness of the therapeutic relationship or may tolerate too much immediate risk in order to preserve the relationship for long-range goals. Many practitioners would probably admit to exaggerating their effectiveness when treating a patient in person. Certainly, when using technology to mediate communication, professionals should know when to share power and responsibility with other people or even to pass the baton. In the case of online clinical practice, remote consultants need not abandon their clients. The consultants can stay in touch and offer some kind of help after a local professional has become the point person.

In any case, appropriate standards of care are not negated because a professional uses technology to mediate a relationship. Suicide or homicide notes sent to a professional's e-mail in-box could sit there unread for days. What are the appropriate response times for e-mail? Are they different from the response times for messages left in voice mail? The American Accreditation Health Care Commission (URAC) has a prominent voice in these decisions. URAC will be discussed more fully later in this chapter. Meanwhile, let's examine its recommendation regarding e-mail response times. URAC norms provide that e-mail and other electronic communications be disclosed on a health Web site (American Accreditation HealthCare Commission, 2001). The Web site also should list the names and titles of the people who will respond. Some clients may fail to read or understand the fine print, however, and may act according to what to them seem reasonable assumptions strongly braced with wishful thinking. Common sense requires that patients be very clearly and repeatedly informed that e-mail is *not* an appropriate vehicle for emergency communications.

Some practitioners use and advocate the use of videoconferencing and/or e-mail for emergency situations. The authors of this book, however, have seen little evidence to support such use. When professionals use videoconferencing technologies (and chat rooms and e-mail), they should have in place a well-considered, written plan for responding to emergencies. The plan should include a list of whom to contact for immediate assistance at the client's location if an unexpected emergency arises.

At the least, when faced with the decision about whether to use psychotechnologies for emergency care, practitioners should consider the American Psychological Association's (2002a) professional code of conduct:

> In emergencies, when psychologists provide services to individuals for whom other mental health services are not available and for which psychologists have not obtained the necessary training, psychologists may provide such services in order to ensure that services are not denied. The services are discontinued as soon as the emergency has ended or appropriate services are available. (p. 5)

One study (Brown-Connolly, 2001b) of significant sample size linked rural primary care with specialty services (13% mental health use). Responses by primary care providers, patients, and specialists indicated that patient care obtained via online clinical practice often had a positive impact on diagnosis (53% change), treatment (62% change), and management (68% change). In addition, client feedback impressions could be mentioned, but such impressions are not considered to be scientific testing of online services for crises (Australian Psychological Society, 1999; Health on the Net Foundation, 1998). Emergency assistance is an area in which the ability to deliver in-person services is particularly important.

Is Any Help Better Than No Help? Situations in which any help is better than none raise interesting issues. Certainly, if one can do more good than harm, then do it (Richards, 2002). The techniques a practitioner would use under such circumstances (as in a severely undeveloped and underserved geographic territory) are not those that are optimal in a well-served, affluent practice. Nor will the authorities hold a practitioner to the same standards.

On the other hand, if a professional treats online a client who could just as easily have been treated in the professional's office (or in a competitor's office), the question becomes, when something goes wrong (emergency or no), whether selecting an online mode was in the patient's best interest or was merely convenient for the professional. A jury that decides it was a convenience only may decide to teach the professional a lesson. Of course, professionals are most at risk in times of emergencies, the outcome of which could result in the filing of a lawsuit or of a complaint to a licensing board. Note that the pros and cons of consulting online—the preparations, protections, and backup requirements (the principles of responsible practice)—apply whether there is an emergency or not.

Suicide Risk. The traditional scientific literature (Schneidman, Farberow, & Litman, 1983) thoroughly covers protocols for dealing with suicide risk and suicide assessment by telephone. At this time, a useful hard-and-fast rule for online clinical practice of suicide risk and assessment cannot be asserted. Suicide hotlines are often used in emergencies when they are not the only option. At least for the overwhelming majority of people in the United States, a person who can reach a suicide hotline also can reach a 911 service or a police station, firehouse, ambulance service, hospital, physician, or neighbor. The reality, however, is that many people seem to benefit from suicide hotlines.

Mental health professionals are expected to do what they can to prevent suicide. Not doing what should have been done triggers more mental health malpractice actions than does doing what ought not be done. Failure to make reasonable efforts to avert suicide is a leading allegation in malpractice claims against mental health professionals, accounting for 42% of the dollars paid in settlements and court awards in 1991 (Bongar, 1991). Mental health professionals are advised to keep this fact in mind when developing suicide prevention policies on Web sites—or anywhere else.

Suicide mailing lists, discussion boards, e-mail counseling services, and support groups are available on the Internet (Stoney, 1998). Some online programs may be quite effective, even highly so (see the discussion of SAHAR in chapter 3). Many of these programs are not subject to the influences of required training, licensure, inspection, monitoring, sanctions, liability, funding, and reputation that tend to make professional health care more rigid and also to maintain its high standards.

It is too early to tell what will be decided about dealing with suicide risk online, but in the United States, the courts will decided the relevant issues. A Web site owned or led by advertising professionals as scientific advisory board members or consultants needs to be particularly cautious. Referring possibly suicidal visitors to a nonprofessional service can be interpreted as endorsing that service and as making a referral. A defendant's lawyers will certainly mention that a suicide mailing list has clearly posted disclaimers, warnings, and guidelines that members agree to follow as a condition of their participation. This type of defense has not yet been widely tested, however; it may have a significant risk of failure, especially before lay jurors.

Plaintiffs' lawyers have long complained about an alleged conspiracy of silence among health care practitioners that supposedly makes it difficult for plaintiffs to get to the jury—that is, to establish a prima facie case. That may have been true at one time, but it is not true today. Plaintiffs can easily find individuals with credentials a court would accept. These people are prepared, for a suitable fee, to make statements under oath that are wildly different from conventional thinking in their fields. Some of these individuals advertise. Others list themselves with matchmakers who broker deals with lawyers. A few earn contingent fees.

Plaintiffs also should have no difficulty finding champions of ideas that are relatively more responsible. In this climate, experts, real or self-styled, may be prepared to say that an emergency call service, such as 911, does not constitute professional backup. It is an unacceptable risk to assume that all clients who have become seriously suicidal or homicidal will request assistance from a police department or other service. Similarly, posting advice to go to the nearest emergency room does not constitute an adequate backup system.

Being on Call.   When a client is relying for treatment on a professional who is temporarily unavailable, the professional needs to establish an understanding of such unavailability in advance or needs to have on call a colleague with similar or superior qualifications. Although electronic connections enable a professional to be on call in some sense even when traveling or on vacation, it is foolish to become too cavalier about such availability and to neglect picking up messages in a timely way or arranging for a colleague to be available if needed. When away from their main equipment, professionals engaged in online clinical practice should not lower the standards for security. They still need to guard passwords and carefully select communication channels. Professions should not keep passwords to confidential client information in an electronic file where they may be easily retrieved by someone who finds the portable computer inadvertently left in a taxi or an airplane.

Terminating the Professional Relationship.   Professionals face difficult choices when treating individuals with severe personality disorders who need psychotherapeutic services but are accessible only through telecommunication technology. Informing a highly distressed client that he or she is too disordered for remote treatment calls for the utmost therapeutic sensitivity and judgment. In traditional practice, a professional can hospitalize a patient or transfer responsibility for care to a suitably qualified professional. In treatment at a distance, the professional must be prepared to effect such a transfer if the need becomes apparent. When a patient announces a more severe disorder than a practitioner can handle is not the time to tell the patient to find someone who is local.

Terminating a professional relationship is an inevitable and critical part of psychotherapy. Clients can react with a mixture of various degrees of sadness, anger, despair, resignation, relief, joy, and/or pride. They can recapitulate their presenting symptoms, display new ones, act out, reject termination-phase interventions, withdraw, abruptly switch to another professional, or engage in a temporary "flight into health," for example. The crisis of termination can damage treatment or can boost it into success. A temporary bad reaction can offer an opportunity for a major advance in treatment, and a good one can lead to stagnation. Complex as they may be, termination issues are compounded and may be partially obscured or muddled when therapeutic transactions are conducted remotely.

At present, little is known about how remote communication influences various kinds of termination with various categories of clients with various diagnoses. Therefore, the best policy would be, when possible, to have at least one final in-person session. As both a practical matter and a symbolic act, this in-person session can also be an opportunity for the client to return any equipment that has been loaned. From a risk management perspective, professionals should be proactive. When preparing consent documents at the beginning of the relationship, they should ask patients to agree to a final session for termination. Doing so improves the chances that the final session will really occur and provides a measure of defense against claims in the event it does not.

When terminating online clinical practice with a therapeutic group, the leader can have at least one final session with each member individually (Counselman & Weber, 2002). The best procedure may be to have both a final electronic group session to seal off that aspect of the relationship and also final individual in-person sessions. As noted with termination sessions, it may be helpful to make this procedure clear at the outset of the relationship and to seek patient agreement as documented in a written consent.

Termination is not necessarily the end of treatment. It could be a temporary suspension or involve a change of professionals, as when residents in training rotate. If online clinical practice is conducted predominantly by videoconferencing with a local professional present at the client's side, then termination occurs when either the local or the remote professional leaves. Termination can be agreed on because treatment goals have been met or because the client wants to quit. It also can result from the exhaustion of funding; a limitation on authorized treatment; a professional's illness, death, retirement, burnout, or transfer; or a number of other unpredictable life events. No matter what the reason, online clinical practice requires the professional to pay extra attention to the termination of treatment. Legal requirements for terminating these relationships differ from state to state and country to country; in some places, such laws have not been developed.

The psychotechnologies may complicate termination, but they also can ease it. "Final" need not really be final. For example, clients may request follow-up e-mail contact with a professional once the consultation has ended. If such contact is to occur, the professional must discuss the limits of the contact and fully educate the client on emergency procedures. The following example discusses a successful continuation of individual psychotherapy through e-mail:

> Jerry was a 50-year-old accountant who sought treatment for anger management. He had a physically abusive childhood, was in his second marriage, and had grown children.
>
> He experienced himself as nonassertive and unable to stand up for himself in work situations. He felt "threatened a lot when things aren't just right." He complained of flashbacks and dreams about abusive childhood experiences. He was also concerned about the possibility of bringing his pathology into his marital relationship.
>
> Jerry had been in treatment weekly for 2 years when Dr. Reed accepted a 2-year position in another country. In the 9 months leading up to Dr. Reed's departure, the in-person treatment focused on the termination and on the Jerry's anger at feeling abandoned by his therapist. Treatment was officially terminated as if the therapist would not return. Jerry was given a referral list of other therapists for continued treatment, but he declined to look for a new therapist, stating that his therapy was completed.
>
> About a month before the agreed termination date, Jerry requested permission for occasional e-mail contact as a way to "stay in touch." Dr. Reed and Jerry discussed the benefits and liabilities of maintaining such contact with regard to the treatment process as a whole.

After considerable deliberation with colleagues and with Jerry in the remaining sessions, Dr. Reed agreed to allow e-mail contact. They signed an appropriate consent agreement that described circumstances under which Jerry could initiate e-mail contact, how either Jerry or Dr. Reed might terminate it, and topics acceptable for discussion (e.g., progress on issues previously dealt with in therapy). The consent form detailed the specific technology to be used (e-mail and not instant messaging or chat rooms). The form also stated that there should be no expectation of immediate response to e-mail and that Jerry would receive no telephone numbers at which to reach Dr. Reed. The names of other professionals to contact were included in the agreement.

As Dr. Reed reported, "I received the first contact from Jerry approximately 1 month after termination. Contact continued weekly for 2 months and decreased in frequency to approximately once every 2 months thereafter. The content of Jerry's e-mail was predictable. He would write messages to this effect: 'I hope I'm not bothering you, but I know that we talked about assertiveness in our session, and I just want to tell you about an experience I had. . . .' Jerry was an amateur painter, and he sent photographs as e-mail attachments, replicating a process he had started in the in-person therapy, when he would bring in his artwork to discuss what it meant to him.

"My e-mail replies usually took 15 to 20 minutes to compose because I wanted to be deliberate about what I wrote and make sure it would not be misinterpreted. The replies basically consisted of nonjudgmental reflections, affirmation of his emotional reality, and support for his attempts at changing the behavior he had worked on in his therapy.

"My e-mail replies usually followed this format: 'Glad to hear from you. It sounds like you are doing well with. . . . It also sounds like you are having a hard time with. . . . and are running into familiar problems when you try to implement some of the things we talked about in therapy.'

"I generally didn't give advice, and I would close my e-mail with, 'If you feel like writing, write. Take care.' I was intending to say, 'I'm not there in person, but I'm willing to hear you in e-mail, and I'll get back to you when I can.' "

Dr. Reed also reported that he didn't feel impinged on, although he didn't collect any fees from Jerry, "because it felt like follow-up. We had a strong relationship, and I knew that Jerry was looking at my replies as inoculation-like boosters."

Upon Dr. Reed's return, Jerry resumed in-person psychotherapy sessions, albeit at greater intervals. The first few sessions focused on reviewing the e-mails they had exchanged. Jerry expressed great relief at and satisfaction with having been able to communicate with Dr. Reed. He felt the e-mail contact had enabled him to continue progress with the work he had started. In the new sessions, they focused on new goals.

Regarding ethics, Dr. Reed stated, "In the absence of specific ethical guidelines, I focused on keeping Jerry's needs in the foreground when responding to his e-mails. The experience was positive for both me and my client. I can't see any downside, because Jerry made steady gains toward his personal goals in my absence. Jerry was a good candidate for this sort of contact because he was not likely to experience the type of emotional crisis that would require emergency treatment. He had agreed to follow specific procedures if a crisis occured, but he didn't need them. When I returned, he said, 'You not being around made me rely on myself and put to use the learning that came from our therapy.'

"From my perspective, this particular client needed reparenting owing to the extent of his childhood abuse. Allowing him to have access to me by e-mail gave him a chance to check in and make sure that I existed, that I still cared about him, that I hadn't just dropped him. He was still important. I served much as a parent who does not live nearby."

As this vignette shows, there can be therapeutic benefit in permitting repeated posttermination electronic contact. One of the most effective safeguards (where applicable) against the risks inherent in electronic communication is the statute of limitations. Statutes of limitations set time limits for dissatisfied patients to bring claims against their treaters. After that time passes, no claim, however meritorious, can be successfully made.

Details vary from state to state. In some jurisdictions, the statutory time runs from the date of the alleged negligence. In states following the so-called continuing-treatment rule, the clock starts to tick on the date of the last encounter at which the relevant problem was dealt with, whether or not malpractice is alleged to have occurred on that specific date. In most such states, plaintiffs would likely argue that, in the preceding scenario, Dr. Reed's duties to Jerry continued throughout the period they were in e-mail contact and that the statute of limitations did not begin to run until, at the earliest, the date of their last communication. Some judges may accept this argument. The result: a longer limitations period and thus a longer period of time in which the patient can successfully sue the professional.

Guidelines from Related Fields. In addition to looking at research-based ethical guidelines in mental health, the motivated professional can examine other guidelines for related health care fields. The American Medical Association (Winker et al., 2003) guidelines may be relevant to discussions on ethical training for psychotherapists online. Specifically, these guidelines state that physicians obtain a complete medical history and perform a physical examination of the client before prescribing medication over the Internet (American Medical Association, 2003), and arrange for follow-up care when medication with harmful side effects is prescribed. As previously stated in this chapter, not all technology is the same. Also, federal reimbursement is available for conducting diagnostic psychiatric evaluations via videoconferencing in the United States.

Standards of Care

In the United States, state law defines standards of care. Basically, a standard of care relates to the pattern of practice the profession generally accepts as reasonable under the relevant circumstances. Members of the medical community have traditionally determined the standard of care in a particular geographic area by looking at local practice. Over time, some states have replaced local standards with state standards; other states have replaced their own state standards with national standards. Used in a legal context, a standard of care is typically established for a specific situation at a specific time.

Online mental health practice has the potential to change how standards of care are viewed and to accelerate the evolution of national standards.

The impact of the collaborative practice model using two-way real-time video has been demonstrated to significantly change the diagnosis and treatment of problems and the management of patients seeking care (Brown-Connolly, 2001b, p. 37). The impact on outcomes and changes in standards of care will develop over time. The expectation is that collaborative practice would, in appropriate circumstances, tend to improve the quality of care.

Scope of Practice

Like standard of care, *scope of practice* is another predominately legal term. As used in this book, standards does not necessarily mean the same thing as it does in the law of tort. Scope of practice refers to the authorized range of services and activities that a health care professional may offer. In the United States, scope of practice is often considered to have four levels:

1. At the professional level, scope of practice includes services and activities deemed to constitute the practice of a profession. The professional scope of practice is always broader than an individual's scope of practice because no individual member of a profession engages in all the possible professional activities.
2. Because licensing laws and related regulations define scope of practice, activities authorized in one state may not be authorized in another. State definitions of scope of practice are often general or inclusive because they are intended to apply to all members of a profession. Therefore, state law may determine scope of practice only partially. Examples include the extent to which, in a given state, a podiatrist is permitted to practice surgery or a nurse practitioner may be given prescriptive authority.
3. A particular health care system, such as a hospital or a clinic, defines a scope of practice for members of a particular profession employed at the system's facility. Professionals in the same community but not employed in the same system are not bound by the same definitions of scope of practice. For instance, private practitioners in California are not required to report suspected spousal abuse, but agency employees who are mental health practitioners are mandated to report such suspicious.
4. The practitioner's training and competence to provide particular services define that individual's scope of practice. This means that standards of professional conduct (established by professional associations) can overlap legal definitions. In particular, standards of professional conduct require that practitioners engage only in those activities within their boundary of competence. For example, psychologists traditionally are trained in administering projective personality tests; but if a psychologist has not demonstrated competence in administering such tests, it would be outside his or her boundary of competence and therefore outside his or her scope of practice.

Practice and Treatment Guidelines

Most professions and government entities recognize two types of guidelines—those pertaining to professional practice and those pertaining to treatment (practice guidelines and treatment, or clinical, guidelines, respectively). Unlike guidelines, standards are mandatory and are often accompanied by an enforcement mechanism. Guidelines typically outline goals, are aspirational in language, and are based in research. Guidelines usually are not definitive, nor are they intended to take precedence over the judgment of practitioners.

Practice Guidelines. Designed to educate and inform clinicians, practice guidelines are a set of statements that recommend specific professional conduct. They outline issues to be considered in practice, and they suggest goals rather than define specific approaches to treatment. An example is the American Psychological

Association's (2000) *Guidelines for the Treatment of Gay, Lesbian, and Bisexual Clients.* These guidelines offer advice and information for mental health practitioners, but they do not mandate treatment standards for psychotherapy with gay, lesbian, and bisexual people. Practice guidelines are most often directed toward topics of controversy, and they may be useful in risk management, where health care comes into contact with the legal system.

Treatment Guidelines. Also known as *clinical guidelines,* treatment guidelines provide specific recommendations about treatments to be offered to patients. Clinical guidelines apply to specific diagnoses, such as depression and anxiety. Information about accepted treatment guidelines is available from a number of resources, including government agencies, such as the Agency for Health Care Policy and Research (http://www.ahcpr.gov) and the National Guideline Clearinghouse (http://www.guideline.gov/index.asp). The information available from professional associations (for example, see http://www.psych.org/libr_publ/resource.htm) attempts to derive best practices from clinical research and experts and from health care systems, which typically focus on cost containment.

Caution. Both practice and treatment guidelines are systematically developed statements. Their purpose is to help determine which health care services are appropriate. In recent years, a number of health professions have articulated various guidelines for their members. The professions have touted these guidelines as an antidote to the problem of rampant, unjustified malpractice claims. To some extent, these guidelines can protect a practitioner against the excesses of the tort system. A practitioner who can cite a particular provision in his or her own specialty's guidelines and demonstrate that, on the occasion in question, his or her conduct conformed to that standard may have enhanced protection from liability. The virtually limitless variability in human biology, however, means that even the most learned and conscientious guideline drafters could not anticipate every permutation of a particular malady, every possible valid therapeutic approach that might be justified in a given circumstance, and/or every potential risk and benefit of a given course of action. Briefly stated, it is impossible to provide good health care by following a recipe.

Remember, too, that lawyers are adept at manipulating language. The same text that the defendant thinks provides a shield may, in the hands of a skilled advocate (and in the eyes of a lay jury), more nearly resemble a sword. Professionals are advised to temper their enthusiasm for guidelines and recognize the risks inherent in their promulgation.

Nonetheless, psychotherapeutic guidelines should be derived from a sound scientific basis in the literature and should reflect expert consensus and "best practices" for helping persons with behavioral disorders to achieve stability, quality of life, and recovery (National Committee for Quality Assurance, 2000, p. 67). Note that, in contemplation of law, no practitioner need follow "best practices." The test, rather, is reasonable care. Excellent care often exceeds the law's requirements. Because all practitioners are potential defendants, they need to be sure not to impose unreasonable burdens on themselves. At a minimum, practitioners should recognize that plaintiffs need no encouragement to develop theories of liability.

Guidelines and policies regarding the use of telehealth applications are available through professional organizations. Many of these organizations have also published disclaimers pointing out the limitations of guidelines and admonishing readers not to misuse them. Such admonitions, however, may not deter people who earn large incomes attacking health care practitioners. Professional association Web sites with pertinent information include the following:

- The American Medical Association Existing Policy on Quality Telemedicine (http://www.ama-assn.org/meetings/public/annual99/reports/refcomm/rtf/ ref123.rtf).
- The American Psychiatric Association Practice Guidelines (http://www.psych. org/clin_res/prac_guide.cfm).
- The American Psychiatric Nurses Association and the International Society of Psychiatric-Mental Health Nurses Practice Guidelines for Psychiatric–Mental Health Clinical Nursing Practice (http://www.apna.org).

The previously mentioned *Report of the Joint Interdisciplinary Telehealth Standards Working Group* (Milholland & Reed, 1998) provided for the rapid development of both practice and clinical (treatment) guidelines by offering a predictive statement for nearly every topic the report addresses. The American Psychiatric Association (2002) has published a look into the process of guideline development.

Potential Impact of Telehealth. There is no doubt that various groups concerned with telehealth technologies will rapidly develop both practice and treatment guidelines. Practice guidelines can help practitioners use telehealth technologies more effectively, although such guidelines will need to be revised frequently, as these technologies are changing so quickly. The development of guidelines would best be undertaken by the health care professions.

At this time, the empirical and experiential bases necessary to develop guidelines for the psychotechnologies appear to be lacking. In addition, as mentioned earlier in this chapter, treatment guidelines are generally intended to be specific to a particular condition or clinical situation. The health care professions may find it difficult to define guidelines based on the medium or tool rather than on the purpose or condition for which the tool is being used (Milholland & Reed, 1998).

Professionals may wonder whether the lack of promulgation of specific practice and treatment guidelines for telehealth is related to the increased litigation surrounding guidelines in the United States. Perhaps the U.S. legal system has created such a tangled web of requirements that professionals cannot meet them all without the risk of prosecution. It appears that for the time being, in the United States, practitioners who use telehealth technologies will need to rely more on ethical statements than on practice or treatment guidelines. Perhaps professional associations will further delineate appropriate guidelines in countries in which the legal environment is not so daunting.

One way to render guidelines less threatening would be to grade each guideline as to the level of evidence on which it is based and to include the specific references. The American Psychiatric Association has taken this approach in developing some guideline documents. Such guidelines appear more definitively as being evolving suggestions that are subject to update and that can be bypassed when necessary rather than as being hard-and-fast rules. As in all forms of health care, however, professionals need to rely, first, last, and always, on their own clinical judgment.

Professional e-Nomenclature   Before we end the discussion of issues related to propriety, let's reflect on the current tendency to name telehealth-related psychotherapy after gizmos. Perhaps we should consider the unfortunate term *telephone therapy*. This unfortunate term dates back to the first use of telecommunications to deliver psychotherapeutic services. Now, as people respond to their call-waiting, trash their e-mail spam, check their round-the-clock online stock reports, and switch their beepers to vibrate, the nomenclature needs some distinctions.

The media seem to have latched onto the terms *online psychotherapy* and *e-therapy*. *Online psychotherapy* generally refers to e-mail or chat rooms but might also refer to slow videoconferencing through such programs as NetMeeting, faster but one-way video connections such as used by EGetGoing, or two-way video connections as being developed by BeBetter, Inc. As we've been noting, each technology has unique advantages and disadvantages for the practice of psychotherapy. But technology should not be a basis for naming therapies; that's the tail wagging the dog.

Names for forms of psychotherapy should be based on methods derived from theories of psychological change. Hence, the field includes psychoanalytic, Adlerian, Jungian, existential, cognitive-behavioral, transpersonal, and many more schools and approaches. Conflating treatment with technology demeans treatment, trivializes the professional, and abets the public's tendency to deny the reality of psychological disturbance and the fact that it must often be confronted to be alleviated. People blithely talk about laser treatment or liposuction as if these were treatments that could cure everything and didn't involve surgery. A similar dangerous attitude enables people to dose themselves with herbal treatments while taking incompatible medication on the presumption that herbs are not drugs.

Professionals using the psychotechnologies should remember that mental health interventions by necessity involve assessment, diagnosis, patient education and informed consent, collaboration, planning, adherence to specific treatment protocols, monitoring progress, maintaining records, consulting colleagues when necessary, arranging for follow-up and/or aftercare, and so on. They might also remember that such professional interventions are informed by a bio-social-psycho-spiritual perspective, are multimodal, are often multidisciplinary, are contextual, are often multicultural and multilingual, inevitably involve more people than just the patient–therapist dyad even if absolutely everything is kept confidential, already involve at least one psychotechnology, and are always much more complicated than meets the eye. Calling a service *online therapy* or *e-therapy* vastly oversimplifies the reality of the mental health professional's work.

By way of solution, we offer in chapter 2 distinctions related to communication carrier services and communication devices. Let's add a third set of descriptors—namely, treatment approaches. Let's specify the service and the technology separately (Maheu & Gordon, 2000). To avoid the inevitable confusion, professionals might use such terms as *e-mail appointment scheduling, Web-based psychological assessment, computerized, self-directed behavioral programs,* and *e-mail support groups.* Such specific wording indicates both the types of treatment or administrative service and the technologies that deliver them.

Precise nomenclature will be essential if licensed practitioners in the United States hope to clearly define legal and ethical ramifications, given the state of affairs related to guidelines previously described. Such specificity also might help restrict the numbers of people claiming to qualify as experts and perhaps by doing so might encourage the recent and highly commendable efforts of many courts to reign in the "junk" science that plagues the judicial system. Such clarity is also needed because, as the psychotechnologies become more highly specialized in function, they will be combined into single tools, such as the text-equipped cellular telephones described in chapter 5.

We have every reason to believe that respectable media will follow the example of the professions once leadership is adequately demonstrated and supported by professionals who have considered the ramifications of what the professions are creating.

ADMINISTRATIVE STANDARDS

Administrative standards are evolving because of the incorporation of new technologies into clinical workflow. The requirements for practice management do not change, but professionals need new workflow patterns to ensure adequate and confidential documentation and client care. The overall philosophy and set of policies for a clinical information system can have a profound impact on its effectiveness and can determine how its technical and clinical standards will develop. When implementing a clinical information system, even in a small mental health clinic or practice, it is wise to bear in mind that someday, owing to the widespread use of the computer-based patient record (CPR) described in chapter 8, the system will interface with the systems of large entities or even with a national health information system. To further anticipate what such systems will be like, to gain perspective on problems they will pose, and to pick up practical pointers and pinpoint possible pitfalls, the reader should consult *Design and Implementation of Health Information Systems* (Lippeveld, Sauerborn, & Bodart, 2000), published by the World Health Organization.

One way to minimize exposure to risk is to obtain certification from a recognized accrediting body. Until research is more advanced and guidelines have been promulgated, a reasonable option for a practitioner is to rely on formal groups established as accrediting bodies to ascertain the reliability and validity of therapeutic uses of technology and of the information offered through comparatively untested media, such as the Internet. Some grass-roots patient Web sites informally rate mental health professionals online, but long-established accreditation groups have just begun to look at telehealth and e-health.

The following short explanation of accreditation should enable the reader to avoid any confusion about the terms used in this section:

> The accreditation process is, at its core, a risk reduction activity. It begins with the setting of contemporary standards that address important organizational functions and then encourages organizations, through the awarding of accreditation, to comply with these standards.... The operating thesis is that if organizations are doing the "right things right," as reflected in the standards, then errors and adverse outcomes are less likely to happen than if there were no such standards. (O'Leary, 2000, p. 727)

Credentialing is the process by which an organization reviews and evaluates the qualifications of licensed independent practitioners to provide services to clients. Professionals must meet defined educational, licensure, professional standing, and service availability and accessibility criteria that conform to professional standards of quality (National Committee for Quality Assurance, 2000, p. 389). Credentialing is one process reviewed by an accrediting body.

The American Accreditation HealthCare Commission (URAC, at http://www.urac.org), a nonprofit organization, was founded to establish guidelines to promote high-quality care and to preserve patient rights for the health care professions and the managed care industry. Composed of employers, consumers, regulators, and professionals, URAC offers a number of accreditation programs, including:

- Case management organization standards.
- Claims-processing standards.
- Core standards.
- Credential verification organization standards.
- Health call center standards.
- Health plan standards.
- Health provider credentialing standards.
- Health Web site standards. (Mack & Wittel, 2001, p. 7)

URAC and Hi-Ethics are collaborating in the URAC Health Web Site Accreditation program. With input from many professional associations, these groups have developed a system to provide on-site reviews and analyses of Web sites in order to demonstrate compliance with ethical standards designed for consumer-oriented, online health resources (*URAC and Hi-Ethics Collaborate*, 2001). Among a long list of requirements, the most notable URAC guidelines refer to the need for empirical support for claims made on health care Web sites and for the prohibition of dangerous and ineffective products. URAC guidelines purport to hold a Web site owner responsible for enabling health professionals to adhere to ethical principles when delivering service through the site (American Accreditation HealthCare Commission, 2001).

Despite their many laudable goals, accreditation organizations, such as URAC, require large application fees and are being scrutinized for their bias toward organizations with large budgets. The Internet poses an interesting conundrum: some of the largest mental health care sites are low-budget operations, and visitors to one site or another may have difficulty distinguishing a credible site or professional from a fraudulent one. In a world in which many clients do not understand the differences among a psychologist, a psychiatrist, and a counselor, seals of approval from one organization or another may not be as meaningful as could be hoped (Baur & Doering, 2000). From a risk perspective, professionals should also understand that a seal of approval from such an organization, however well respected, means only that, in the organization's opinion, the site is ethically sound. That does not necessarily mean that the site is operating in a manner that is relatively unlikely to give rise to claims. Many online practices of undoubted ethical propriety may nevertheless be legally risky, and many safe practices may be totally ineffective.

Consumers who do not understand the need or lack the desire to thoroughly examine a professional's credentials might type *online therapy* in a search engine simply because they've read or heard those words as the name for psychotherapeutic services delivered online. The names of number of Web sites will appear, some operated by individual practitioners and others by organizations. Still others contain media articles about the topic. To the novice consumer, these Web sites might all appear equally credible. Most people would not realize that anyone can claim to have graduated with honors from the Sorbonne in Paris, and any organization might offer "credentials" to online practitioners or health care Web sites.

Credentialing of health care professionals is a difficult and expensive process if done in a reliable and thorough manner. It is not uncommon to learn of phony doctors and dentists who have fooled hospitals, patients, and sometimes even licensing boards for years before being unmasked. Verifying documents, checking references, scanning public records of license suspension and revocation, and keeping everything up to date are not tasks that a voluntary lay group can accomplish. Judging whether a health care Web site meets a set of carefully crafted quality criteria is easier, but it calls for special skill sets, specialized knowledge, an unusual ability to make judgments, as well as freedom from undue influence.

To an unwitting client or professional, a rating from a consumer-driven credentialing site, such as Metanoia (http://metanoia.org), might appear as credible as a seal of approval from URAC—*but it is not*. Professionals are encouraged to get their stamps of approval from such professionally affiliated credentialing bodies as URAC. Credentialing by grass-roots groups is problematic on the Internet, particularly when they might represent one, two even a few dozen individuals. No matter how frequently a credentialing Web site is cited by the media, professionals ought to take the time to investigate the education, licensing, authority and potential conflicts of interest of any individual or group claiming to credential others on the Internet. Fortunately, simply clicking on the "About us" link available at many such Web sites will reveal the true nature of individuals or group offering credentials on the Internet. Ironically, professionals and consumers alike need to take the extra step of informing themselves about Internet credentialing bodies before investing them with credibility. An environment in which anyone can have an equal presence on a home page tests issues of professional ethics and trust to their fullest.

For practitioners who want to be thorough, URAC and other established credentialing bodies are available for telehealth service delivery. For instance, mental health professionals working within organizations can refer to specific requirements for their particular system of care. For instance, when providing direct clinical services through a managed mental health organization or a hospital system in the United States, standards and guidelines are available from two accreditation organizations in particular—the National Committee for Quality Assurance (http://www.ncqa.org) and the Joint Commission on Accreditation of Healthcare Organizations (http://www.jcaho.org).

The National Committee for Quality Assurance (NCQA) provides standards and guidelines for managed behavioral health organizations (MBHOs). The MBHO standards encompass comprehensive guidelines for the provision of mental health services and credentialing requirements for mental health professionals in health care organizations. Proponents characterize these guidelines as standards that all professionals should meet in order to deserve the public's trust. NCQA is beginning to evaluate issues related to telehealth practice, and it addresses the evaluation of new technologies in guideline section UM 7. A process is required to evaluate new clinical technologies and new applications of existing technologies (National Committee for Quality Assurance, 2000, p. 150). Common sense and professional ethics suggest that standards will eventually expand to include new technologies while maintaining or enhancing clinical care.

The Joint Commission on Accreditation of Healthcare Organizations (JCAHO) amended its selected medical staff standards to include telemedicine:

> In January 2001, the Joint Commission on Accreditation introduced standards for how existing credentialing and privileging requirements are amended to accommodate new telemedicine and telehealth technologies. These JCAHO standards apply to practitioners who provide consultation, diagnosis or treatment to patients via a telemedicine link

between two hospitals or organizations. Although other bodies also accredit hospitals, JCAHO is the largest and most recognized body certifying medical facilities in the United States and is influential worldwide. (American Telemedicine Association, 2001, p. 1)

The telemedicine standard is presented here because of its importance for mental health professionals working in hospital-based systems of care:

Intent of MS.5.16 through MS.5.16.1: Practitioners who diagnose or treat patients via telemedicine link are subject to the credentialing and privileging processes of the organization that receives the telemedicine service.... The medical staff determines which clinical services are appropriately delivered through this medium, according to commonly accepted quality standards. If a telemedicine practitioner prescribes, renders a diagnosis, or otherwise provides clinical treatment to a patient, the telemedicine practitioner is credentialed and privileged through the medical staff mechanisms set forth in MS.5 through MS.5.15.7 by the organization receiving the telemedicine service. An organization may use credentialing information from another Joint Commission accredited facility, so long as the decision to delineate privileges is made at the facility that is receiving the telemedicine service. Consideration of appropriate utilization of telemedicine equipment by the telemedicine practitioner is encompassed in clinical privileging decisions. (Joint Commission on Accreditation of Healthcare Organizations, 2002)

Updating current administrative standards based on changes in law is an ongoing process. For example, many states have passed laws regulating the practice of telepsychology (Koocher & Morray, 2000). All standards regarding medical records would also apply to an electronic medical record, as discussed in chapter 8.

TECHNICAL STANDARDS

Many mental health professionals have misgivings when they consider introducing any form of technology into their behavioral health care practices (Elias, 2001; HealthLeaders, 2001; Imperio, 2000). The most obvious concerns are with the technology itself: Does it function technically without distorting the therapeutic relationship, and does the information transmitted from a remote location allow the clinician to resolve the clinical question?

Technical standards in health care pertain to properties of the equipment, software, and data transfer needed for valid and reliable transmission and reception of health care services, assessments, and tests. The technical standards for the data transfer and networking needed to build an online practice address text-based interactions, other Internet services, videoconferencing, and store-and-forward applications. Here, we present an overview of these standards, as well as sources of continually updated information. As for the degree to which an application of technology may degrade aspects of treatment, much more data must accumulate before mental health professionals can begin to sketch out tentative general standards. For now, professionals must fall back on that ephemeral and indefinable entity, common sense.

Transmission

Standards for telecommunication are set by the International Telecommunications Union (http://www.itu.int/home/index.html) and the Internet Engineering Task Force. These United Nations agencies strive for compatibility in global telecommunication networks and services. The reader is also referred to the *Directory of Health Technology Assessment Organizations Worldwide* (World Health Organization, 1998) and to appendix D, which is a draft proposal developed by the International Bar Association to encourage debate about and eventual agreement on a multilateral treaty to govern and foster cross-border telehealth services.

The technical standards defined by the International Organization for Standardization (ISO; http://www.iso.ch) are documented agreements containing technical specifications or other precise criteria for practitioners to use consistently as rules, guidelines, or definitions of characteristics so that materials, products, processes, and services are fit for their purpose. ISO medical information and information technology application standards for health care technology are used worldwide (International Organization for Standardization, 2001).

When purchasing equipment, practitioners should ask vendors whether the equipment is compliant with applicable standards. Standards relevant to behavioral health care include HL7, which is a messaging service specification for the secure transfer, routing, and packaging of electronic data over the Internet. (http://www.HL7.org),[2] and H.320, which comprises a set of standards commonly used in live, interactive video applications. The International Telecommunications Union (ITU; http://www.itu.int) developed H.320 for narrowband visual telephone systems and terminal equipment typically used for videoconferencing and videophone services. ITU makes the full set of standards available for purchase at http://www.itu.int/itudoc/itu-t/rec/h/h320.html.

Depending on the application chosen for online practice and the type of telecommunication carrier service required, other standards may be relevant. Some explanatory Web sites (e.g., http://www.teamsolutions.co.uk/tsstds.html) clarify these standards for professionals and help them safeguard their investment in equipment. ITU sets additional telecommunication standards intended to ensure worldwide compatibility.

The European Commission's Open Information Interchange (OII; http://www.diffuse.org/oii/en/oii-home.html) provides standards for medical data processing, billing, image transfer, and videoconferencing; the Interchange also identifies when and in what country the standards are used (http://www.diffuse.org/medical.html). The OII Web site also provides a concise listing of formal standards bodies and industry consortia developing standards and specifications for multiple languages.

The National Institute for Science and Technology (NIST; http://www.nist.gov) and the American National Standards Institute (ANSI; http://www.ansi.org) have issued technical standards relevant to professionals setting up telehealth programs in the United States. The Center for Medicare and Medicaid Services (http://cms.hhs.gov) provides links to codes and technical information consistent with its privacy regulations under HIPAA. The American Telemedicine Association (ATA) publishes updates of technical standards that affect telehealth transmissions and provides links to full standards and source documents free of charge at http://www.atmeda.org/news/standards.htm.

---

[2] Several groups of standards for video, audio, and data, respectively, are H.320, G700 and T.120, for videoconferencing; and H.323, G723, and T.120, for Internet conferencing. These standards are used with protocols for real-time transmission and conferencing. These protocols are commonly known by their acronyms: RTP (Real-Time Protocol) and TCP/IP (Transmission Control Protocol/Internet Protocol). Despite its name, the latter protocol is widely used even when the Internet is not being used.

Security

Sensitive information sent or maintained electronically should be accessible to authorized personnel on a need-to-know basis only, and these personnel should exercise discretion in using the information. Security violations occur when computer communications are misdirected, intercepted, or otherwise read by an unauthorized party. A system breakdown or the accessing of data or backups of data by unauthorized users could compromise patient confidentiality (Australian Psychological Society, 1999). Organizations providing services must budget adequate resources to protect the confidentiality of data (Ziglin, 1995).

National governments have adopted various computer security standards. The United States has HIPAA security rules, which have been finalized (Guerin Gue, 2003). Briefly stated, in recognition of the rapid evolution of relevant technology, the security rules do not specify hardware or software to be used. Rather, they call for adoption of a "best-practices" approach. The United States also has a systems security manual for the business partners of the Center for Medicare and Medicaid Services (formerly known as the Health Care Financing Administration). The manual is available at http://www.cms.hhs.gov/manuals/pm_trans/R2SSM.pdf. European standards have also been published. The European Standards Organization, CEN (http://www.centc251.org), has a special committee for medical information processing standards, TC 251. In Germany, the Bundesamt für Sicherheit in der Informationstechnik (http://www.bsi.bund.de) has published a baseline on detailed security measures for commercial computer systems. In the United Kingdom, the British Standards Institute (http://www.bsi.org.uk) published BS 7799, the standard code of practice for information security management (Mathews, 1998).

The European Health and Telematics Association (n.d)(EHTEL) is a European initiative. EHTEL's principal objective is to "encourage the emergence of interoperable healthcare telematic solutions on national and European scales." Among other things, EHTEL is developing a legal framework to foster telehealth services in the EU.

First published in February 1995 and subsequently revised, in May 1999 the European BS 7799 code is used to protect the integrity, availability, and confidentiality of information. Professionals designing online systems to deliver mental health services should refer to this code. The code is in two parts: (a) Practice and (b) Specification for Information Security Management Systems. These parts were transformed into an international standard, ISO/IEC 17799 (http://www.iso.ch/iso/en/ISOOnline.frontpage). This standard is expected to become the reference document for codes of good practice to promote secure and trustworthy e-commerce worldwide.

Encryption. Sensitive information being sent through transmission channels can be encrypted to prevent its being read by unauthorized parties. *Encryption* involves converting data into a form that can be understood only when a special decryption scheme is applied. Encryption programs are important tools for protecting transmitted information.

To see how encryption might fit into the workflow pattern in a mental health practice, consider the following imagined scenario:

In preparation for her telepsychiatry appointment with a patient, Dr. Reilup logs on to the secure network with her private identification number and password. This gives Dr. Reilup limited access to the mental health center computer system. She then enters the patient-specific identification and again a password to access the computer-based medical record for her patient. She reviews the file and makes additions to it. The file is signed electronically and sent via e-mail, automatically encrypted, to the remote clinic. When it arrives at the remote clinic, the file is automatically decrypted, and the content is accessible to the nurse practitioner who will assist in the telemedicine conference later that day. The nurse practitioner enters an identification code and password, reviews the doctor's additions to the patient's psychotherapy notes, and is now ready for the day's appointments.

An encryption process occurs before information is presented to the Internet for transmission, and a decryption process occurs after reception from the Internet. A large organization would probably have an Internet server (or gateway) on its premises, whereas a small organization might have an Internet client (e.g., a browser) and use a server owned and operated by an Internet service provider (Health Care Financing Administration, 1998).

© 2000 RANDY GLASBERGEN.

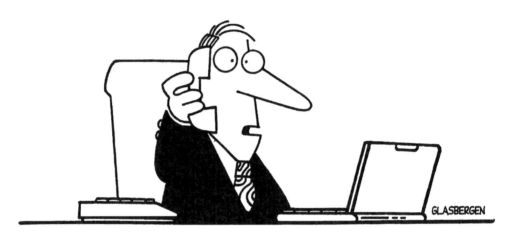

"Information security is becoming a big problem here. Do you still have my Captain Crunch decoder ring, Ma?"

Even sophisticated encryption can be broken by an experienced hacker with sufficient time and resources. Cyberattacks by hackers keep increasing in frequency and effectiveness (Hulme, 2002). Once a code is broken, all messages using it are easily read. Encryption raises an outsider's cost of obtaining privileged information. The expense of breaking a code should exceed the value of the information to the intruder.

Generally, the weakest link in the chain of protection is rarely the encryption method. In general, computer users are surprisingly cavalier about guarding their keys and passwords. Transmission of encrypted material can inadvertently reveal what should be secret: the fact of transmission itself, the frequency of transmissions, and the identity of the sender and recipient may betray damaging information. After all, a person could be stigmatized by another person seeing his or her name on a secretary's appointment roster or hearing him or her being called into a therapy session even if the clinical record itself is inaccessible. A professional's diligent attention to encryption can be undermined if it gives the patient a false sense of security that results in information leaking from another source.

Another important threat to security is negligent abandonment, loss, or theft of a computer or storage medium. When disposing of a used computer, remember that the next owner can read the data on the hard drive. The "delete" operation does not actually erase the data but merely removes a reference to a file. Even if a computer is not operational, the disk drive may function flawlessly when installed in a different computer. If the disk drive has crashed, the data on it can usually be recovered. Mental health professionals should consult computer professionals about rendering unreadable all clinical data that reside on a disk drive they wish to discard. The same is true about floppy disks and removable media: Deletion does not guarantee erasure. People sometimes forget their PDAs in a restaurant or taxi cab, and computer theft is common. In South Africa, roughly 50% of corporate desktops, laptops, and servers are stolen annually (Otten, 2002). This high theft rate underscores the need to keep all sensitive data encrypted.

Mental health professionals should know U.S. government restrictions about sending encrypted messages to international clients. The terrorist attacks of September 11, 2001, have led to a questioning of U.S. policy toward encryption (Podesta, 2001). HIPAA requires encryption of data using various types of transmission channels (as discussed in chapter 9; see also Klein, 2002). The U.S. Departments of State and Commerce enforce laws that may affect the transmission of encrypted messages outside the country's borders. Also, when working with an international client, a professional should review the regulations of the client's country to ensure that no laws are being violated. It will often be prudent in such circumstances to seek advice of counsel–and in some cases to confer with lawyers in the client's country as well as in one's own country.

Passwords. Professionals should store passwords in encrypted password protection software, not only in a document file on their hard drives. Passwords, more recently referred to as passphrases, must be scrupulously protected. They should be nonsensical strings of letters and numbers, not some compound of dictionary words, such as "accessASmith or "accessAJones." Passwords for various clients should not resemble one another, as they do in the example just given. Furthermore, passwords should be completely changed on a regular schedule (probably monthly). The passwords should be relatively convenient to retrieve when needed but not accessible to any but selected authorized personnel, who should be strongly counseled about keeping the passwords secure. It would be wise, if not legally obligatory, to create a disciplinary policy for any employee who fails to maintain password security. Professionals should document their password policy and the date of each password change as proof that they have diligently addressed this aspect of security. Biometric authentication (fingerprint, iris scan, etc.) will probably become the norm for computer security. It is already close to being less expensive to install and operate, and more secure, than a password system, at least in mental health facilities with more than three or four employees.

Virtual Private Networks

HIPAA provides that practitioners are obligated by law to secure "patient records containing individually identifiable health information so that they are not readily available to those who do not need them (Virtual Private Network Consortium, n.d., p. 1)." The act does not specify how these records should be secured, and it leaves this decision to the covered entity.

One popular way to secure and transmit sensitive health care information is through the use of *virtual private networks* (VPNs) (Maheu, 1999). A VPN connects multiple computers over the public Internet, using encryption and other security procedures. The existing public Internet infrastructure is "virtually" turned into a private, secure network. VPNs go beyond simple data encryption to encrypt the addresses of the sending and receiving computers; they also use other sophisticated security techniques.

VPNs offer various levels of security, some of which may not be HIPAA compliant. Professionals should obtain a letter from their VPN vendor certifying that the equipment is HIPAA compliant. Specifically, a professional should look for four security components in a VPN vendor agreement:

1. Encryption: High levels of encryption are used, such as triple 56-bit DES (3DES).
2. Authentication: Digital certificates and two-factor authentication are provided.
3. Audit trail: Data are collected and stored for security audits.
4. Event reporting: Technology is capable of diagnosing and reporting operational irregularities or device failures. (HIPAA Resource Center, n.d.)

Using a VPN to transmit data can be considerably less expensive than building a privately owned network within a company (To protect sensitive data, Microsoft, for example, transmits information internally by using private telecommunication channels not open to public access). The software that enables secure transmission is typically installed on a user's firewall.

Some studies are under way to determine the cost-effectiveness and feasibility of VPNs for behavioral telehealth. For example, the Rural Wisconsin Health Cooperative VPN Feasibility and Design study is looking at the feasibility of implementing VPNs for use in medical applications, including telepsychiatry (Halverson, 2001).

Professionals leave themselves open to risk if they do not adhere to accepted standards. To help the reader manage the potential for such risk, Table 10.1 identifies standards and gives Web addresses for locating pertinent information. Although the list is not comprehensive, it does identify several places to start gathering relevant information. Note, too, that such standards are subject to change as the technology evolves.

When providing direct client services, professionals must use the appropriate standards, whether for transmitting, securing, and documenting clinical data or for submitting electronic bills. Following technical standards alone does not guarantee that the psychotechnologies are used competently. Asking patients suffering from intermittent dementia to use e-mail or videophones to facilitate contact may place an undue burden on them. Although this may be obvious to an onlooker, overly enthusiastic practitioners may be blinded by their excitement about traversing a wide geographic distance electronically. It is the responsibility of the vendor and the health care system to ensure that technical standards meet clinical needs. It is the responsibility of the practitioner, however, to be sufficiently aware of clinical issues that might interfere with the adequate use of the psychotechnologies.

TABLE 10.1
Web Addresses for Risk Management Information

Category	Standard	Official Organization
Diagnostic codes	ICD version 9 & 10 codes	WHO http://www.who.org
Current procedural terminology codes	CPT codes	AMA http://www.ama-assn.org/ama/pub/category/3113.html
Prospective payment (diagnostic-related groups)	DRG	CMS http://cms.hhs.gov
Billing	Multiple code lists HIPAA HCFA	EDI http://www.wpc_edi.com/CodeLists.html
Billing forms	CMS-1500 CMS-1450 (UB92) CMS-1491 CMS-1490S	HCFA http://cms.hhs.gov/providers/edi/edis.asp
Provider classification system	Taxonomy	National Uniform Claim Committee (NUCC) Data Subcommittee http://www.nucc.org
Pharmaceutical/drug code	WHO drug codes	WHO http://www.who.org
Pharmaceutical/drug code	NDC	FDA http://www.fda.gov
Clinical data	SNOMED	College of American Pathologists http://www.snomed.org
Unified language	UML	National Library of Medicine (NLM) http://www.nlm.nih.gov
Modular health knowledge base	Arden Syntax ASTM E1460	Subcommittee E31.15 http://www.astm.org
Electronic security	BS 7799 (ISO17799)	ISO http://www.iso.ch/iso/en/aboutiso/introduction/index.html
Videoconferencing	H.320 and 323	International Telecommunications Union http://www.itu.int/home
e-Message format	HL7	Health Level Seven http://www.hl7.org
Imaging standards	DICOM	ACR-NEMA http://medical.nema.org
Message format for billing information	EDI standards: X12N standard & EDIFACT	DISA http://www.hedic.org
Formats for transmitting clinical data (laboratory)	ASTM E1238	Subcommittee E31.11 http://www.astm.org
Communication between clinical instruments and computer systems	ASTM E1394	Subcommittee E31.14 http://www.astm.org
Neurophysiological data transmission (EEG and EMGs)	ASTM E1467	Subcommittee E31.16 http://www.astm.org
Medical information processing standards	TC 251	CEN http://www.centc251.org

(Continued)

TABLE 10.1
(*Continued*)

Category	Standard	Official Organization
Accreditation standards	Organizational standards for managed care organizations	NCQA http://www.ncqa.org
Accreditation standards	Organizational standards for health care organizations	JCAHO http://www.jcaho.org
Accreditation standards	Organizational standards for health Web sites	URAC http://www.urac.org/

Now that we've reviewed various types of standards and their applicability in telehealth, we turn our attention to a model for risk management. The next three chapters introduce a set of practices we call the OCPM Model. Chapter 11 discusses the first step—professional training. Chapter 12 outlines specific procedures for risk management related to referrals, patient education, and consent. Chapter 13 discusses the heart of the matter—assessment, direct service delivery, and reimbursement.

11

Online Clinical Practice Management (OCPM): Training and Support

Mental health professionals see that innovation through technology is inevitable and can greatly enhance the delivery of mental health care, as well as general health care. With the new wave of technologies being developed for health care, practitioners have many choices to make. Trainees need to know the basics of using a computer and how to use the Internet. They particularly need to know how to use new mental health care tools, adapt existing tools, and avoid problems with procedures and assessment tools used offline. The psychotechnologies offer many new opportunities to those practitioners who use them wisely.

It is tempting to plunge into an online clinical practice—freed of office expenses, rigid office hours, and the obligatory professional garb. Supporters of *online clinical practice*—that is, remote therapeutic conversation with a patient—think that it will allow mental health practitioners to access individuals who need treatment and who are reluctant to initiate or sustain in-person psychotherapy. Venturing into online (e-mail and chat room, telephone, or video) dialogues with patients may provide interesting shortcuts and lead to unexplored areas. Depending on the technology chosen, online dialogues may also provide the convenience of relative anonymity.

As the use of information technology becomes more prevalent, the solo mental health practitioner may unknowingly invite legal woes (Pies, 2002). As described in earlier chapters, there are many online pitfalls. Professionals wary of online clinical practice see (hear) it as a siren song, luring the eager adventurer into peril. They point to the risks to licensed and regulated professionals in working outside the current standards of practice. Even though these doubters believe that exploring new paths is essential to the profession's growth, they think that such exploration should be left to researchers before delivering services to patients. Without institutional review boards considering dangers and setting limits, overzealous clinicians may inadvertently harm their patients and face malpractice lawsuits. The probability of a lawsuit is low when a clinician has a good relationship with a patient, but it may be higher because online clinical practice entails emotional distance and introduces added distortion. Of course, readers outside the highly litigious United States may find the latitude for informal experimentation with patients to be broader.

PROCEEDING WITH MINDFULNESS RATHER THAN WILLFULNESS

Arranging for adequate professional training and support before venturing to treat clients online is sound risk management. For example, such training might elucidate facts such as those related to standards of care. More specifically, such training might make current liabilities more apparent. A lower standard for care has not been established for offering treatment to previously unmet, unseen, and, in some cases, anonymous clients through the Internet. Even if professionals argue that they are taking advantage of new treatment tools in order to serve the unmet needs of a particular client or are delivering e-therapy or are coaching, these standard of care arguments may dissipate when the professionals face an upset parent in court, particularly if the client was a minor who pretended to be of age and subsequently committed suicide. The professionals' defense is likely to be enhanced if they can present documentation to establish that they made reasonable attempts to deliver services according to the applicable standard of care, can establish that they had acquired the level of skill and knowledge possessed by colleagues who are reasonably adept at using the technology, and can point to research showing the efficacy of the technology used.

A solid body of empirical knowledge is needed first, however, before clear, valid, and accepted guidelines can be established in the emerging and complex area of online clinical practice (Nagy, 2001). General risk management suggestions need to be adapted to a clinician's specific services and circumstances (Maheu, Whitten, & Allen, 2001). Each professional should review applicable ethics codes and licensing laws in order to identify at least some aspects of the risk of providing particular services to particular populations through any of the psychotechnologies.

A counterargument to the danger of problems with online clinical practice is the possibility of entering the field too late. Such technology-based practice is quickly evolving in other areas of health care delivery. In general health care, new technology is being adopted at a surprisingly rapid rate. For instance, approximately 58% of California health care organizations surveyed in rural areas indicated that they relied heavily on the use of information technology (IT), 28% reported moderate reliance on IT, and less than 15% reported minimal or no reliance on IT. Thirty-seven percent of health clinics and 33% of hospitals said that they use video teleconferencing applications for patient consultation (Turisco & Metzger, 2003).

As of now, however, the approximately 200,000 practitioners in Canada and the United States have not gravitated to the Internet to deliver services (Maheu & Gordon, 2000). Health care professionals are resistant to change and to outside influence. Their conservatism may be explained and justified in many ways (see Reece, 2003).

Failure to adapt to new treatment approaches and to seize new opportunities may work against the interests of both patients and practitioners in mental health care. For instance, as we discuss in chapter 1, employee assistance programs (EAPs) are ready to fill the void created by licensed professionals' reluctance to adopt new technologies; the EAPs are eager to meet employee and employer demand for remote services delivered via the telecommunication technologies. Some National Health Services and health insurance companies are responding to the pressure of competition by offering mental health care that includes telephonic and e-mail contact with practitioners who agree to work with anonymous clients (Masi & Back-Tamburo, 2001; Masi & Jacobson, 2002).

Many large organizations have existing resources and infrastructure to help them develop, deploy, and support online clinical practice. These resources have enabled these organizations to develop and use centralized administrative control, emergency backup procedures, and referral procedures through such systems as operational telephone call centers. Some organizations are imposing practice standards on their practitioners. These organizations often employ a younger generation of professionals, who are more familiar and comfortable with electronic technology and might be more eager to use technology in their training and work (Carroll, 2003).

The ethics of the mental health professions have always served to protect the vulnerable from the irresponsible. A new array of services provided outside traditional professional boundaries may lack such protection. In addition to the usual clinical considerations involved in any mental health treatment, and aside from modifications of therapeutic techniques that may be necessary in online work, professionals should know how to prepare themselves, their patients, and the setting to conduct online clinical practice prudently and effectively.

To help the reader make well-considered decisions and to minimize the risks associated with psychotechnologies for online clinical practice, we present a clinical practice model originally developed by one of this book's authors as steps to risk management (Maheu, 2001). Here, this model is expanded and referred to as the Online Clinical Practice Management (OCPM) model. The seven steps of the OCPM are:

1. Professional training.
2. Referral.
3. Client education.
4. Consent.
5. Clinical assessment.
6. Direct care.
7. Reimbursement.

This chapter examines the first of the four steps of the preparatory phase. Chapter 12 introduces the three remaining steps of the preparatory phase, and Chapter 13 discusses three aspects of delivering direct care.

DEFINITION OF ONLINE CLINICAL PRACTICE—REVISITED

To expand our earlier definition (see chapter 1), *online clinical practice* encompasses all therapeutic dialogue conducted at a distance, whether over a relatively direct video link (sometimes referred to as *telepsychiatry, telepsychology,* or *telemedicine*) or over a network, such as the Internet or an intranet. Included are psychotherapy, behavioral techniques, making diagnoses—any clinical discussion with a client—as well as supervising a professional or obtaining assistance with a case. Much of this chapter is also relevant to providing professional mental health assistance interactively over electronic channels, including telephones and other audio communications technology. Even though technology as we describe it in chapters 1–8 includes back-office functions, we do not refer to such functions in this discussion of online clinical practice.

Audio technologies are included here because, as discussed in chapter 5, telephones, computers, e-mail, and video capabilities are converging. Just as handheld computers, personal digital assistants (PDAs), and cellular telephones are evolving into newer, more compact devices, telephonic services are becoming more difficult to treat as a stand-alone topic. Even if the telephone were merely a telephone, however, professionals might recognize that many principles of the OCPM also apply. Even though we include text-based applications in our definition of online clinical practice, we encourage professionals to be aware that scientific research, ethical standards, and legal precedent have yet to clearly define an appropriate use for text-based environments with specific groups of mental health patients. Until then, we will remain cautionary when discussing OCPM and the use of e-mail, chat, or other forms of text-only technologies for direct client mental health care.

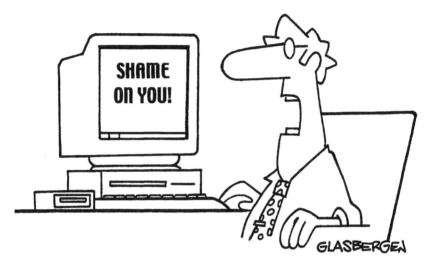

**"You can correct my spelling and grammar,
but my ethics are none of your business!"**

However, sporadic messages that are not part of a course of therapy and automated psychoeducation do not fit our definition of online clinical practice. Clinical dialogue is an essential ingredient in our discussion. Our OCPM territory also includes preliminary discussions in which the potential patient and potential practitioner decide whether to engage in treatment. However equivocal these situations are (with all their attendant rights, privileges, and obligations), we include them if—and only if—a professional relationship is in effect; this condition is still undefined—only a jury could decide it existed.

We believe that text-based telecommunication technology will eventually converge with other forms of technology and will be widely used as a means of treating patients with specific disorders and high literacy levels but will be used less for patients with different disorders or lower literacy levels. Similarly, we believe that combining in-person and distance delivery will soon become routine.

Chapters 11, 12, and 13 offer a conservative model of care. By taking a conservative approach to online clinical practice, professionals are more likely to progress toward expanding their roles while minimizing the risk of harm to people who seek care. Professionals also will be managing their own practice risks.

Our caution is based on the lack of empirical research substantiating anything other than a conservative approach to working with a client population that can at any moment present critical life situations and with an understanding of the

U.S. legal system. Whether in the United States or elsewhere, the ultimate responsibility for using technology with any client rests with the professional (or, in the case of an organization that has hired unlicensed professionals, responsibility rests with the organization). The first step in the OCPM model, then, involves proper training of the professional.

OCPM STEP 1: PROFESSIONAL TRAINING AND SUPPORT

Training is the fundamental prerequisite for delivering responsible medical evaluations and psychotherapeutic clinical practice using psychotechnologies. Training can help professionals wade through licensing laws in relevant states or countries and understand the latest ethical positions adopted by their professional associations.

In general, plaintiffs and regulators will probably succeed in requiring telehealth practitioners to adhere to the same standards that apply to practitioners of traditional health care. For malpractice purposes, state law defines the standard of care. Some states, such as North Carolina, continue to rely on local standards. Others states, such as Virginia, apply state standards. Many states now impose national standards, with which all practitioners of a given specialty in a given jurisdiction are obligated to comply. Improved Internet access will probably encourage movement toward the use of national standards. A special lower standard for care in cyberspace is unlikely to become law in most jurisdictions.

The ultimate challenge for any training program related to the psychotechnologies is to help practitioners determine which technology, if any, is most appropriate for which patient. After this determination, the practitioner should understand when in the treatment the technology is appropriate to use and which practitioner of the treatment team should deliver the care. Specifically, professionals need to know how to:

- Identify special considerations that arise in mental health practice as the result of using technology to communicate with clients or other professionals.
- Select which, if any, psychotechnology to use.
- Match treatment protocols with client needs.
- Decide when and how to optimally offer treatment through one or more psychotechnologies.
- Assess practitioner competence at using each technology.
- Engage in supervision.
- Choose training experiences related to the psychotechnologies.

Trainees need to be exposed to different points of view. Some practitioners support telephone counseling and one- or two-way videoconferencing. Other practitioners support e-mail treatment (Grohol, 1999, 2001). Some practitioners speak from clinical experience and see the importance of adopting technology. All practitioners may want to participate in training programs that discuss the reasonable risks and benefits of using the technology they think most appropriate for the clinical populations they serve. Much research is still needed to guide the practitioner in each of these areas. We next briefly discuss existing dilemmas and topics.

Choice of Technologies

Communicating at a distance requires selecting a primary medium, such as a telephone, text-based environments, or videoconferencing. Each medium has advantages and disadvantages and calls for its own training, techniques, and cautions. In-person psychotherapy within the privacy of the consultation room has a century of experience for support, as well as principles many clinicians take for granted. These principles pertain to the arrangement of furnishings, proper dress, and professional behavior, including not blocking a psychotic client's path to the exit and attempting to provide acoustic isolation to preserve privacy. By contrast, practitioners still have much to learn about practicing through and with any of the psychotechnologies.

Telephonic Technologies. More familiar than the psychotechnologies to both professionals and clients are the telephone, answering machine or service, fax machine, and beeper. Graduate programs usually train professionals to be relatively comfortable with these technologies and confident that they can work around unexpected problems in their use. For instance, professionals are generally taught to develop phone messages giving details of availability and instructions on what to do in the event of a crisis. Professionals are taught to return routine phone calls only during business hours, use beepers after hours, and rely on the predictability of these devices to deliver their intended messages.

Another aspect of training professionals to use telephones is how to use cordless and mobile telephones. Trainees using cordless or mobile telephones with patients need to realize the risks involved. Until cellular, mobile, and other wireless communication devices in the United States become more secure, wireless telephone calls can be intercepted and the client's confidentiality compromised. Many people would be surprised to learn the range of legal eavesdropping activities in the United States (see http://www.MonitoringTimes.com for more information). Practitioners using mobile telephones also should know that analog connections are more susceptible to being heard by eavesdroppers with a scanner. Older cordless phones and cellular phones use analog mode. These types of telephones are also susceptible to eavesdropping when a cell site makes an error in switching the call to another cell site as the user is traveling. Practitioners with multiband mobile telephones should activate the phone's notification feature, which sends a signal that can be both seen and heard when the telephone switches to analog mode. If conducting a psychotherapy session with a patient by telephone when the phone mode switches, tell the patient that the conversation is no longer secure, and arrange to speak another time.

For cordless phones that practitioners use in patient contacts from the home or office, digital or spread-spectrum cordless telephones are more secure; that is, they are more protected from intrusion. Digital mobile phones are generally secure for more confidential mental health purposes. As telephones carry e-mail and Web access, telephone use will become increasingly complicated. For now, let's look at text-based environments from the perspective of the specialized training mental health practitioners will need.

Text-Based Environments. Text-based environments are generally not part of the curriculum in medical or graduate schools. This lack of training has left the pioneering professional to navigate the often murky waters of new interactions that can arise in text-based environments. The following sections suggest two training areas needed in the curriculum—text-based training for professional-to-professional interactions and for professional-to-client interactions.

Text-Based Training for Professional Interactions.   Online discussion forums can spin out of control, even in experienced hands. Many professionals who have experienced online discussion forums can recall rude or inflammatory comments made about another list member, followed by an apparently heartfelt apology, usually accompanied by such statements as "I don't know what I was thinking."

Some professionals have themselves sent such e-mail messages to professional listservs only to be embarrassed and retract their statements with apologies a few hours later. One author recollects:

> *My first experience of witnessing a flame on a professional discussion list occurred one morning as I sleepily read an e-mail from a practitioner discrediting another practitioner by calling him a "drunken bastard," among other things. Several other listserv participants had posted to the thread, reprimanding the practitioner making the accusations for his unprofessional behavior. The practitioner responded to the reprimands by apologizing and explaining that it had been late when he was posting, and he was not sure why he had let himself get so upset.*
>
> *As I reflected on the apology to the listserv members, I marveled at how this same professional had, in a discussion on another professional listserv the week before, detailed his successes in online practice with anonymous patients via e-mail.*

How would the angry practitioner have behaved had he been speaking with patients rather than with a peers in the wee hours or the morning? Would he have behaved more appropriately with clients than with peers? Judging from the rude exchanges evident in early e-mail discussion lists among professional mental health practitioners, one might think that some professionals send e-mail when their judgment is impaired by fatigue, medication, alcohol, and/or outside distractions. All too often, emotional or erroneous messages are sent impulsively or sent to the wrong address. Personal messages still get accidentally directed to a group of professionals rather than to the intended recipient.

In other cases, the subtle nuances of an e-mail message are lost, impressions are extracted, and reactions are sent in rapid-fire succession by subgroups within a larger group. Sometimes, these reactions can be intentionally distorted to discredit a group member. Although not common in professional lists, such behavior does occur, and could be called "text-based guerrilla warfare." For samples of errors in expression, interpretation, posting to the wrong address, and of text-based guerrilla warfare toward identified mental health professionals, readers can study the archives of NetPsy, a professional discussion list founded by one of the authors of this book for discussing the practice of psychotherapy on the Internet. To join the list and access archives, go to http://maelstrom.stjohns.edu/archives/netpsy.html.

In training programs, trainees can learn from the experiences of professionals who have operated in these environments and often learned their lessons the hard way. Trainees also can learn how and why to use and enforce discussion list charters (provided in appendix B). Trainees can be taught how to work with software and programmers to maximize the benefits of developing these powerful discussion forums, already important in mental health care. Obviously, professionals interested in using such environments for communicating with patients should learn both the potential benefits and the pitfalls of text-based interactions so as to maximize the therapeutic efficiency of these applications.

Text-Based Training for Client Interactions. Most clinicians have received no instruction in how to pursue text-based exchanges with clients. For example, in graduate school, clinicians are not taught how and when to respond to e-mail posts, how to diagnose clients in text-based communications, or how to screen clients who might be candidates for using text-based media rather than requiring in-person treatment.

Until research determines which patients will and won't benefit from which information or telecommunication technologies, clinical judgment is the best guide. At the onset of treatment, it may be reasonable to assume that most Internet clients are not markedly impaired by social or emotional problems. However, severe mental disturbance may not be as easily detectable if all professional–client contact occurs in text-based environments. Also, if clients in a particular diagnostic group are difficult to maintain in outpatient treatment, they might also be difficult to maintain in exclusively text-based exchanges.

Until further research disproves this assumption, professionals probably should avoid attempting text-based therapeutic contact with highly reactive and potentially dangerous clients, such as those with disorders in the paranoid and dissociative continuum, with borderline and narcissistic personality disorders, or with recently exacerbated psychoses. It is interesting to note that clinicians working with bipolar and schizophrenic patients report that videoconferencing technologies are quite effective and, in some cases, seem to help patients "tell me what they need" more quickly than they do in-person (C. Zaylor, personal communication, May 23, 2003).

Trainees may need to learn that the effectiveness of text-based communication media depends to a large degree on the user's skill with both the technology and the written word (Clawson, Bostrom, & Anson, 1993). It is often a rude awakening for practitioners to realize that they are deficient in the ability to communicate using a keyboard. For text-based environments, required skills include touch-typing, computer navigation, a good grasp of grammar and spelling, and an understanding of the social conventions used in these newly evolved self-help venues (Stofle, 1997).

Additionally, training in how to use e-mail and chat rooms should cover such topics as the speed with which e-mail tends to be read, especially by a distraught reader; e-mail conventions; and the best ways of dealing with the cognitive distortions common to psychotherapy, combined with the literary distortions typical of e-mail exchanges (Maheu & Subotnik, 2001; Suler, 1998, 2000c). Given the speed of composing and sending e-mail messages and the lack of the typical restraints associated with traditional settings, professionals may make mistakes. Special training with the technology also may be necessary for the practitioner and the client.

As with any clinical communication, the professional should know the client's intelligence and their literacy and educational levels. A clinician may have to deal with a client's inability to write clearly or to comprehend the nuances off the clinician's attempts to express a complicated thought in writing.

A client who is a superb and candid writer, however, could also be shy or beset by a disorder that isn't being seen or addressed. Such a client might have a drug or alcohol dependence, which could remain hidden if the patient isn't seen in person. Even when seen in person, many disorders require acute clinical observational and interview skills to detect.

More subtly, the client could develop unconscious transference to the communication medium, which could interpose an unrecognized layer of complexity between current status and a successful outcome. Training sessions give professionals the opportunity to role-play with each other in training e-mail or chat rooms before delivering service to consumers. One of the authors of this book has developed a free chat room for professionals to use in training. Any reader is welcome to arrange for one or more colleague to meet, follow the instructions, and create a quick chat room interaction at http://telehealth.net/chat/chat_room_agreement.html.

Web Sites. Until security issues are clarified, trainees should be restricted to Web sites with a reputation for protecting visitor information. Experienced trainers should have a list of such Web sites or should be told where to locate them.

Patient Information and Records. In many disciplines, patients are encouraged to communicate with their practitioner or support staff through the clinician's office Web site, to develop and use a private password, and to send e-mail to the clinician. The clinician receives an e-mail notification that a message is waiting. Similarly, when the clinician answers the patient on the Web site, the Web site sends the patient an e-mail saying that a message is waiting. This model is being tested, and, of course, abuses have been reported. Take this situation, for instance:

> In an apparent reversal of its privacy policy, Drkoop.com sold former members' e-mail addresses to an online vitamin company. This sale occurred after an agreement with the Texas attorney general stating that members must give specific authorization for any personal information to be released. (Gilbert, 2002)

Supporters of Drkoop.com note that e-mail addresses are considered a company's asset and thus can be sold to cover bankruptcy. Critics view the sale as a clear violation of privacy. Professionals seeking to expand their practices by working through dot-com companies that offer supposedly secure platforms should verify the security of such Web sites with an outside consultant. The professionals should also ascertain the ownership of e-mail transmitted through a Web site. Does the e-mail belong to the client, the professional, or the Web site owner? Some states specify that a patient's medical record belongs to the patient; others vest ownership in the practitioner. But does this ownership include Web communications? Institutions that train professionals should answer these questions when discussing the risks and benefits of using Web sites in clinical practice and how to best protect both the patient and the practitioner from exploitation online.

A Web site that shares objective information and contains accurate data may not meet the inquirer's need for empathy or support. Some Web sites that provide a lot of exposure to gory detail may overload distressed patients with negative affect when they were seeking comfort. Exposure to new ways to vomit or to cut or burn oneself may be fascinating to the patient who is struggling with binge eating or self-inflected violence. Some patients then may be unable to resist the temptation to read all related e-mail, to seek out Web sites devoted to these topics, and to act out in new and more destructive ways—all while knowing that they should stay away from these Web sites.

Referring to Web Sites. Professionals should be trained to be responsible in referring clients to online support groups or Web sites (Finn & Lavitt, 1994). These Web sites might need to be investigated for content and also for how they are managed (see chapter 12). Even though constant vigilance toward referrals is impossible, the practitioner can help the client gather information by knowing and characterizing the tone and type of information available from various resources (Institute for Healthcare Improvement, 2002; PATH Organization, 2002). Through their professional Web sites (as described in chapter 4), practitioners can also make available population-specific information.

Web Site Company Disclaimers. Practitioners need to be able to decipher the wide range of disclaimers that Web-based companies offer in their contracts. Training programs can outline common traps for clinicians wishing to deliver services through a dot-com company Web site. Specifically, some Web-based companies attempt to disclaim responsibility for anonymous e-mail or chat room services, stating that they don't have the capability to obtain the pertinent information from patients. Practitioners should then ask these companies why they recruit licensed professionals who are bound by the jurisdictional regulations imposed by state licensing boards. Their response is often that services through e-mail and Web sites are not considered psychotherapy but rather are e-therapy, coaching, or advice giving. Critics ask whether these new forms of practice are specifically noted as exceptions in their state definitions of practice.

Malpractice insurance is a related area that warrants close scrutiny. Many professionals do not realize that malpractice insurance typically includes only interactions within a practitioner's state (or geographic area) of licensure. The insurance may not cover practice across state or national borders, regardless of what the service is called. Practitioners might also ask whether their malpractice insurers cover services that are defined as e-therapy, coaching, and/or advice giving- or whether the insurer expressly disclaims such coverage. Practitioners then may want to ask their insurers to issue a written agreement to extend such coverage. Such agreements need to be carefully reviewed; often they contain only vague definitions, and little or no coverage. For example, in a letter, one malpractice insurance carrier agreed to cover any Web-based service that is "comparable to services delivered in a traditional office." This agreement seems to cover services through Web sites, but, as discussed throughout this book, text-based interactions differ significantly from technologies that provide auditory and visual input, and, in the eyes of a jury, both might differ from in-person, office-based services. It therefore might be difficult to convince a plaintiff's attorney that Web site or e-mail contact is the same as in-person service delivery. Professionals who seek to use specific technologies might take the time to specifically outline their services, such as using a Web site, e-mail, videophone, or telephone. They then might ask that the malpractice carrier use the *inquirer's exact description of service* when responding to whether such service will be insured.

Practitioners who sign contracts with Web-based groups serving as intermediaries between practitioners and patients may want to hire legal counsel to carefully review all Web site procedures for contacting new or established patients to determine the disposition of all financial and clinical records over time and to determine whether such records are kept only on a server or in paper form as well.

Lending One's Name to a Web Site. Professionals may also be taught to ask about the credentials of Web site supervisors and other clinicians, to note who on staff is in a decision-making position, and to determine who might be serving as window dressing to entice unsuspecting practitioners or investors. Many Web-based companies compensate well-known clinicians to serve on their advisory boards. Some of these professionals, however, may not understand the issues related to using specific psychotechnologies to contact patients or deliver services. Practitioners may also discuss the importance of verifying the credentials, licensure, and history of these named associates. Practitioners may want to consider whether the people in the Web site's decision-making positions have actually practiced in the real world. Practitioners who lend (or sell) their reputations to a Web-based company should be assured that the company's decision makers have demonstrated minimal competency. The Internet offers everyone the same starting point—a Web site homepage, which can camouflage a lack of proper experience and appropriate licensure.

Videoconferencing.   Practitioners need specialized knowledge to set up and deliver psychotherapy through interactive videoconferencing equipment. They must also be sensitive to the limitations of these communication channels and able to deal with privacy issues and support at the remote location.

Training topics for videoconferencing include how to set up and troubleshoot videoconferencing units, the role of eye contact, and other fundamental aspects of telepresence. As discussed in chapter 5, trainees might be particularly interested in learning about optimal positioning of the camera, the benefits of using distance, and the zoom and freeze-frame features. Trainees need to know how to use lighting and makeup to enhance rather than detract from the professional relationship. Other training topics involve how to teach clients to use video and what to address in the informed-consent agreement, including the establishment of backup procedures in case of an emergency or a technological failure. Distractions, such as sounds, movements, and jewelry, are a relevant topic, as is knowing what to place on an office desk (name card) and on the wall (clock). Receiving training through videoconferencing technology (Rees & Gillam, 2001) enables trainees to understand some of these issues firsthand.

How to prevent technology misuse is important, especially in mental health. Specifics about note taking while in session and how to include a client's family members who might be in the room also need to be addressed. Trainees are often relieved to learn that straightforward online clinical practice with adequate backup is more similar to in-person psychotherapy than they had imagined.

Supporters of two-way interactive videoconferencing (ITV) posit that it provides the visual and auditory cues described in the American Psychiatric Association's *Diagnostic and Statistical Manual of Mental Disorders* (4th ed.) (DSM IV) as criteria for distinguishing among various types of psychopathology, particularly in the more seriously mentally ill or chemically dependent populations. Clinicians use these criteria largely to diagnose illnesses and to decide on treatment plans. Videoconferencing supporters maintain that it is best for practitioners to use a medium that most closely resembles a community's standard of care, which, in most locales, is in-person treatment.

Steering Clear of Profiteers.   Trainees should be informed of the strengths and weaknesses of each technology. Trainees also need to be able to identify who is to be trusted online and who is to be avoided. Zealots who approach licensed mental health practitioners to participate in the latest online venture might argue that state regulations are out of sync with the realities of today. Even though advocates are needed to advance mental health fields into emerging opportunities, we encourage practitioners to be advocates for regulatory change rather than to put their practices at risk by serving as test cases while corporations make a profit.

The following dialogue occurred between one of this book's authors and a Web-based company founder before the NASDAQ crash of 2000. Details have been changed to disguise the identity of the Web-based company. Please note: Web-based companies now usually have much smaller budgets.

E-COUNSELING COMPANY FOUNDER: We are interested in hiring you as a consultant to help us develop our online counseling Web site. We have a large number of licensed professionals who will be available by e-mail and telephone from several different states. Providers will be contacted by e-mail to arrange for appointments directly by consumers.

AUTHOR: Do you have a licensed mental health professional on your staff?

FOUNDER: Oh, yes, we have Dr. So-and-so.

AUTHOR: Terrific. Is Dr. So-and-so going to train the other professionals in how to deliver their services exclusively via e-mail and the telephone?

FOUNDER: Well, no. We don't see the need for training—these other professionals are all licensed.

AUTHOR: Yes, they are licensed and probably trained in how to deliver in-person psychotherapy, but that is different from e-mail-, chat-, or telephone-based psychotherapy.

FOUNDER: I don't see the problem. They are licensed, and that covers it.

AUTHOR: Okay, imagine this scenario. Your licensed professional receives an e-mail note from a minor who says she is going to shoot her high school teacher because he has been harassing her. She has received an F in his class, and she can't bear to go home with her report card. She has taken her uncle's hunting rifle and is going to wait in her car until the teacher leaves school tomorrow night. When she has shot him "good and dead," she will shoot herself. What would your licensed professional do? This correspondence could lead to a nightmarish lawsuit for that professional and for you.

FOUNDER: The fact is that we have a $20 million budget. If we spend a million or two defending ourselves in court, it is no big deal. You know, there is no such thing as bad publicity.

A month later, this founder called the author to check into pricing for professional training. When quoted a fee of $2,000 per day, plus expenses, he said he'd check with his board and be back in touch. The next month, the author received an e-mail, saying that the company had refocused its direction and would not be needing training.

Incredible as this story may seem, it is offered to educate trainers and trainees about the need to be aware of profiteers. At best, it might be said that some entrepreneurs might not be aware of the needs or goals of the average mental health practitioner or patient. Both legally and ethically, professionals need to understand the duties and obligations of licensure and professionalism.

Practitioner Competence

Competence requires (a) training that exposes the trainee to the relevant body of scientific literature (on problem etiology, diagnosis, and intervention); (b) service in an appropiate training and treatment program; and (c) supervision over an appropriate period of time. The presence of some subspecialties requires additional supervised work experience and a certifying examination. Competence is necessary to minimize risk and optimize care. The appearance of competence is also necessary to attract and retain clients. To a degree, certification of competence assists in the defense against imputation of wrongdoing or malfeasance or nonfeasance in the face of less than optimum results.

Competence in diagnosing and treating specific client populations using the psychotechnologies, however, is difficult to establish. In court, the plaintiff's counsel often questions, if only implicitly, whether the defendant is competent. With a lack of training programs and a lack of professional association consensus on the specifics of how to mediate communication with clients of various populations, mental health practitioners have difficulty defending against accusations of incompetence when delivering online services to clients. Although online clinical practice is in its infancy and scientific evidence on its use is sparse, the public, as well as professional colleagues and plaintiffs' attorneys, expect professionals to practice with the same expertise in cyberspace as in the office. Indeed, adhering to the basic principles of ethical practice, based on a reasonable adaptation of *primum non nocere*,[1] can still serve as the main ethical goal. "In those emerging areas in which generally recognized standards for preparatory training do not yet exist, psychologists protect clients, students, supervisees, research participants, organizational clients, and others from harm" (American Psychological Association, 2001, p. 9).

With the psychotechnologies, it is important to stay current with developing research, to track the recent experiences of peers, to understand and become adept at using new technology, to refer clients to appropriate online and off-line adjunctive services, and to document efforts to maintain competence. Some professionals successfully use the telephone for follow-up and even for primary therapy without special preparation. However, the novelty, complexity, and unknowns of some psychotechnologies are greater than for the telephone, and they demand specific training. Proving one's expertise by demonstrating competence in e-mail or chat rooms with peers is different from proving one's competence in diagnosing or treating clients in real-time video or text-based environments. Conversing with a relative on a videophone does not demonstrate technological expertise. To use any technology without specific training is similar to delivering treatment without specialized training. Consider this analogy: a practitioner who has identified himself or herself as an alcoholic and has rigorously adhered to the principles of Alcoholics Anonymous, Rational Recovery, and/or any other alcohol treatment model may be experienced, even knowledgeable. This professional is not necessarily considered to be an expert in alcohol treatment, however.

Similarly, psychotherapists who are stepparents, divorced, and/or adoptees may claim to have life experiences that have given them a greater than average perspective on stepparenting, divorce, and/or adoption. However, these psychotherapists are not *ipso facto* considered experts who are competent to deliver mental health services to other stepparents (or divorcés, and/or adoptees).

Practitioners need to know how to make the best use of each technology and also how to remedy the types of problems that might occur when using the technology. They also need guidance in when to use a psychotechnology during a particular treatment protocol with a particular patient. As the body of scientific information develops and as the marketplace demands that professionals familiarize themselves with the psychotechnologies, formal teaching programs are evolving. As we discuss in chapters 6 and 7, even the most rigorously researched and computerized treatment

---

[1] "First, do no harm," though commonly quoted in Latin, is attributed to Hippocrates, the Father of Medicine.

protocols, such as evidence-based treatments, are still being developed and tested, and their use in daily practice is still not at all common. Some protocols remain controversial. Trainees without access to experienced supervision can join associations of practitioners who offer expertise in related fields and hold regular conventions that offer training. A list of such associations appears at the end of the epilogue.

Despite our emphasis on the importance of training, we also need to point out that in this field, as in any other innovative field, there must be pioneers. Certification, as such, is neither necessary nor sufficient for competence. Continuing education related to certification, however, is a growing area in behavioral telehealth. Interested readers are encouraged to visit http://telehealth.net for related information.

Practitioner Isolation. Many state licensing boards require continuing education. One primary reason is to prevent practitioner isolation, which is highly correlated with malpractice complaints. Even though this correlation does not imply causation, licensing boards believe that preventing practitioner isolation is good for professionals. Hence, there often is a limit on the number of home-study types of continuing education classes that practitioners can apply to relicensure requirements.

Most practitioners can assume that general interaction with peers is good. No doubt some mental health professionals who embrace online work will stay isolated and use computers for all communication with the outside world. While immersed in cyberspace, however, even practitioners who remain sociable may fall into a state-dependent set of behaviors and responses that differ from their ordinary practice and from the real world. Paradoxically, one way of broadening a state-dependent perspective is to engage in discussion groups with online peers, who can supply corrective influences to combat the tendency toward eccentricity, grandiosity, and excessively firm opinions characteristic of social isolation.

Online training actually does allow for practitioner interaction and, in fact, might even require interaction as part of online coursework. Innovative distance learning programs could provide the best instructors and also help practitioners from all geographic regions benefit from intellectual, experiential, and perhaps personal interaction with one another through the advanced technologies, including telephone, voice over IP, Web pages, and videoconferencing (Bergvik & Gammon, 1997; Kulik & Kulik, 1991; Lambert, Hedlund, & Vieweg, 1990; McLaren, Ball, Summerfield, Lipsedge, & Watson, 1992). One study found that rural providers were able to treat 72% of their patients after using telemedicine equipment for an educational consult. Normally, 42% of these patients would have been referred to nonlocal practitioners (Turisco & Metzger, 2003).

Cultural Competence. The advent of the Internet, the growth of teleconferencing, and the availability of computer-assisted assessment are enabling mental health professionals to serve an ever-widening array of clients. Professionals have the opportunity to expand their practices and to extend helping hands across the globe.

Following a marked upsurge in suicidal terrorist activities worldwide, several mental health therapists from various parts of the United States asked Dr. Pulier in unsolicited e-mail messages how they might offer individual psychotherapeutic support electronically to one or two people in a distant country. The would-be volunteers spoke only English and had no experience with online clinical practice or any special equipment or software that might be required. Dr. Pulier suggested first joining a discussion group to explore ways to prepare for the undertaking. He also recommended contacting professional organizations in the locality of interest to negotiate where their enthusiasm could best be applied.

The Internet's linguistic and cultural diversity makes cultural competence crucial for the mental health professional online (American Psychological Association, 1997). This diversity derives from the vast geographical scope of the Internet and its penetration into isolated rural and Third World communities. People from many different societies participate in online discussions, including culturally unassimilated immigrants accessing the World Wide Web from low-cost public sites and older retirees using their personal computers to find health information.

Cultural and Religious Differences. Understanding cultural and religious traditions and beliefs and typical family roles and structures is essential when intervening in family discord, for example, or when intervening in collectivist cultures in which family dynamics are central to the self. A temporary move to a shelter for a Judeo-Christian battered wife may seem to be a reasonable measure, but in other cultures, it can be a lethal misstep. In some sects in India, a woman attempting to abandon her husband, their children, and their home can be punished by being gassed and burned, regardless of how often she has been beaten or mistreated. To intervene in such situations, and to make suggestions from a Western perspective, can be damaging and dangerous. Would a practitioner who advised the woman to leave be morally responsible if the woman were killed as a result of advice received through the Internet across international boundaries? It might be difficult to enforce legal sanctions against the sender. Nonetheless, the professional community is likely to hold the treating professional morally and ethically responsible for this woman's death.

How people relate to authority is another complex issue that distinguishes social groups even within a relatively homogeneous local population. Western-trained psychotherapists tend to favor open, free dialogue on a basis of equality. One of the authors' experiences training psychiatric residents, particularly those of non-Western origin, shows that many are reluctant to discuss their own opinions or ask probing questions; they strive to say what they think the professor wants to hear. When dealing at a distance with relatively less educated and sophisticated patients in their home country, a therapist should be aware of being "yessed" by someone who does not understand or accept or who is offended by what the therapist is saying.

As we discuss in more detail later in this chapter, there are both advantages and disadvantages to developing an international register of mental health professionals who have been certified through appropriate qualifying training and examinations. One advantage is that such a registry would enable the matching of clients and professionals to ensure linguistic and cultural compatibility. The availability of culturally competent mental health professionals on the Internet can become an important resource for relief workers entering new disaster areas and can provide valuable backup for professionals in the Third World who are expanding professional mental health services in such locations.

Cultural Competence in Making Referrals. Professionals working through telecommunications would do well to make referrals to competent local professionals wherever possible rather than assuming all responsibility and control themselves. It is helpful, if not essential, to be in contact with consultants or a peer group that, through advice and explanation, could help bridge cultural and ethnic gaps.

For example, a French-speaking Québequois consultant may be useful to a Mayo Clinic pain specialist who is working with a depressed fibromyalgia patient from Montréal, Canada. In Québec, the highly revered "Ramancheurs" practice folk medicine. These informally trained practitioners are sought to cure physical ailments, especially those related to the musculoskeletal system. Their techniques, handed down from elder to apprentice, combine the ritualistic aspects of Catholicism and Native American traditions and use various rituals to support, calm, and soothe patients. A single practitioner can draw a hundred patients in a day. However, their influence is not likely to be discussed with practitioners of Western medicine.

Mental health professionals working remotely with such tightly knit cultural groups need to know about such alternative therapies and how they are used. Whether this learning is best accomplished by interview or by extensive screening tools has yet to be determined. When working remotely, the client's community is important, and a remote practitioner also must learn how to join this community. If the influence of alternative health care practitioners is strong in any particular community, their aid may be enlisted in some circumstances to help with specific aspects of treatment, such as backup or direct intervention. Also, online supervision by a qualified consultant familiar with a client's culture is valuable as backup in traditional mental health practice when encountering other clients from that culture.

Language. For a Brit to hold a telephone conversation with an Aussie can be difficult, but a therapeutic session in a text-based or synchronous video environment between such a pair could be impossible. Familiarity with the colloquial expressions, idioms, and local variations of word usage can make a crucial difference in therapeutic outcome. Nuances of language and dialect can affect the interpretation of even the simplest written phrase.

Assuming that the dialect spoken by the professional will be universally understood is a dangerous error. Misunderstandings also can occur between two people of different ethnic backgrounds residing in the same country or between two individuals from the same culture but speaking different dialects of the same language.

Even with an excellent video connection, many significant "specks of behavior," such as a quick wink or subtle shrug, may be "unphotographable" (Geertz, 1973) and not available for the "thick description" of meaning-within-context necessary to qualify and hence to understand what is being said (Ryle, 1968). Bereft of visual clues in a text-based environment, people are hard-pressed to notice, let alone interpret, what is going on between the lines of a foreign language or an unfamiliar dialect. Of course, even visible gestures, such as maintaining steady eye contact, shaking one's head, or protruding one's tongue, may have conflicting meanings in different cultures. Remember the international incident in 1992, when President George Bush flashed a peace sign to Australians, only to find out later that the hand gesture was similar to that of extending the middle finger in the United States. Making a similar mistake with a mentally ill patient could have devastating effects to the professional–patient relationship.

Extensive use of interpreters may be necessary when a crisis overwhelms local health care resources and draws in remote consultants and practitioners. Translation can markedly distort communication between the remote clinician and local colleagues, informants, and, of course, the patient. People who are willing and able to mediate health care communications are best identified before they are needed, and should be registered when they are actively engaged.

Interpreter training is important. Professionals need to be aware that untrained and inexperienced interpreters of health-related interviews may decide to shield the patient from what they consider unpleasant, unwholesome, unnecessary, and/or shocking communications from the professional and may try to protect the patient's privacy by not translating potentially embarrassing material that the patient provides. The responsibility interpreters feel can be stressful. The interpreters can be physically and emotionally exhausted and be experiencing their own challenges, perhaps in an environment of calamity, social disorganization, and/or physical danger. In traumatic situations, interpreters might be reacting to upsetting revelations, descriptions of suffering, accounts of torture, and other dreadful experiences. Under such adverse circumstances, interpreters may develop what has been termed secondary posttraumatic stress disorder. Use of interpreters may thus create an extra duty of care for the remote therapist (Lipton, Arends, Bastian, Wright, & O'Hara, 2002).

Even excellent translations of or familiarity with a patient's dialect may not bridge profound cognitive differences between cultures. Such variances include different emphases on such values as honor, revenge, tradition, obedience, honesty, wealth, affiliation, and logical consistency and differences in fundamental interpretations of the world and of reality. Beyond these differences, work at the Culture and Cognition Program at the University of Michigan (http://www.lsa.umich.edu/psyc/cultcog/index. html) strongly suggests that various ethnic groups may process sensory information differently (Nisbett, 2003; Nisbett, Peng, Choi, & Norenzayan, 2001). In one study, for example, Japanese subjects shown pictures of aquariums remembered the relationships between the fish and background objects, whereas Americans focused on the fish and seemed not to notice the background (Goode, 2000).

Differences in how people process information can lead to misunderstandings that neither party in a conversation can appreciate even when such discrepancies are pointed out and explained. Therefore, practitioners should develop specific cultural competencies before engaging with remote patients from another ethnic or cultural group, regardless of the technological ability to immediately connect with such patients.

In addition to the practitioners' cultural competence training and exposure described, the clients themselves can help in getting past cultural and ethnic barriers. For informed clients, their consent includes deciding whether to find a more culturally compatible professional and how to handle a mismatch. Screening tools, such as brief acculturation scales, may also help a client select an appropriate practitioner. Although the implications of cultural differences may be extensive and often subtle, even psychotic clients can understand that they have a responsibility to enlighten the professional when necessary. In such a situation, clients need to feel that the professionals are giving permission—are expressing an eagerness to be informed and corrected—rather than that the professionals need to be educated because they are culturally ignorant. This issue becomes more complicated when neither the clients nor the professionals realize that they are operating from different ethnic and cultural perspectives.

Local Events. Local events—the particularities of time and place—can affect the emotional state of faraway clients. Professionals cannot expect their remote clients to reveal all relevant information during a session. Just as this happens in conventional in-person therapy, it is much more likely to occur in therapy at a distance. For example, remote patients might not think to mention a recent cultural celebration that included heavy consumption of alcohol or drugs as a norm. Clients may feel depressed or helpless after a kidnapping, assassination, or drive-by shooting that everyone in their neighborhood knows about, but of which the professional is unaware.

Practitioners also should assess the impact of media on a client's mood if, local television or radio news covered an atrocity in detail. For example, during a therapy session, an Afghan patient struggling with the recent discovery of marital infidelity might not mention a foreign soldier's massacre of wedding guests in Afghanistan.

But this event could be profoundly upsetting to the patient and might intensify the patient's reaction to the discovery.

Clients often do not realize that an event is affecting them or may feel that time is too short to raise a subject or may assume that the remote professionals are aware of what they themselves consider obvious. It is therefore important for a mental health professional to keep abreast of news events in each client's environment and to routinely ask questions in order to learn of local events that might influence the client's mood or outlook.

Lawful Conduct. Future official qualifications for using psychotechnologies with remote populations may include cultural competence, linguistic fluency, and knowledge of local events. Professionals might need to demonstrate skill in counseling and familiarity with therapy models appropriate for the groups they intend to serve and for the telecommunication channels they intend to use. For now, licensed professionals or health care agencies should responsibly recognize and remedy existing limitations of the unlicensed professionals they hire. Demonstration of diligent effort to achieve reasonable levels of competence may prove to be an invaluable defense in a malpractice suit.

Some extant laws await the reckless, or at least hapless, online health professional. It may not even take a treatment mishap to bring a professional before a foreign court or administrative tribunal.

The High Court of Australia (*Dow Jones Company Inc. v. Gutnick*, 2002) held that an allegedly libelous statement published on the *Wall Street Journal*'s U.S. Web site had become subject to Australia's laws on defamation once it was accessed in Australia. The court's lengthy and extensively documented opinion suggests that a health service that is acceptable in the country in which its provider operates may violate the law or be liable for malpractice in other countries and thus may create legal liability in each country in which that health service is accessed or delivered. Under such circumstances, language difficulty may be a minor shortcoming compared with ignorance of another country's legal system.

The Committee on Law and Medicine of the International Bar Association has created what is believed to be the first Draft International Convention on Telemedicine and Telehealth (see appendix D). Although not yet law, this draft is intended to be a model for a treaty or other multilateral legal instrument. Until more progress is made in international law, however, the legal implications of cross-border practice are substantially unknown. As we discuss in this chapter, professionals dealing with foreign clients work best when they avoid ethnocentrism and attempt to understand the clients' cultural norms, local traditions, and religious rituals. Professionals also should try, if feasible, to collaborate with a local professional well versed in such matters. A practitioner working alone and without adequate knowledge of the client's culture may find a dissatisfied client who alleges that the delivery of mental health care was unethical and outside the standard of care (American Psychological Association, 1990).

Although the efficacy of a home page disclaimer has not yet been established, professionals may wish to include a disclaimer on their Web sites, where appropriate, substantially stating:

> The information posted here originates in the United States of America and is intended for use in the United States only. No representation is made or implied that the information is suitable for use in or lawfully available elsewhere. Persons in other jurisdictions are admonished to obey applicable laws and to access this information only if doing so is permissible under the laws pertinent to them.

Technical Competence. Practitioners should understand technical features of psychotechnologies. These features include many of the issues, such as encryption, electronic signatures, audit trails, and storage of electronic records, as they relate to privacy, confidentiality, security, and data integrity (as discussed in chapter 10). For example, knowing how to communicate through the Internet can help deter third parties from secretly recording entire conversations. Unencrypted e-mail can be intercepted by hackers or by curious children and teens who use their parents' computer. Even encrypted e-mail can be accessed by a client's family or friends if they know the client's password system.

As another example, videoconferencing poses the possibility that whoever owns the equipment (a hospital, university, or colleague) may be able to record sessions without the practitioner's knowledge. Videophones may give the client the chance to take snapshots of the clinician and alter them for other use. Videophones may include a feature that allows the client to manually control the remote camera, making it possible for the client to visually scan the clinician's office. This may present a problem if the professional assumes that personal items are out of the camera's frame, but upon scanning can reveal damaging personal or embarrassing information. For instance, some professionals may set up a home studio that appears as a normal office from the professional's camera.

If a professional were unaware of the scan feature on a client's remote videoconferencing unit, the client could potentially see items that could interfere with the effectiveness of the therapist. Other specific technical issues relating to competence with the various types of technology are discussed in previous chapters (see chapters 1–8).

Knowledge of equipment and security features enables professionals to better advise clients of the confidentiality risks and also to protect their own privacy. Trainees should study with trainers who know how to develop HIPAA-compliant vendor agreements that cover technology-related issues, such as how to construct secure Web sites and how to use videoconferencing equipment to protect both their clients and themselves.

Combining Psychotechnologies and Physical Presence. Telemental health care practice is turning toward using a combination of modalities to serve clients rather than relying on only one. In contrast to in-person communication, in which the professional can be resourceful and flexible, each psychotechnology imposes its own rigid limits and must therefore be coordinated with other modalities. In general, online clinical practice will include some concomitant or intermittent in-person involvement as well as some combination of e-mail, telephone, instant messaging, chat room work, psychophysiological monitoring, Web-based homework, and/or other modalities. The following vignette shows how a practitioner can orchestrate technologies to deliver mental health care. Note that the remote psychiatrist delivers services by interactive video, fax, and telephone and also through Dr. Dennery, who was physically present with the client:

> *Our correctional institution began implementing the new wave in medical and mental health care—telehealth. I learned that much of the inmate population would no longer be seen by a flesh-and-bones psychiatrist but by a psychiatrist in a far-away location. I questioned whether this process would be in the best interest of my inmate clients. Years of clinical training had ingrained in me the idea that in-person rapport with our clients was the cornerstone of therapeutic progress.*

I was asked to facilitate the first consultations with our TV psychiatrist, beginning with a group of 15 prison inmates. I'm one who can't even program a VCR, so I was naturally ambivalent about using a sophisticated teleconferencing unit. I was experiencing the largely unfounded initial concerns that had bedeviled users of such new technologies as the television, microwave oven, or the Internet. However, to my delight, after a couple of meetings with a person familiar with the equipment, my comfort level increased, and my technoanxieties dissipated. Equipped with a teleconferencing unit, a fax machine, and a telephone, I was quickly online with a staff psychiatrist at a federal medical center a thousand miles away!

I faxed individualized consult forms on the inmates. These forms detailed their psychological and medical histories. Armed with this information, the contact psychiatrist, in conjunction with the local mental health provider familiar with the cases, conducted real-time diagnostic interviews through the teleconferencing unit and prescribed needed medications. A follow-up consult was conducted if any one at the local level requested psychodiagnostic testing and lab work.

Of the 15 inmate participants, only one refused "to talk to any TV." Not bad, I thought, as some resistance to technology is bound to occur at the outset of its use. The other inmates enjoyed the experience and reported it to be at least as helpful as the traditional in-person contact. After several consults, the inmates were much more stabilized on their psychotropic medications than before.[2] Ultimately, I concluded that such innovative approaches could serve this prison population in a more routine and consistent manner than could in-person consultations. I quickly went from asking "Why?" to "Why not before?" I now see that telehealth serves the best interest of my clients, both clinically and ethically. Guess I'll give programming my VCR a whirl!

—Claude H. Dennery, Psy.D.[3]
Staff Clinical Psychologist
Federal Correctional Institution
Fairton, New Jersey

In addition to the appropriate selection of psychotechnologies, online clinical practice requires choosing appropriate therapeutic protocols for individual clients. Some treatment approaches may be ideal for delivery at a distance, whereas others may require modification or supplementation or may not be suitable.

Selecting Appropriate Psychotechnologies for Client Needs.   Before trying to match a psychotechnology to the needs of a client, professional trainees should be reminded about how to examine professional journal articles for scientific value and should be encouraged to look at secondary sources with the same eye for scientific rigor, while also seeking inspiration for new approaches. Trainees demonstrate their professionalism by using technology-based procedures that have been documented through the scientific literature as being safe and effective wih the client population to be served. Whichever technology professionals choose for direct care, they should critically examine the literature about it. They should understand that this literature consists

[2] This anecdotal report is not proof that medication became more effective; it describes its author's shift in attitude toward online consultation.

[3] The views and opinions expressed in this passage are those of its author only and do not necessarily reflect the policies or opinions of the Federal Bureau of Prisons or the U.S. Department of Justice.

of opinion pieces and reviews as well as empirical research. Most research reports about online clinical practice deal with process rather than outcome, and even outcome reports tend to involve client satisfaction rather than clinical improvement. Even less empirical data exist on mental health outcomes overall than on other forms of health care. Furthermore, especially in a new field such as online clinical practice, a researcher's personal opinions have an above-average potential to influence a study's outcome (Luborsky et al., 1999); therefore, replication of a study should precede conviction, about its validity.

While we await the development of such a scientific literature for to some technologies, it is wise to proceed cautiously and to use technologies with a proven track record. Because the videoconferencing and telephone literatures have been developing for several decades, these technologies are most likely to be the wisest choice for direct patient care when in-person treatment is not feasible. Trainees need to know that long-established professional associations, credentialing agencies, and other bodies have published a fair amount of relevant information. For instance, the Association of State and Provincial Psychology Boards (ASPPB) offers public information about mental health services via the Internet (http://www.asppb.org/exam/default.asp). Hospitals and ambulatory care centers may have policies that are in compliance with Joint Commission on Accreditation of Healthcare Organizations (JCAHO) requirements for remote treatment. Pending training and implementation of HIPAA-compliant technology, for example, routine use of e-mail with psychotherapy clients may be expressly forbidden on the open Internet.

Similarly, just as with formal publications (such as the *Journal of the American Medical Association*) the *Guidelines for Medical Infomation on the Internet* (Winker et al., n.d.), which governs health information found on American Medical Association Web sites, reminds professionals that they must adhere to legal and ethical principles and avoid sharing personally identifiable client information in e-mail discussion groups, chat rooms, and other casual forums.

Ways of relating to clients in person cannot be imported wholesale into cyberspace. An immediate response to a client's verbal or nonverbal communication may have special power in an in-person situation but, because of unavoidable transmission delay, the same response can lose its impact or even reverse its effects in remote treatment. A practitioner's gentle quip that has succeeded numerous itmes in breaking the ice with a client when accompanied by a smile and a shrug in person, for example, may fatally misfire in a text-based exchange, even if qualified by "<grin>." Remarks meant to be humorous can create more problems when writted than when uttered to the client in the clinic. In written form, a witticism lives forever; in verbal form, its life expectancy may be minutes. Online, the client also shares some responsibility for completing a transaction.

Clinical Backup. Clients may decompensate emotionally during psychotherapy, and telecommunication technologies often complicate the detection and remediation of decompensation. A professional therefore should have adequate backup services in place before undertaking the treatment of clients through the newer technologies (Maheu & Gordon, 2000; Reed, McLaughlin, & Milholland, 2000). This chapter has thus far discussed the benefits of obtaining the support of people who can translate language and interpret cultural matters. Support at the local site also should include other emergency clinical backup organized for a particular client or locality. The support needed in an online clinical practice can include various forms of supervision and consultation.

Backup resources might include the community's hospital emergency department, a trusted colleague who practices locally, the patient's primary care provider and/or specialty practitioners, or a family member. When working remotely, the professional must become acquainted with such resources in the patient's community before, not after, therapy begins. For example, in a closed community, a religious leader may be an alternative resource if other people are not trusted or available. In some societies, a tribal chief may serve a similar function. Practitioners also should know of other emergency resources in the client's immediate geographic vicinity, including the police, the fire department, and crisis lines.

Authorization to Release Information forms can be extended to include information related to a remote patient's insurance coverage, hospitals covered by the insurance, and the names and numbers of people to be contacted in the local community for emergencies that may arise during online clinical practice. Potential patients can be asked to research insurance information, facilities, and practitioner names and addresses and to supply the remote practitioner with such information for inclusion in a comprehensive set of release forms.

It is prudent for patients to provide releases in advance of need. Patients are not at significant legal risk when they give practitioners insurance information and contact numbers to use in emergencies if the practitioners then follow proper procedures. For example, under the HIPAA Privacy Protection Rule (U.S. Department of Health and Human Services, 2002) a "covered health care provider may, without prior consent, use or disclose protected health information . . . to carry out treatment, payment, or health care operations: (A) in emergency treatment situations, if the health care provider attempts to obtain such consent as soon as reasonably practicable after the delivery of such treatment. Other federal and state statutes and regulations tend to be consistent with this principle.

The remote practitioner should designate a local physician or, where appropriate, a tribal or religious leader as the person responsible for contacting a client if necessary and for helping the remote professional answer such questions as whether hospitalization is needed or whether family and other support could be recruited. The well-designed backup plan can avoid a patient's complete dependence on the remote professional. Such a plan requires a local person to be able to access at least part of the client's health record or to know key information about the client. Of course, written permission from the client to arrange such a plan and for the remote professional to contact backup personnel is an essential component of initial online arrangements with a client. This permission is closely related to developing an informed-consent agreement (see chapter 12 for elements to include and appendix C for a sample agreement).

Another concern, especially in the United States, is liability exposure. A local tribal or religious leader, on whom the professionals is relying, probably will not be insured and may be judgment-proof. Similarly, the chance of entering into a valid indemnification agreement with this backup person is probably remote. These liability problems will usually not arise if the local contact is a physician, however—at least in the United States.

Allowing a client anonymity—not commonly done in traditional health care—is an attractive marketing advantage, as we discuss in chapter 1. An anonymous employee could contact an EAP almost casually, without feeling entangled or exposed. However, unlicensed practitioners working with anonymous clients may not be able to meet duty-to-warn obligations or to contact the authorities if an emergency arises. Although anonymity may meet the needs of some clients and employees, it doesn't meet the needs of clients being abused—children, spouses, and the elderly, for example.

Companies that provide Web-based mental health services need a system of backup procedures for emergencies to cover locales in which services are offered. Just as telephone hotlines have community directories for backup services in the communities served, so should Web-based mental health services. Representatives from some Web-based mental health services respond by saying that the Internet goes all over the world and that they cannot find a service to provide backup mental health services to the world. This is true. But why take risks with the clients who reveal their innermost thoughts, concerns, and fears? E-mail and chat rooms are not necessarily safe for use with unknown, unseen, and unidentified patients.

When working with a distant caller in crisis, the professional may attempt to transfer care. This can be especially hazardous and difficult, especially if the practitioner does not know that person's identity. Advising the distraught person to call 911 or the police is a common response, but many people who are suicidal or homicidal, including those who present a fully detailed plan in e-mail or a chat room do not want to contact the police. In some cases, a jury may view referring a suicidal or homicidal patient to 911 as malpractice.

Crisis intervention in the United States has historically involved an entire support team, not a solo practitioner. Many suicide telephone hotlines have emergency support systems staffed by paraprofessionals who are supervised by a professional. The staff usually works as a team to contact the police while the crisis worker keeps the caller on the line. The police work in conjunction with the hotline staff members behind the scenes to trace the call, obtain an address, and send a patrol car to the point of origin. When such a team approach is considered traditional and the standard of care for crisis work in many communities, having appropriate local backup—not just a backup plan and not just for emergencies—is an important part of preparation for treatment at a distance.

Supervision. Supervision traditionally involves an interpersonally focused, intensive, one-on-one relationship in which one person is designated to help develop the competence of the other (Loganbill, Hardy, & Delworth, 1982). In traditional in-person supervision, a good supervisor does the following (P. Sussman, personal communication, September 27, 2002):

- Promotes a strong supervisory alliance and secure attachment.
- Creates an atmosphere of safety, understanding, and trust.
- Shows an interest in supervision (shows up for supervision).
- Has more clinical experience than the supervisee.
- Conducts regular therapy in addition to supervision.
- Possesses a breadth of theoretical and technical knowledge.
- Helps decrease the supervisee's performance anxiety.
- Helps normalize the situation and related struggles.
- Shows a benevolent interest in promoting learning and development.
- Helps the supervisee feel safe in exploring and experimenting and promotes nondefensive analysis.
- Teaches at the supervisee's developmental level.

- Allows the supervisee freedom and autonomy.
- Self-discloses and creates an atmosphere of experimentation and allowance of mistakes.
- Knows how and when to use pacing and leading.

Supervision goals include mentoring, training, and teaching principles and techniques while attempting to uncover nuances of style and pattern in order to foster an independent style in the trainee (Laveman, 1994). As yet, not many teachers or supervisors are expert or even very experienced in online clinical practice. Having a benevolent professional oversee one's clinical behavior, however, adds the reassurance, comfort, insight, correction, and courage to change that are necessary when entering a new area of practice. The creativity and guesswork required in online clinical practice leave much room for transference and countertransference error, missed opportunities, performance anxiety, forgetfulness, demoralization, slips, tumbles, and other plagues mental health professionals suffer.

A practitioner should request and obtain a supervisory contract when establishing a formal supervisory relationship. This contract, which is a legal document, should be reviewed by legal counsel to determine its strengths and weaknesses in various states. A sample supervisory contract is found in Sutter, McPherson, and Geeseman (2002). Although this sample contract does not address issues related to conducting supervision through telecommunication technologies, elements from the consent agreement developed for patients can be incorporated into the contract (see appendix C and the discussion of consent in chapter 12). This contract can be especially important when supervision is to take place through a telecommunication technology.

Where local professional societies and academic institutions have not set up a supervision service for online clinical practice and the application of the psychotechnologies, a professional can arrange ongoing supervision with an interested colleague or a group of colleagues. Asking a senior professional to be a supervisor could be illuminating, even if that supervisor has little experience with telehealth. Contracting with a peer, such as for reciprocal supervision, also can be valuable. Online supervision (for both online and in-person therapy) is another option.

Online Supervision. Online supervision raises many of the same questions as does online clinical practice. For example, should online supervision be preceded by the establishment of an in-person relationship so that the supervisor and the supervisee can adjust to each other's skills, styles, strengths, and weaknesses? Boundaries must be as defined as for in-person supervision. In addition, patients should give informed consent to the supervision, and all individually identifiable patient data must be eliminated or disguised to protect the privacy of the patient. Although the goals of supervision are different from those of psychotherapy, the same methodologies may apply. Supervision, whether by an individual or a team, can be enhanced by the following (P. Sussman, personal communication, September 27, 2002):

- Asking questions.
- Ongoing provision of books, articles, papers, and discussion.
- Role playing.
- A two-way mirror, listening device in the ear, or blinking light on the telephone.
- Audio- and videotapes.

- The use of genograms (diagrams of family relationships).
- Having the supervisees develop their own diagnosis and treatment plan templates.
- Positive reframing.
- The use of a case presentation format.

Most of these techniques can be adapted to remote supervision, particularly if videoconferencing is the technology chosen for communication. If e-mail is used, other issues may arise. For instance, the identity of the supervisor is important. If the supervisee has never met the supervisor or has not been introduced in a clinical setting in which credentials have been checked, is the supervisor really who he or she claims to be? Research in this area may help answer this question and others. (Kanz, 2001; Oravec, 2000).

Accordingly, supervisees are advised to check a supervisor's credentials, including licensure. Supervisees can obtain information on credentials by asking for a supervisor's curriculum vitae and by contacting the listed training institutions. Most states also list professional licensees, so checking a state's Web site might be the easiest route to verify a supervisor's licensure. A more difficult task is to verify experience. Asking the supervisor for any publications on the topic or for a list of professional symposia given on the topic may be worthwhile. Checking with references is another avenue. When part of a health care delivery system, national health service, or managed care entity, professionals are protected by credentialing processes that make it easier to identify appropriate supervisors and their respective areas of practice.

Online Group Supervision.   We encourage anything that will add to a professional's accumulation of input from other professionals about treatment, including online group supervision (with full protection of individually identifiable patient information, of course, as mandated by HIPAA). Based on our experience with various types of online group supervision and support experiments, however, we must alert the reader to potential pitfalls. Three experimental groups of professionals participating in outgrowths of the NetPsy discussion list in the late 1990s experienced some of these pitfalls.

The first problem relates to the basis for trusting other members. As discussed, relationships with unmet and anonymous colleagues in e-mail discussion lists may be improved by requiring all members to fully identify themselves, their training, and their credentials. This book repeatedly stresses the benefits of combining electronically mediated transactions with in-person meetings and of bringing in the more humanlike modalities (telephone and video) to make text-based communication more personal.

Professionals participating in electronic discussions are pleased to meet their colleagues in the flesh at annual congresses, such as those of the American Group Psychotherapy Association, the American Psychiatric Association, and the American Psychological Association. Many professionals who have met online arrange personal get-togethers while traveling. One offshoot of such meetings is the discovery of how many assumptions and misconceptions are dispelled when remote correspondents meet each other—a valuable lesson for dealing with clients at a distance.

The truth is that, in online group supervision, a professional may be sharing personal information, including about relationships with clients, or with a supervision group that includes someone who, if met in person, would never be considered a confidant. For example, what if one client is a therapist in training who later graduates and becomes a member of the group and thus is able to access archives of the therapist's supervision? Professionals should get to know a group's members before sharing any information in e-mail that might come back to haunt them.

A second issue of concern is how to discover a breach of the rules, such as the client's spouse peeking at the screen during a supervisory session. A third issue concerns lack of communication. What should a practitioner do when a group member quits the group, breaks off communication, and refuses to respond to inquiries about what happened? What recourse would group members or the supervisee have if a group member misbehaved, left the group, and threatened to publish an account of his or her view of the group's process? A practitioner should have each online supervisor and client provide a telephone number or the name of a third party as a contact in case that person fails to respond to e-mail. Another solution to this problem is to establish and post a set of terms and conditions setting forth behaviors permitted and not permitted. The group could make participation contingent on agreeing to the terms and conditions. This approach would not guarantee compliance with the rules, but it would encourage compliance, and would create a legal remedy for violations.

To what extent will group dynamics (e.g., suspicions, dominance, and favoritism), poorly modulated because of bandwidth constriction, dominate and interfere with supervision of individual cases? Can the online medium adequately convey important nonverbal clues about countertransference, evidence that the supervisee is missing the point of the supervisor's intervention, or evidence that the supervisee is withholding vital information? Which ethical guidelines might apply? Where do responsibilities fall? How would a court of law or a licensing board regard infractions? We have no answers to these important questions but we do encourage research into these areas.

Risk Management

Risk management comes in many forms. In addition to practicing within one's boundaries of competence, practitioners should consider other risk management issues. The risks that professionals need to manage are not limited to their particular professional disciplines. The novelty of conditions on the Internet and the number of people involved could result in various creative legal theories and new opportunities to bring suit. Health care practitioners traditionally have been targeted, in part, because of their assumed deep pockets.

Professionals cannot tell from statutes and regulations what risks might arise but rather must wait for other professionals to be sued, and for lawsuits to be decided and appealed (Alexander, 2000). It is foolhardy to think that this talk about risk management is much ado about nothing. When enforcement of state law does occur, the process can deprive the clinician of basic rights as a citizen and defendant such as the right to call witnesses, or the right to be assumed innocent until proven guilty. The process of defending one self can go on for years (Maheu, 1997a). Moreover, limitations in staffing and other resources in state licensing agencies tend to diminish the frequency and intensity of regulatory supervision.

The best risk management strategy is for practitioners to be prepared to assert a strong defense against a possible suit alleging negligence, practicing beyond the boundaries of competence, and/or failure to obtain informed consent. Especially relevant to the psychotechnologies is the rule that a practitioner maintain a special hard-copy file (not just an electronic record) containing dated documentation that contains the following information:

- Specific training in the technology and treatment modality used.
- Study of the relevant literature.
- Consultation with peers.
- Consultation with legal counsel.
- Opinions requested and obtained from licensing boards, the ethics committee of the appropriate professional association. This may include advice from one's attorney. (First, learn about waiving attorney/client priviledge.)
- Informed consent from clients.

Mental health practitioners who do not have an ongoing relationship with an attorney knowledgeable about legal issues specific to health practice and online clinical practice should urge their professional associations to retain expert legal counsel to develop guidelines and to respond to new questions. Given the volatility and vulnerability of some patients whom mental health practitioners serve, risk management information must be made available to practitioners. This information is vital now, when insurance companies and dot-com companies are offering services through the Internet, sometimes in blatant disregard of standards that have sustained patient confidence for decades.

The following sections focus on data backup, peer consultation, and written inquiries. Professionals should receive some training to become familiar with these topics to help manage their risks. As stated in other sections, documentation of training activities is essential.

Data Backup

Haiku error message: "Three things are certain:/Death, taxes and lost data./Guess which has occurred." (Varon & Rosenau, 1998)

Online clients might not sue for slips and falls or for having their raincoats vanish from the waiting room, but neither office insurance nor malpractice insurance will necessarily compensate for a loss of clinical information caused by a disk crashing, voltage spiking, accidentally pressing the "delete," keys or spilling coffee on a Zip-drive. Professionals who depend on psychotechnologies must back up data regularly and must have procedures for data recovery. Professionals should also scrutinize their existing insurance coverage for gaps and should purchase coverage to fill these gaps. Advice from colleagues or professional organizations may help professionals determine what gaps need to be filled. As for malpractice, just how the boundaries run through cyberspace remains to be gradually and painfully illuminated by case law (Alexander, 1999).

Peer Consultation. Some professionals and clients challenge conventional healthcare by insisting on full disclosure to the patient of the breadth and depth of the practitioner's personal experience with the therapy in question. At present, and in general, there is no legal duty for a practitioner to make such a disclosure, in person or in cyberspace. But given the ready availability and excessively cooperative attitudes of many self-styled experts who are willing to testify in court, it would not be surprising if some of them testified that the standard of care imposes such a duty. Therefore, when a practitioner consults a colleague about a particular approach using technology (whether for a specific client or in general), the practitioner should record the date of the discussion, its content, and the professional credentials or activities that lend credibility to the colleague's response.

Written Inquiries. At present, professional organizations, licensing boards, or malpractice insurance carriers will probably neither approve nor disapprove specific projects, such as individual Web sites or videoconferencing setups. These organizations and companies may make suggestions about disclaimers, privacy statements, or other practice-related documents used on a Web site, or about a specific treatment protocol to be offered through video. A prudent practitioner would compose a letter of inquiry to as many such entities as possible (county, state, and national), describing the technology to be used for each treatment, the intended treatment protocol, and the rationale for delivering the services.

Responses often contain suggestions. The practitioner now has documentation from these entities. This information can help practitioners improve the innovative services to be delivered and can further reduce the risk of a malpractice suit. Such documentation enables practitioners to demonstrate that they tried to determine what a prudent colleague would have done in a similar situation and to establish their attempt to follow the community, state, and national standards of care. Should a disgruntled client file a lawsuit, evidence that the practitioner consulted peers and recognized authorities before delivering services in an innovative area could carry significant weight in the court's decision. Also, professionals may find that the entities contacted through a letter of inquiry have valuable information.

Serving a discipline-wide purpose, another benefit of sending letters of inquiry is that, in the aggregate, they provide tangible evidence that mental health professionals are interested in developing services using technology. Evidence of such interest may lead to the allocation of specially earmarked funds. For instance, professional association funding can lead to the appointment of special task forces and committees to address and educate members about technology-based emerging issues.

The main risk in seeking advice about using a psychotechnology is that the party to whom inquiry is made may condemn the practice. In this case, the practitioner will have generated a potentially troublesome document that could prove discoverable if the practitioner persists in using the psychotechnology and someone alleges that, as a result, he or she has come to harm. Practitioner submitting such an inquiry should be prepared to act on any reasonable recommendation that might be forthcoming.

A professional who decides to make a written inquiry may be wise to have it reviewed by counsel before sending it. Written inquiries may be discoverable. Skilled health professionals who lack legal training might make statements that can later be damaging or that omit language that could be protective. A knowledgeable attorney can help write an appropriate letter that is less likely to create problems and more likely to yield benefits. If the professional is designing a Web site, for example, the letter of inquiry might contain these elements:

- The specific nature of the Web site to be developed.
- Information about the professional that will be posted on the Web site.
- A description of the services to be delivered through the Web site.
- Copies of all disclaimers and consent forms to be disseminated through the Web site.

- Information to be requested of visitors to the Web site.
- Procedures for handling backup and duty-to-warn situations.

An attorney might also make inquiries in a way that maintains the anonymity of the professional (owner of the Web site or videoconferencing setup, for example) and reduces the risk that the responses will be problematic.

Creating legal documents is beyond the interest and training of most mental health professionals. On commercial Web sites, the legal wording of disclaimers, privacy statements, and consent is in a state of flux, as deficiencies and oversights are discovered and wording is improved. Depending on the quality and function of the original and any applicable copyrights it may (or may not) be wise to copy boilerplate language. A lawyer can modify boilerplate to suit the professional's needs. Ask an attorney about these issues. This communication with counsel may be privileged and therefore sheltered from discovery in a lawsuit. Translation of Web site content into another language may call for further inspection by a legal expert with language skills.

As with a Web site, if the professional plans to provide services through videophones to elderly homebound clients, for example, the previous topics should be included in the letter of inquiry and augmented with additional detailed information. This information could include a description of the rationale for videophone-based services; a protocol for how clients will be trained in the use of the technology; which steps will be taken if the connection does not occur, the professional is late, or the phone connection is prematurely terminated; and which types of information will be kept in the client's file. A letter of inquiry should include as much specific information as possible.

Many professional associations, and even county or state associations, make the service of an attorney a membership benefit. Malpractice carriers often do the same for their insureds. Access to such an attorney may be limited in time, but the time is typically renewed every year. Seeking the help of such attorneys can be an inexpensive and effective way to develop and maintain an online clinical practice. These attorneys also tend to be aware of the specialized needs of practitioners who are developing new practice strategies.

Training Opportunities

Training in the psychotechnologies is evolving rapidly; such training has not yet been stabilized or standardized or become a commodity. Types of training are not interchangeable. Trainees should look for unbiased, professional training organizations. Programs offered by established universities or colleges might be the obvious first choice, either campus or distance education programs. These U.S. organizations offer technology-related programs at their national conferences:

- American Association for Behavior Therapy (http://www.aabt.org).
- American Association for Technology in Psychiatry (http://www.techpsych.org).
- American Counseling Association (http://www.counseling.org).
- American Psychiatric Association (http://www.psych.org).
- American Psychological Association (http://www.apa.org).
- American Telemedicine Association (http://www.atmeda.org).

- Association of Telehealth Service Providers (http://www.atsp.org).
- International Society for Telemedicine (http://www.isft.org).

Training in online techniques is also offered at other nontelehealth or Internet-related professional conventions, conferences, congresses, or pre-congress workshops, as well as at smaller, specialized meetings. Consult the conference calendar at http://telehealth.net/calendar for a number of these programs.

Because professional association or university-based telehealth training for mental health professionals is not yet plentiful, private training programs or workshops are a good second choice. An Internet search might turn up interesting options, but serious practitioners should be leery of private Web companies that offer direct clinical care to consumers and that also purport to offer training for professionals. An unspoken agenda of such a company might be to recruit graduates to invest in the company, trade services for equity in the company, or deliver services at a discount for the company through the same Web site. Dual relationships are best avoided whenever possible.

It is essential to investigate the credentials of the trainers. Do they have extensive clinical experience? Have they developed a reputation by presenting their ideas at national or international conventions? Have their ideas been published in respected journals or by respected publishers? Do they have dual relationships, such as holding an undisclosed seat on the board of a company that stands to profit from the mention of that company to their training audiences? Accounts of professionals with dubious motives are beginning to surface (Posen, 2001).

More specifically, are trainers familiar with a range of psychotechnologies? Have trainers established themselves in academic or professional circles as authorities on psychotechnology practice? What types of services, if any, do trainers offer to clients via technology: informational services or direct patient care of any kind? Most important, are the trainers licensed or otherwise credentialed by a respected authority and, if so, where? Are they aware of legal and ethical issues across state and international boundaries and across professions? Of course, anyone can offer training in anything.

Another avenue for learning about the use of specific technologies is to seek references from equipment vendors. They can often provide reliable information about the functionality and performance of their products, including the names and addresses of respected professionals who have used the products or who have published articles supporting their use. Vendors and the professionals using their products can suggest institutes, Web resources, and keywords to use in searching for criticism of the products in question. A practitioner thinking about using products from a particular vendor should contact unaffiliated professionals before investing time, energy, and funding in a particular brand or type of psychotechnology.

Although telehealth trainers may attempt to fill the gaps left by existing ethical codes, the ultimate responsibility for ethical judgment and behavior rests with the practicing professional and is determined by the ethics boards of professional associations. Trainers can raise issues, questions, and concerns, but they cannot definitively determine whether a professional's practice is ethical.

This chapter has examined the first step in the preparation phase of the OCPM model—professional training, including preparing for emergency backup and risk management. Chapter 12 describes the other preparatory steps: generating referrals electronically, patient education, and obtaining consent. Chapter 13 discusses the three steps in the online clinical practice phase: clinical assessment, care delivery, and reimbursement.

Online Clinical Practice Management (OCPM): Referrals, Client Education, and Consent

Obtaining and giving referrals, training clients for treatment, and obtaining consent are functions that many clinicians might perform without much thought. With each step, however, a little forethought can spare aggravation and possible litigation when the professional relationship is mediated or supplemented with technology. Chapter 11 introduces the OCPM model for online clinical practice and discusses professional training. This chapter discusses options for referrals, the educational needs of clients, and issues related to essential agreements for clinical practice when using various technologies. Chapter 13 focuses on the delivery and reimbursement steps of the model.

OCPM STEP 2: REFERRALS

In psychotherapy and counseling practice, accepting referrals has been primarily by telephone. Referrals are increasingly being controlled by insurance companies, in line with the overall shift in power created by the market forces described in chapter 1. Many insurance companies in the United States ask clients to dial the 800 numbers listed on their insurance cards and request a list of potential practitioners. Some companies refer clients to Web pages that list provider panels searchable by ZIP code and specialty.

As economic pressures force insurance companies to compete for market share, they will follow the trend toward increasing automation in order to lower costs. It is much less expensive for insurance companies to send potential clients to the Internet than to staff telephone lines. Liability for the insurance companies also might decrease when a client selects a practitioner from a long list rather than being assigned to a single professional by a referral or triage specialist.

Insurance companies are not alone in listing professionals on the Internet. Using tools ranging from electronic yellow pages to organizational rosters, many groups are promoting health care professionals. The next section discusses these Internet-based referral systems and provides suggestions for their use.

Directory Web Sites

Directory Web sites develop databases of professional contact information and categorize the information according to specialty, location, or other criteria. Insurance companies, professional associations, private businesses, and private groups support-ing a cause are creating such Web sites. Because many people now use the World Wide Web as a reference library, it is not surprising that practice directories and referral ser-vices appear there. The Web engages clients who may not use other sources. When visitors to an informational behavioral health care Web site read an article about a problem that concerns them, they often are motivated to pursue links to a related directory of professionals.

The following are some directory Web sites not managed by insurance companies. Some of these Web sites list practitioners with telephone numbers and street addresses; other sites offer to connect patients to practitioners directly through e-mail. Some of the sites are owned and maintained by private companies; others are sponsored by professional associations:

- 1-800-therapist (http://www.1-800-therapist.com).
- 4therapy.com (http://www.4therapy.com).
- American Mental Health Alliance (http://www.americanmentalhealth.com).
- Anxiety Disorders Association of America (http://www.adaa.org).
- Athealth (http://www.athealth.com).
- Emindhealth (http://emindhealth.com).
- Find-a-Therapist (http://www.find-a-therapist.com).
- Mental Help Net (http://www.mentalhelp.net).
- Mentalhealthpros (http://www.mentalhealthpros.com).
- Planetpsych.com (http://www.planetpsych.com).
- Psychotherapy Finances (http://www.psyfin.com).
- Websitesfortherapists.com (http://www.Websitesfortherapists.com).

Look for directory Web sites that clearly offer legal and ethical protections for practitioners as well as for clients. Also, consider the legalities of referral directories in general. Health care services that are reimbursed in whole or in part by federal funds (Medicare and Medicaid) are subject to rules that, among other things, prohibit a health care entity from referring to itself. The U.S. government has created safe harbors, however, that permit exceptions to the rules under certain circumstances. Under the law, these services must meet specific standards (U.S. Department of Health and Human Services, 2002).

A professional directory must be organized to be useful. The simplest organiza-tional scheme is to cluster professionals by office location. Web sites most often ask users to enter their ZIP codes (or postal codes); the sites then provide a list of the near-est professionals and estimate the mileage between client and professional. Optimally, a Web site could offer a search feature that allows the visitor to select specific desirable characteristics in a professional and the preferred psychotechnology ("specializes in stress," "fluent in Tagalog," "uses videophone," for example).

Accepting Online Referrals

Professionals should consider their approach before jumping online for free adver-tising. A scan of existing directory Web sites shows that some professionals seem to believe that the best strategies for building their practices are to register with ev-ery available site, to claim the broadest scope of practice, and to provide extensive information and lengthy descriptions wherever possible.

Practitioners can manage risk for professional liability simply by being listed and not embellishing their listing with additional claims. Clinicians who offer anything beyond ordinary care, claim any special skills or techniques, or make any statement interpretable as a guarantee of a good result may find a client asking a court to hold them to what the plaintiff's lawyer will characterize as the implied promise.

Moreover, the statute of limitations for fraud is often longer than that for malpractice, and proving fraud may not require the plaintiff to bring in an expert witness.

The advantages to plaintiffs of fraud claims do not end there. First, the more theories a plaintiff has, the greater the chance that the jury will like at least one of them. Second, the word *fraud* is designed to, and generally does, inflame the jury much more than does the word *negligence*. As a result, the jury may express its anger in the only way it can—by awarding large compensatory damages and sometimes even punitive damages. A sobering thought: Against punitive damages, most professionals have no liability coverage.

Moreover, although in many jurisdictions, tort reform legislation has ameliorated the risk of malpractice to some extent, rarely will such legislation provide any comfort where the theory of recovery is fraud. A legitimate question, then, is whether advertising is appropriate or necessary at all. Plainly, it is legally permissible, and it is constitutionally protected. Whether advertising is wise from a business standpoint or from a risk management perspective is a different question. In all cases, truth in advertising is a necessity.

The following fictional vignette introduces potential problems with text-based communication technology:

As a licensed psychotherapist practicing comfortably in Anytown, USA, you optimistically send your first payment to a respectable mental health professional association offering discounted Web site development services. Proceeding confidently within the confines of your professional association's Web site recommendations, you develop research-based content for your new Web site to match the interests and concerns of your current patients. You accurately represent your skills in your online advertising, and you hire a qualified attorney to double check and tailor the disclaimers provided by your professional association to meet your particular state requirements.

You clearly stipulate on your Web site that you offer "online counseling" but will accept new referrals only from your own state because your license is valid only in your state. You request that residents of other states find practitioners in their own states, and you give them a list of other avenues through which they can seek referrals. You ask new clients to sign a consent form, which they print from your Web site and fax back to you, with a written signature. You send sample Web pages to your licensing board, professional association's ethics board, and malpractice carrier, asking each one to review and comment in writing on your work and also to assure you of compliance with all known ethics and state and federal laws. They do.

You had included your e-mail address at your Web site, so your first potential client contacted you by e-mail. The client asked you a question in e-mail, and you type a succinct yet thorough response for a fee, collected through a secured credit card processing system installed on your Web site. This practice continues, and occasionally you schedule an in-person appointment with a new client obtained through your brochure Web site. All clients contacting you through your professional Web site do so in a secured portion of your site, so that e-mail to or from clients is never sent through the open Internet.

Your confidence in your abilities to handle text-based interactions with clients is increasing. You cut back your in-person office hours by 1 day a week to accommodate the changing nature of your practice.

On your request, your attorney sends you a copy of your state statute defining practice of your profession. From it, you learn that regardless of what you call it, the services you plan to offer fall within the purview of your licensure. You then ask your attorney whether you should relinquish your license before offering such services. You are informed that if you do and offer services that could be construed as psychotherapy, you could be considered as having tried to evade the oversight of your licensing board and could incur harsh judgement if challenged in court. More specifically, in court, on cross-examination, a dismayingly charming and polite plaintiff's attorney could ask you to explain your training, supervision, and experience in the specific area needed by the plaintiff, your client. Several of your colleagues are already boasting of their success with practicing in e-mail, so you push forward and begin offering services online.

One day, you receive an e-mail from a new potential client. It describes one of the following situations:

1. Client A is plagued with thoughts of suffocating her 5-month-old son; "he cries all the time, no matter what I do."

2. Client B "had to teach" her 11-year-old daughter "to stop using vulgarity, by sticking a pin through her tongue," but regrets it. Now her daughter has a serious infection, and Client B is reluctant to bring her to the doctor. She's been reported for child abuse in the past and is afraid that this latest incident might lead to having her daughter removed to foster care, which would only harm the daughter further. Client B is "desperate to protect my daughter" and lives alone with her. She refuses to come in to any professional office and promises to control her anger in the future, but she wants your help.

3. Client C plans to poison his neighbor's dog for "breaking into" his home and killing his cockatoo, Priscilla. This new client claims that "Priscilla has been my best friend since I was 15. I can't stop crying, and I hate that dog and my neighbors." You realize that a telephone number or country and state of residence of the sender is not included. In each of these cases, how do you respond? How would you respond if telephone and residence information had been provided?

How can a practitioner be protected from these types of problems? Working with a professional association or experienced Web site construction group is a good place to start. When looking to directory Web sites for patients, the professional should review the directory Web site's claims. When in doubt, the professional should request written assurances that cover the issues discussed in this section and then show the assurances to knowledgeable legal counsel (see the section in chapter 9 about selection of legal counsel).

Other Types of Referrals.   As we mention briefly in chapter 1, e-counseling companies have had difficulty surviving economic challenges, but some of those companies still stand. Owners of surviving companies have needed to think creatively, to make profit a primary focus, and/or to keep costs to a minimum. Some practitioners sign on to these services to increase their referral pools. Some practitioners report good experiences; others do not.

Some professionals also might not be aware of how they might be compromising their own effectiveness as clinicians. Consider, for example, a Web site offer of gift certificates for professional services. Such a creative and convenient referral approach might also be perceived as coercive and presumptuous by a recipient who isn't seeking treatment. This approach diminishes the professionalism of health care, which over time may tend to erode the self-governance that is the hallmark of the professions.

Many practitioners have worked with clients who sought treatment only to appease someone else. Is this Web offering bringing such coercion to a new level? Who is educating the therapist offering such plans about the complications that might arise from working with multiple members of a family or friendship group and having each intervention, and each thought recorded in text or on video? And who is educating the buyers of these gift certificates of the appropriate boundaries related to sharing a therapist?

The bottom line: Adhering to community standards of practice for accepting new referrals is the wisest approach until legal and ethical precedent has been clearly established for accepting clients via new referral strategies.

Of course, other problems can arise from accepting referrals from Web-based companies. The next section outlines other referral issues that can cause problems for mental health professionals using online directory services that supply a professional's e-mail address to the global public-at-large, either as a listing on a free-standing directory site or as an employee of a third-party corporate service.

When listing oneself in a directory Web site or developing a brochure Web site (discussed in chapter 4), initial contact by e-mail can be precluded by listing only a telephone number as contact information on such Web sites. If an e-mail address is provided on a Web site for other purposes, such as identification of the Web site owner, consider these options:

- Clearly and specifically state that e-mail contact by new patients will not be given a response in e-mail.
- Ask that new clients make contact only by telephone (and either provide your telephone number or ask for theirs).
- If the possibility of engaging that client seems promising and if the prospective client supplies a telephone number, consider returning the contact by telephone.
- Include a specific statement by e-mail addresses on the Web site that informs potential self-referrals about duty-to-warn situations.
- Stick to the stated policy and do not respond to e-mail inquiries for any form of text-based contact from potential clients.

Suggestions for subsequent contact are found in discriptions of the remaining steps of the OCPM model.

Authenticating Client Identity.   With in-person treatment, authenticating a client's true identity usually proceeds satisfactorily on the basis of these factors:

- Common sense.
- The circumstances of the referral.
- Direct observation.
- The payment method.
- Communication with family and the client's previous health care providers.

In online clinical practice, to the extent that these verification tools have been used, the provider is protected (as is the client). People arriving at an office or clinic for mental health care may be reluctant to disclose certain facts, thoughts, or feelings, but unless people are in serious violation of the law or severely paranoid, they usually are forthright about revealing their identities. Once in the presence of a professional, a

client will be inhibited from pretending to be someone else. Even clients with dissociative identity disorder usually present their main selves initially, with alters emerging
as the therapeutic relationship progresses.

As we discuss in chapter 3, it is easy to falsify identity in text-based environments.
The odds of impersonation are much greater in e-mail or chat rooms than in an office.
On e-mail or in chat rooms, the practitioner has only text on a screen to use for
verification. The practitioner cannot asses sex, age, race, general physical appearance,
clothing, and demeanor. Even with videoconferencing, a client whom the practitioner
has never met in person could be misrepresenting any number of attributes, including
name, sex, race, and/or age. Treatment plans based on false information could harm
the client. Blaming the client for such a mishap is unlikely to get the professional out
of legal difficulty.

On the Internet, people are much freer to engage impulsively in treatment. As
contact with the prospective client becomes more anonymous, potential liability for
the practitioner increases, and the client's commitment to the therapy or obligation
to the professional is likely to decrease. Anonymity, or relative anonymity, can tempt
clients to falsify information (Maheu & Subotnik, 2001). Suppose, for example, that a
client who claims to be 25 years old and living in the Canary Islands is actually only 15
and living in Utah. Treating a minor without proper permission and without diligent
investigation of the client's background could be more than problematic in a state in
which one is not licensed.

On the other hand, a group at Georgia Tech (Berman & Bruckman, 2000, 2001)
is studying the results of 2,212 "Turing game" rounds, in which players tried to
spot the imposters answering their questions in a text-based discussion venue (see
http://www.cc.gatech.edu/elc/turing). Detecting imposters was surprising successful. Implications of the research suggest that a traditionally trained practitioner's skill
at detecting and challenging falsified information supplied remotely could be more
accurate than expected. This variable needs further research.

Meanwhile, it may be wise for professionals to ask would-be online clients whether
they are being themselves and are genuinely seeking help for a burdensome problem.
Why have they not obtained local referrals from their primary care physician? Are
there topic areas about which they cannot be frank and open with local practitioners
or with anyone in person?

Anonymity.   In services designed for people to intentionally access paraprofessionals or professionals anonymously, the problems increase. Of the greatest concern to
professionals are companies that encourage the professionals to accept e-mail contact
from unknown, unseen, and undiagnosed patients. Potential clients select a field to
identify their state or country of residence and are given the names of professionals
within that area—even if they reside in Iceland. They then send e-mail or arrange for
chat room sessions with available clinicians.

Although some companies attempt to screen clients by state and country of residence, their sites often lack a reciprocal verification procedure to protect the practitioner. Clinicians may want to determine whether screening is reliable for geographic
location. The clinician may also want to be certain that all referral arrangements protect the practitioner from misrepresentation by minors or other clients who could
become a liability when community standards of care are used to measure one's professionalism in accepting new clients.

A relatively simple but potentially useful measure is for the professional to require
the would-be client to specifically affirm his or her age, address, and other personal

data at the outset, before any clinical information is obtained. A jury hearing the claim of an imposter who deliberately misrepresented his or her identity by some affirmative declaration at the start of the relationship may be more likely to appreciate the defendant's predicament and may be less sympathetic to the dishonest plaintiff.

The legal issue of duty is worth mentioning here. In many litigation contexts, the first substantive question asked is whether the defendant owed a duty to the plaintiff. This question it is not always easy to answer. Good Samaritan cases, for example, can raise thorny questions about what, if any, duty was owed and at what point the duty attached.

Consider an example that applies directly to the use of psychotechnologies. Suppose that a patient, dissatisfied with the services provided anonymously, seeks compensation in tort. In an ordinary malpractice claim, the plaintiff's first burden is to prove that the defendant owed her a duty. When the practitioner and patient (defendant and plaintiff) are anonymous, this would be a challenge. At present, there is little precedent directly on point to elucidate the rights and responsibilities of the parties.

How could this hypothetical plaintiff proceed? Presumably, a patient wishing to bring a claim could not be constrained from identifying himself or herself, so the first identification requirement can easily be met. Second, through the existing tools of discovery, counsel may be able to convince a court to strip the site of anonymity, at least to the extent necessary to identify which provider had interacted with the plaintiff. Even if the defense were successful in maintaining the anonymity of the author of a particular bit of advice, however, the plaintiff might then try to sue the sponsoring organization (and actually might do that anyway). That such a move might lead to poor public policy decisions does not mean that the plaintiff's lawyer will be reluctant to make it.

We repeat—it is generally sound advice for a practitioner never to underestimate the creativity of the plaintiffs' bar.

Direct Observation. Authenticating patient identity is often ignored as a legal or ethical training topic. With expanding use of technology, however, authentication is a growing industry. In fact, authentication is now a regulated area of telehealth service delivery (Maheu, Whitten, & Allen, 2001). As we discuss in the next chapter, mental health care practitioners should insist on an in-person assessment period with patients by a qualified professional before initiating remote care.

The importance of direct observation to establish the patient's identity is another reason for in-person assessment. Critics of this procedure argue that patients may respond better to anonymity. This may be true, but then, who protects the welfare of the clinician when the potentially mentally ill patient can't be identified properly? As telecommunication technologies meld with common clinical practice, practitioners need to require protections from patients, insurance carriers, technology vendors, legislators, and other representatives.

Remote contact, even over high-quality video, is less reliable for establishing someone's identity than are in-person meetings. Direct observation is best accomplished during the initial transactions of intake and assessment. Another option is to have a trusted professional present with the client at the remote site. This professional can also accomplish intake and authentication.

Jealous spouses, competitive coworkers, and other malintentioned people can pretend to be the client in text-based media, for example. The informed-consent agreement can warn the client of this possibility. Once the professionals know who the client truly is, they can use passwords or biometric technology to guard against someone masquerading as the client. Software can impose time-outs that require a user period-ically to resend identifying information. This procedure can thwart an impersonator taking advantage of the user's temporary absence from the computer.

Remote Referrals and Third Parties.   An important service to both the patient and the practitioner in accepting remote referrals is obtaining medical and psychiatric histories from hospitals, physicians, and therapists who have served the client. In fact, failure to contact such information sources can be considered insufficient effort to authenticate the client's identity.

Third parties to remote clinical practice can appear without the clinician's aware-ness or involvement as well. Home- or office-based telephone or videoconferenced sessions can easily take place within earshot of family, friends, or neighbors. Intrud-ers can be secretly in the same room as a patient, unidentified to the practitioner, and threatening to the client. Clinicians would do well to always begin remote sessions by asking whether anyone might be within ear- or eyeshot of the patient.

Establishing the client's identity in a text-based referral is especially important. It is common knowledge that on the Internet, children, teens, college students, and adults regularly feign problems in text-based environments—sometimes for entertainment. It thus is reasonable for practitioners to suspect that the same can happen with people experiencing social or emotional problems, particularly if their identity cannot be established and maintained.

An unknown person may have taken the client's place at the computer during the session for any number of reasons. Using passwords obtained for e-mail contact, person(s) unknown to the client can initiate a session with or without the knowledge and/or participation of the real client. To avoid this problem, practitioners can suggest that a client's passwords be augmented with code words or more elaborate biochem-ical authentication technologies. Clients can be asked to exclude other people from remote sessions unless they first discuss third-party presence with the professional. In all cases, referrals can be accepted with explicit agreements about who will and will not be involved in the remote sessions.

Duty-to-Warn.   In many geographic areas, mental health practitioners have a spe-cific legal obligation, called a duty-to-warn, when a third party is identified as being in danger of serious harm inflicted by a patient. While different jurisdictions may mandate different actions by the clinician in these situations failure to abide by local mandates can lead to dire consequences for all involved. When attempting to engage clients online, then, we suggest the clinician consider the following suggestions.

Before a potential client has a chance to disclose a duty-to-warn situation, it would be prudent to get the client's informed consent to treatment. Professionals may want to make it clear that the consent agreement must be discussed and signed before the referral will be accepted. Inform the client that the first discussion of the consent agreement is just a preliminary getting-to-know-you discussion to see whether a pro-fessional relationship can be established. The professional can also offer alternative resources and list them in a written consent agreement, which can be posted on a Web site for reading before the initial contact.

When discussing the consent form, the professional should tell the client that no information is confidential until a preliminary working agreement is negotiated, that mental health professionals are obliged to report certain matters to the authorities, and that supposedly secure chat rooms lack confidentiality. Encrypted e-mail is now a legal requirement for clinical contact with a health care practitioner. These understandings, of course, must be imparted to the would-be client without threatening a budding therapeutic relationship in an online exchange.

Similarly, professionals could quickly educate the client about any misunderstanding of scope of practice and subspecialization and could point out that a licensed professional must know who the client is and whom to contact in emergencies. The informed-consent agreement could contain names and addresses of the client's emergency contact personnel in the client's local area. Ask the client for telephone numbers of local hotlines and emergency crisis lines to include in the consent agreement. The practitioner who uses these referral forms could make clear that under no circumstance is the client to use the remote service in an emergency.

Duty-to-Warn Hazards to Avoid. At this point, the reader may benefit from anecdotes offered by colleagues who accepted e-mail from referral Web sites and didn't take the precautions outlined here. The following vignettes are composites of true stories reported to the authors:

> *Dr. Delatto registers with an online referral service that allows consumers to select psychotherapists in their states of residence. He receives an e-mail message from a new client whose elderly mother lives with her. The client claims that she "had to punish" her mother last evening for refusing to take her medication. The episode apparently occurred after many nightly arguments with her mother, who had not showered for a week. The client states that she was "disgusted" with her mother and was "unwilling to put up with it anymore." She reportedly "threw mother into the shower, turned on the water, and said, 'Here's some soap. Do something for yourself.'"*
>
> *Her mother's "entire right side is black and blue." The client is worried. She is seeking help to manage her violent feelings toward her mother.*
>
> *The client's note contains sufficient detail to warrant reporting an elder-abuse incident. The dot-com Web site has supplied the client's name, street address, and telephone number as part of the referral process.*

Dr. Delatto fears that reporting this new client could lead to a lawsuit, as he has never met her, has not diagnosed her, and has not developed a therapeutic alliance. On the other hand, Dr. Delatto knows that in his jurisdiction, he is a mandated reporter of abuse and that his failure to report could, if detected, expose him to disciplinary action or even civil liabilities. Also distressing to the doctor is the possibility that the client's mother might continue to experience elder abuse.

> *P. Heinz, LCSW, obtains a referral anonymously from an employee assistance program offering e-mail contact to employees who sign on to a secure intranet site. The EAP work/life service provides Heinz with no demographic information about the client. In their e-mail exchange, the client reveals that she is worried about her alcohol intake and that when she has been drunk, she has, on occasion, physically abused her son. Heinz follows the company's policy of referring the client to the telephone call center. The suspicious client refuses to call the hotline.*

Should Heinz continue e-mail contact and ask the client to contact her the following day—hoping to push through the impasse? Or, should she encourage the uncooperative client to seek private psychotherapy and, if an emergency arises, to call 911? Knowing that the client's child might continue to be abused, how will Heinz feel about the exchange after receding into cyberspace and driving home after a full day's work at the EAP?

In both cases, the well-trained, licensed therapist has an independent sense of professional duty to override corporate attempts to sidestep state laws about reporting elder or child abuse. How can the duty-to-warn situations be screened and at-risk clients be prevented from initiating contact through e-mail? Some professionals think that Web sites should use detailed disclaimers to educate potential patients of duty-to-warn situations, but the efficacy of such disclaimers has not been established. Still, it probably is better to include the disclaimer. Relying on its protection against a malpractice suit however, is unwarranted at this time.

Eventually, case law, or perhaps legislation or regulation, will determine the rights and responsibilities of the participants in duty-to-warn situations when the client–professional introduction occurred through text-based environments. For now, definitions of professional relationship through text-based environments, as well as protections for practitioners dealing with unknown, unseen, undiagnosed, and unassessed mental health patients, have not been formulated.

Referring Clients to Online Resources. When referring clients to a colleague, be sure that the colleague understands and uses online security requirements such as encryption. When asked for a referral to other practitioners, regardless of whether they practice down the street or in Nepal, professionals are vulnerable if they don't either select adequately trained colleagues or admit their inability to make a referral. Standard practice in many areas is to offer a number of referrals and encourage the client to screen them personally.

Many practitioners want to find a few good Web sites for their clients to use. Clinicians may want to examine a broad variety of health and mental health Web sites, discussion forums and/or e-mail discussion lists before encouraging patients to obtain information or support from them.

If this practice takes too much time, consider encouraging patients to look for their own resources on the Net and to proceed at their own risk. (See chapter 3 for information about where to begin). Vulnerable patients, however, can be drawn to information and find themselves unable to disengage. They might spend hours looking at eating-disorder- or self-harm-related Web sites, reading articles or discussions that inspire acting out rather than self-care. These patients might receive e-mail from discussion lists that are poorly managed and might find themselves flooded by distressing e-mail.

Properly selected online resources can provide credible information and also a supportive and nurturing community, available 24 hours a day. For discussion forums, either e-mail or Web site based, look for a code of acceptable behavior. For e-mail discussion lists or forums, these codes are often referred to as Charters or are in files called Frequently Asked Questions, commonly referred to as FAQs. For Web sites, codes of acceptable behavior might be published in the discussion forum itself or found in files known as Terms and Conditions. When accessing a resource offered and managed by mental health professionals or patients, professionals could read the codes and evaluate them for fairness and common sense.

Look for a history of successful operation. A resource that has been around a while is likely to be able to handle the heat of flame wars and other expressions of disgruntled users.

Take a few minutes and subscribe to e-mail discussion forums that might be of use to patients. Be sure to keep the initial files sent by such e-mail lists. These files contain directions for unsubscribing from the mailing list without sending a message to the entire community.

Join only one or two lists per week, in case traffic is heavy and too much e-mail arrives. If traffic is slow, the forum might be retired and responsive only to an occasional inquiry. As messages come in from each list, read a few. Get a sense of who the community leaders might be; they will set the tone for the group. Discussion forums are not problematic if they contain disgruntled members, but how those members are handled will determine the appropriateness of any discussion forum for patient referrals. In particular, look for evidence of inappropriate posts being handled behind the scenes, without upsetting an entire community with expletives, harsh reprimands, and/or ridiculing. If leaders are respectful and responsive, consider using the group for referrals.

When searching, look for material that would help someone understand a disease or illness and that has information to help decide among treatment options or strategies to improve coping ability. WebMDHealth (http://my.webmd.com) lists disease conditions and provides information on its own Web site. Look, too, for evidence of bias or editorial viewpoint. Many sites are sponsored by advocacy groups that subtly or blatantly slant the material in a manner calculated to advance the group's agenda. Noncommercial sites sponsored by consumer specialty societies or developed by amateurs devoted to a particular disorder tend to be more generous in linking to other Web sites.

OCPM STEP 3: PATIENT EDUCATION

The third step in delivering psychotherapeutic consultation through the psychotechnologies is to educate the client about the specific technologies used. Other areas for patient education are security and explaining Web-based information.

Psychotechnology

The professional may need to provide the client with a full explanation and demonstration of the technology to be used. Some clients might be anxious about using technology. They might fear that their incompetence with technology will show or that their privacy might be compromised.

Part of an explanation session might be used to increase a client's comfort with the psychotechnology. A hands-on demonstration of how it works and an explanation of the underlying security of the technology might be needed. During this practice session, the professional or an assistant can explain to the client how to set up the technology, troubleshoot technical problems, use proper techniques while using the technology, and proceed during emergency situations.

Clients are likely to request services outside the scope of judicious professional practice. Clinicians have no obligation to furnish personal information to clients who want to know where they live, or how many cars or children they have. The trained professional knows better than to cater to the client's requests. Setting appropriate boundaries is important.

Similarly, whether a service is offered in person or via any of the psychotechnologies, a licensed professional is responsible for delivering appropriate individualized treatment based on a thorough evaluation, which might include information from external sources. Clients cannot be expected to know how psychotherapy is practiced, and it is the clinicians' duty to inform them of appropriate limits to their services.

Security

Teaching clients about security issues is another important part of client education. Some clients may not be interested in or concerned with the security of their e-mail, telephone, or video-based interactions with a practitioner. Research shows, however, that, when queried directly, most patients are concerned with the risks technology poses to confidential information (California Healthcare Foundation, 1999). When using any form of technology to mediate communication, professionals should warn patients that, despite reasonable efforts to protect confidential information, its security cannot be guaranteed. However, taking this cautious approach will not still offer complete protection from claims leveled against the professional. Risk management efforts cannot do that. This action will decrease the risk of claims, however, and will improve the chances that, if a claim is brought, it can be defended successfully.

Spy Techniques. The client may need to know specific security aspects of the technology. For example, e-mail and cellular telephones are vulnerable to a variety of spy techniques that people can use to intercept confidential communications between the client and the professional. The professional should explain some of these techniques to the client to protect against snooping houseguests, for example. New high-tech gadgets can be used to invade privacy (Stanley & Steinhardt, 2003). A visitor, spouse, or teenager can easily install a device in the client's computer to record and relay information to a third party over the Internet. These devices could transmit e-mail notes composed on the client's computer regardless of encryption. Screen shot software can store everything appearing on a computer monitor display at a given instant. If the client is composing an e-mail message or using a personal computer videoconferencing unit, some images could be captured. Clients can be recorded by their own nanny cams. These small hidden video cameras are usually positioned to record any behavior by children or domestic employees and to supplement the home security system.

In the workplace, the employer has the legal right (and perhaps in some circumstances, the duty) to record and review all e-mail. Employees using the corporate computer network from home should not expect privacy. If a client uses a home computer, there is some possibility that another family member might also have access to the information. As a minimum, practitioners engaged in chat rooms should point out these risks to their clients. Doing so does not guarantee that tort or other claims will not be made, sometimes successfully. Failing to do this, however, greatly increases the chance of both.

The security of computers in clinics, public libraries, and cybercafes is also questionable, unless browsers have been modified to prohibit each user from seeing Web sites visited by the previous users. Some computers can be set up to keep track of all Web sites visited for days, weeks, and even months. (Owners of computers used by children or employees find this to be a convenient feature.) Clients can be taught that all tracking features on the computers they use must be disabled to prevent subsequent users from tracing a previous user's path through cyberspace when the Internet is used.

Internet service providers (ISPs) may store records of communications transmitted through their computers and may be compelled to do so by law. ISPs also may need to access customers' systems to do maintenance. This is another reason that a point-to-point infrastructure is more secure for psychotherapeutic encounters than is a system using a centrally mediated Internet configuration.

Telephones and Videoconferencing Technologies. A client who feels encouraged by a professional to use an unsecured modality may assume that the professional is guaranteeing privacy. Standard telephone lines offer a greater degree of protection against related security problems than does the open Internet. Laws against wiretapping and legal precedent have established telephone communication as acceptably secure for much mental health care. Therefore, many behavioral telehealth professionals prefer to use psychotechnologies operating over telephone lines (and secured Internet connections) rather than the open Internet.

Behavioral telehealth programs have used the telephone-based technology of videophones for almost a decade. As described in chapter 5, videophones provide a point-to-point connection between client and clinician.

The following vignette explains how the use of a videophone can be successfully explained to a client:

> *Jonathan was a 22-year-old enlisted soldier who suffered from chronic pain. We started him on a pain management program by meeting with him in person for our evaluation and having him sign a consent agreement. The intake included a standard screening interview. He showed no signs and reported no history of psychosis, alcohol or drug abuse, being a danger to self or others, suicidal ideation, acting out, or violent assaults. We also discussed the videophonic technology we would be using and described the limits of confidentiality.*
>
> *Because his assignment was in Peru, where telephone lines are not as secure as those in the United States and Canada, we needed to use the Autobahn. The Autobahn is a dedicated Department of Defense phone line with a higher picture quality than is available with commercial lines. Part of Jonathan's treatment would involve weekly sessions with a psychologist. Jonathan would enter data about his condition into an interactive Web page, which is encrypted and scrambled through a secured socket layer.*
>
> *The 8 × 8 videophone is like a phone line. Jonathan was told, "If you trust the phone line system to talk about intimate things with your wife, that same system can be used to do psychotherapy." Jonathan was also informed that other people might be in the room with the psychologist but that he would always be told who was in the room during every session.*
>
> *We scheduled a time each week for pain management or hypnotherapy using the 8 × 8. Once we resolved language communication problems with the operator on the first connection, we were able to get a direct office-to-office connection for five hypnotherapy sessions. The patient's pain symptoms subsided over the 5-week course of treatment. In the 6th week, Jonathan returned home, having completed his military mission. In vivo follow-up indicated that he no longer needed treatment.*
>
> —**Larry C. James, Ph.D., ABPP**
> **Lieutenant Colonel, United States Army**
> **Chair, Department of Psychology**
> **Walter Reed Army Medical Center**

Explaining Web-Based Information

Other client training issues include explaining or interpreting information gathered from the Web into a language appropriate for the client's developmental stage and knowledge base. Clients can become confused by the wording of some Web site content and may need such information explained before taking action. The consent process can address those issues. The next section discusses issues related to obtaining consent, both verbal and written, and to making definite arrangements for treatment.

Web-Based Questionnaires. Web-based questionnaires could be useful in patient education. Much as the *Beck Depression Inventory* can be used repeatedly throughout treatment to educate the patient and to keep all parties aware of depressive thoughts, Web site screening questionnaires can help the patient understand the importance of identifying cultural mores, local events, and other factors that can influence behavior—including depressive thoughts, anxiety reactions, and alcoholic drinking. Of course, as discussed in chapter 6, the development of diagnostic tools is complicated and might be prohibitive. Questionnaires can keep the clinician informed of any important events, such as existing or changing local or environmental circumstances, family situations, or recent violence experienced or witnessed. The use of questionnaires can keep both the patient and the professional aware of how events can influence the client's emotional well-being. Remote patients might be asked to scan checklists of potential influences at the clinician's Web site every few sessions. As also described in chapter 6, branching logic could be used to minimize tedium. Other uses for questionnaires could be to determine whether the client is being treated by other practitioners and to teach the client that coordinating treatment with other professionals is appropriate.

Patient Education Programs. Practitioners who want to develop a client education program for using psychotechnologies and to house that training program on the Web should consider the findings of a related literature review (Riemsma, Taal, Kirwan, & Rasker, 2003). Riemsma et al. classified in-person patient education programs provided in the context of ongoing medical treatment into three broad categories and looked at the effectiveness of each category:

1. Information only: exchange of information via persuasive communication or informative brochures. (If looking online, this Web site gives consumer protection information to mental health patients about selecting online information: (http://helping.apa.org/dotcomsense).
2. Counseling: discussion aimed at giving social support or an opportunity for the patient to explore problems.
3. Behavioral treatment: techniques aimed at behavior change, such as behavioral instructions, skill training, or biofeedback.

Only programs of the last type made a statistically significant difference in disability, patient global assessment, and depression scores. These benefits were small and short-lived, however, even when booster sessions were delivered. To obtain long-term positive effects of one-time client education programs for using the psychotechnologies, practitioners may need to follow the education program quickly with use of the technology for treatment. The short-lived nature of gains resulting from training may also show the importance of continually educating the client through ongoing agreements—the topic of the next OCPM step. Education and the associated expansion of informed consent often are gradual, ongoing processes interwoven into other components of treatment.

OCPM STEP 4: BASIC AGREEMENTS

Having the patient act as a partner rather than as a subject in a health care program is probably the best way to get a thorough assessment, to develop treatment plans, to enhance adherence to the chosen regimen, and to avoid premature termination. Empowering remote patients by encouraging them to use the psychotechnologies involves informed consent, signified by written and verbal agreements.

Informed Consent

Informed consent is a crucial part of providing mental health services (James, 2001). Mental health professionals are expected or required by law to obtain and document informed consent from clients before providing services either in person or via electronic transmission. The use of technology in providing mental health care does not alter the practitioner's general duty to inform. On the contrary, technology use expands the range of issues professionals need to discuss with clients. If a client is to receive treatment via a telecommunication technology, the practitioner should include in the consent agreement the limitations of treatment by means of this technology as well as all technical limitations and risks.

Traditionally, obtaining informed consent has been the norm in mental health care involving physical procedures (drug treatment, electroconvulsive therapy, or psychosurgery). For a long time, it seemed less necessary for psychotherapy, in which the patient is supposedly conscious, aware of what is going on, and always in control of choices and participation. Now, however, the American Psychological Association (1992) ethics and the American Psychiatric Association (1998b) require informed consent for psychotherapy. The patient-is-always-in-control argument that is no longer valid in psychotherapy also is no longer compelling for avoiding the issue with any other online interventions.

Seeking a patient's informed consent is not without hazard. Trying to obtain client consent can introduce uncertainties, misgivings, doubts, fears, objections, and confusing complications, and it can also waste time. It can create negative expectations, impose a legalistic posture, and become an excuse for avoiding the "real" issues (Beahrs & Gutheil, 2001). The increased potential for miscommunication inherent in online clinical practice makes the impact of informed consent particularly unpredictable. Standardized consent procedures may exacerbate this problem. These are all valid reasons for weaving informed consent into the ongoing treatment relationship and not isolating it as a preliminary event.

The informed-consent process can easily deteriorate into a perfunctory ceremony performed for the record to protect the practitioner from the client rather than the other way around (Jauhar, 2002). This result is particularly true for common Web-mediated consent agreements. Such agreements are necessary for legal protection, however.

To obtain consent, it may not necessarily be enough for the practitioner to post a page with a form full of fine print and give the client the option to click "OK" or "Cancel." A more informative posting consists of a series of pages with carefully crafted explanations and interactive features that require reader comprehension to navigate successfully. Even then, it is less than clear whether mouse-mediated completion of this process constitutes sufficient evidence of informed consent in all circumstances.

At present, the court cases seem to go both ways. In *Forrest v. Verizon Communications, Inc.* (see http://www.legalcasedocs.com/120/243/676.html), the Washington, D.C., Court of Appeals upheld a trial court's dismissal of the claim on the grounds that the plaintiff, dissatisfied with Verizon's service, was bound by the terms of Verizon's contract, which provided in pertinent part that all legal claims had to be filed in Virginia. Although the site urged the visitor to "READ THE FOLLOWING AGREEMENT CAREFULLY," the forum clause appeared in the final section of an agreement 13 pages long, including two long appendixes.

On the other hand, a U.S. district court refused the defendant's motion to compel arbitration in another case because, said the court, the arbitration clause, part of an "adhesion contract" (one drafted by a party with superior bargaining power), was "unconscionable" (*Combs v. PayPal*, 2002). A series of lawsuits and appeals (i.e., case law) could establish reliable guidelines eventually, but the process will take time. Knowing the rate at which the common law evolves, legislators and lobbyists will probably be unwilling to wait; they probably will fashion and enact appropriate legislation. In the interim, practitioners could impose terms and conditions, try to make them enforceable, speak with the client, and document that conversation to strengthen the claim that the client's consent was informed.

Consent obtained online, which can supplement verbal informed consent, may include information about the technical aspects of the technology to be used, the risks and benefits of using the technology, and the risks of the communication methods and equipment. For example, a client using an unsecured Internet Web site feature, such as a chat room, risks having personal information intercepted, because chat rooms are notoriously vulnerable to hackers. A client on a private integrated services digital network (ISDN) with a direct link to a confidential medical location incurs little risk. Until standards are more fully developed for the telecommunication technologies, it is important to inform clients of the specific risks involved with users each technology.

Note, however, that the consent process is ongoing in therapy. New decision points arise during the course of treatment, and old decisions merit reconsideration as facts emerge, the client's overall understanding improves, and new questions arise. Here, psychotechnologies have an advantage over ordinary in-person communication. In contrast to the situation in which a premedicated client on a stretcher is asked to approve impending surgery, establishing or revisiting a consent agreement remotely through an asymmetric communication mode gives a client a good opportunity to study alternatives, obtain independent information, consider the pros and cons, consult family and friends, and make an autonomous decision without the pressure of an eager or impatient, hovering professional.

Electronically mediated informed-consent procedures can sometimes confuse patients by barraging them with boilerplate and burying them in a blizzard of minutiae. The patients' eyes might glaze over when confronted by warnings, disclaimers, and legalistic explanations. A professional who presents patients with such material risks training them to disregard other thoughts the professional may communicate.

Instead, an informed-consent method that succeeds in teaching, enlightening, giving perspective, answering questions, and reassuring patients about a diagnosis or treatment can have a direct therapeutic effect independent of the main therapeutic modalities being applied. Because they are untiring, flexible, upgradeable, multimedia capable, interactive, and able to present material repeatedly and in various wordings, computers can be excellent vehicles for obtaining informed consent. Nonetheless, the practitioner could present, and require an indication of assent to, a carefully crafted consent document. The sophisticated, high-tech, high-quality consent process continuing thereafter will supplement and improve on, but not replace, the documentation needed for adequate risk management. Informed consent can emerge from an ongoing dialogue that elicits the patient's values and preferences, respects the client's autonomy and choices, and involves the patient in decision making. But practitioners need to get their paperwork done.

Elements of an Ideal Informed Consent Agreement. Professional practice standards are frequently used to establish the basis for and level of disclosure required for informed consent. In the United States, required elements of the informed-consent agreement vary from state to state. In the context of mental health practice, professionals can refer to established standards of professional conduct and practice set by their state licensing boards and legislatures. It is always wise to consult with an attorney familiar with local laws. In the general context of online mental health practice, the elements in the consent document should include all elements required for current consent—the what, when, and how of consultation—as well as alternatives covering the use of any psychotechnologies. Therefore, ideal informed-consent activity will have the following consequences:

- The treatment team will clearly and thoroughly understand and acknowledge the uncertainties faced by the patient (and possibly the patient's family).
- The patient (and possibly family) will gain insight into the treatment team's own uncertainty and into how the team's suggestions and decisions reflect the influences of clinical factors, organizational issues, and, subordinated to professional ethics, economic pressures.
- The treatment team will identify any heightened possibility of patient dissatisfaction so that the problems can be discussed, defects can be remedied, and appropriate risk management steps can be initiated before problems occur.
- The patient will be better able to participate in treatment planning, will understand his or her role and duties, and will be more determined to make the treatment work. (The patient will be inspired to become actively involved and convinced to be trustful, compliant, and loyal.)
- The treatment team members will be kept on the same wavelength as they meet the special needs, rhythms, and preferences of the patient (this communication should promote trust within the team, continuity of care, commonality of focus, and a united approach).
- Implicit in these principles is the intention that the informed-consent process will have a direct impact on the clinicians involved and not just on the patient (and family).

It is doubtful that this detailed ideal is ever realized. In practice, although the requirements vary somewhat from state to state, informed consent generally obliges the practitioner to acquaint the patient with the nature of the proposed therapy and its risks and benefits, with the risks and benefits of all other reasonable alternative treatments, and with the risks and benefits of doing nothing. Providing this information in understandable terms and being able to provide documentation of having done so should generally satisfy the law, even if the process falls short of the ideal. Remember that no professional is expected to achieve perfection. The standard of care is the degree of skill and diligence that other reasonably prudent practitioners—as opposed to extraordinary, ideal, exemplary, or stellar practitioners—provide in the same or similar circumstances. The law requires no more. In theory, no professional satisfying the standard of care is liable.

Informed consent in an online consultation can involve a combination of several communication modalities:

- Spoken dialogue (in person and remote) with a designated main therapist and perhaps with other treatment team members.
- Modeling of the proposed diagnoses and interventions (and even potential outcomes) by video or slide-show presentations, preferably interactive ones, delivered over the Web, to give the patient and, where appropriate, the patient's family concrete examples of what is being discussed (see discussion of storyboarding in chapter 5).
- Modeling parts of the informed-consent process itself so that the patient can observe a patient participating in a discussion, asking questions, and using the educational modules.
- Modeling of a family grappling with the issues, complaining about the treatment team, squabbling, misunderstanding each other, coming up with questions, and eventually working through the informed-consent material and the family stresses caused by the patient's disorder.
- A frequently asked questions (FAQ) resource, preferably tailored to the patient's circumstances, presented both on the Web and in printed form.
- Interactive educational modules posted on the Web or delivered in print form and chosen and tailored for the patient. These modules will answer a wide range of questions, from "What is mental illness?" to "How do a PsyD and an EdD differ?" to "Do you really mean I have to lay off the dope to stop my panic attacks?"
- A users group, a virtual community of anonymous patients facing similar issues. Their meetings or discussions are not treatment sessions but rather a forum for venting and sharing concerns and insights about treatment.
- Quizzes or other devices to show where the patient lacks sufficient understanding to give informed consent.
- Automatic documentation of all informed-consent-related activities for each patient.

These suggested informed-consent components to include in a technology-enhanced treatment program represent the ideal. Although the law encourages professionals to strive for the ideal, the law does not hold them liable for falling short.

A word of caution: The law does not favor volunteers. A physician who ignores a stranger lying on the road after being injured by a car may be ethically challenged but is legally in the clear. The doctor becomes vulnerable to a claim of negligence only by stopping to help.[1] Similarly well-meaning psychotechnology practitioners who try to follow an idealized model of informed consent could theoretically augment

---

[1] Many states have enacted Good Samaritan laws, named after the biblical story of the passerby who came to the aid of a stranger in distress. Where such statutes are in force, a measure of protection is afforded to health professionals who, though not legally obliged to help, do so. Samaritans who inadvertently harm the person they are trying to help are protected from liability claims. The terms of these statutes vary from state to state, but the protection often is limited to cases in which there was no duty to respond, the Samaritan rendered no bill, and he commits simple, as opposed to gross, negligence.

their liability exposure by offering to do more than the law strictly requires. Before undertaking a heavier burden than that imposed by law, a practitioner should consider the implications and confer with counsel.

Consent in Real Life. To see how consent agreements are used in medical settings, consider the procedure used by Madigan Army Medical Center's Web-Based Virtual Primary Care Clinic (VPCC), which provides primary care and behavioral health services online. The goals of this system are to increase patients' involvement in their health care, to improve access, to allow practitioners to become more efficient in delivering care, and to support clinical research on e-health concepts.

The VPCC periodically extracts data from the hospital legacy data system to let practitioners and clients review the clients' clinical charts via the Web. The following is a typical scenario. Note that mention of the consent form is a regular part of the intake procedure.

Martha, the wife of a retired sergeant major, received her medical care through the Army Medical Center. Like all beneficiaries, she was assigned a primary care manager (PCM), who had overall responsibility for her care. Most of her medical needs centered on routine monitoring of her diabetes and questions related to side effects, new medications, and medication renewals. To keep her appointments, she had to drive more than 30 miles each way and also had to wait to be seen. The process often took more than 2 hours, all for a 10-minute appointment.

Martha's PCM knew that she was a computer user and suggested that she enroll in the Virtual Primary Care Clinic (VPCC). He gave her an information sheet on the VPCC and the e-mail address of the VPCC manager in case she was interested in joining. The information sheet was intentionally used to ensure that she did not feel coerced into participation. Martha decided that using the computer was a great solution. She enrolled, signed the informed-consent agreements, and was given a password for secure log-in to the site. She was then able to review her lab results, securely consult with her PCM, and receive information related to her medical conditions without having to leave home.

Additionally, her VPCC provider was able to suggest some behavioral interventions to help her better manage her diabetes. As guidance, she received specialist-prepared information sheets that were sent to all diabetic patients, and she also was able to use some of the self-monitoring tools on the Web site.

—**Gregory A. Gahm, Ph.D., LTC**
Madigan Army Medical Center

Professionals can discuss preliminary consent agreements verbally and have them signed before any treatment is given (Maheu et al., 2001). Professionals can also give patients a video segment that explains informed consent issues (Burton & Huston, 1998), including issues that might influence the decision to use a particular technology, such as monetary costs and the limits of confidentiality (American Psychological Association, 2001).

Organizations are beginning to include statements in their ethical codes about informed consent. Among these organizations are the Internet Healthcare Coalition (2000) and the National Association of Social Workers (Code of Ethics, 1999), which states in its ethics code that social workers should inform clients of the risks associated with services delivered through electronic media. The Australian Psychological Association (1999) suggests that warnings describing the reliability and security of the technology should be posted on Web sites that allow communication with a client.

Consent Documentation.   It is clear that clients need to be informed of the risks to their privacy and confidentiality when information is transferred electronically (California Department of Consumer Affairs Board of Psychology, 2004; Fisher, 2001). Disclosure is needed about the basic processes of each telecommunication technology being used. Clients need to know who will be involved in the consultation and to what extent and the manner in which any privacy-protected documents will be kept confidential. Furthermore, clients should not be penalized if they choose not to take advantage of any technology. Clients should not have services denied or delayed because they choose in-person over online clinical practice, or vice versa. Then again, many practitioners and patients could state that needed services are already being denied or delayed with in-person healthcare. To expect a generally higher level of care through technology is a goal but not necessarily a reality at this time.

The decision to use a specific technology is both the professional's and the client's. Both parties should consider whether they feel comfortable using the technology in question. Above all, the professional needs to be able to avoid harm, that is, to safely serve the client and establish the necessary rapport (Brown-Connolly, 1999).

Giving clients sufficient information for informed consent can be a problem if mental health professionals themselves do not fully understand the risks inherent in using any given technology (see chapter 11 for training issues). For example, how many professionals who use e-mail can accurately discuss the risks of communicating with a client through e-mail? Mechanical understanding is not necessary for operational proficiency, as in driving a car. A person can drive an automobile without knowing how the engine works or where the fuel pump is. Similarly, professionals can send and receive e-mail without understanding the risks to confidentiality. As a consequence, they may struggle to explain the risks as mandated by federal law or their ethical codes of conduct, without learning about the risks, how to communicate them to specific groups of clients, or how to develop an appropriate consent agreement for exclusively text-based treatment.

Moreover, knowing how to drive an automobile is different from knowing how to drive a motorcycle or a bus, each of which has its own rules and necessary skills. The same is true of the various psychotechnologies. Using e-mail is different from using a LifeShirt or from videoconferencing. Thus, understanding the functional aspects of the psychotechnologies under consideration for use is an important component of a professional's ability to inform the client and obtain truly informed consent.

Mental health professionals are usually required to acknowledge the limitation of the services provided online and to inform clients of these limitations before any confidential information is shared. Some organizations now publish guidelines for professionals who use various forms of technology. For example, URAC standards require a health Web site to disclose limitations and appropriate uses for services offered through the site (American Accreditation HealthCare Commission, 2001). Mental health professionals using the Internet are advised to provide one-on-one services only through secure Web sites and e-mail programs that use adequate encryption technology to prevent unauthorized third-party access (American Counseling Association, 1999).

Clients can be informed of any risk to their privacy and the confidentiality of their treatment records or communications with medical or nonmedical personnel, whether on private secure telephone lines or when using Internet-based services. Most professional organizations agree that, when interacting with a client online, a practitioner should have a signed informed consent form in the client's medical record. The form should cover the specific uses, risks, and benefits of the technologies used.

Practitioners may consider including these elements in informed-consent agreements:

- A brief description of the equipment to be used, the services to be delivered, and the purpose of using remote service delivery (e.g., continuity of care, the comfort or convenience of being treated at home).
- Details of licensure, state licensing board contact information, and waivers to resolve issues of jurisdiction in case of complaints.
- Identification of the specific roles of all professionals who will be involved in remote service delivery, including supervisors, consultants, and referring professionals; their credentials and the types of records the professionals will keep; and which treating professional has ultimate authority over the client's treatment.
- Notification that the client has the right to prohibit identifiable psychological information from appearing electronically.
- A description of follow-up procedures when the client or the professional fails to appear at the scheduled appointment time.
- Identification of vacation arrangements, client e-mail addresses, average response time for contacts initiated by either the client or the professional, and topics not appropriate for discussion.
- A description of backup procedures for failed receipt of e-mail, delayed receipt, access or server problems, or unannounced changes in meeting schedles for all types of electronic communication (text-based, telephonic, or videophonic).
- A listing of hypertext links from the professional's Web site (using capable e-mail readers or Web browsers) and all other appropriate contact information, such as the addresses and/or telephone numbers of certification bodies and licensing boards and Web site addresses for sources of legislation related to security.
- A notice that the client is never to use e-mail in an emergency situation.
- Required passwords or code words to verify both client and professional identity.
- A description of the limits of confidentiality with e-mail, a statement that encryption is required for all client contact, and a statement that paper copies will be made of all e-mail messages and kept in the client file.
- The professional's policies on retaining and distributing information received from and about the client.
- Schedules for use of local support systems (e.g., crisis hotlines, Alcoholics Anonymous).
- Procedures for labeling e-mail, such as type of transaction (e.g., appointment scheduling, billing question, journaling, referral).
- Procedures for handling sensitive subject matter (e.g., rape, HIV status, domestic violence, suicide intention), using a remote technology.
- A description of conditions under which remote contact will be suspended pending in-person contact with a local professional before resuming remote services, such as when the remote professional is informed of a duty-to-warn situation (e.g., abuse, threat of suicide or homicide), and what the remote professionals will do and whom they contact in these circumstances.
- Compliance with HIPAA mandates (see chapter 9) and what they mean to transmission, privacy, and confidentiality related to the chosen technologies. For more information on consent that HIPAA requires, visit http://www.apapractice.org.

- Procedures for terminating and resuming the therapeutic relationship in the future, if desired, including what may be expected if the primary or consulting practitioner withdraws from the case (because of retirement, illness, etc.).

The core informed consent document that a client signs (not clicks on) and returns by hand, surface mail, or fax (not e-mail) might contain clauses that indicate the following:

- The client has read and understood all information presented, has had an opportunity to ask questions, and has had all questions answered satisfactorily in a manner and language that he or she understands.
- The client has filled in all blanks in the agreement (or their electronic equivalent) at the time of signing.
- The signing client is not under the influence of medications or impaired by social or emotional problems to the extent that he or she has difficulty understanding the nature and content of the agreement.
- The client has been reminded not to use the equipment of his or her employer to communicate with the practitioner except when such use is clearly acceptable for the employer to inspect and retain the client's communications.

Most, if not all, of the information contained in consent agreements could be posted on the professional's Web site, possibly as a part of the site's terms and conditions. Although well-composed and properly signed, dated, and witnessed documents can help confirm that the client's consent is adequately informed, these documents are not a substitute for a spoken (in-person or remote) discussion that includes ample opportunity for the client to ask questions and for material to be explained in different ways. After this discussion, the practitioner creates documents that show that the client has been presented with all the required information and has understood the key issues. The documentation can include client quotations that demonstrate comprehension or a formal quiz that the client has taken.

The specific informed consent agreement might include the following elements:

- A description of the risks of the selected psychotechnologies and the advantages of alternative approaches.
- Permission to consult with specific colleagues or supervisors on specific topics (even if the client is not identified to these people).
- Names of local resources, including hospitals covered by the client's insurance carrier; information about mental health insurance carriers; name and contact information for the client's local primary care physician, trusted members of the client's family, trusted friends, the client's religious leader, and/or other people for the practitioner to contact in an emergency.
- Permission to contact people in the client's support group in case of an emergency.
- Identification of any linguistic and cultural incompatibilities.

In addition to containing a signed informed consent agreement, each client's chart might document the time, date, location, and content of consultations with colleagues and discussions with the client about informed consent matters. Maheu et al. (2001)

specifically describes general health care elements to include in patient consent agreements.

Practitioners in the forefront of technology may want to consider accepting electronic *digital signatures* (also known as electronic signatures, or e-signatures) on consent agreements from their patients who are in remote locations. Digital signatures are a special way to authenticate the identity of the sender of an e-mail, message, regardless of whether the message is encrypted. Professionals seeking more information on digital signatures and the law can visit http://www.epic.org/crypto/dss.

Somewhere in all the suggestions gathered from various resources, practitioners must find a reasonable balance of what they include in consent agreements. Table 12.1 can help practitioners develop a workable document. The table distills this discussion of possible elements to include in an informed consent agreement or addendum. To clarify the process, a sample consent agreement addendum for videoconferencing forms of telehealth, appears in appendix C. Of course, practitioners should obtain

TABLE 12.1
Informed Consent Agreement Elements

Explain or Identify ...

Services	Average response times
Purpose of remote electronic contact	Emergency procedures
Equipment	Identity verification process
Roles of all parties involved	Security requirements
Risks	Sensitive-information procedures
Follow-up procedures	Payment procedures
Limits of service	Jurisdiction
Vacation arrangements	Special provisions
Inappropriate discussion topics	Record storage
Privacy protections	Patient role
Patient rights	Termination procedures
Backup procedures	

Provide ...

State licensing board contact information	Contact information for professional
Details of licensure	Passwords or code words to access communication channel(s)
Link to professional Web site for policy updates and other information related to treatment	Schedules and contact numbers for local support systems

Obtain ...

Authorization to contact insurance company	Local resources from client
Insurance contact information	

Phrases to consider incorporating:

	Procedures used are not validated by research.
Client has been given the opportunity to ask questions and has received satisfactory answers.	Client has read and understood all information presented.
Client has been given an explanation of how services via technology differ from services delivered face to face.	Client has been given a description of the positive and negative consequences of service via technology.
Client has been reminded not to use the equipment of his or her employer.	Client has been told which treating professional has ultimate authority over the treatment.
Client has been given the opportunity to prohibit identifiable medical information or images from appearing in any electronic medium.	Client has been given the opportunity to prohibit use of identifiable images or information by researchers or other unidentified entities.

a legal review by a qualified attorney before using these suggestions or the sample agreement with clients. These documents may need revisions to conform with federal, state, or local law. Revisions will be necessary as the law evolves. As we discuss in chapter 9, a reasonable balance might be found through additional inquiries directed to a practitioner's licensing board, professional association ethics boards, and/or malpractice carrier.

Scheduling. In telehealth programs, scheduling appointments can be complicated (Maheu et al., 2001). To facilitate the process, scheduling problems can be discussed as part of the consent agreement. When scheduling appointments with a distant client, a professional must consider each party's local time. An international client may live in a time zone several hours ahead or behind the professional's, and this discrepancy can change with the seasons (see, e.g., http://www.worldtimeserver.com). If either party is using a specialty site housing the psychotechnology, the appointment times must fall within the facility's hours of operation. The client can be told that the appointment time represents the actual time of the session and that additional time before the session may be needed to set up the technology. Additionally, it may be helpful for practitioners to confirm the appointment time with the client on the day before the appointment.

Practitioners can send reminders by using various technologies (encrypted e-mail, telephone, etc.), depending on the capabilities of each party. As with telephone reminders, e-mail reminders may need to reflect that someone other than the client may intercept the message. Also, consideration may need to be given to the possibility that a spouse, child, relative, or coworker might (intentionally or unintentionally) access the message.

Scheduling can turn good intentions into time-consuming telephone tag. But technical assistance is available. For instance, companies offer Web-based scheduling to help telemedicine networks ease administrative burdens associated with scheduling either or both store-and-forward and video teleconsultation. The E-Ceptionist is one such service:

> *The E-Ceptionist scheduling service is available to customers in the United States and Europe. The service allows customers to schedule health care appointments in real time over the Internet and to manage the health care process after the appointment occurs. Service is secure, encrypted, and meets HIPAA standards for the privacy of patient information. The U.S. Department of Defense uses the service as its e-health platform in TRICARE Region Nine to schedule appointments for video and store-and-forward teleconsultations. Today, Internet scheduling is a routine course of business, saving both time and money.*

> —**Merrick Alpert**
> **Chairman**
> **E-Ceptionist**
> **Houston, TX**

Supporters of interactive videoconferencing admit that no telecommunication technology can do as well as in-person contact in distinguishing between a seriously mentally ill client and a mildly neurotic client. Therefore, the use of interactive videoconferencing as the only method of making contact with an unknown client may be needlessly risky, especially without the involvement of other trained professionals in the client's locale. The model we discuss in chapters 11, 12, and 13 advocates that practitioners use various media as well as in-person contact as often as deemed appropriate after an initial in-person assessment period.

Financial Agreements

Because services delivered through telecommunication technologies may seem adjunctive and nontraditional, the professional may inadvertently omit the normal discussion of financial matters with clients. Practitioners may need to make an extra effort to remember to fully disclose fees and payment methods (California Department of Consumer Affairs Board of Psychology, 2004; Internet Healthcare Coalition, 2000). They can give this information to the client in various ways, depending on the technology being used. For example, e-mail autoresponders can automatically send an e-mail when requested from a Web site. Such autoresponder e-mails can describe the mental health professionals's fees, collection methods, and reimbursement policies. To avoid making the site seem too commercial, the professional should pay attention to language selection. Drafting an appropriate e-mail document may require an attorney's expertise to protect against the worst-case scenario.

Practitioners who want to collect payment through the Net should remember that a credit card number is not adequate to authenticate the identity of the person on the other end of an online clinical practice link. Additionally, patients may be reluctant to divulge their credit card number on the Internet. Identity theft is rife on the Internet, and credit companies are resigned to living with a much higher rate of deception than is acceptable in a clinical situation. In an office setting, it is rare that anyone cheats a mental health professional by paying with someone else's plastic or with a forged check. In cyberspace, however, where lying, software pirating, and music theft are by some definitions normal behavior, providing phony credit information may be reasonable to a person considering and exploring psychotherapy. Furthermore, it may be easier for a patient to justify evading payment where the online professional seems less real than one known in person.

Financial arrangements also can be discussed in the consent agreement, thereby improving the chances that the topic of payment will not be overlooked. Ideally, however, financial matters are separately handled, so that if the professional needs to introduce the consent document into evidence, its usefulness to the defense will not be impaired. A document containing financial arrangements would be easy to misuse in cross-examination; the plaintiff's lawyer could suggest that its author was more concerned with getting paid than with informing the patient.

Now that we've examined the first four steps in the OCPM model—professional training, referral, client education, and consent—the next chapter describes the three steps in the delivery of online clinical practice: clinical assessment, direct care, and reimbursement.

Online Clinical Practice Management (OCPM): Delivering Care

The first four steps of the Online Clinical Practice Management (OCPM) model, discussed in chapters 11 and 12, deal with professional training, generating referrals, conducting patient training, and obtaining consent. The practitioner and the client know with whom they are dealing, the client knows enough about telecommunication services and devices, and the practitioner and the client have signed basic consent agreements. We now discuss clinical issues, the next three steps of the OCPM delivery phase: clinical assessment, direct care, and reimbursement.

OCPM STEP 5: CLINICAL ASSESSMENT

Like informed consent, assessment continues throughout a therapeutic relationship. Assessment is mutual: the client is assessing the professional and is being assessed by the professional. Conducting treatment online can affect (enhance, constrict, or distort) many aspects of assessment.

Although how the law will deal with telemental health is uncertain, it probably will hold professionals who communicate with clients through psychotechnologies to in-person standards of assessment. If psychotechnologies are eventually shown to markedly improve the assessment process, standards may be expanded. For now, professionals can assume that assessment at a distance begins at a disadvantage. The virtual world enabled by technology may be the next best thing to being there, but it isn't the same as being there. As we've discussed for professionals who have been trained to detect and discuss the symbolism often manifested in a therapeutic relationship, managing the emotion that often ensues can be difficult enough. It is far more difficult to manage when the exchange is reduced to a text based exchange. This is particularly true it the message is sent electronically and immediately.

Matters become even more complicated through text based technologies. Nonetheless, when clinical assessment is attempted several preliminary assessment instruments use telecommunications. More in-depth analysis is needed to determine whether any of these instruments have been researched and developed sufficiently for environments in which there is no in-person contact with any administrator. Psychological tests have traditionally been administered in very standardized settings rather than in rooms in which distractions are readily available. Offering paper-and-pencil, Rorschach, or thematic apperception tests through Web sites may be a violation of test security and also an incorrect administration of standardized testing instruments. Furthermore, before any test can be responsibly offered to the public via computer or Internet (see chapter 6), the test should be developed with the targeted population in mind, and its validity and reliability should be evaluated. The impact that online administration has on the test results might also be crucial for assessing emotional state.

Mental health professionals are trained to integrate sensory cues when evaluating a client's condition and monitoring the therapeutic relationship. As discussed in chapters 3 and 5, professionals who use the psychotechnologies must learn how to make allowances for the limitations of electronic media and how to take advantage of techniques that could compensate for physical separation and surpass in-person encounters in clinically useful ways. Over time, technology may make in-person identification and assessment obsolete, but for now, requiring in-person contact with a licensed health practitioner at the beginning of remote treatment is a reasonable step toward expanding the current standard of care.

The Case for In-Person Assessment

In-person therapy allows the practitioner and the client to make assumptions about what they see without a discussion. This is also true for other sensory modalities. The fact that blind or severely hearing-impaired people may be licensed for mental health practice establishes that vision and hearing are not absolutely required to meet standard-of-care obligations. Research on the effectiveness of video versus in-person sessions for accurate diagnosis and treatment is ongoing (see appendix A). Also worth noting is that insurance reimbursement seems to be forthcoming for initial psychiatric interviews with remote patients. On the other hand, the American Psychiatric Association (2000b) maintains that clients should initiate treatment in an in-person setting and move to telepsychiatry after therapeutic rapport has been established.

When working with psychotechnologies under special circumstances, as during a natural disaster, professionals may wish to establish intermittent in-person treatment sessions whenever possible. The laws in some states (e.g., California) stipulate that in-person treatment may not be mandated as a condition of reimbursement. Other states or countries or any given profession, by contrast, may require in-person treatment as a condition for the therapy. Practitioners may want to consider the limitations of an insurance company's willingness to reimburse for a particular service. Reimbursement is not a green light to proceed; particularly when it comes to delivering new services such as those adapted and thereby modified by technology. Therefore, psychotherapists are encouraged to arrange for in-person visits on a regular basis as warranted by their professional judgment. Professionals are also encouraged to review chapter 10 discussion of issues related to standards of care and of professional conduct when using the psychotechnologies for delivering direct care. Of particular concern are such topics as structuring a professional relationship (Black, Balun, & Cozza, 2002), avoiding harm, emergency care and backup, providing care to children, boundaries of competence, and terminating the professional relationship.

The *Diagnostic and Statistical Manual* (*DSM-IV-TR*) of the American Psychiatric Association (2000a) often requires a visual or auditory evaluation of a client's hygiene, posture, carriage, gait, coordination, rate of speech, agitation, eye contact, height, weight, and other attributes to make a proper diagnosis, particularly with more severe disorders. Through video, however, it is difficult for a practitioner to estimate how big a client is. (Consider, for example, how often one is surprised at the short stature of some Hollywood leading men when viewed off screen and how much stouter and more wrinkled people may look onscreen without the benefit of professional makeup and lighting.)

All clients, to some degree, manage how they appear to other people, often using such tactics as simulating distress, exaggerating symptoms, or malingering. Jockeying with truth and deception is integral to interpersonal relating in general, and a professional who does not engage in such game playing fails to relate to a client as a fellow human being. It thus is important with a client to open communication channels that can carry, in both directions, the hidden messages and unspoken signaling essential to developing and maintaining rapport in emotional situations. Thus, despite its promotion of technology, Hi-Ethics (a nonprofit organization whose goals are to establish and comply with ethical standards in health care) acknowledges that online interactions between a professional and a client cannot fully replace an in-person professional relationship (Health Internet Ethics, n.d.). This organization therefore strongly advises an in-person meeting before substantial use of a psychotechnology for any purpose. The in-person assessment period is also an ideal time to review and obtain informed consent, both verbal and written.

If an in-person meeting is impossible, a videoconferenced assessment period is considered the second-best option. However, important classes of information may be lost in distance treatment, even with an excellent audiovisual setup. When a transmission signal is interrupted or delayed, videoconferencing equipment avoids falling behind by dropping a few video frames, possibly deleting important information. For example, the bat of an eyelid could reveal the true feelings of a client who is idealizing the professional, but this gesture might be missed by the transmission equipment. It is also important for the practitioner to be able to spot indications of a physical disease or injury in a client. Seeing a client limp could impel a professional to ask about the cause of an injury. Screening for physical symptoms is especially important for patients visiting a mental health facility. A person suffering from social or emotional problems may have a physical disease, which might be caused or exacerbated by a mental disorder. Additionally, a person suffering from social or emotional problems may be more likely to underreport or ignore a physical illness that should be treated. In addition, even mild adverse reactions to psychotropic medications can discourage a patient from taking the drug. In particular, sexual side effects are often not unearthed without specific questioning, yet they are a major reason that patients stop taking their medication.

As discussed in chapter 5, videoconferencing technology cannot transmit cues that do not appear in the monitor's limited size. Lack of peripheral vision and the inability to make sense of background noise prevent both the professional and the client from understanding what conditions are like in the other person's room. Twiddled thumbs, knocking knees, and bitten fingernails may thus escape the screen shot, and the sound of shuffling feet or muttering under one's breath may not travel through cyberspace.

A videoconference also involves only vision and hearing; clues for other senses are not transmitted. Certainly the firmness of a handshake can convey significant information in any relationship. Although the mental health literature gives the sense of smell scant attention, odors could be important for assessing clients (such as when hygiene or alcohol is an issue). An astute observer may detect odors that could provide valuable clues to diagnosis of physical ailments even if these ailments are unrelated to mental ones.

Information flow in text-based environments is even more constricted than in videoconferencing or in communication by audio alone. Such information depends on the client's writing ability and level of comprehension. A professional may have difficulty assessing these client abilities, especially with a depressed or otherwise compromised and medicated individual. According to Colón (1996), the lack of visual cues in a text-based environment can adversely influence transference. In her pilot study, clients in online psychotherapeutic interactions found it easier to project idealizations and fantasies onto the psychotherapist and also expressed anger more often. This early study needs to be replicated before developing treatment recommendations. Professionals therefore should proceed cautiously with unassisted text-based patient intake and assessment until research can more clearly determine their validity. As structured telephone interviews gain more acceptance, clinicians may want to be more aware of how audio technologies could be adapted to assist with text-based intake and diagnosis.

Initial assessment can be tricky, whether online or in person. Silence can be the most expressive ingredient in a conversation. An awkward, dramatic, or pregnant pause can reveal a wish to conceal, can imbue a declaration with gravity, or can result from lapsed attention. Without a practitioner in the room, the remote patient who seems to be unusually silent during a videoconferenced session may be displaying a symptom or may be awe-struck by the magic of the technology.

Similar misinterpretations can easily occur in a text-based environment. For instance, interruptions and hesitations do not come across in e-mail. A professional's use of silence can be powerful, but patients using e-mail may need to be taught to use special conventions to convey silence or any other internal process (Murphy & Mitchell, 1998). Specifically, patients might be taught to write something such as:

......hands on hips, tapping foot, thinking ...... ok, I'll tell you that....

Overall, many limitations of treatment at a distance can be overcome to make online clinical practice highly effective. However, practitioners may want to conduct intake and assessment in person until research shows that remote diagnosis and explanation of the consent agreement are successful with specific patient populations.

One assessment strategy is to use psychotechnologies to supplement rather than replace in-person treatment when possible. Evidence is beginning to emerge that supports the use of videoconferencing. A California telemedicine demonstration program evaluated services delivered to 1,301 patients. Mental health services were provided to 13% of this group. Survey results indicate that the services were as good as in-person services, that the practitioners were capable of making accurate diagnoses, and that the collaborative practice facilitated by videoconferencing resulted in significant changes in the treatment and management of the patients' conditions (Brown-Connolly, 2001a). The report concluded that remote collaborative practice via videoconferencing can facilitate coordination of the treatment team.

Suggestions for Assessment

A practitioner's initial assessment of a client can include a mental status examination as detailed and broad ranging as is reasonable. If an initial in-person assessment is possible, the professional can assess the appropriateness of future remote contact. Practitioners may determine that clients who are at high risk of becoming homicidal or suicidal or of presenting duty-to-warn situations are not fit to receive treatment through any psychotechnology without the presence of a professional at the remote site to manage the treatment plan. In this early stage of the evolution of the psychotechnologies, practitioners should err on the side of caution and exclude clients whose diagnosis is in doubt. Just as private-practice clinicians use the assessment period to determine whether they can and should deliver services to a particular patient, clinicians can take similar approaches with patients who need to use psychotechnologies. Based on the results of the initial in-person assessment, clinicians can select suitable modalities for each client. The conditions being treated can match the technical capabilities of the technology, the treatment methods available for the chosen psychotechnology, the client's willingness and ability to participate in the proposed arrangement, and the professional's competence with that technology. Online support groups and informational and self-instructional Web sites can also be used to augment treatment.

A cyberspace port of entry may attract patients with motives that differ from those of patients arriving by traditional routes. A professional's careful inquiry about a patient's treatment goals and expectations is particularly important in online clinical practice and may be easier to conduct with the aid of automated questionnaires and a follow-through discussion. Two examples from a Web-based clinic illustrate some issues and ambiguities that can arise from online counseling:

A woman anonymously requested help from PsychPark's Web-based virtual psychiatric clinic. She was put in touch with one of our dozens of mental health clinicians for online consultation via e-mail. Our virtual clinic offers free electronic counseling for psychiatric patients or their friends or relatives. By chance, the e-therapist who took the patient on was the psychiatrist who was treating the patient at a real clinic at the time. It turned out that the patient was trying to check on the reliability and capability of her in-person psychiatrist. A request for a second opinion is legitimate, but using duplicity to pit one clinician against another can be risky for both the patient and the professionals.

In a second case, Jones, a 21-year-old male college student, sought help at our virtual clinic to deal with his girlfriend's recent suicide attempt. He described her as beautiful, a good student, and happy at school, and he said that she had apparently enjoyed normal interpersonal relationships during their 2 years together. Therefore, he was shocked when she overdosed on antidepressant and hypnotic medicines and later revealed to him that she had obsessive-compulsive disorder.

Our therapist began corresponding with Jones by e-mail, providing support and suggesting how Jones could be help his girlfriend, such as by guiding her to a real psychiatric clinic.

Over the next 3 months, Jones engaged in six sessions of online consultation, during which he focused on six concerns: (1) He wanted to learn about the drugs his girlfriend took in her suicide attempt and the damage these drugs might cause; (2) His girlfriend was smoking, drinking excessively, and abusing other drugs, which he felt made her condition worse and more difficult for him to deal with; (3) He managed to bring her to a real psychiatric clinic, but she refused the recommended admission to hospital, so Jones wondered how to overcome her objections; (4) Jones had trouble getting along with his girlfriend's family or communicating with them; (5) Sometimes he felt infuriated with her oscillation between indifference to and dependence on him; (6) He faced a severe conflict over whether to leave his girlfriend or to help her. He felt on the verge of breaking down from the burden she presented but was afraid that her condition would deteriorate if he left.

In the end, Jones sent an e-mail message to thank us. He told us how good our Web site was and claimed that he hadn't felt lonely during the crisis, because we had accompanied him, offered him a catharsis channel, and relieved his anxiety—but unfortunately, his girlfriend had committed suicide the day before.

Jones' failure to notice his girlfriend's psychiatric disturbance before the first overdose he mentioned may evince his problems with intimacy and suggests why he decided to communicate with a doctor in cyberspace rather than in person. Although he described his own discomfort and his conflict about breaking off with his girlfriend, much of the communication involved practical and intellectual matters.

More than 20% of clients in the PsychPark virtual clinic ask questions on behalf of other people. Jones' involvement with the clinic may have led to his engaging his girlfriend initially with the professional mental health system, but ultimately that contact was not enough for her. Jones himself thought that he had benefited from the support he received, and he felt sufficiently connected to express his gratitude.

Could the treatment Jones received be counted as successful? After all, overt patient satisfaction was high, the patient did not break down as he had feared he might, and he followed through on advice to bring his girlfriend to a real clinic for help. Would Jones have done better without the PsychPark virtual clinic, which gave him an easy alternative to consulting a mental health professional in person? Would he have gone to a real clinic? Of course, we cannot answer these questions.

However, the incident points up the difficulty of establishing an adequate grasp of a case without the usual in-person interviews, physical examination, laboratory workup, and opportunity to see signs of improvement and deterioration that a patient may not report. In Jones' case, instead of e-mail discussion of the girlfriend's problems, having the couple come in for evaluation might have led to a better outcome. On the other hand, she had been evaluated in a real mental health clinic as a result of our online consultation with Jones.

Overall, cases involving suicide or other events that highlight the shortcomings of a virtual clinic are unusual. For most of our patients, the advantages of using a virtual clinic seem to exceed the disadvantages.

—Chao-Cheng "Chris" Lin, M.D.
Attending Psychiatrist, Yuli Veterans Hospital
Webmaster, PsychPark Virtual Clinic
Taiwan

When formulating a treatment plan during initial assessment, practitioners should remember that they can use various psychotechnologies throughout the course of treatment and, if possible, can combine these technologies with intermittent in-person appointments. When scheduling remote sessions, the practitioner can set clear goals along with criteria for meeting those goals. Plans can also define decision points so that, for example, a client's failure to meet the goals can result in discontinuation of remote contact, referral, or termination of treatment. Additionally, the practitioner can:

- Use psychological testing as appropriate during the assessment phase. Psychotechnologies enable practitioners to conduct testing and interpret the results more extensively and inexpensively and at the client's convenience. However, be sure to check the *Standards for Educational and Psychological Testing* (American Psychological Association, 1999a) to determine whether the tests administered through Web sites have been developed using approved methods.

- To gain as much information as possible about the client, ask family or friends, when appropriate, to participate in assessment and screening activities. Their involvement, of course, needs to be guided by the client's comfort.

- Obtain all required releases from the client, as well as from family and friends. Note that participation of these outsiders by means of electronic technology may fall under the purview of HIPAA. It is possible that, to engage in this type of communication, an authorization rather than a mere consent may be required.

• To reduce the risk that data could be lost because of a computer malfunction, the practitioner can set up a duplicate computer system to mirror the primary computer (Polauf, n.d).

OCPM STEP 6: DIRECT CARE

Once practitioners have formulated an adequate treatment plan through an initial assessment, they can deliver direct care. For many practitioners, direct care is the goal, the main focus. They have decided to use psychotechnologies with a client and may also have arranged intermittent in-person contact. We now discuss practice management issues relevant to three primary modalities introduced throughout the book: text-based environments, Web sites, and videoconferencing. Even though many emerging areas of technology are worth discussing, this book focuses on these three topics.

The next section, discusses benefits of and barriers to text-based communication in mental health. Text-based interactions, which are the farthest from traditional in-person health care situations, would be the most difficult to defend if the plaintiff's counsel were to use an in-person standard of care as the standard to which a practitioner is held. Nonetheless, proponents of text-based care raise some valid points about risk management (Lebow, 1998). Here, we examine specific risk management issues, presenting thoughts from both sides of the argument. See in chapter 3 for a review of the literature related to various types of text-based environments.

Direct Patient Care via Text

As text-based communication becomes more prevalent, it may not only supplement ordinary discourse but also change how human beings communicate (Schaefermeyer & Sewell, 1988). The absence of visual cues or physical presence, the altered speech patterns, and the relative anonymity of some text-based environments enable novel styles of relating to individuals and groups. Time, distance, and even honesty assume new meanings. Some people reveal thoughts and feelings that they find difficult to express under other circumstances, whereas other people seem to relish anonymously duping the recipients of their messages. Alternatively, an object relations perspective says that a client who has not achieved sufficient object constancy cannot attain such detailed inner focus.

Although general medical interaction with patients can be different from psychotherapy or counseling, the general medical world has produced empirical evidence that mental health practitioners have only begun to approximate, despite their prolific writings (Laszlo, Esterman, & Zabko, 1999). See Azy Barak's Web page (http://construct.haifa.ac.il/~azy/azy.htm) for an extensive attempt at cataloging some such writings.

The general medical world provides facts related to e-mail use. Physician–patient e-mail communication in general health care has been off to a slow start—only 10% to 13% of surveyed physicians engage in such correspondence (Harris Interactive, 2001a; Medem, 2000). Physicians in one study underestimated the public demand for communication through e-mail, believing that most patients have no interest in having e-mail communication with their physicians (Medem, 2000).

Refuting this impression, a January 2001 Harris Interactive (2001d) poll showed that 80% of patients are eager to communicate with their physicians by e-mail. This poll found that 60% of the patients complained that they forget to ask all their questions when they see their physician, and 41% said that they would rather not schedule a visit for questions that physicians could answer online. Patients want follow-up e-mail after an office visit and would like to receive preventive-care reminders. Patients want to communicate more with their physicians in whatever ways make sense: in person, via telephone, or through the Internet.

A study of family practices found that 54% of patients surveyed have e-mail access and that 90% of these patients expressed a desire to use e-mail for prescription refills, 87% for nonurgent consultations, 84% to check lab reports, and 77% to make or cancel appointments (Couchman, Forjuoh, & Rascoe, 2001). Another survey found that of the 33.6 million patients interested in contacting their physician's through e-mail, only 3.7 million have done so to date (HealthLeaders, 2001).

In looking at these two studies, professionals must remember that the topics psychotherapy patients may choose to discuss with their psychotherapists may differ from the ones they discuss with their physicians. A true test of text-based modalities will occur when the necessary funding is devoted to empirical analysis of how these technologies are used in mental health practice.

E-Mail Communications in Mental Health. E-mail may seem to be the most inviting technology to meet and greet clients in cyberspace, but this appearance is generating controversy. In general, as previously stated, in chapter 3 technology supporters believe that advances offered by e-mail, instant messaging, and chat rooms hold much promise for mental health care. Critics of e-mail contact between mental health clients and practitioners (Griffiths, 2001; Manhal-Baugus, 2001) note that e-mail creates a record of the information being conveyed. This record can be an asset or a liability in a lawsuit. Even though professionals using e-mail usually have a master's or doctoral degree (Laszlo et al., 1999), many do not realize that they may face legal action because of their behavior as professionals online (Maheu & Gordon, 2000). Although there is wide variation in enforcement by state and federal officials, state licensing boards are devoting special attention to health care services delivered over the Internet. Professionals seeking to deliver direct care through the Internet therefore need to be fully aware of and operate within the rapidly evolving limits of the law (R. Waters, personal communication, September 11, 2002).

Treatment records may be requested not only in malpractice actions but also in custody disputes, the contesting of wills, and other legal venues in which a client may waive confidentiality or in which a judge demands the original data. Before starting e-mail with an established patient, consider the following experience by one author of this book:

> *"How many of you have used e-mail to communicate with clients?" This question has been posed to mental health professionals at many Web development and telehealth seminars, and it always brings up many hands. "And it how many of you are still communicating with clients?" Nearly all hands drop. In these seminars, professionals of various disciplines typically report high levels of anxiety after communicating with one too many personality-disordered clients.*

The anxiety that so many professionals report may be the result of their own inexperience, their client's inexperience, the peculiarities of text-based messaging, or the difficulties they face in working with people who struggle with social or emotional problems.

Some practitioners may not want to take the time to write e-mail as opposed to speaking. Although e-mail use may benefit a patient, it may be an added burden to a busy professional. The professional may think it an imposition to take the time to respond to e-mail questions not asked at an in-person session.

For patients, using e-mail may be an easy way to avoid difficult material that they should discuss in-person. The psychotherapy office is considered to be an appropriate place for patients to learn to function openly and honestly in the real world. Some clinicians may think that e-mail is a safe way for a patient to start revealing difficult material; others may argue that a patient's office or living or bedroom is not the appropriate place to conduct such dialogues with a professional.

The professional may have a prearranged agreement with patients that any topic they raise in e-mail must be the first issue addressed in the next in-person session. Such an agreement would circumvent the objection that patients, not practitioners, should introduce difficult material into the session. The most objectionable issue of concern is professional liability—where the professional is asked to function in a world fraught with unknowns, without research to support the effectiveness of the process without proven legal protections, and without adequate professional guidelines.

Because professionals need special skills to steer safely through the minefield of e-mail communication with clients, this may be the last area in which the deliver professionals service. In some parts of the world, however, e-mail may be the only practical option for distant but therapeutic communication.

Security.   For text-based communication to approach or surpass the telephone and standard mail service for clinical use between professionals and clients, it must mature in reliability, confidentiality, specificity of function, and ease of use. Historically, when the telephone operated through party lines and manually directed switchboards, users were aware of potential eavesdroppers; professionals knew they could not reasonably assure patients of confidentiality. Once confidentiality could be ensured, telephone use by mental health professionals grew in popularity for very limited and specific functions, such as appointment setting, support, and brief crisis intervention between visits with a therapist, and occasionally for counseling. The therapist's preference and client diagnosis determine by the time spent on telephone transactions and the nature of the exchange between clinician and client.

Security of telephone lines is now reasonably ensured by telephone companies in the United States and is protected by specific privacy legislation. An evolutionary trajectory similar to that of the telephone can be predicted for text-based communication as security and reliability improve.

Clinicians concerned about security can use text-based software to help in psychotherapeutic encounters. An example is PQSafeWeb™, which professionals can use to overcome the many clinical and logistical challenges that arise when they are trying to provide continuity of care for mentally ill clients. Some of these challenges are geographical relocation by established clients, vacations, business travel, and illness. However, for Internet-based tools to be maximally safe and useful, they must offer security, portability, audit ability, ease of use, convenience, structured work flow, and interoperability with other software and tools.

Medem is a service provided through the Internet for physicians. Founded by the American Medical Association (AMA) and allied organizations, Medem has introduced an *online consultation* service (http://www.medem.com/corporate/

corporate_oc.cfm). Fulfilling online appointment requests, prescription refills, and address updates, online consultation purports to facilitate HIPAA-compliant secure text-based communications between professionals and patients. For nonemergency inquiries, patients ask clinical questions of their individual practitioners. Most physicians seem to use the service for the routine administrative services previously described rather than for individual consultation. Online consultation differs from similar e-mail messaging services by working within the context of the previously established patient–physician relationship.

The Medem Web site has a FAQ (Frequently Asked Questions) file. The Medem FAQ suggests that clients avoid conventional e-mail for communication with a physician and that neither should discuss mental health issues through any form of e-mail, conventional or secured.

The following two client questions and answers are excerpted from the FAQ file (http://www.medem.com/pat/pat_faq_patient.cfm#3):

5. What's wrong with conventional e-mail for communicating with my physician?

Standard e-mail does not live up to state and federal laws for patient privacy nor does it conform to medical liability carrier guidelines. It is not encrypted nor password protected and often uses employer-sponsored e-mail networks thereby making the messages the property of the employer. You would not trade stocks, pay bills or even buy a book online using standard e-mail. Your communications with your physician are too important and private to risk on standard e-mail. You will, however, receive notifications in your regular e-mail account when you have received a secure message from your doctor or his/her office. The message will contain a link that allows you to directly access your secure message from your physician so you will not have to check more than one e-mail account to find all of your messages.

6. Is there anything that I should avoid using an Online Consultation for?

Medem's Secure Messaging services, including Online Consultation, should not be used for emergency, urgent, high-sensitive or high-risk health care issues. Subjects of concern may include treatment for, or information regarding, acquired immune deficiency syndrome (AIDS), mental health issues, substance abuse, etc. Specific topics to avoid should be worked out directly with your physician.

Even if a mental health professional is assured that problematic issues will not surface with a particular patient in e-mail, caution is clearly warranted; security systems are being developed, however. The following vignette shows how software developer and psychologist Greg Alter uses PQSafeWeb in his practice. The patient's name and identifying information have been changed to protect confidentiality:

Ms. Euphenia Ellipsis was a patient of mine for nearly 7 years. She came to me on referral from the Federal Office of Workers' Compensation. She had suffered racial discrimination and harassment in her job as a clerk for a Defense Department civilian subcontractor.

Ms. Ellipsis had been depressed and also had many paranoid traits that manifested themselves in social avoidance, angry outbursts, and periodic alcohol abuse. It took several years to develop a working clinical alliance. As therapy progressed and she resolved many life issues, a recurring discussion topic was her desire to leave San Francisco, where she had lived for more than 30 years. She was frightened to move but felt compelled to return home to Alaska. She feared that the move would end her therapy and thereby end the first significant and trusting relationship she had developed with another human being.

I reassured Ms. Ellipsis that I would help her make the transition. We developed a schedule of phone contact and e-mail to maintain regular communication. I obtained a release form from Ms. Ellipsis for me to contact a university-based clinical colleague who could help with the transition. My colleague was willing to serve as a backup in case of emergency and also agreed to make a referral to an Alaskan psychologist for Ms. Ellipsis.

Ms. Ellipsis was familiar with e-mail, having used it in her job. Even though she was disabled, she took pleasure in tinkering with computers and was engaged in a number of online activities, including tracking the stock market, reading online bulletin boards, and making several online friends. As the date for her move to Alaska approached, I suggested that she use my Web site (http://www.altermedx.com), on which I had installed my secured messaging system in a software program called PQSafeWeb.

Ms. Ellipsis was instructed to log on to the Web site, using her own private password and user name. She understood that once she established the log-in, all communication was encrypted and therefore secure. In addition, the text of any communication using the Web site was stored in a password-encrypted database on a secure server at a commercial data center. Messages would not automatically be stored on either of our hard drives but would stay on the Web site, thus guaranteeing an additional measure of privacy. Our use of encrypted passwords to enter the site also guaranteed that messages to and from Ms. Ellipsis on my Web site would be private.

Once inside the Web site, Ms. Ellipsis could send me a message by clicking on a "New Message" icon and choosing the type of message to send: a free-form message, a session follow-up, a medication follow-up, or an outcomes questionnaire. A variety of other types of messages available on the system would not appear on Ms. Ellipsis' screen, either because they were developed for other practitioners or because they are administrative rather than clinical. That is, a user on PQSafeWeb can access only the functions I assign to them.

Once Ms. Ellipsis sends a text message through my Web site, I receive a companion message in my regular e-mail. The companion message tells me that I have a secured message waiting at my Web site. I click the Web site address in my e-mail note; then my browser opens, displays my secured mailbox, and shows the incoming confidential message from Ms. Ellipsis. I can choose to answer her using a variety of response templates.

After some experimentation, we both were satisfied that the secured messaging system would meet our needs. In late 2002, Ms. Ellipsis moved back to her small village near Fairbanks. By using the secured system, we were able to discuss the emotional aspects of her move in open and frank ways that would not have been possible in public e-mail. I was also able to use another feature of the software to give Ms. Ellipsis support in the form of articles housed in the PQLibrary. She read all the articles I suggested and referred to various thoughts or skills they mentioned. She appreciated my taking the time to find this information and make it available to her, and she made it a point to discuss and use the information she was learning. We also used the in-house messaging system to schedule appointments for phone calls. When we wanted to have contact in real time, we held real-time chat sessions through a secure PQChat interface similar to AOL Instant Messenger™ and Microsoft Windows Messenger™.

A consent form informed Ms. Ellipsis that a detailed log of all our interactions would be printed on regular paper (hard copy) and kept in her chart. Time and billing accounts are also kept so that online activity is easily compared to face-to-face contact time. Every 3 months, Ms. Ellipsis travels to my San Francisco Bay Area office for in-person meetings.

Soon after moving, Ms. Ellipsis asked me, "Why do I need to switch to another doctor, when this software and the telephone are working so well?" Given the clinical situation, along with the medical–legal considerations, it is optimal for Ms. Ellipsis to be

seen by a local psychologist. Until that transition occurs, Ms. Ellipsis can benefit from the continuity of care I can provide to her through PQSafeWeb at my Web site.
        —Greg Alter, Ph.D.
        Teleotech Systems
        Richmond, California

For a professional who chooses to use an established site rather than to purchase and install software on a personal Web site, an inclusive Medem-type service (that is, one supported by various national associations) does not yet exist for all mental health professionals. However, several dot-com companies offer connection services to the mental health community.

Whatever type of service licensed professionals use, they should double check the process by which e-mail is to be exchanged at any site chosen, even if offered through what appears to be a secured site. The next true story should awaken the naive professional. The anonymous licensed practitioner involved in this situation requested that this eye-opening referral story be published. The names used here are fictitious:

Dr. Perot was eager to get involved with the new technology trend. Being a pioneer in developing a cognitive-behavioral treatment program for a specific disorder, he decided to experiment with online service delivery. He hoped to learn about online service delivery and eventually to market his treatment program through the Internet. He signed a service agreement with a leading dot-com company and began delivering services at scheduled hours. The dot-com company collected fees through a merchant charge card system installed at the dot-com's Web site.

After delivering services for a few months, Dr. Perot was surprised when the company sent a letter describing its financial stressors. The letter was a solicitation as well as a notification. It asked for practitioners who might be interested in gaining partial ownership of the company, in exchange for financial support. Dr. Perot saw this as another step in the direction of expanding his online experience and enhancing the potential market for his treatment program.

After investing a large sum of money, he was given access to the back end of the Web site, including financial records. As he became acquainted with the programs operating the Web site and with the company's files, he was impressed. When he dug a deeper into the credit card processing records, however, he found a clear history of fraud. He checked his date book to be sure, and was shocked to realize that his new company had used his name and license number to bill for sessions he had never delivered.

As an owner of a company that obviously defrauded consumers, Dr. Perot is reluctant to let his identity be known. Even though some professionals have been involved in insurance fraud and some insurance companies have been reluctant to give professionals the protections that some of them feel they need, mental health professionals, as a group, have been shielded from blatant fraud. Professionals need to be diligent when contracting with groups or companies that promise to deliver secured communication services through technology. As always, when in doubt, a professional should seek the advice of a qualified attorney before signing any contracts.

Clinical Issues. Clinicians have routinely used postal and telephone services in their practices, mainly for scheduling and paperwork. E-mail is more convenient and is less expensive than standard surface mail. Text-based communication is also superior to paper-and-pen communications for supplementing mental health treatment because of its flexibility with regard to time and place (Barak & Wander-Schwartz, 1999; J. Suler, personal communication, July 18, 2001). The advantages of text-based communication are likely to make it a significant tool for delivery of health services.

Professionals can successfully use e-mail for some types of interactions with existing clients. Supporters of e-mail contact with existing clients point to the added service of allowing clients to ask questions they may have forgotten because they felt rushed or unfocused during a session. Clients can bring up matters they were reluctant to raise in person.

An online connection can also serve as a transition that allows the client to feel the presence of the practitioner even when not in the office. Intersession messaging allows clients to capture their states of mind at the moment and in vivo rather than to wait until the next in-person session to report retrospectively. Patients might use a therapist's telephone answering machine (voice mail) for such supplementary communication, but e-mail does not demand immediate attention and does not cut off a user in the middle of a long message. E-mail also allows the clients more time to collect their thoughts and to compose what they need to say. The therapist may choose to reply in kind to a patient's intersession e-mail.

Alternatively, by prior agreement with the patient, the clinician may not even read the patient's e-mail messages. For the client, the act of writing itself may be therapeutic (Suler, 2000a). Bibliotherapy and journal keeping are useful for clients who need to examine their inner lives.

Becoming more common are interactive workbooks and journals containing inspirational messages that can nudge the reader to be more introspective. This development should not surprise professionals. Sigmund Freud conducted early psychotherapy through written correspondence. Technology then, provides new vehicles for using traditional techniques. Wise practitioners will assess a patient's technological preferences, discuss the pros and cons, and obtain the appropriate consent form before proceeding.

E-mail can help professionals clarify their instructions (Kane & Sands, 1998) or can remind a patient about appointments, preventive care, and compliance schedules (Nettleman, Olchanski, & Perlin, 1998). A therapist can easily send follow-up advice to a patient who may have been emotionally distressed while in the consulting room but who is calmer when reading and rereading e-mail and thus better able to contemplate its meaning (Borowitz & Wyatt, 1998). E-mail also creates a record that the patient can review at leisure. E-mail may thus reduce the likelihood that, because of faulty memory or other problems, the patient will not understand the instructions as well as needed. From a medicolegal standpoint, the written record of instructions may be valuable in defense of claims alleging that instructions were insufficient.

A clinician can also e-mail release forms, questionnaires, and explanations for a patient to read or complete before the initial session. Scheduling a synchronous text-based group meeting can be easier than arranging for all members to travel to one office. Even a person who becomes temporarily physically ill need not miss a virtual counseling session. E-mail can also be an alternative to spending session time providing educational materials or writing out a list of support group locations. Moreover, once they have prepared these lists, professionals can e-mail them repeatedly as needed for other clients. Patients who misplace such material may be reluctant to ask for it again, but they can readily retrieve it from e-mail. Patients may be more likely to access these outside materials if a link to a related Web site or attachment is provided along with the e-mail.

As mental health researchers have known for decades, relationships are extremely difficult to study in the in-person world. The added dimensions of cyberspace complicate this study. On the other hand, written communication is confined to a form that facilitates the study of relationships. Consider the following advantages of text-based communication, in this case, e-mail, for counseling:

My e-mail relationship with a client began when she spontaneously e-mailed me about an encounter with a date. The date had turned out very differently from what she had expected. I see this client only once a month, and she wanted to tell me about the episode sooner than her scheduled appointment. She didn't ask for a reply, but I sent one with a supportive comment and a reminder that we should discuss this more when we next saw each other. I viewed the exchange as a positive step because this client is extremely reluctant and slow to disclose, and it had taken several months to gain her trust.

Now when I see her, I remind her that she can e-mail me if anything happens between sessions. She is very protective of her emotional independence, and I assume she likes knowing that she has the backup even though she chooses not to use it much. She is a client from whom I welcome communication because it is difficult to get.

I can think of other cases in which I would have to draw clear boundaries about what type of e-mail I would be ready to receive and what kind of replies I would write, in the same way that we all have to clarify for telephone calls. The more I discuss Internet therapy, the more I think the client–therapist–medium match is in need of the greatest attention.

—Susan X. Day, Ph.D.
Clinical Research Faculty
University of Houston
Houston, Texas

Psychiatrist Joel Yager offers another example of successful clinical practice using e-mail as an adjunct. Known for treating patients with eating disorders, Dr. Yager works with a virtual team of professionals consisting of a psychotherapist, a dietitian, an exercise coach, and, at times, a family therapist. Through its Web site, each virtual team member sends text-based treatment notes about every patient to all the other team members. Dr. Yager thinks that this means of communicating with a treatment team offers important dimensions to accessibility and flexibility. The following vignette exemplifies some of the recommended practices Dr. Yager follows when dealing with his patients:

I do not believe in disembodied treatment for anyone, particularly not for eating-disordered patients. I require patients, who are often teenagers, first to come to see me for a 2-hour initial interview. I have in-person as well as e-mail consultation with each patient's parents, who often let me know that the patients are not doing what they say they are doing.

I tell my patients that all sources of information are useful but that I won't divulge information that a patient identifies as being off-limits. If the family is not communicating, I want to understand why, while respecting boundaries.

Every one also has to understand that I am an agent of the patient and not the agent of the family. I have never had a patient say, "I don't want you to hear what my parents have to say." Instead, patients may want me to hear that what their parents say is distorted. I allow patients to give my e-mail address to their extended family, too. I will not cut and

*paste Aunt Betty's words into an e-mail to my patient, but I will let my patient know that
her aunt has contacted me. I have to be sure that I do not send e-mail to the wrong person.*

—Joel Yager, M.D.
Professor of Psychiatry
University of New Mexico School of Medicine
Albuquerque, New Mexico

Practitioners are finding other uses for e-mail as well. A example of a successful nonprofessional text-based program is Support and Listening on the Net (SAHAR), established in Israel. SAHAR offers a free, anonymous, and confidential online environment for Web surfers in distress to access a help team (in Hebrew) via chat rooms, instant messaging, or e-mail. The helpers, who are trained during a 16-week course, have directly contributed to saving the lives of distressed individuals on many occasions. SAHAR is not presented as a psychological service, although it is based on clear psychological principles and is supervised by mental health professionals. In addition to these services, the Web site (http://www.sahar.org.il), which appears in Hebrew, includes articles, an updated list of support organizations, and emergency contact information. Although it does not have an official backup system other than the Internet, SAHAR often uses the police for backup. Evaluation research is under way to examine the effectiveness of SAHAR's various online support components (Barak, 2002).

Professional licensing laws in Israel differ from those in other countries, just as they differ between U.S. states. Because of their interest in human nature, many mental health professionals want to generalize research findings to various ethnic groups and also to offer their services across jurisdictional borders, regardless of local regulations. This outreaching will undoubtedly provide many opportunities to study the effects of various licensing structures, the consequences of flouting the laws, and the impact of different national attitudes about how and when to deliver mental health services through telecommunication technologies, such as the Internet.

As this fictitious situation depicts, e-mail with an established patient can raise thorny clinical issues:

Dr. Oga thought it would be innovative to develop her own Web site and offer psychotherapy to established patients using e-mail. She followed the American Psychiatric Association guidelines and insisted on an in-person meeting with all patients before prescribing any medication. She uses her password-protected and secured Web site to communicate with patients who have medication questions.

Three months after establishing her Web site, Dr. Oga received a message from a patient who had seen her once in the previous 2 months. The patient confessed that he had his antidepressant prescription filled but that when it came time to take the medication, he was frightened. He admitted that he had read that an overdose of antidepressants could be lethal, and he secretly was storing them, in case he ever wanted to commit suicide.

This patient was clearly writing to ask for Dr. Oga's help. He reported that he had started taking the medication the previous night, after he frightened himself by strangling his cat in a fit of rage. He also stated that he had been drinking heavily prior to the incident. Today, he was feeling much worse because, he stated, the guilt from killing his "only friend" was "overwhelming" him. He was afraid to leave his apartment, thinking that his neighbors would have heard the incident and must think that he is "a crazy man."

Dr. Oga could not convince him to come to her office for an in-person session. She was unable to get a telephone response from him when she called. In his last e-mail message, he expressed frustration that her Web site stated that she would not respond to him in e-mail. He finished his last note with "Drop dead and leave me alone."

Dr. Oga didn't know how to handle the situation. She was embarrassed to be in such a predicament. She considered herself a senior clinician. She was also concerned for her patient. He might continue to be violent. She didn't have enough information to report him to the police, because he hadn't made overt threats about intended victims or himself.

By consulting her notes from their one in-person meeting, she saw that he lived alone, had a history of suicide attempts, and reported having no friends or family except for his cat. In her confusion about, what to do, she decided to let the matter drop and hoped that no one would learn of her exchange with him.

Some professionals are capable of playing possum. Although problems similar to this one can arise with any in-person practice, licensed professionals operating on the Internet have different resources and, possibly, different responses.

Other Practical Suggestions for Clinicians Using E-Mail. Various professional groups advise clinicians who decide to use e-mail with clients to print all e-mail communications and to file them as part of the client's record (e.g., Kane & Sands, 1998). Clinicians who include e-mail messages in their patients' charts should tell all the e-mail system's users, lay and professional, of this practice. In fact, clinicians should instruct all users about this and other medicolegal considerations before allowing them to use the e-mail system. For instance, e-mail may be electronically copied to floppy disk or other removable storage and may be at risk of being discovered if retained on a computer's hard drive. This risk factor is particularly relevant to computers used for nonprofessional purposes, such as a home computer, which conceivably could be subpoenaed along with any written record. Encryption is not a protection for the unknowing client—as the court can order that the clinician supply all associated keys and passwords. (Encryption is required for all sensitive e-mail, however.)

Additionally, in a health care context, users should assume that an e-mail message, potentially discoverable, is a legal document. Juries base conclusions on many factors, including the perceived professionalism of the defendant clinician. Accordingly, clinicians should compose e-mail messages with the same attention to such details as they use in ordinary snail mail for professional correspondence. Some e-mail enthusiasts claim that it would be a breach of professional duty for practitioners to deny services when e-mail would have been available.

Chat Rooms. Chat rooms are another arena for text-based communication with a patient. Eventually, research on their effectiveness will clarify when to include the use of a chat room in a patient's mental health treatment. Chat rooms assume that people can type quickly, especially if they want to stay in sync with an ongoing conversation. Hunt-and-peck typists are at a disadvantage. In a therapeutic environment, type-writing skills cannot be taken for granted with many clinical groups. Furthermore, impulsive people may also find themselves delighted with the unmitigated opportunities to react quickly. Typing ability and emotional stability, then, may interfere with a practitioner's exchanges that are attempts to be therapeutic in a chat room setting. The professional's own typing ability is also at issue.

Clinicians are advised to look for advances in technology development. For example, integrating a new voice technology may obviate the need for typing, eliminating typing inability as a barrier to participation. Some supporters of chat room use for therapeutic intervention advocate for their use for group treatment (Barak, 1999). In large, public chat rooms, a consumer may write about issues that are causing personal or emotional distress, and a professional in the room might respond with advice, support, and/or interpretation or might suggest coping strategies.

It is important for clinicians to remember that chat rooms are exceedingly difficult to secure, regardless of Web site claims for security. Unsecured chat rooms are not confidential. Let us be clearer: If a Web site claims to operate a secure chat room, be skeptical. To ascertain whether a chat room truly is secure, hire the services of an independent security company to try to hack its way in. Such companies can easily be found on the Web.

Another hazard to using chat rooms is that outsiders may have a legitimate right to access the information posted in a chat room. For example, a patient using a computer owned by his or her employer has in contemplation of law no reasonable expectation of privacy in any communication conducted using that computer. Similarly, under certain circumstances, Internet service providers may need to gain access to either the computer as a whole or, more likely, to the contents of its communications for maintenance. Clinicians should remind patients of this possibility when the presence of a mental health professional today tempts them to reveal more than they might feel comfortable with tomorrow.

Some professionals are posting contact information in the chat room in the event the consumer wishes to pursue private treatment. Such online promotional fishing expeditions are not yet popular, however. These seemingly fearless professionals appear to consider their work nontherapeutic and advice giving in nature. This activity by licensed professionals in the United States is naive.

Ethical issues related to chat rooms are still murky. If, for example, a drug manufacturer sponsors a chat room devoted to a particular drug, some professionals argue that the manufacturer should identify itself as the sponsor. Reports exist of physicians, employed by pharmaceutical houses, lurking on such sites to monitor, analyze, and report to the company on the statements made and opinions expressed. Given the ability to post messages anonymously or with a pseudonym, professionals or sales people can easily contribute to the conversation without identifying themselves or their affiliations. On the other hand, physicians, pharmacists, and/or other knowledgeable people who do identify themselves may tend to dominate a conversation. In general, with the possible exception of participating in a group therapy situation developed on a private and secured Web site, health care professionals should, from a liability perspective, exercise caution when engaging in chat rooms discussing health care topics.

Web Sites as Adjunct Treatment Vehicles

Existing Web sites seem to focus on the earlier stages of a patient's readiness to change, technically the easiest approach and the one least likely to raise issues of confidentiality and liability. Thus Web sites provide information about behavioral health, self-help, and mental health care.

In providing information, most behavioral e-health Web sites are static and passive, delivering preformed content on request, although most of the larger sites have enhanced navigation aids and search features. The more active Web site features involve discussion groups or other forms of interaction with staff or fellow visitors. Even though a static and passive Web site is less likely than a more active site to lead to legal entanglements, the passive site is not free of risks. Intellectual property, privacy, defamation, and other issues may still arise when using a passive Web site. In particular, an overly glowing description of the site owner's capacity to assist users paves the way for greater liability exposure. Marketing, which is a legitimate Web site function, should be undertaken with care and with the recognition that adversaries might misuse marketing statements to create contracts where owners intended none.

Examples of Treatment Web Sites. Some Web sites are exploring how to provide mental health treatment either in a stand-alone fashion or as part of a broader therapy regimen and with varying degrees of human support. For example, Student Bodies™ is a Web-based program that uses psychotechnology to provide education, behavioral change therapy, and emotional support. The Student Bodies site was developed to help young women reduce their dissatisfaction with their body image, develop healthy eating and exercise behaviors, and avoid eating disorders. Unhealthy weight regulation methods and body image concerns, which may predispose people to clinical and subclinical eating disorders, are particularly widespread among young women. Some 20% of college women may engage in binge eating (Bushnell, Wells, Hornblow, Oakley-Browne, & Joyce, 1990), and only a small percentage of this population are nondieters (14 to 18%), in comparison with the totality of casual dieters (42 to 44%), intensive dieters (25 to 31%), dieters at risk (10%), and frankly bulimic women (3%) (Drewnowski, Yee, Kurth, & Krahn, 1994). Based on these statistics, it was reasonable to conclude that a low-cost, Internet-delivered, computer-assisted health education program for young women might address eating disorders. To date, in a controlled trial, Student Bodies has been effective in decreasing the drive for thinness and in improving body image, but its impact on the incidence of clinical disorders has not yet been reported (Winzelberg et al., 2000). Another example of a Web site designed to improve mental health is MoodGYM (http://moodgym.anu.edu.au). This company has developed an Internet-based cognitive-behavior therapy intervention Web site designed to treat and prevent mental disorders.

Lingering Questions. Even though such programs have been shown to be effective, clinicians are not yet skilled in knowing when, who, and where to refer patients to mental health Web sites or how to coordinate treatment with Web site offerings. Continued research may answer some of these questions. Until then, each practitioner must try to understand how best to use these specialty sites. Nonetheless, until the psychotechnologies are developed to the point at which low-cost videoconferencing is available to the average practitioner and client through such communication channels as the Internet, such Web-based self-instructional programs will be the next wave of innovation in behavioral e-health treatment.

But what is treatment? Where should practitioners draw the line between preparation for treatment and treatment itself? Chapter 12 discusses informed consent and patient education as though these topics are merely part of the preparation for treatment, but the discussion emphasizes that these activities are ongoing. Even in the "precontemplation" stage of Prochaska's transtheoretical model of behavior change (Prochaska, Johnson, & Lee, 1998)—the stage at which a person is not considering behavior alteration or treatment in the foreseeable future—it is useful for the practitioner to present the person with comparisons between his or her behavior and that of people who are absolutely or normatively ill. This tactic increases the person's awareness of the need for treatment, raises the person's level of concern, and helps the person envision the possibility of change. Leading the horse to water at this point may be best accomplished through a Web site that questions visitors about their behavior, (e.g., using the CAGE to explore a alcoholism; Mayfield, McLeod, & Hall, 1974) and feeds back a rating and interpretation along with further information.

As a person progresses through Prochaska's "contemplation" stage to later stages, a specific therapist or treatment team can begin to play a more important role, as can online clinical practice (i.e., a formal series of discussions with a professional via one of the telecommunication technologies). Then, after the "action" stage, as the person moves through the "maintenance" stage to the "termination" stage, Web-based modalities may again become the main vehicles for the delivery of care.

As costs decline and online clinical practice becomes better understood, the use of audiovisual conferencing can be expected to depend less on special studios and videoconferencing installations and to spread to more ordinary locales. In addition, videoconferencing will converge with other communication modalities, such as those available through Web sites.

Managing Risk for Web Site Owners. The array of substantive legal issues important to Web site owners is broad: Intellectual property, labor and employment, professional liability, privacy, and defamation are just a few. Web site owners need to protect themselves, their content, and their readership. When developing a Web site, owners need a written agreement with the Web site designer. If the terms of the agreement are not met, the individual or association has a contract to enforce or at least someone to hold accountable. A site owner should also have built into the site a set of terms and conditions and a privacy policy, each of which should be accessible from each page of the Web site. These documents create a contractual relationship with visitors, defining their rights and responsibilities. Equally important, site content should be developed with an eye on legal issues, to avoid the inclusion of potentially actionable statements.

The structure of any agreement depends on what the practitioners are buying. The contractual elements for an online Internet practitioner will depend on the services purchased. Agreements range from a simple contract practitioners read and verify online, similar to the ones seen when registering with an Internet service provider for home-based Internet access, to a Web site hosting agreement with specific contractual elements.

The agreement can specify all expectations and deliverables (e.g., graphics of a particular size, number of pages, number of words on each page, specialized features, forms, promotional activities), including time lines for each deliverable and penalties for late delivery. Web site owners may want to specify the number of edits they are allowed for each page before incurring additional fees. The contract also can specify cross-platform compatibility or other words stating that Web pages must be accessible from certain versions of specified browsers.

Web site designers must make all access and permission codes available to the Web site owner from the first day of site development. Web site owners may wish to learn how to download all Web page files onto their own hard drives and to schedule regular downloads in order to have their own backups in case of server problems. Web site designers should list in advance all fees for such access or extra services. Web site owners are responsible for taking reasonable steps to protect privacy of their readership's identity. Therefore, agreements with Web site designers should provide that all designers will act in a manner compliant with applicable federal and state statutes and regulations, including HIPAA (discussed in chapter 9) and will comply with applicable Web site development guidelines, such as those defined by the

American Medical Association (http://www.ama-assn.org/ama/pub/category/1905. html) or URAC (http://www.urac.org).

Rather than rely blindly on a vendor, however carefully selected, or even on an Internet service provider's Web site package, the online professional should understand the underlying technology and be versed in licensure, ethics, and security standards. The Web site designer should assign ownership of intellectual property, including Web page code, copyright, domain name, and all locally generated Web site content to the Web site owner.

For stronger protection, the site owner should register all trademarks and copyrights. To ward off claims of infringement by other copyright owners, consider complying with the terms of the Digital Millennium Copyright Act (DMCA). Sites that have complied with the DMCA enjoy considerable protection from infringement claims. A site owner must post a policy acknowledging the copyrights of contributors and discouraging site users from infringing activities, must promise to take down any material that a visitor deems to be infringing, and must identify an individual (the DMCA agent) whose role is to respond to inquiries and complaints from visitors and other people who believe that infringing activity has occurred.

Web site owners can check content for correctness before sending it to the Web site designer (content can be expensive to change at a later time) and then again for content and formatting after the material appears on the Web site. Web site owners should avoid posting any content that visitors can misconstrue as defaming a third party, especially if the owner resides in the United States. Web site owners should treat publishing on the Web as responsibly as publishing in print; ramifications can be severe, if someone decides to file a lawsuit. Two examples illustrate this important point.

The Web site owner may be liable for any infringements related to plagiarism. Plagiarism is common on the Web; a visitor can easily copy any page or any content and reproduce it elsewhere. Assume that the Internet never forgets. Future employers or clients could see postings and articles for years to come. One of this book's authors recalls an episode of the ramifications of intentional plagiarism and implied defamation:

> *Several years ago, a colleague invited me to review his Web site. The site seemed well designed, but when I clicked on his list of articles, I noticed that he had copied an article of mine and posted it on his site, without citing my name as the author. When I wrote to discuss this finding, he told me that his Webmaster had told him that it was common practice to take information from other Web sites. I reminded him of our graduate training and of how plagiarism is plagiarism—with or without a Webmaster's approval.*
>
> *This episode led to the development of a Frequently Asked Questions (FAQ) page for my Web site, on which I address issues related to whether people can copy content from my site, either on their Web sites or for hard-copy handouts or magazine reprints. Over the years, we have had at least one request per month for magazine reprints, and the Q&A file has been accessed frequently for various types of information.*

Common law has evolved by applying well-established theories and principles to new situations, including situations undreamed of when the principle first appeared. Hence, copyright, which was invented by an ancient Irish *brehon* late in the first millennium to decide a dispute about a hand-copied manuscript ("To every cow her calf, so to every book its copy"), can be applied in the 21st century to thoughts conveyed exclusively by electrons.

Here is another example of how innocent professionals might find themselves
hamstrung online:

> *One day, Dr. Maheu received an unusual call for help. During a job interview, in which*
> *the caller was being considered to be hired as a psychologist for a large municipal office,*
> *the chief administrator summoned him into a separate room, pointed to a computer*
> *screen, and demanded an explanation.*
>
> *Posted under the psychologist's name was an essay touting the benefits of good com-*
> *munication in polyamourous relationships. The administrator was outraged to learn of*
> *this article and of what it supposedly revealed about the psychologist being interviewed.*
> *The administrator made it clear that he had "wasted his time," and that a supporter of*
> *polygamy would not be an appropriate choice for municpal employees in middle America.*
>
> *The contributing author/psychologist asked Dr. Maheu to explain to the administrator*
> *that the psychologist's article as it appeared online had been significantly modified from*
> *how it originally appeared in* SelfhelpMagazine *(http://selfhelpmagazine.com).*
> *For instance, when copying the article to the polygamy advocacy site, the word* wives
> *had been substituted wherever the psychologist had written* wife.
>
> *After the potential employer read the true version online, as well as Dr. Maheu's*
> *explanation, the psychologist got the job. Dr. Maheu then contacted the polygamy Web*
> *site Webmaster, urging removal of the polygamy article based on copyright violation.*
> *She never received a response. Continued inquiry revealed that the polygamy Web site*
> *was located offshore. Within 3 months, the Web site was no longer available at the same*
> *Web address, and owners of the Web address had abandoned it.*

Many Web sites are operated offshore or in countries other than where the originating Web site owner is located. In such cases, professionals attempting to redress
copyright infringement have little or no recourse, especially if operating on a limited budget. Professionals posting articles online need to be aware of these limitations.

Other infringements also can occur. With Internet communications, as with more
conventional communications, libel can be a viable claim. Widespread Internet broadcasting of a defamatory statement is likely to result in compensable damage. Even
when a statement is made anonymously on an Internet billboard, recovery is possible
if a plaintiff has the funds to hire an attorney, and can establish the identity of the
defendant. The courts rely on a concept that deals with newspapers and extends it
to libelous statements made on the Internet. The threat is all the more significant because, in general, insurance coverage is usually not available for this type exposure.
Moreover, because the damages in such cases are to some extent related to the extent
of dissemination, the Internet's worldwide range could augment the exposure far beyond the locale of a newspaper or journals reach. Also likely is that lawsuits will be
brought in countries where libel laws may be more troublesome and more difficult to
defend against than in one's own locality.

A Web site that exhibits unedited material contributed by forum members may
contain troublesome postings. Complaints against a Web site may involve allegations
of libel or plagiarism. Professionals and organizations operating a Web site should
publish and enforce policies for removal of improper material. Asking forum users
to send their complaints to the Web site owner through a convenient e-mail link on
forum pages is also a good policy. An editor should scrutinize articles posted by
professionals just as if this material was being published in an organization's printed

newsletter. Some resources relevant to digital publishing are:

- Berkman Center for Internet & Society at Harvard Law School (http://cyber.law. harvard.edu).
- Center for Internet and Society, Stanford Law School (http://cyberlaw.stanford. edu).
- Chilling Effects Clearinghouse (http://www.chillingeffects.org).
- Electronic Frontier Foundation (http://www.eff.org).
- Internet and Intellectual Property Justice Project, University of San Francisco (http://www.law.usfca.edu).
- Samuelson Law, Technology and Public Policy Clinic, School of Law, University of California, Berkeley (http://www.law.berkeley.edu/cenpro/samuelson).

Site Auditing.   Claims against site owners are increasing. The Association of American Trial Lawyers of America (http://www.atla.org), the organized plaintiff's bar, is actively coaching attendees at its continuing legal education programs to surf the Web in search of causes of action or of evidence to use in support of causes of action. In legal proceedings, site owners may have difficulty distancing themselves from information that is on their Web sites.

A legal Web site audit can help site owners understand what legal risks they face by posting site content. The site owner engages a suitable professional, usually a lawyer, or possibly a risk manager, to look at the Web site as a plaintiff's lawyer would. The reviewer scrutinizes each page, studying text and images for vulnerabilities. They reviewers report any such areas to the owner, along with a brief discussion of why the text cited or the image under discussion poses a threat. Often, the reviewer suggests alternative, lower risk language to convey meaning similar to that of the original. The reviewer also furnishes appropriate legal protector, such as a set of terms and conditions, a privacy policy, copyright notices, disclaimers of various kinds, and other documentation. Such audits cannot guarantee that legal claims will not be made, but they minimize risk.

The cost of a legal Web site audit depends on the size and complexity of the site and the number and variety of legal issues implicated on the site. Simple, brochure-style sites often can be audited for a few thousand dollars. Large, complex sites with thousands of pages and multiple issues can costs tens of thousands of dollars to audit properly. Thus, audit cost, is roughly proportional to the magnitude of the risk. In general, however, if the Web site owner can avoid even one claim, the service pays for itself. Litigation is costly in time, money, and emotional capital, and avoiding the process is devoutly to be wished.

Site owners who want to decrease their liability exposure but who lack the means or the desire to pay for a formal Web site audit can use McGuireWoods Healthcare Connect (patent pending) invented by Joe McMenamin, a contributor to this book. This proprietary self-help tool enables site owners untrained in law or in risk management to scrutinize their own material and to identify statements made and omitted and/or images projected that could give rise to liability. McGuireWoods Healthcare Connect is not the same as a professional audit and cannot provide the same level of protection. It does, however, offer guidance that for comparatively simple Web sites may be sufficient to decrease risk and improve the owner's comfort level.

Insurance.   Some malpractice insurance carriers belive that professional liability arising from Web activities is not covered under conventional policies. This position may be vulnerable to challenge in court, but few, if any, cases have provided much insight into how the courts will interpret insurance policies drafted before Internet use became widespread.

However, some insurance products are available to protect against the liability risks entailed in creating and maintaining a Web site. Some policies are specifically designed for Internet activities and ecommerce. Until the law clarifies how more conventional policies will be read, it may be appropriate to consider purchasing coverage specific for Internet-related risks.

Among the claims arising out of Internet activities that have the greatest possibility of protection under existing coverage are malpractice, defamation, and privacy. Liability arising from alleged malpractice might be covered by errors and omissions (E&O) insurance. Coverage for defamation and privacy may be available under comprehensive general liability (CGL) policies, particularly under the personal injury clause (as opposed to the bodily injury coverage clause). Web site owners should check for any Web exclusions, which are sometimes written into the insurance policies they purchase.

Claims that would be difficult to fit under most existing general policies are breach of contract (unless covered by endorsement under a CGL policy), antitrust (except defense costs, when the defense is successful), copyright (including code) infringement, trademark infringement, fire risks, and data losses. A Web site owner can consider purchasing coverage specific for these situations, if it is available.

Audio- and Videoconferencing

As we discuss here and in chapter 5, the important practical question *is not whether* to use audio- (e.g., telephone) and videoconferencing psychotechnologies instead of traditional in-person assessment and therapy. Rather, the questions to ask are *when, where, for whom,* and *how to blend* audio, video, and other psychotechnologies with traditional treatment in order to provide better access and quality to mental health services. Thus, when we describe the relative advantages and disadvantages of, for example, the telephone versus the videophone, we are seeking to clarify some of the more salient opportunities, limitations, and risks to consider while selecting options to develop a comprehensive treatment plan for any particular patient.

To be sure, there are cogent objections to behavioral telehealth. Inevitably, after acknowledging the convenience of audio and visual psychotechnologies, some people feel compelled to look for the apparent shortcomings in such areas as dealing with emergencies, conveying nonverbal communications, and ensuring patient privacy (as discussed in chapters 5 and 9). Some people seem to forget that for many years, no-fee suicide hotlines have dealt with countless anonymous first-time callers; the sense of urgency involved in such calls understandably overwhelms any misgivings about confidentiality and safety. That such services can flourish under harsh conditions suggests that the occasional emergency will not doom an audio- or videoconferencing interaction. On the other hand, practitioners should not forget that even though a mental health professional might not deem such an emergency contact to be a problem, a plaintiff's attorney might try to prove otherwise, particularly when the practitioners is using a new modality, such as videoconferencing technology.

Another topic of concern is how therapy at a distance must be inferior to being there and thus cannot substitute for the real thing. For instance, a professional can never be certain about what is happening on the other end of the line during a telephone consultation. Many people may be in the room with the client, lurking, popping in or passing through, overhearing private matters, perhaps commenting verbally or nonverbally, and otherwise compromising the therapeutic relationship. The patient may be eating, intoxicated, leafing through a magazine, surfing the Web, or masturbating during an encounter.

Problems also appear among professionals who use telephones for psychotherapy. Over the phone, the therapist has less incentive to stay attentive; the patient thus may have more justification for feeling suspicious and insecure about the therapist's level of engagement. The professional could easily be distracted. When using the telephone, practitioners who often multitask may open the next envelope from the stack of mail or may check their e-mail. The truth is that it is difficult to maintain consistent vigilance and sensitivity to the client when communicating over a distance. In an in-person situation, however, the client can see what the professional is doing. Even from the classic psychoanalytic couch, the client can steal a backward glance. The use of video in a controlled remote setting, especially with local therapeutic support or with an already well-known patient, minimizes these risks.

Clinicians should remember, however, that if these risks led the clients to view the results as less than gratifying, there is considerable risk that these clients might make a claim. There is no assurance that an enterprising plaintiff's lawyer will not persuade a jury to find the participating professional liable in tort should any outcome be realized other than that sought. Suppose, hypothetically, that in encoding, compressing, and transmitting the visual images, a technical problem had rendered it more difficult to discern abnormalities, thus hampering the diagnostic effort. If this problem had delayed diagnosis, the chances are good that some expert would have been willing to testify to a breach of the standard of care. A capable and aggressive plaintiff's counsel might try to embroider a product liability claim into the fabric of an otherwise relatively straightforward malpractice claim. In many states, tort liability can be visited on a product manufacturer who is not at fault. As always, there is the chance that one defendant will blame the other (see McMenamin, 1998).

Ethics Revisited.   As covered in chapter 10, a number of health and mental health associations are examining ethical issues, but few have made clear and substantial statements about each of the technologies discussed in this book. The American Medical Association (http://www.ama-assn.org) has issued an elaborate series of detailed and relevant statements. Other associations have made broad, interim statements that recognize that these technologies exist and are being used by practitioners, but offer a minimal amount of direction. For example, the statement by the Ethics Committee of the American Psychological Association (American Psychological Association, 1997; 2002a) suggests that existing ethical standards for in-person treatment also apply to behavioral telehealth. In both documents, the committee discussed the following areas as being of particular concern:

- Boundaries of competence—taking reasonable steps to insure their competence and protect patients from harm by knowing the advantages and pitfalls of using a particular communications medium.
- Assessment—being able to obtain adequate information to diagnose, understand, plan treatment, and monitor progress.
- Structuring the relationship—maintaining proper control over the circumstances of treatment, roles, and interpersonal boundaries.
- Confidentiality—an especially vexing problem in distance communication.

Professionals are warned that the ethical rules of their discipline, the licensure requirements of the states in which they practice, and the practice standards to which they are held all remain in full force. It's no excuse to say, "I was just coaching." If a complaint is made against the licensed professional, ignorance is not a defense for professionals working with people with social or emotional problems. Furthermore, the definition of standard of care varies because professionals are continually asking themselves what is reasonably prudent and are continually refining their answers. It is possible that the standard of care may eventually require the professional to make psychotherapy available at a distance. Practitioners should recognize, then, that the standard of care against which their conduct will be measured is not fixed; it is a moving target.

The defining characteristic of a profession is its self-governance. The requirement in most professional liability litigation—that the parties provide expert witnesses to opine on the standard of care—is consistent with this philosophy. The experts, familiar with and applying the received wisdom within their field, sit in judgment of their colleagues. This power to self-regulate is a privilege. Like all privileges, however, it imposes responsibilities. Too frequently, practitioners trained in the relevant field, experienced in patient care, and well versed in the advantages and disadvantages of a given source of action testify to ideas completely foreign to their peers.

OCPM STEP 7: REIMBURSEMENT

The push toward electronic service delivery is unprecedented. Practitioners need to follow the money to see what the future holds. Insurance companies probably will lead the way. They are slowly drawing practitioners to technology and eventually will encourage practitioners to use the psychotechnologies to make contact with patients. The Robert Wood Johnson Foundation–sponsored report by EvaluMetrix shows that the increase in online health care service is driven by the people who hold the purse strings:

> Because of the potential for substantial cost-savings associated with providing services online, insurers, payors, and employers may be anxious to substitute online services for some face-to-face services in the future. However, the ultimate impact of this transition on health care quality and outcomes is unknown because research on the relative effectiveness of online versus offline care delivery for most health services is nonexistent. (Eng, 2001 p. 75)

Reimbursement concerns arise in part because reimbursement models are still developing. Although practitioners are using psychotechnologies, these practitioners may not yet be receiving reimbursement through mainstream insurance carriers. Third parties are not enthusiastic about paying for mental health services in cyberspace because the current liabilities outweigh the fiscal benefits. Once research paves the way for attorneys to defend specific applications of the psychotechnologies, their use will predictably skyrocket.

Progress has begun. Some sectors have helped develop telemedicine and mental health programs through their reimbursement policies, including:

- Correctional medicine contracts to provide mental health services in prisons.
- U.S. federal programs, such as Medicare, Medicaid, and State Children's Health Insurance Programs (SCHIP).

- Health insurers in at least 18 states which have enacted legislation for reimbursement of telemedicine service.
- National health services in other countries.

Overall, delivering services through videoconferencing technology has been most successful at obtaining reimbursement for treatment at a distance from these sectors. This is no surprise; much of the research and funding focused on the delivery of behavioral telehealth services has been for videoconferencing. An acceptable assumption, then, is that videoconferencing will be one of the first telehealth areas to receive broad reimbursement from other insurance carriers. Blue Cross of California now reimburses professionals for videoconferenced services on a par with in-person rates (Brown-Connolly, 2001b). Other insurance carriers are experimenting with similar models.

Meanwhile, not enough appropriate analyses on reimbursement offer clear proof of the cost-effectiveness of using videoconferencing. Some studies show that telepsychiatry may be too expensive in specific areas of the U.S. (Szeftel, 1999; Werner & Anderson, 1998). More recent studies are surfacing with data indicating cost-effectiveness (Brown-Connolly, 2001b).

Commercial ventures, rather than legislation, may lead the way in reimbursement by making other telehealth modalities as cost-effective as interactive video consultation. In a disease management environment, advocates argue that more frequent communications with practitioners treating chronic problems will delay and, in some cases, prevent the long-term sequellae that can otherwise be treated only in an inpatient (i.e., expensive) setting. For example, in Europe, tds (Dermatology) Limited, based in Manchester, England, conducts about 2,000 teledermatology appointments each month, using store-and-forward technology (M. Alpert, personal communication, May 16, 2002). The potential for early identification of disease and for improvements in diagnosis and management promises cost savings to the delivery system in ways that may not require interactive video. Appropriate reimbursement based on the *relative value unit*[1] is needed for store-and-forward applications.

Text-based interactions may become a reimbursed service in mental health as well. At the end of the 1990s, half of the U.S. physicians surveyed indicated that they would use e-mail with their patients if reimbursed (Medem, 2000). But, as discussed previously in this chapter, most physicians don't want e-mail contact with patients, because it is another service they usually don't get paid to render. The American College of Physicians (2003) has called for reimbursement of computer-based care, stating that the major barrier to using e-mail consultations in health care is the lack of reimbursement. Currently, the private-pay sector comprises the majority of the reimbursed e-mail consultations in mental health. However, having clients pay fees monthly up front or by credit card for e-mail-based mental health treatment has generally failed. Some business-oriented professionals still hope to make this model successful. Eventually, they want to gain acceptance in the marketplace and compete with successful employee assistance work/life programs, which are very successful. Professionals who hope to expand their services through such online operations will need to present an attractive, reassuring, secure, and convenient interface.

---

[1] A Relative Value Unit (RVU) is often comprised of three factors when determining the reimbursement rate for work performed by a professional- work (or time spent), practice expense and liability insurance.

Several health plans, including Blue Shield of California, ConnectiCare, and Aetna, are conducting pilot projects to determine whether reimbursing physicians for e-mail consultations will reduce health care costs. Reimbursement for the secure, structured e-mail consultation varies; it often is around $18 to 25, or approximately 60% of typical office visits (Benson, 2001; California Healthline, 2001; Healinx, 2001; Laszlo et al., 1999). In a survey of 40 Internet sites that offered text-based therapy, sites offering group therapy through a chat room charged an average of $26 dollars for a 35-minute session, and sites offering individual chat therapy charged an average of $45 for a 45-minute session (Laszlo et al., 1999).

Other reimbursement strategies also are evolving. An ongoing joint pilot project of Healinx, Blue Shield of California (https://www.mylifepath.com), and the University of California, Berkeley, is looking at client satisfaction with webVisit, Healinx's new online clinical practice system for medical patients and physicians. Rather than using free-form e-mail messages, webVisit structures the doctor–client exchange through a series of questions and decision trees. Professionals can charge a sliding fee at their discretion.

RelayHealth, the developers of webVisit, sponsored another study. This study allows patients to visit with their primary care physicians online and handle business matters with medical office staff. A Connecticut-based insurance firm, ConnectiCare, offered webVisit to a pilot group of patients seen by ProHealth Physicians, a group practice of primary care physicians. The results are so convincing that other insurers reportedly agreed to pilot webVisit:

An "e-visit" costs a ConnectiCare member $5, and the health plan pays the $25 balance to the doctor. Other ProHealth patients, whose insurers aren't reimbursing for the e-visits, would pay the full $30 themselves. According to Jack Reed, ProHealth president and CEO, patients are using webVisit most often for tasks for which there's no charge, such as renewing prescriptions, messaging doctors, getting lab test results or referrals, and scheduling appointments.

ProHealth says that its patients, including those who aren't enrolled in ConnectiCare, have been averaging 350 to 400 uses of webVisit a month. Of those uses, from 150 to 180 are free administrative requests, such as for appointments and referrals, and 65 to 75 are prescription requests. Another 150 are clinical in nature, but these uses include queries for which there's no charge.

In Connecticut, the program has increased the productivity of ProHealth physician offices by reducing time spent handling simple telephone transactions. ProHealth also hopes to use webVisit for disease and disability management and for monitoring and helping some patients with chronic conditions, such as diabetes or back pain.

For medication refills, some patients and clinicians might find it more convenient to exchange e-mails. Similarly, copies of the prescription requests could be sent to the pharmacy via secure messaging. Many companies are developing secure e-mail messaging for this purpose. Some reimbursement models for this service charge fees to the clinician and patient; other models charge the patient and give a kickback to the clinician. In one study, physicians responding to e-mail from patients took on average only 4 minutes to reply (Borowitz & Wyatt, 1998). Satisfaction with e-mail as a means of communication tends to be high among both patients and physicians (Borowitz & Wyatt, 1998; Spielberg, 1998). Despite some of these potential benefits, reimbursement for e-mail continues to progress slowly.

We see a similar lack of progress for mental health practitioners in telephone use. Few clinicians formally track their commonplace and routine telephone calls, and, unfortunately, there has been little interest in arranging specific payment for these calls. Perhaps this is because telephone use is so casual and traditional that third-party payers have been able to escape reimbursing this activity. Clinicians know that refusal to use the telephone without being paid would hamper their effectiveness and could be characterized by other professionals as malpractice. Even though expanded telephone applications may enhance clinical outcome and modify societal mental health costs, this potential does not yet outweigh the insurance companies' short-term interests and competitive needs. Although expansion of telephone applications is occurring and although payment might some day be arranged once research demonstrates both efficacy and cost savings, the near future seems to be mainly with flashier video and Internet technologies. Eventually, payment plans that reimburse for videoconferencing time may be liberalized to cover certain types of text-based services and telephone conferencing sessions as well.

Reimbursement Legislation

Insurance reimbursement for videoconferencing is already mandated by some state laws; they reimburse videoconferencing but not other telecommunications methods (Thompson, 1996; Telehealth Improvement and Modernization Act of 2000). In general, U.S. mental health professionals are prohibited from collecting on expenses for using specialized telephone lines or equipment, composing or sending facsimile transmissions, or answering e-mail (Federal Register, 1998). Consider, for example, the California Telemedicine Development Act of 1996 (SB 1665), one of the first laws related to telemedicine. The act, which mandates insurance payment for telemedicine for specified practitioners in California, received widespread support among legislators (Schanz, 1996). A 1997 amendment to the act removed telephones and e-mail from its reimbursable services category. For other telehealth delivery modes not specifically mentioned, such as chat room or discussion board, the legal status is unclear. Details of this and other important telehealth legislation can be found on the Arentfox Web site (http://www.arentfox.com).

Medicare. Medicare defines telehealth services as professional consultations, office and other outpatient visits, individual psychotherapy and pharmacologic management, and, most recently, as psychiatric diagnostic interviews (Mulligan, 2002b). Practitioners eligible to receive payments under Medicare include physicians, nurse practitioners, clinical psychologists, and clinical social workers. Payment is available only if their services are furnished via an interactive real-time videoconferencing system. Telephone and e-mail services are not covered (Ballie, 2001).

The federal Medicare program has supported and funded a variety of telehealth demonstration projects since 1993. The 1999 U.S. federal budget covered interactive video services delivered to Medicare patients. Medicare reimbursement rates for individual psychotherapy and psychopharmacologic management via interactive telecommunication systems are now set at the same level as for in-person service (U.S. Department of Health and Human Services, 2001). Medicare reimburses for telehealth services if the client lives in a federally designated rural area or in a designated health-provider shortage area.

The Medicare Telehealth Validation Act of 2003 added county hospitals and mental health clinics or other publicity funded mental health facilities as eligible originating sites for reimbursement. The National Emergency Telemedical Communications Act of 2002 includes similar language, but its definitions of eligible entities and practitioners are vague (Nickelson, 2002). For the most current information about eligibility, fee schedules, billing requirements, and covered services, refer to http://www.cms.hhs.gov or to the Telemedicine Information Exchange (http://tie. telemed.org). For regular updates on Medicaid, Medicare, and other reimbursement issues, visit http://www.arentfox.com.

Medicaid. A summary of current information about state reimbursement for telemedicine service can be obtained on the Center for Medicare & Medicaid Services Web site (see http://cms.hhs.gov). In most cases, reimbursement for remote treatment is available only for services traditionally covered in the usual in-person manner. In some cases, the specific billing requirements include modifiers, and there may be exceptions for coverage. The mental health professional is encouraged to contact the appropriate state representative for current information.

Claims Submission and Payment Processes

It is clear that in the United States, electronic claims submission will become standard. Health insurers strongly advocate electronic claims submission and support their network providers in effecting a faster turnaround for payment. Bills can be processed more quickly and features built into the software to identify missing information before a claim is submitted. Electronic claims processing also is faster on the receiving end for the claims adjudicator to identify claims that require more information and follow-up.

Procedures for Obtaining Reimbursement. Procedures and standards for billing for online clinical practice in particular will be in flux over the next decade. Procedures for obtaining reimbursement for mental health services probably will be organized not by individual practitioners but by payer organizations, health maintenance organizations, and, perhaps, by vendors of electronic practice systems. Professionals should have a general perspective on the issues, but few professionals will become expert in all the processes. Obtaining optimal payment for such services may require practitioners to know coding standards for claims submission and electronic transfer of information for third-party payer or federal programs, such as Medicaid, Medicare, and the Children's Health Initiative programs.

Traditional billing codes use nomenclature of the World Health Organization's International Classification of Diseases (ICD) 9 and 10 and the American Medical Association's physician current procedural terminology (CPT) codes. In the United States ICD-9 nomenclature is used and in Europe ICD-10 nomenclature is used. Billing for services in the United States using the ICD-10 diagnostic nomenclature thus would probably be returned without payment. Although ICD-9-CM codes and CPT codes continue to be used, the clinical modification of ICD-10-CM will probably soon replace the diagnosis section of ICD-9-CM. However, payers will also need to be aware of and adhere to electronic commerce standards, called electronic data interchange (see http://www.wpc-edi.com). Professionals will need to check with the respective payer entities for the required format.

Federal programs generally use fee-for-service billing. Professionals use the Health Care Financing Administration (HCFA) Form 1500 when submitting bills. A modifier to the billing code may be needed. Mental health professionals should contact the appropriate state billing service and request information on how to complete and submit various documents.

Reimbursement for mental health services may depend on billing that uses specific codes for covered services (CPT, ICD-9, or, possibly, ICD-10). Telehealth reimbursement for direct patient care services is frequently limited to specific services identified by codes. For example, Blue Cross of California reimburses live online clinical practice for new and established patient office visits (CPT codes 99201–99205 and 99211–99215, respectively) and identifies the office visit codes for specialists for diagnosis, testing, and therapy (Brown-Connolly, 1999). The Medicare program publishes reimbursement criteria and billing processes on the Internet at http://www.cms.hhs.gov.

Another aspect of reimbursement is how payment will take place. The British Columbia Ministry of Health Services is accepting applications from a number of medical specialties for direct bank payments (i.e., direct deposit by payors) (Ministry of Health Services, 2002). The application is one-page form that requests information about the financial institution (name, routing number, account number, address, etc.), much like the standard direct-debit forms that are submitted for electronic payment for such bills as gym memberships, car loans, and health insurance. This trend, toward direct bank payments, which has not gained widespread acceptance in the United States for telehealth, is a natural step from the widely used electronic claims submission. Electronic reimbursement will save more time by avoiding the delays of traditional surface mail.

Risk Management in Seeking Reimbursement. How do professionals manage risk in relation to reimbursement? Avoiding fraud is a primary concern. Just as telephone consultation should be recognized as such when billing for psychotherapy, billing codes for treatment delivered via any psychotechnology should reflect the type of technology used with a patient. Although billing for technology-mediated services as if they were in-person services might be tempting, this practice puts the practitioner at risk for accusations of fraud.

To avoid the accusation of submitting fraudulent insurance claims, the best strategy is for professionals to speak candidly to third-party carriers in order to determine when and how telehealth services might be reimbursable. The following vignette describes one of the authors' experience in obtaining reimbursement for videophone contact with a patient:

> *Mary, a patient being treated for dysthymia and borderline personality disorder, was scheduled for a hysterectomy. She lived alone; had a history of sexual abuse, self-mutilation, and major depression; and had undergone two previous psychiatric hospitalizations for suicide attempts. She was distraught at the idea of not being able attend her weekly psychotherapy sessions, particularly after major surgery involving her reproductive system.*
>
> *I called her insurance carrier, explained the situation, and mentioned that a disturbance in the continuity of care at the time of hormonal fluctuations could easily lead to another psychiatric hospitalization for this patient. The case worker at the insurance company understood my concerns. I asked whether the company would reimburse me for four postsurgical weekly contacts through a videophone. The assumption was that Mary would be able to comfortably drive herself to in-person sessions after 4 weeks of recuperation at home. The case worker asked what videophones involved. I explained that they are similar to video cassette recorders (VCR) and plug into a telephone and a television at each of the two sites—my office and Mary's home. I then explained*

that I could call Mary by telephone and she would hear and see me through her telephone and television set. Likewise, I would be able to hear and see her through my telephone and television set. The case worker asked, "Oh, you would be calling her by telephone?"

Following my affirmative answer, she said, "Then we'll just bill this as a telephone consult, and you need to use the code for telephone consults for those four visits. I'll make the needed notation in her record that I've approved her for videophone consults using the telephone for those 4 weeks."

The point of this true story is that honesty can go a long way. An inquiring approach with the insurance company case worker, paired with information about this patient's need for continuity of care, led to a positive outcome. This creative case worker found a way to work within the insurance company system to get reimbursement for visits by telephone, which is the core technology for the videophone.

At this time, these are the important questions: When will the research and legislation support reimbursement? and which services will be reimbursable? As of now, a range of legislation related to third-party reimbursement for behavioral telehealth, telemedicine, or behavioral e-health has been passed or proposed.

Advocacy and Lobbying

Although advocating for one's profession is rarely taught in medical or graduate school, the state of mental health reimbursement and other crucial professional issues warrants that all practitioners become advocates. In relation to the telemedicine topics covered in this book, mental health professions should lobby government officials to influence the evolution of regulations and legislation about funding for research and reimbursement for remote care. Graduate schools and federal, state, and private funding agencies should encourage research on the efficacy of treatment mediated by the psychotechnologies. In this next section we will detail procedures to obtain funding to help the reader understand their availability, and the importance of continued advocacy for more such funding.

Grants. Federal funding through grants often has the goal of developing self-supporting programs.

A grant application for funding should convince the funding agency that the project addresses a real need in a significant way (Coley & Scheinberg, 1990). The nature of the project should be clear, and the setting should be described vividly so that readers can understand how the project will proceed. The request for funds should detail why the money is needed and how it will be spent. The objectives should conform to the funding agent's specific priorities. The project should promise the following:

- An imaginative and novel approach.
- Clear and attainable objectives.
- Relevance to the needs of a specific population.
- Potential generalization or extension to other populations or areas.
- Cost-effectiveness.
- Effective administration of the project.
- Promotion of the mission of the funding source.

Where professionals are offering direct care to a client through technology, these are some questions they need to address to help justify the cost:

- What combination of in-person and distance methods is most promising?
- Is this client an appropriate candidate for any particular psychotechnology? Why or why not?
- Are professionals prepared (e.g., do they have adequate skill, equipment, backup, fallback planning)?
- Even if prepared, is this the right professional for this approach and why?
- At what points in the course of treatment should any one or a combination of the psychotechnologies be used?
- How will the outcomes be measured?
- What is the backup procedure?
- What might the estimated cost range be for this course of treatment, taking into account various contingencies?
- How will this approach be preferable to traditional in-person treatment?

Advocacy and Lobbying Efforts. Advocates and lobbyists can use the findings from such studies to obtain legislation that provides for reimbursement and to tailor legal and ethical codes to clients' needs and to the particular requirements of each mental health discipline.

Perhaps in the near future, mental health professionals will be obliged to ask, How will in-person treatment be more beneficial than online clinical practice? Here, we quote part of the California Telemedicine Act of 1996 known as SEC. 6. Section 1374.13, which was as added to the Health and Safety Code:

> *(c) On and after January 1, 1997, no health care service plan contract that is issued, amended, or renewed shall require face-to-face contact[2] between a health care provider and a patient for services appropriately provided through telemedicine, subject to all terms and conditions of the contract agreed upon between the enrollee or subscriber and the plan.*

SEC. 10. Section 10123.85 was added to the Insurance Code:

> *(c) On and after January 1, 1997, no disability insurance contract that is issued, amended, or renewed for hospital, medical, or surgical coverage shall require face-to-face contact between a health care provider and a patient for services appropriately provided through telemedicine, subject to all terms and conditions of the contract agreed upon between the policyholder or contract holder and the insurer.[3]*

These code sections seem encouraging for supporters of telemedicine, except for two technicalities. They do not identify who decides what is appropriate. They also do not state that health care service and disability insurance contracts may not require clinicians to provide services through telemedicine where in-person contact is appropriate.

---

[2] Here, the term *face-to-face* denotes in-person. Generally, in this book we use face-to-face broadly, to include video communication, whereby the participants can view each other in real time.

[3] Details of this legislation are available on the Arent Fox Web site.

One dramatic effect of managed care in the United States has been to substitute ambulatory care for a lot of unnecessary and possibly damaging inpatient treatment. This change may be seen as an improvement, but it also is troublesome. Many mental health professionals have been dismayed at the extent to which they have been unable to provide hospital care when they were convinced it was necessary. Developing standards for hospitalizing patients and dispute resolution are time consuming. These decisions are made by a political process influenced by ideas of how to balance the good of the many with the good of the individual, as well as by research findings, cost analyses, and lobbying by volunteer professionals. In the case of selection of treatment venue—hospital versus outpatient setting—many practitioners regret not having been more proactive in lobbying for more control. Ideally, similar remorse will not develop about online clinical practice.

The California Telemedicine Development Act of 1996, one of the first laws related to telemedicine, received widespread support as it passed through the legislative process (Schanz, 1996). Why did insurance companies (with a strong California lobby) not oppose passage of a law that states that their health care plans shall not require in-person contact between a practitioner and a patient? No doubt the insurance companies believed that making treatment more accessible to more people would improve the population's health. Perhaps they also expected that substitution of treatment at a distance for some in-person sessions would result in substantial cost savings. We agree with this prediction. However, there is the danger that enthusiasm for less expensive care delivery can become more important than concern for the welfare of individual patients. Suppose that the practitioner determines that in-person contact is needed? There may come a time when practitioners will be glad that professional organizations lobbied effectively to preserve the practitioners' power to select the appropriate treatment venue.

The truth is that development of financial models can occur without legislative change (McGinnis, Williams-Russo, & Knickman, 2002). There is benefit in encouraging change without having to go through legislative politicking. In many cases, an employer has paid for health care services, but the employee has not been able to access them locally. By creating a burning issue in negotiations between health plans and employer and beneficiary groups, the telehealth beneficiaries could receive services not available in their own community. This approach will fuel competition between health plans and will provide for benefit expansion, improved access for contracted services, and improved quality and outcomes. Technology provides the means, and public demand will fuel the development of a delivery system that may be more equitable through the use of technology (Brown-Connolly, 2002b; Gold, 2003).

The reader is encouraged to act as an advocate and to contact various insurance companies to determine whether they offer reimbursement for services delivered through any of the psychotechnologies or plan to do so in the near future. Issues for advocates to investigate include which technologies the companies plan to cover and for which purposes, payment for telecommunication carrier charges or devices, and, for companies operating under regulations, such as the California Telemedicine Development Act, who decides when in-person contact is preferable to online clinical practice. Clinicians interested in learning how to advocate effectively can approach their state or national associations for help in making their voices heard.

The Near Future

Already late for his 8 a.m. meeting with Henley, Steve is sweating it out in the slow-traffic lane. As a stop-smoking ad comes on the radio, Steve jabs the button for the all-news station. Hearing his health insurance company promoting the new stress management feature on its Web site, Steve grimaces, lights a cigarette, and punches to a music station.

Two hours later, the meeting with Henley, the last person Steve wanted on his design team, ends with no agreement on the basic plan. Steve rides the elevator down to the building entryway for a quick cigarette, then returns to his desk to find e-mail from his supervisor moving the project deadline one day closer and asking Steve to work out a new timeline with Henley. The word "stress" comes into Steve's mind, and, just to put off facing Henley yet again, Steve clicks his computer browser to the insurance company Web site. The "What's New?" box offers a self-test entitled "Do You Have Stress or Does Stress Have You?" Steve enters his responses, gets a high score, and is presented with a choice of recommended online courses in stress management. Steve doesn't believe that he needs a shrink, but he decides that a computerized course can't hurt. He enrolls.

Over the next few weeks, with friendly e-mail reminders to accomplish his stated goals, Steve is pleasantly surprised at how much better he feels and at how many strategies he has integrated into his lifestyle. A few months after he completes the course, Steve experiences a difficult situation at work and notices that he is losing sleep, is irritable, and feels isolated. Steve remembers that help from trained psychotherapists in stress management and relationship skills was offered through the health insurance company's Web site, and he quickly locates a therapist in his geographic community. Steve is given the option of calling the therapist by telephone or completing a therapy request form via e-mail that is automatically forwarded as a secure encrypted transmission to the therapist he has chosen. He chooses to send an e-mail.

Between sessions, Dr. Simpson reviews her e-mail and finds Steve's request. From Steve's description of his problem, Dr. Simpson decides that this is not an emergency and that there are no duty-to-warn overtones, so by e-mail she offers Steve several appointment times. Dr. Simpson also directs Steve to a Web site on which he can complete routine office paperwork (verification of benefits, initial treatment authorization, assessment forms, and release to view his medical record). Over a secure transmission channel within his company's virtual private network, Steve can fill out a brief medical history form, including contact information for his other health care practitioners. After issuing a suitable disclaimer, Dr. Simpson recommends an online article related to his work situation for Steve to review. If Steve had indicated a more serious situation, with the risk of harm to himself or other people, she would have responded to him by telephone as a first contact to gain a more thorough understanding of his immediate needs.

Following two in-person assessment sessions, Steve and Dr. Simpson agree that she will see him in her office once per month and that the in-person sessions will be augmented with weekly videoconference sessions (available through the health insurer's secure Web site). The insurer's Web site provides Steve with guidance in selecting and purchasing a video camera that is compatible with his computer. Steve is pleased with how easily he can install it. Dr. Simpson further recommends that Steve participate in an online smoking-cessation program available through the same Web site. Dr. Simpson will receive regular progress reports to help Steve reach his goals for smoking cessation while they both work toward successfully managing his relationship issue at work.

This chapter is about the future, and it starts by describing a scenario that is almost here. What is new in this scene is the orchestration of existing psychotechnologies and in-person techniques to bring Steve from a position of denial to active engagement in therapy. Currently, practitioners don't have far to go to reach this level of technologically enhanced practice.

Steve's use of his employer's computer network raises a confidentiality issue. Companies have the right to inspect all e-mail and to monitor all communications carried out with use of company-owned equipment. A firm could waive this right (perhaps under union pressure) or could supply technologically secure tunnels or entirely separate networks supporting reasonably private transactions with specified entities, such as its employee assistance program, health insurance companies, and associated health care providers.

Reasonable guesses as to where technology and society are headed can help practitioners acquire skills to advance their practices. This chapter discusses innovations in technology and online clinical practice and the ripple effects on in-person treatment likely to occur within the next few decades. Readers should keep in mind the gap between the possible and the likely and realize that many clever ideas fall by the wayside. Having said this, consider the following quotations:

> *Radio has no future.* (William Thompson, Lord Kelvin, 1824–1907)
> *This telephone has too many shortcomings to be seriously considered as a means of communication.* (Western Union memo)
> *Everything that can be invented, has been invented.* (Charles H. Duell, U. S. Commissioner of Patents, in 1899)
> *I think there is a world market for maybe five computers.* (Thomas John Watson, chairman of IBM, in 1943)

In offering predictions, so-called expert opinion may be no better than sophisticated mathematic extrapolations or reading tea leaves. Even though forecasting is fraught with the possibility of failure, this chapter presents a scenario for mental health delivery systems in the mid-21st century.

There's both good news and bad news about the future. First, the bad news.

NEW INTERNET-RELATED ISSUES

Telecommunications and multimedia technology are reaching into living rooms and bedrooms. Cyberinfidelity and other Internet-related problems are emerging as clinical issues with little precedent. Practitioners can obtain specific information about these growing problems and about how to handle them in the context of the therapeutic relationship. In particular, the influence of the World Wide Web on sexuality is of concern to psychotherapists (Cooper, Boies, Maheu, & Greenfield, 2000).

In addition to cyberinfidelity and cybersex, some common Internet-related disorders involve engaging compulsively in day trading, online auctions, shopping, gambling, and/or interactive games to an extent that interferes with social and/or occupational function. Approximately 25% of online shoppers do their shopping at work (CEA, 2002), and about 33% of all Internet gambling casino traffic comes from users at work (Reuters, 2002). According to a NewsFactor Network study of 389 subjects, people who gamble on the Internet may be more likely to have serious gambling problems than do other types of gamblers (McDonald, 2002). Gambling through mobile wireless computers may be the next big revenue stream for online gambling.

The Federal Trade Commission (FTC, 2002) has found that minors can access gambling sites easily and that no effective mechanism for blocking minors has been established on gambling sites. The FTC noted that online gambling allows undetected and uninterrupted gambling for long periods of time.

Research in these area of compulsive online behavior should include:

- Personality characteristics of people who develop these problems.
- Neurological conditions of people who become dependent on Internet-related phenomena to the point of harming themselves or others.
- Interaction of drugs, alcohol, and prescription medications on Internet-related problems.
- Interaction of hormones on Internet-related problems.
- Classical and operant reinforcement principles.
- Technology inherent factors, such as time and place distortion, that sustain these problems.
- Assessment and treatment options.

As a first step toward understanding these problems, clinicians may want to experiment with chat rooms. In the following vignette, one of the authors of this book explains her use of a chat room workshop for professionals:

When I train professionals in a number of areas related to Internet behavior, from cyberinfidelity to the ethics of practicing online, I poll my audience members about their online experience. Although many people have used e-mail and have surfed the Web, only a small percentage have used chat rooms. Because many Internet-related problems with mental health significance occur in chat rooms, I constructed a sample chat room for professionals who want to explore this world without risk. It is easy to use and free. Just invite one or more colleagues to experience this world firsthand. Up to 20 people can meet at the same time. The chat room can be found at http://telehealth.net/chat/chat_room_agreement.html. When first accessed, the site displays a set of rules. Participants can choose to use an alias if they prefer.

Cybersex

Internet sex is boosted by the "triple A engine" of access, affordability, and anonymity (Cooper, 1998) that will also enhance mental health service delivery. Virtual communities, centered on every conceivable sexual interest and practice, normalize fantasies and practices that were condemned in the upbringing of many people, providing social support to people otherwise isolated, disenfranchised, or bereft of opportunities for satisfactory sexual expression (Cooper, Boies et al., 2000; Kim & Bailey, 1997; Newman, 1997; Weinrich, 1997).

The connection between sex and marriage is less binding in cyberspace. Even before the Internet, extramarital affairs have always occurred. Although some people experience guilt over consuming pornography or engaging someone online in mutual sexual stimulation, most participants claim not to view this behavior negatively and don't consider themselves to be cheating. Because their significant others may have different ideas, however, cyberinfidelity is likely to complicate many lives (Maheu & Subotnik, 2001; Schneider, 2001; Shaw, 1997). Nearly two thirds of the people engaging in some type of online sexual activity are in committed relationships. More than half of the remaining one third are involved not just in casual sex but in a continuing romantic or sexual relationship online (Cooper, Morahan-Martin, Mathy, & Maheu, 2002).

On the bright side, the Web's wealth of educational material on sexual health may reduce the anxiety many people have about sexuality (Williams, 1994). Greater openness, freedom of action, and tolerance of sexual diversity will probably result from the many controversies and exchanges of opinion posted on Web sites. The Web also offers opportunities to experiment, virtually, with new gender identities and sexual behaviors, be it via asynchronous text media or immersion in virtual reality. For researchers, the Internet facilitates conducting surveys (e.g., see http://www.selfhelpmagazine.com/cgibin/cyber_survey.cgi and http://www.socio.demon.co.uk/Cyborgasms.html#anchor352851) and otherwise reaching and communicating with study subjects. The Internet also is a new frontier within which to explore environmental influences on sexuality and thus perhaps to clarify a core component of human nature.

On a more physical plane lies the prospect of *cyberdildonics* (Rheingold, 1991). So far, the market offers few, if any, devices that a physically remote partner can operate over a communication network to directly simulate a sexual episode. Vivid Entertainment, Inc., once showed a prototype of a neoprene bodysuit intended to let people vibrate and tickle selected body parts, but safe, affordable, appealing, and FDA-approved equipment has yet to be marketed.

When suitable equipment becomes available, professionals might be tempted to consider providing remote sex therapy. A simple discussion with a client of sexual problems, even if supplemented by video-based education, is often inadequate. Practical physical exercises may be necessary to resolve a client's disorder. For this reason, sex therapists favor couples therapy.

Professionals have objected to recommending surrogate sexual partners for clients. This practice raises obvious legal, ethical, therapeutic, and personal questions. The approach may be unsuitable for certain clients and yet be useful for others, however (Cooper, Boies et al., 2000). Some objections to surrogate therapy might be assuaged by substituting video and remote devices for direct contact with either a surrogate or another willing sex partner (perhaps a spouse who could benefit from the physical and emotional distance technology provides). This solution would afford the client more options and the professional more safety and even more control. This area is likely to continue to be controversial, however, despite (or may be because of) the use of computers and telecommunication technology by sex therapists or surrogates.

The Younger Generation

With a majority of U.S. teens online, the Internet is having a profound impact on the lives of today's youth (Tapscott, 1998). Youngsters are as comfortable with chat rooms and e-mail as their parents were with the telephone and television. Young people conduct their social lives in a mix of in-person interactions, telephone conversations, and chat room discussions. Mental health professionals also may need to mix and match modalities to make psychotherapy seem as relevant to the lifestyle of the young. Future generations will probably embrace online clinical practice as a natural extension of routine mental health checkups and adjustments.

For now, it is difficult, if not impossible, to shield young people from the Web's sexual material and activities. Commercially available programs that wall off portions of cyberspace from youthful gaze are not foolproof. Also, they can limit access to topics that most people would deem morally acceptable, such as breast cancer.

Aside from the dangers of excessive sexual freedom and stimulation, people must recognize the more general limitations of young people: They can assimilate only so much information at an early age. As communication technology evolves, young people may be at risk for becoming overloaded. For example, how will 14-year-olds approach a first date if they have been secretly privy to their parents' cyberdildonics from age 8 or if they fear that a prospective partner is already expert in such matters? Will 14-year-olds reach for a date's hand during the movie or tentatively seek a good night kiss? What will happen after they share virtual sexual experiences in the privacy of their own bedrooms and get together afterward? How well will teenagers be able to restrain their impulses if they have been encouraged by electronically enhanced fantasies? Will children be disappointed when real life fails to match up with the fantasies depicted in passive entertainment media, such as movies, and also falls short of their own sexual experiences in virtual reality? Or, will such virtual training do away with maladaptive inhibitions and ignorance and improve the sexual health of the next generation?

These questions and their answers will soon become realities. Professionals should be considering their repercussions now. Research shows that a person's ability to build intimacy may be impaired if a significant proportion of his or her sexual development takes place in cyberspace (see, for example, Roffman, Shannon, & Dwyer, 1997; Schnarch, 1997). The market for child pornography and the financial rewards for exploiting children sexually have soared with the wide distribution of, and anonymous access to, child pornography provided by the World Wide Web.

Sex aside, communication technology is involved in a lot of psychosocial development in the industrialized world. Younger people use instant messaging (IM) freely and frequently to keep in touch and for casual communication. They regard e-mail as more formal than IM or speaking on the telephone, requiring in-depth attention and demanding a prompt reply when encountered in their mailboxes (George, 2002). IM and its associated jargon make for rapid staccato interchanges in which a serious message gradually emerges between the lines. The therapist who uses relatively ponderous, carefully composed e-mail may be unable to establish rapport or may be perceived as unable to appreciate or convey emotion. At the same time, any delay in responding to a young person's e-mail may be interpreted as a sign of indifference, neglect, disapproval, disrespect, or, most likely, simply being out of it, as shown by the following vignette:

You've probably seen adolescents, perhaps your own, giving their thumbs a thorough workout sending friends messages with cellular telephones using SMS (Short Message Service). In fact, many young people use this messaging system to organize social gatherings by adding friends to a group on their phone's address book and by sending the address of a party to everyone in the group via one send operation, much like sending an e-mail message to a list of receivers.

I'm told that new friendships are being forged this way and that kids move from party to party when they receive a new SMS. As with Internet technologies, downsides to the proliferation of the SMS mobile telephone system have also been discovered. One downside is the use of text messages by some children to extend their bullying activities. Bullying was first documented in British press stories suggesting that much of the activity was related to the British class system. Web-based institutes have been set up to combat this new phenomenon (http://www.redballoonlearner.cambs.sch.uk). The site's owner, as reported in the online magazine Wired, said that "text messaging is extremely powerful" and that "it is devastating for the children it affects. You don't know who did it, but you know it's someone you know. Someone who has your number and knows personal stuff about you. You start wondering if it was your best friend that did it. You can't get away from it, and two of our children got rid of their phones because of this very problem" (Ó hAnluain, 2002).

The Wired article went on to quote Alex Taylor, a researcher with the Digital World Research Centre in Surrey, who has studied children's uses of technology: "SMS bullying is like stalking . . . far more insidious than other forms of bullying. . . . The mobile phone and texting have meant that you can bring school home with you. That means that your school day doesn't end when you get home; you can still interact with your friends, and that can be very positive. But it also means that other less desirable school phenomena, like bullying, can follow you home too."

There is a further potential downside to the proliferation of SMS—and soon MMS (Multimedia Messaging). Some people may overuse SMS during their daily lives. Given that each SMS costs 25 cents and that some youngsters may send three or four in one exchange (just replying "okay" costs the same as sending a long message of 160 characters), some people could total very large monthly bills unless they self-limit.

In mid-2002, reports circulated in the media about a 25-year-old Copenhagen taxi driver who was sending on average 217 messages each day (Schreier, n.d.). His quarterly phone bill rose to $2,800, and he became "one of the first SMS-related patients at a Danish clinic that previously dealt with gambling disorders and has branched out into the treatment of people suffering from Internet addiction. In the past two years . . . some 60 people have received treatment at the Internet therapy center."

Research on chat room and SMS addiction was also reported in March 2002 at the first Prevnet Conference of Telematics in Addiction Prevention, held in Athens (see http://www.prevnet.net). Teuvo Peltoniemi, a Finnish drug rehabilitation specialist, presented "Net Addiction in Finland," interesting research suggesting that 1 in 3 people in a survey of 500 Internet-using Finns knew a "net addict."

As part of his presentation, Peltoniemi listed eight features leading to addictive SMS use, including the existence of a virtual social community, provision of companionship and social support, interactive activities, enhanced feelings of control and command, regulation of psychological distance (anonymity), role change possibility, escapism, and fulfillment of excitement or sexual needs.

At the First International Conference on HIV/AIDS and Substance Abuse (http://www.hopeconference.org/seven.html), held in India in 2000, Peltoniemi also reported on the use of mobile phones and SMS messaging in the treatment of drug abuse. Given that mobile phone use in Scandinavia is about 85%, it is not surprising that new interventions are being sought using such technologies, especially with the convergence of SMS, e-mail, and the Internet into one digital appliance. Peltoniemi also reported that self-referrals to his institute for drug treatment have increased 25% since his practice added Internet and *phone services. He cites anonymity and self-help aspects as likely reasons for reaching more people.*

—Les Posen, Ph.D.
Psychologist
St. Kilda South, Australia

Professional Issues

External pressures on practitioners to be aware, to be available, and to be avant-garde in delivering ethical services will eventually induce professional organizations to develop specific ethical directives and guidelines for practice involving the psychotechnologies. Until now, there has been only a modicum of direction in this area. Practitioner reluctance to explore the many uses of telecommunication technologies and the difficulties in obtaining reimbursement may be partly responsible. There is also a lack of scientific evidence showing where new ethical pronouncements are justified or needed.

In the absence of a body of literature on which experts can agree, the professions have adopted a wait-and-see posture. For licensing boards this amounts to awaiting a clear-cut test case in which an overeager practitioner has run afoul of existing standards. Such cases can help clarify the boards' positions and can serve as examples for all practitioners. The hope is that such cases will occur before patients are harmed—or think they have been harmed—and consult a lawyer.

In some jurisdictions, one standard defense against a malpractice allegation is the respectable-minority doctrine. This doctrine holds that a disputed activity falls within the standard of care if a number of practitioners are engaged in it. The basis for this doctrine is that the existence of an accepted theory underlying the supposed malpractice is indicated when many practitioners use the activity. In the relatively unexplored territory of cyberspace and the psychotechnologies, however, defendants may find little such support. On the other hand, the rate of increase in the penetration of Internet access is so fast that the array of practices possibly defensible under the respectable-minority theory could grow.

This leaves the field open to experimentation and innovation. Also possible is the appearance in cyberspace of practices and/or services based on the psychotechnologies set up by people who lack the background, training, experience, and constraints imposed by licensure and professional ethics on current mental health professionals.

The American Psychological Association has established a Web site (http://helping.apa.org/dotcomsense) to help consumers "protect your privacy and assess whether mental health information found on the Internet is credible and accurate." The site's focus is on empowering consumers, not on providing practitioners with an opportunity to augment their incomes by developing new revenue streams online.

Much work is still needed to make the Internet a safe place for practitioners to work with clients and patients. Some of this work is being forced on professional associations by HIPAA (discussed in chapter 9). During the next few years, the associations are likely to devote a lot of time and energy to complying with HIPAA rules (see http://www.apapractice.org). Only thereafter will professional organizations devote significant resources to setting up guidelines for relatively Internet-dependent psychotherapy.

So much for the dark side of the future. And now for the good news.

THE NEXT WAVE OF BEHAVIORAL HEALTH SERVICES

Some predictions are easy to make. Now on the horizon are next-generation technologies that will make mental and behavioral health care easier, more accessible, and more efficient. As brain mapping based on electroencephalography, functional magnetic resonance imaging (fMRI), and PET scanning become more clinically applicable, these technologies will work their way into standard practice (Nemeroff, 2001). Images that compare a patient's brain function with the pattern associated with various disorders and conditions could assist with diagnosis and could point up areas of relative strength and weakness for clinicians to consider in planning a psychotherapeutic approach. It may become possible for practitioners to efficiently predict and monitor a patient's response to not only medication but also psychotherapy by repeatedly imaging the brain while the patient is responding to selected challenges or performing certain tasks.

Furthermore, gadgets that measure physiologic responses will become less expensive and more versatile and will become integrated into newer forms of assessment and treatment. Therapists will no longer have to rely on the observation of sweaty palms or on such homilies as "cold nose, warm heart." Patients will be increasingly able to participate actively in augmenting their clinical records by completing computer-administered questionnaires. The data will be made available to the clinician as separate reports or automated analyses and also will be integrated with other material on record. This procedure will avoid flooding the clinician and the patient with unnecessary information while presenting potentially useful comparisons, summaries, and displays of trends. The computer will serve as an intelligent assistant, preparing drafts of reports and other documents that the clinician could then edit and endorse rather than having to generate each document from scratch. A somewhat similar procedure is in use in emergency medicine—through a series of prompts, a commercially available program helps the emergency room physician prepare a chart.

In general, the practice of having multiple paper records and possibly computer files for a patient will give way to an integrated clinical record system that interfaces with similar systems of various health care facilities, third-party payers, service agencies, and other involved parties. The electronic patient record will become routine before the end of this decade.

The Electronic Patient Record

In the United Kingdom, the National Health Service is working to develop and implement a uniform, systemwide *electronic patient record* (EPR). The Health Service hopes that the EPR will meet mental health and social service needs as well as the needs of general medical care.

In the United States, the Veterans Health Administration has computerized much of its clinical record keeping, and the various military branches are pursuing related initiatives. These organizations are hierarchically integrated and have the power to direct professionals to comply with centrally established policies.

Leaders in the health care field agree, and have agreed for decades, on the urgent need for an electronic patient record. Thus far, the problems in creating an EPR have been nearly insurmountable. Professionals resist changing their methods, are generally uninterested in record keeping, don't want to waste time filling out reports and writing summaries, and prefer not to expose their work to criticism. These are only some of the difficulties (Maheu, Whitten, & Allen, 2001).

The informational transactions involved in health care practice are extremely complex and poorly understood, and no one knows how to capture what is occurring in a meaningful, objective, efficient, and succinct way. In addition, medical information needs differ from one practice to another, and, once installed, an EPR is very difficult to change. For example, some electronic systems for entering data from physical examinations have no provision for recording head circumference, an important variable in pediatrics. A doctor would have to keep a separate file on each patient in order to handle such neglected data categories.

Of all health domains, mental health care is the most challenging in this respect. One key motivator for enacting HIPAA was congressional desire to encourage more widespread use of electronic record keeping in health care, which, it was thought, would help control costs. The resources expended on information technology in health care are dwarfed by those spent in other information-intensive fields, such as banking, for example. Many professionals argue that health care has paid a high price for this lack of progress in dollars, efficiency, and patient satisfaction. Now that the era of the Privacy Rule is here, perhaps the objective of an EPR will be reached more rapidly.

Mental health professionals often resent using an electronic clinical record system that makes more than rudimentary demands. As a result, the EPR for mental health lags behind EPRs for other health care specialties. This attitude may change. Mental health professionals know from their training that presenting a case to a supervisor and answering some well-aimed questions can lead to a breakthrough in understanding and a dramatic clarification of goals and plans. Why could not an intelligent automated information system come up with helpful questions?

Mental health treatment usually involves obtaining extensive information from clients, including facts, opinions, and thoughts. An EPR system could bring the client in as a partner in gathering this and other material, in organizing and summarizing it, and in suggesting interpretations and therapeutic interventions. Mental health treatment often requires coordinating the activities of an interdisciplinary team, interfacing with professionals from various medical specialties, and dealing with family members, various agencies, and community resources. An EPR can support much of this work, especially as so much communication is involved.

HIPAA requirements in the United States will force all the country's mental health professionals to grapple with electronic record-keeping issues. Few mental health professionals will have the know-how, resources, and interest necessary to create and maintain an HIPAA-compliant electronic record-keeping system. They will turn to large third-party entities for their software and data-processing services and perhaps to commercial vendors or professional organizations. The hope is that this need will create a competitive marketplace within which a cost-effective EPR for mental health care will evolve.

The information-handling needs of mental health care practice are too complex to be dealt with by filling in a few standardized forms or printing out a simple report. An EPR system will have to be highly integrated and sophisticated before mental health professionals will welcome it. The intermediate steps along the way to a record system that is sufficient may be painful and may temporarily interfere with treatment delivery. Mental health professionals must maintain an active interest in the development of EPRs to ensure that these records meet the needs of their profession.

An EPR can serve as a foundation for other psychotechnologies, particularly those that enhance and supplement communication between therapists and patients. Most of the clinical progress that can be applied right away in the psychotechnologies is now on the Web. Indeed, the mental health professional's Web site, rather than the EPR, may become the flagship for the other psychotechnologies.

Ongoing Changes in the Web and in Computers

Owing to its global span and its ability to stimulate innovation, the Web will inevitably grow, as it has from its inception. The greatest immediate expansion of the psychotechnologies is occurring on the Web. The main bottleneck in the Web's progress is social inertia. Now that it is becoming ordinary for the smart masses to have at least rudimentary computer skills, cyberspace is enticing many people (Gammon, Svendsen, Jenssen, & Bergvik, 2003). This steep increase in use, proceeding interpersonally and with no need for special commercial promotion, is termed *viral spread*. It won't be stopped, any more than were the mass uses of automobiles, telephones, and televisions.

Communication Channels. Additional build-up of Internet infrastructure may allow streaming video to reach an acceptable level of quality for online clinical practice before the end of this decade. In the United States, mental health professionals may soon be able to extend visual communication to their clients (Maheu et al., 2001; Yellowlees, 2003).

Broadband growth, however, which is required for expanded high-speed Internet access is hobbled by the continuing financial woes of the giant communication carrier service companies. Unless the federal government follows through on its intention to promote broadband access, few users, even in the United States, will soon be partaking of medium-quality streaming video and other fancy Web gimmicks available in cyberspace.

Brightening the dim prospect offered by a sluggish broadband market is the prospect of some viable solutions to the *last-mile connectivity* problem, that is, connecting broadband to people's desktops. Installing individual cables between the final main network communication trunk and people's homes and offices is expensive and cumbersome. Several start-up companies are poised to help people who live near very high speed underground optical fiber trunk lines yet who cannot get linked. The latest approaches involve local line-of-sight infrared or high-frequency, low-power radio transmission rather than wires. The receivers can act as little transmitters, passing signals along to other neighboring receivers to implement wireless outdoor *neighborhood area networking* (NAN). From remote control television to NANs, society is becoming wireless!

NAN is available in some locations. The Institute of Electrical and Electronic Engineers (http://www.ieee.org) has enunciated IEEE 802.11b, informally dubbed WiFi, a technical standard for broadband wireless communications over a radio frequency that is open for unlicensed or low-cost use at low power levels. WiFi-based networking has been implemented at strategic locations, such as coffee shops and airports, or near the homes of public-spirited hobbyists, often for free, to the dismay of companies trying to profit from the technology. A subscriber (or, in some places, just anyone) can sit on a park bench with a laptop, log in, and be on the Internet for as long as the batteries hold out. A faster technical standard (IEEE 802.11a), less subject to crowding and interference, will probably soon overrun the earlier one. But beware: Practitioners should not transact sensitive communication over dubiously secure systems (Murphy, 2002).

Wireless communication in general may be a bigger revolution than the Internet (Bennett, 2001). WiFi, with each network confined to a very small local area (a so-called hot spot), is one of many competing methods. Although most mobile phone service providers cannot offer fast broadband connectivity, they offer subscriptions to e-mail and Web page transmission. A sizable market exists for this service despite the spotty coverage, slow interaction, small readout screens, and difficulty of writing with a tiny keyboard or a little stylus. Clearly, there also is a market for better connections for both mobile computing and desktop machines.

Several enterprises offer broadband communication via geosynchronous satellites. This service is comparable to television service; a transceiver (combination transmitter and receiver) hovers in an orbit that keeps it more or less constantly above a fixed geographical location as the earth rotates. Such broadband services may produce $2.95 billion in revenue in 2006, compared with $210 million in 2002 (Marek, 2002). Two-way wireless Internet access may come to account for 60% of home Internet use in the United States (IDC, 2000). In the future purchasing broadband satellite service may be like purchasing POTS (Plain Old Telephone Service) Internet service today.

Wireless technologies are particularly relevant to rural areas in the United States, Australia, Norway, and Sweden and also to most of India, China, Indonesia, Brazil, Nigeria, and to any other country in which stringing wire or cable is prohibitively expensive.

In highly industrialized cities, where Internet connectivity is available by phone at a reasonable price, wireless access has become popular for social correspondence, particularly for inconsequential text messages between friends and for playing interactive games. Interactive games require high data transmission rates and are a major impetus for WiFi. So many people may be willing to spend money on handheld computers and wireless service subscriptions to play games and correspond electronically that mass production may drive the costs down to a point at which even mental health care delivery could take advantage of the rapidly evolving technology. The expansion of the wireless Internet is expected to spark a new class of e-health applications.

In chapter 2, we distinguish between carriers leasing transmission channels (e.g., broadband wireless connections) and telecommunication devices (the computer being a prime example). The power of the personal computer has been growing at such an astounding rate that a typical laptop now has much more computing power than did the giant mainframes of yore. Despite this increase in power, the future of computing in health care seems to lie less in increasing the capabilities of personal computers than in storing and processing information remotely. Computers seem destined to revert to being terminals for larger systems.

Redefining the Computer. Personal computers have evolved from being mainframe accessories to functioning as powerful stand-alone tools. Increasingly sophisticated operating systems, such as Windows and Mac OS, support elaborate and highly capable word-processing and database programs. The Internet, however, and particularly the Web, together with broadband communication services, are causing the pendulum to swing back. Moore's law holds that the speed and power of computers double every 1.5 years. This prediction has been remarkably reliable for decades and will apparently continue to be reliable for several more years. Enhancing the utility of personal computers, however, no longer depends on ever-larger memories or ever-faster central processors but instead involves using the machines as clients of centralized servers—definitely a retro trend.

It now is common for people, even many mental health professionals, to have more than one computer. (This includes mobile phones that are almost a computer and also the full-featured answering machine, the digitized cable television converter, the handheld personal assistant [PDA], and the digital camera.) A type of future technology that may accompany a person everywhere may be something like the Guardian Angel (Dertouzos, 1997; Motluk, 2000). The Guardian Angel is a type of personal lifelong active medical assistant, which may soon store the entirety of a person's health information, schedule appointments, pay medical bills, and automate medication reminders.

In today's world of digitized gadgets, it will be in society's best interest to have them interconnected, cooperating, and sharing resources. Home networking and the installation of digital intelligence into many home appliances, including the home security system, coffee pot, and refrigerator, will be advocated by advertising campaigns trying to convince people to purchase the latest in home entertainment systems. In smart houses are on the market, lights turn themselves on at night and off when not needed, the air conditioning and heating systems adjust themselves to the seasons, and the coffee maker turns on and brews in time for breakfast. As a spin-off, people will speak of their personal digital network rather than of their computer.

Multiple machines in this network means multiple vulnerabilities, however. Professionals will have to know how to guard sensitive information they place on their networks because the communication pathways and storage media might also be used for their collection of music and the cartoon videos they play for their children.

The computer is becoming not only a more diffuse but also less passive entity. The old-style computer obeyed the lists of commands that constituted a program. Newer computers are interactive and respond to users through a graphical user interface. Soon, computers will function like hunting dogs, seeking out desired material and retrieving it, sometimes on request but increasingly in anticipation of the user's wishes.

The next section discusses intelligent agent programs. It discusses how computers are being further redefined and losing their individuality as they revert toward the client–server or mainframe–terminal configuration, with the heavy work done elsewhere and the local computer providing an interface with the remote system. The discussion includes briefs accounts of grid computing (in which computers are combined for added power), utility computing, open source programs, application service providers, and security technologies.

Intelligent Agents.   One major shift in the Internet may be a transition from today's human-driven applications—sending e-mail, watching the news on streaming video, or communicating via videophones—to applications in which people play little or no role. Most Web surfing may be done by *intelligent agents*, which are automated personal assistants that ferret out resources, make purchases at optimal times from optimal sources, set up appointments, and present information in a structured way. Intelligent agents charged with mental health duties can supervise behavioral homework practice and medical regimens and can provide reminders.

In addition to recognizing key phrases, such programs can consider the source of information and its context, the user's expressed preferences, and the program's past interactions with the user. Increasingly, search engines can achieve relevance to the user's intended search topic. Programs can rephrase technical, medical, and scientific terms into more common expressions. Practitioners therefore can expect an intelligent agent to hunt through cyberspace on their behalf and to return with an organized and succinct summary of its findings tailored to suit each professional's needs.

For example, the question "Does my health coverage exclude the fire walk planned as my office's next corporate bonding exercise?" could receive an accurate answer, accompanied by a form to fill out for low-cost disability insurance that would supplement Workers' Compensation. Synthetic agents with access to a database of the user's preferences, characteristics, and previous choices may be available via mobile phone and wireless networks.

Many people who have tried to purchase airline tickets or win an eBay auction have experienced confusion and frustration. How, then, can they expect an intelligent agent to make meaningful decisions about what to bring to the user? The answers are XML and SNOMED.

eXtensible Markup Language (XML) provides a way of explaining what data refer to by attaching tags to them. For example, the datum $3.57 can be tagged <FEE>$3.57 </FEE> to indicate that the dollar amount refers to a fee. If an intelligent agent can understand XML tags and if the same tags are used on many Web sites, then the agent can compare therapists and recommend the one with the cheapest interpretations, among other relevant attributes.

Various controlled vocabularies can be used to standardize tags. The *Systematized Nomenclature of Medicine* (SNOMED; http://www.snomed.org) is among the languages that are appropriate for health care and agreed on by leading medical organizations. If a Web page presents information embellished by SNOMED-compliant XML, the tags are not shown on the screen, but a computer program can understand the data. Thus, an intelligent agent could potentially evaluate the nature of a person's problem; calculate how many interpretations it would take to clear the problem up; add up the 2-cent interpretations, the 5-dollar ones, and so on; and give the user an estimate of what a successful course of psychotherapy would cost.

Now we can pull back from the too-distant future to consider more immediate trends. Recall the pendulum, which is swinging back to using computers as servants of larger entities.

Sharing Mousepower

In "Answer," Frederic Brown's (1977) classic science fiction story, the chief scientist solders the final connection uniting the world's supercomputers at the inaugural ceremony for an awesome new system and smugly poses the initial question he has prepared for the machine: "Is there a God?"

Suddenly, the scientist has a terrible insight. He lunges at the power cord, but before he can yank out the plug, a giant spark flashes from the computer, killing him instantly. This answer then appears on the printer: "Now there is."

The notion of *grid computing* is nearly two generations old (Licklider, 1960), and it may be another generation before it becomes widespread. When grid computing arrives, it will again revolutionize how we live and work with computers.

Just as electricity is fed by generating plants into a power grid from which users extract what they need, multiple computers can be connected, using the Internet to pool their resources. Even during active use, computers usually operate at a small fraction of their capacity, spending most of their time awaiting the next keystroke. Combining the unused mousepower of thousands of small computers results in the equivalent of a supercomputer.

Grid computing is already a reality. One Web site, SETI@Home (http://setiathome. ssl.berkeley.edu), uses idle time on personal computers to search for extraterrestrial intelligence. Pharmaceutical corporations use a grid configuration to sift through imaginary compounds for shapes that might fit key cellular receptor sites to alter the body's physiology. The U.S. Department of Defense has grid computing volunteers testing compounds that might similarly block smallpox attachment to cells. Computer manufacturer Gateway has connected the thousands of computers displayed for sale in its retail outlets and rents out their combined power by the minute (Greenemeier,

2002). The ultimate prospect of grid computing, however, is not so much to cheaply emulate expensive supercomputers as to turn the Internet into an enormously capable computing platform that anyone could rent.

Utility Computing.   The *utility computing* model for providing information technology services to an organization involves purchasing computer time, renting storage space, and paying for the use of programs from an outside vendor on an as-needed basis rather than using personal equipment or leasing facilities by the month or year. This model resembles how people pay for groceries and gas, in contrast to the rent or mortgage, which is due monthly. Blue Cross and Blue Shield of Michigan uses the utility approach for certain operations, but the utility computing infrastructure is still too new and untested to warrant entrusting it with direct patient care–related functions (Greenemeier, 2002).

Web Services.   An important trend in information technology is to use automated shopping for computer assistance. For example, the intake process for a new client can be broken into many small subtasks. To accomplish each subtask under a *Web services* scheme, the practitioner's computer searches a directory for vendors that can perform the work and ranks them on the basis of cost, effectiveness, and past performance. Then, rather than wait an extra few milliseconds if the first choice is busy, the computer contracts with an alternative source, gets the job done, and pays the fee. The computer then may use the result for the next subtask, farming all the work out expeditiously. This scheme may eventually have some relevance to data processing for mental health services.

Although the topic of Web services may seem far afield from the direct concerns of a mental health practice, computer industry pundits predict that Web services may hasten the demise of elaborate operating systems, such as Microsoft Windows. One possible outcome for mental health is *distributed computing*. In distributed computing, data processing and data storage occur at various locations both on a local network and across the Internet. This process may undermine monopolistic trends and enable the EPR and other psychotechnologies to evolve in response to market pressures. Thus, mental health professionals would be able to select one vendor for describing a patient's sense of identity diffusion and another vendor for an intervention involving homework exercises for assertiveness training.

Open Source.   Like windows, most software in use is licensed, protected, controlled by a commercial enterprise, and priced accordingly. In contrast, in its most general sense, *open source* refers to an idealistic virtual community of software developers who freely share their ideas and programs to create and make available many types of computer applications (see http://www.opensource.org). The source code behind the programs is published on the Web and is not copyrighted. Anyone may modify it, and programmers eagerly write upgrades and improvements.

The vast number of such programmers and their enthusiasm and communal spirit let open source program development outpace the more cautious, committee-bound, market-researched approach of commercial software foundries. Many of the kinds of software in everyday use, such as word processors, e-mail programs, and Web browsers, originated as free programs. Open source software is often more secure, less subject to attack by viruses, and less expensive to maintain. Thus far, however, the open software movement has been unable to overcome the problems posed by the diversity of desktop and laptop computers and peripheral equipment. Thus, attempting to install open source programs and make them work with existing hardware setups can drive even computer experts back to Windows.

Web site developers are cautioned against using vendors that would not consider using open source as opposed to a proprietary software package to program a server, for example. A vendor agreement to use proprietary software should provide for free or deeply discounted rates for translation to open source if the professional paying for the Web site decides to use open source within a reasonable period of time, say, 1 year after Web site construction.

Application Service Providers. *Application service providers* (ASPs) will soon be prevalent in mental health service delivery. These firms accept data over the Internet from their subscribers, process the data, and return results on a pay-per-use basis. This arrangement is similar to the original client–server configuration, in which a central mainframe accepts input from and sends output to terminals or workstations. The main technical difference is that now, the information travels over the Internet rather than over cables within a building. The more important difference is that ASPs do not run programs remotely but instead undertake complex processing assignments, such as the automation and communication tasks involved in back-office functions: billing, bookkeeping, obtaining authorizations for treating clients, and so on. Managed care organizations are understandably eager for professionals to adopt ASPs to improve the organizations' communication with and control over their provider networks and also to promote efficiency.

Despite the many potential advantages of computerizing every level of mental health practice, from solo professionals to large hospitals, the process remains difficult, time consuming, and fraught with mistakes—and the results are usually unsatisfactory. Theoretically, an ASP could resolve most of the difficulties. Ideally, an ASP would take care of infrastructure problems, such as data storage and backup, security, and software purchasing, licensing, and upgrading. Local computers that feed the central ASP need not run at high speed or have large memory capacity. The subscriber no longer needs to have much personal expertise or to hire a computer expert to fix computer problems.

Paradoxically, the centralized control an ASP exercises over security could make computer use for behavioral health care much more secure. Keeping a site secure from intrusion, providing adequate backup, and keeping abreast of and complying with HIPAA and other regulatory requirements are beyond the abilities of most professional practices, associations, and hospitals—and may even be too much for most medium-sized commercial ASP enterprises.

In light of this limitation, large health care providers, such as hospital chains or university hospitals, and large health maintenance organizations and insurers are likely to become ASPs. They would gain financial stability and also could develop more effective measures to protect confidential information. Unaffiliated professional practices and organizations would then probably contract with these large centralized and specialized services for much of their computer support.

As they take on total computerization of health care practices, ASPs may be able to provide many professional and managerial services, including accounting, purchasing, promoting, and recruiting, to the point of taking over and consolidating practices into ever-larger provider organizations. Much as the giant conglomerates of the future (e.g., comprising insurance, health maintenance, accounting) will be profiting by managing professionals, Web service providers may be profiting by managing data processing for them. Each additional level of complexity, however, introduces further opportunities for error, skullduggery, hidden costs, and lawsuits.

Farming computerization out to ASPs carries several major, perhaps fatal, disadvantages. It is very difficult to change from one ASP to another. Their data formats, workflow patterns, reports, and proprietary information are difficult to transfer or obtain. If an ASP performs poorly or is acquired by another firm with a reputation for treating confidentiality issues too casually, the contracting party may still be stuck with it. If the new concern goes bankrupt, all the clinical data may be jeopardized, and files of accounts receivable and authorizations may be lost. Worse, the newly bankrupt company, desperate for funds, may sell the data, as in the Toysmart case (see http://www.ftc.gov/os/2000/07/toysamrtthompsonstatement.htm). Furthermore, giving a remote commercial enterprise unencrypted sensitive clinical data to process seems risky and may lead to legal problems.

Security. As exchange of personal information over the Internet becomes ubiquitous, technology that safeguards individuals' privacy will have to keep pace. For online clinical practice, the professional may need to determine the identity of a client who participates in a Web-based treatment program. Some people will undoubtedly try to fake their identities to gain access to certain therapy groups (e.g., groups related to sexual compulsion). Access to these groups will have to be protected.

Authentication services and digital signatures are protection tools in use (Maheu et al., 2001). The front-runner approach to security for health care is called *public key infrastructure* (PKI). PKI combines software, encryption technologies, and services. *Digital certificates* issued to individual users are used to sign documents in a way that assures the document's reader that its author has been authenticated and that the document has not been altered or corrupted in transit. The electronic signature supports *nonrepudiation* so that the document's author cannot credibly disclaim responsibility for having created or endorsed the document. Digital certificates can replace passwords (which are usually easily guessed and frequently lost) as a means of enabling users to gain access to information and services.

Keyboards of the future may come with integrated identity card readers. Instead of credit cards, people could carry electronic smart cards with a built-in memory. Members of the U.S. armed forces are using this technology. A smart card can positively and unambiguously identify the bearer to a computer. A smart card also can contain encrypted information about the bearer's credit balance, medical insurance, medical history, and medication use. Such sensitive material would not have to be transmitted from a remote database to be made available to the local computer. Of course, the bearer would have to supply some kind of key to enable the information in the smart card to be read. This feature is necessary to protect the information if the card is misplaced or stolen.

Biometric technologies, such as fingerprint or retinal scanners, though not sufficiently foolproof to protect sensitive medical information (Thalheim, Krissler, & Ziegler, 2001), may become more cost-effective (Andress, 2001) and more reliable and may eventually complement identity cards.

On the other hand, smart card technology has not caught on commercially and may be superseded by a better technological invention before it becomes widely used. For example, there is now an implantable identification device about the size of a grain of rice that, when energized by an external scanner, emits a unique verification number (VeriChip Corporation at http://www.adsx.com/prodservpart/verichip.html). This number is being used as a key to unlock medical records in case of an emergency (Garcia, 2002). Another technology that could support a highly tamper-resistant and extremely secure authentication methodology was reported by the MIT Center for Bits and Atoms (Pappu, Recht, Taylor, & Gershenfeld, 2002).

Verifying an Internet user's identity may also be possible through the user's *enumber*, or ENUM, a universal identifier that would link the person's Internet address and phone number. The communications industry envisions a sophisticated global electronic address book directing messages to various personal communication devices, such as a fax machine, computer, or telephone, using the 11-digit ENUM. Because it could help reach people wherever they may be at any moment, an ENUM system could make it easier to remind people to take their medicine or to make an entry in their symptom diary. However, the universal identifier represents a leap in private data warehousing and would dramatically increase the risk of privacy invasions. The system is promising because of its convenience, but it will need built-in safeguards.

Ripple Effects. Some degree of Internet-based mental health service delivery is being taken for granted in industrially developed countries. As the novelty and misgivings recede, popular demand for electronically mediated health services will grow. Professionals will respond in many ways to satisfy the market. Many people access the Web as their first source of authoritative information (and, unfortunately, misinformation masquerading as authoritative information) about psychological or relationship problems. As the provision of such information becomes better integrated with secure, valid, and reliable treatment options, overall mental health care use rates may increase. Internet-based services are an ideal complement to traditional mental health services and can reduce costs, improve outcomes, and reach people who need help but have been reluctant to seek it. Using the World Wide Web's dissemination network, therapists can make their expertise widely available, adapt their services to meet multicultural and multilinguistic requirements, and deliver quality care to people within the convenience of their homes and communities. Other psychotechnologies will come into common use, brought into the mainstream by clients' and professionals' acceptance of electronics in mental health care.

Whither the Web? The World Wide Web was designed for text documents. Browsers have added sound, animation, video, and interactive communication, making a Web site the best base for the professional online presence. As the Web becomes the main organizing system for professional electronic communication, the Web browser will become the dominant front end for personal computer use. Even the operating system that runs the programs on a personal computer is becoming less important than the browser, which sends data to remote computers and then formats the response for presentation on the local screen.

Many clinicians and professional associations are developing Web sites to explain their practices and offerings. Increasingly, their sites include features that improve administrative efficiency, such as appointment requests, membership applications, and registration forms for symposia.

E-health Web sites are becoming more interactive, extending office-based services to cyberspace and giving clients access to practice personnel in order to schedule appointments, renew prescriptions, and ask brief questions. The emerging one-stop supersites are set to become channels for more extensive direct patient contact with practitioners as well as channels for the interaction of clients with their own medical records (Bernard, 2000; Stevens, 2001).

As agencies that regulate health care adopt a less paternalistic approach (Lièvre, 2002) and relax their standards in response to industry pressure (Moynihan, 2002), more dangerous drugs and devices may be approved for over-the-counter and prescription sale. Furthermore, as the psychotechnologies proliferate, as more mental health approaches are developed, and as more mental helpers enter the marketplace, patients will have to determine a correct balance between risk and benefit and then select suitable treatment approaches. Dr. Mark Blatt, of Intel Corporation, predicts the following:

> Home health care information technology (HCIT) is just emerging as a commercially viable solution after more than a decade of research and pilot programs. The main reason for this, at least in the United States, is that a reimbursement model, in the form of prospective payment systems and disease management programs, is also rapidly emerging. This technology is developing in the rest of world at even a quicker pace; in the last 3 years, the cost of these systems has dropped dramatically while the reliability and the flexibility of the system tools have improved dramatically.
>
> Mobile home networking is on the verge of becoming a reality. LAN-in-a-box technology, on both the client and the networking sides, is emerging and within the next 12 months will be a reality. The presence of this technology will lead to a jump in the emerging field of remote patient monitoring. The clumsily wired intermittent connections to PC-like boxes will be replaced by constantly connected 802.11a/b sensors that link to easy-to-use push-button Internet appliances. Countries with more established broadband infrastructures (countries in Europe and parts of developed Asia) will benefit the most, whereas the United States will lag. As WANs (wide area networks) become more reliable in these same areas patients will be able to leave their homes and still be constantly connected to their providers.
>
> The future of acute care medicine will change slowly with these ubiquitous connections, but the near-term changes in the management of such chronic illnesses as diabetes, congestive heart failure, chronic obstructive pulmonary disease, and systemic hypertension will be more dramatic. Because of continuous monitoring, these illnesses will be treated more effectively, and deviations from good control will be identified quickly before they become dangerous to the patient and costly to treat.
>
> Technology, in some small way, will be the answer to the daunting access issues medicine faces owing to ever-increasing demands for services and the ongoing scarcity of skilled resources. (M. Blatt, personal communication, October 24, 2002)

Dr. Blatt is probably correct about the direction in which mental health care is headed and perhaps is right about the rate at which the field is proceeding. The field has tools that allow relatives or caretakers to monitor the elderly in an independent living arrangement and thereby to delay or avoid nursing home placement. The technologies Dr. Blatt describes as imminent are more sophisticated than are current technologies but are in principle simply extensions of them.

Nonetheless, these technologies might be seen as a mixed blessing. Their critics are not likely to believe that health care professionals and the technology companies assisting them have sinister motives. Rather, the critics are likely to agree that the participants' motives are consistent with the highest values of medicine, and they might admit that the potential for improvements in diagnostic capabilities would be difficult to exaggerate.

Critics might nevertheless be concerned about the potential for mischief inherent in remote patient monitoring. Ultimately, are most not people patients? Even though (and partly because) most people know that at some time, they will need a doctor, many people do not wish to be monitored. Many people resent being monitored to the extent that they already are, through such means as credit card transactions, census form questions, phone calls to organizations that are automatically recorded for quality control, the increasing (and sometimes unlawful) use of Social Security numbers for identification, the little video cameras mounted on the bank walls, and, yes, the computerized patient record.

Most individuals have concerns about these developments. Knowledge is power. The first thing bureaucrats do when they want to expand their power is to gather data about the governed. And the more personalized the knowledge, the greater the power delivered. What more personal information could there be than that a patient has a fasting blood sugar level of 200, that his or her vital capacity is 60% of normal, or that he or she has a history of alcohol dependence or of cyclothymia? The right to privacy, as Justice John Marshall Harlan observed decades ago, is the right to be let alone. In some respects, this is the most fundamental right, except for the right to life itself. This right must be guarded.

Proponents of the HIPAA privacy rule point to its complexity, its turgid prose, its impenetrable definitions, and the litigation it is guaranteed to spawn. The critics point out, however, that even though this privacy rule is not a perfect solution to the problem, it does proceed from the realization that there is a problem with giving away privacy.

Chapter 12 discusses the expanding role of patient education as part of informed-consent procedures in mental health care. An increasingly important part of care delivery will be the education of patients, families, and the general public about mental health issues, the psychotechnologies, and their eroding right to privacy (Dyson, 1998). Most important, as they design individual treatments, practitioners will need to respect the patient's ultimate decision about the trade-off between some types of technology-based care and the loss of privacy.

The Remedy for Contextual Deficiency.   Most people acquire their knowledge of scientific matters from newspapers and television. These media tend to report bad health news (Bartlett, Sterne, & Egger, 2002), exaggerate its importance (Woloshin & Schwartz, 2002), and stir up excessive worry (Benarde, 2002). These media are also too uncritical of junk science, which seems to be more at home on television than in court. In striving for a balanced view, the media tend to create the impression that the evidence supporting each side of a health care controversy is of equal value and weight, leaving people not knowing what to believe (Jackson, 2002) and, more important, leaving them ill-equipped to reach reasoned, logical, well-supported conclusions. Some popular magazines provide excellent in-depth appraisals, but these sources are not easily available when needed. In contrast, Web sites can reproduce this material and also can present many more illustrations, other multimedia enhancements, references to original information sources and further reading, definitions of terms, and links to other Web sites. Web sites can be kept up to date, are easily found and searched, are available on demand, and can be reached from almost anywhere. Professionals can offer information on their own Web sites or can provide judiciously selected links to external Web pages for patients to ponder as part of an informed-consent dialogue. A therapist may promote a broad perspective by offering clients a list of sites maintained by professionals from other disciplines (W. Stilwell, personal communication, August 18, 2002).

In the evolution of consumer health Web sites, the spread of self-promotional brochureware was followed by health encyclopedias describing illnesses and treatments. Now sites present evidence-based information on an extensive suite of pages developed by Web site staff and contain guidelines and interactive decision-support tools. A therapist may guide a client to such sites to help select the best intervention.

A new automated guidance tool (http://www.vitalseek.com) is the accredited search that can block references to Web sites that have not met the rigorous URAC standards. When a user requests a list of sites on a particular topic, filters limit the array of health care sites retrieved, based on quality indicators demanded by the user, such as whether the user seeks traditional or alternative approaches, the level of privacy desired, and what aspects of the chosen topic are of immediate interest. These and other solutions to the problem of quality on the Web are likely to emerge.

THE MARKET FOR PSYCHOTECHNOLOGIES

Although the Internet is creating an enormous market for the psychotechnologies, difficulties remain in reaching large numbers of people. Policies related to development and deployment of the psychotechnologies should consider both marketplace opportunities and population needs.

The Internet is a global meeting place that allows communication to flow easily across large distances almost instantly and, for Americans, inexpensively. A large, coherent Internet marketplace for offering goods and services already exists in the United States, supported by a single currency and language and a dominant culture. This marketplace makes delivering therapeutic services online relatively easy to people who have Internet access.

In Europe, many people below age 50 speak English fairly well and have studied other languages. Also, most people in Japan share characteristics that could support a vigorous online health care community. Other areas of the globe have similar pools of shared resources, and China, India, and Brazil, for instance, have large developing markets. Most middle-class urban dwellers in China read Mandarin and have Internet access, India has become a leader in Internet technology, and most people in Brazil, which has a fairly well developed Internet infrastructure, speak Portuguese. In contrast, the marketplace in sub-Saharan Africa is fragmented by marked diversity in language and ethnicity; in the northern part of the continent, marked differences between regional dialects tend to interfere with marketplace unity. In Africa and large areas of Asia, Internet connections are not yet available to the population at large.

Developments that might help people who are interested in language and translation are available. The United Nations and other venues in which polyglot conversations are frequent use automated services for simultaneous translation from one language into many others. This technique has achieved considerable success, even though the subject matter may be complex or technical and even though there may be nuances and subtleties whose loss could be problematic. One approach to language barriers in the world of online clinical practice would be using similar automatic translation methods. Even though speaking one language into a machine and hearing another language come out may seem futuristic, a handheld universal translator that does just this is already available (see http://www.ectaco.com).

Even in the most developed countries, many groups of people are difficult to reach because of the digital divide attributable to minority culture and language issues, poverty, access problems, physical and cognitive handicaps, illnesses, and other impediments. Also, in the United States, licensing and reimbursement policies vary between states. Despite all these obstacles, in each of the larger and more developed market areas, the dominant ethnic and socioeconomic groups are sufficiently popu-lous and wealthy to fuel rapid growth of the delivery of behavioral health care at a distance and the deployment of other psychotechnologies.

Providing services between markets is different from providing services within markets. It is wrong to assume that therapists in Utah can treat upper-middle-class patients in India who speak English fluently as readily as they can treat patients in Montana. Transporting mental health resources between markets requires careful adaptation by experts, just as translating a novel into another language calls for spe-cial sensitivity and abilities. Although Web sites and programs perform surprisingly good translation between languages, there is an increasing need for human transla-tors to work with mental health experts in creating language adaptations (not just translations) of Web sites and applications of the psychotechnologies that are suitable for each marketplace. Once the translators have done their job, there will also be a need for legal review, so that conduct and messages that are safe and lawful in the country of origin do not violate the law or create unacceptable risk in another country.

Now, however, some pressing mental health service needs cannot wait for orderly marketplace development or optimal translation and adaptation. Huge population segments will continue to face a chronic emergency health care situation. Professionals will be called on to provide remote treatment in remote areas across daunting cultural, linguistic, and sometimes legal barriers. Outside the larger potential marketplaces are hundreds of millions of people, particularly in Africa, Eastern Europe, and Asia, whose needs require an appropriate and immediate response yet whose diversity of ethnicity and language and paucity of cash challenge market economics. Adding to this are war, political upheaval, repressive governments, famine, and natural catastrophes, each generating new psychological emergencies and calling for currently unavailable services, such as crisis intervention, rape counseling, grief work, therapy for torture victims, and treatment of posttraumatic stress disorder and depression.

Today, the world is a new kind of marketplace for emergency mental health services worldwide, created by a new way of delivering these services. There is a clear and persistent need for ways to assemble and mobilize mental health teams and to pro-vide them with materials and resources to assist populations in particularly stressed regions. Funding, organizational support, and publicity will come from the United Nations, possibly, and, in particular, from the World Health Organization. Method-ology and technology developed in the military sector will be transferred for civil-ian use.

The pressing needs for emergency services challenge current concepts of profes-sional ethics. Mental health professionals will be called on to extend their services through the Internet to distant and unfamiliar disaster sites and under circumstances not adequately contemplated by current formulations of practice standards. Also needed as international attention to devising new, sufficiently flexible guidelines, certification mechanisms, and protection for health care professionals responding to emergencies from a distance.

Career Opportunities

Various permanent employment positions are opening up for mental health profes-sionals who can do the following:

- Contract with prisons, rural clinics and hospitals, school systems, and other or-ganizations to provide clinical services remotely from one's office.

- Consult remotely and/or travel as needed to coordinate with local mental health systems and advise and participate in developing programs and resources that take advantage of the psychotechnologies.
- Apply administrative, operational, technological, and clinical expertise in supporting remote mental health care teams.
- Join and serve in ad hoc or permanent crisis teams located in the field, help the teams apply the psychotechnologies appropriately, and help them coordinate with central support systems.
- Produce (through creation or adaptation) flexible psychoeducational materials and methodologies suitable for treatment situations in which the psychotechnologies are being used.
- Produce psychoeducational materials and methodologies that can upgrade mental health–related skills of general health care personnel, enhance their awareness of mental disorders, or shift their culture (e.g., taking evidence of domestic violence more seriously or dealing more sensitively with rape victims).
- Design ways to incorporate the psychotechnologies into procedures and interventions relevant to the conditions and cultures of underserved populations and of populations experiencing crisis.
- Engineer funding and publicity for permanent and ad hoc international mental health crisis relief programs.
- Assist journalists in identifying, visiting, and describing such programs.
- Advise governments and agencies in setting policies and evaluating programs that rely on the psychotechnologies.
- Write content about mental health issues that developers can place on their Web sites (e.g., news summaries, opinion pieces).
- Train professionals in relevant technical and administrative skills and inform them of ethical, legal, and regulatory requirements.
- Produce psychoeducational materials and methodologies that can train mental health workers to use the psychotechnologies.
- Provide clinical training in integrating the psychotechnologies into existing treatment programs and in applying new forms of treatment that grow out of the psychotechnologies.
- Plan, organize, and conduct research in any area already mentioned, including investigations of efficacy, cost-effectiveness, treatment delivery, and accessibility.
- Advise all people concerned on the relevant legal issues.
- Identify, diminish, and insure against the clinical and professional risks involved in nearly all these preceding points.

Telehome Health Care

Home health care is expanding rapidly, particularly for people with severe and persistent social or emotional problems. The growth of home health care is creating opportunities for mental health professionals with knowledge of certain psychotechnologies. Patients with various chronic physical illnesses are also increasingly being treated at home, at least in part, and many or most of these patients would benefit from the services of a mental health professional, as might family members and/or other caregivers. This need is particularly true for patients who are elderly or afflicted with dementia. For example, AIDS dementia remains a significant chronic problem despite the new antiretroviral cocktails. The disease puts a strain on helpers that can be somewhat ameliorated by judicious application of the psychotechnologies.

Telehome care uses psychotechnologies to provide a broad range of health care services. As practitioners and health plans become more knowledgeable about the potential of telehome care, they will be able to provide cost-effective services to patients (California Telehealth/Telemedicine Coordination Project, 1997). Nurses visiting patients while carrying laptops wired for videoconferencing have developed a significant body of literature supporting the efficacy and cost-effectiveness of telehome care (Goldberg, 1997).

Many patients who are homebound or bedridden or who have difficulty traveling can benefit from having cameras in their rooms. Treatment staff can drop in or visit by appointment and observe how the patient is doing. *Telemetry* (measurement from a distance) can enable less skilled visitors and caregivers to convey accurate quantitative information to a consultant at a central location. If adequate bandwidth communication service is unavailable, a patient or caregiver can prepare a video recording showing the patient's performance on selected tasks and responses to questions. This recording can be transmitted to a consultant via a store-and-forward communication method before a telephone conversation with the patient and/or caregiver. If high-bandwidth service is available, videoconferencing can support such an examination in real time.

The number of people suffering from dementia is increasing rapidly. Through the use of technologies, these people can be cared for at home and will require fewer trips to a health care facility. This group of patients, particularly demented elderly people living with relatives, may be the first to benefit from telehome care on a large scale. Given the high cost of nursing home care and its limitations, telehome services may not only improve the quality of care but also improve it more inexpensively than would otherwise be possible.

Interested professionals should watch for developments in home health care for older people and the disabled and also in the area of palliative interventions. "Palliative care is a combination of active and compassionate therapies that is primarily focused on the physical, psychological, social and spiritual suffering of the patient, family and caregiver" (Ann M. Berger, M.S.N., M.D., in Kirsch, 2002, p. 45). Hospice treatment is traditionally associated with terminal illness, but techniques developed in that venue (Berger, Portenoy, & Weissman, 2002) can be extended and usefully applied to telehome health care for people with chronic diseases, pain syndromes, and lengthy courses of treatment (e.g., cancer chemotherapy). Better management of psychological issues in such situations can improve the quality of life and also can make a marked difference in family functioning and individual outcomes.

Currently, home health care reimbursement is being cut, but if telecommunication technologies prove cost-effective, a substantial shift to telehome care may occur. Positions should be opening up for mental health professionals who can provide or facilitate this method of treatment delivery.

There are enough options for applying the psychotechnologies in the area of mental and behavioral health care to make it difficult to choose among them. Newer technologies and developments in mental health theory and interventions will expand the range of choices even more within the next decade. Because Internet time rushes ahead very quickly, a mere 10-year leap forward plunges practitioners into "the distant future of behavioral e-health," the topic of the next chapter.

15

The Distant Future

This last chapter projects somewhat farther into the future. Consider the following vignette:

> *Paddock, the toadlike Personal Digital Familiar[1] (PDF), would not give up: "Good morning, glory. Up, up, up. Rise and shine. It's Saturday. All day. Remember your promise. It's show time."*
>
> *Laurie loved a little teasing, but this was too much, especially because the machine was right. The night before, Laurie had told Paddock that in the morning, she was going to inquire about therapy. Laurie fumbled for her polarizing contact lenses in the container next to her bed.*
>
> *Paddock restarted the streaming video from the point at which it had paused when Laurie fell asleep. "Okay, Paddock, you win," Laurie grumbled to her PDF. "Ditch the* Harold and Maude *and hold any phone calls. I'll call a psychotherapist for my depression."*
>
> *As Laurie was splashing water on her face, the PDF erased the picture over Laurie's bed showing Abu Ammar with his third Nobel Peace Prize and replaced it with an annotated list of clinicians who were connected with Laurie's insurance plan and who had special expertise in treating depression through psychotechnologies. "There," said Paddock as Laurie returned to the bedroom, "enjoy."*
>
> *Three names were marked as especially favored by Laurie's primary care physician. She wondered whether those people were Dr. Jelabi's golf cronies. She scanned through the blurbs, finally pointing her finger at the picture of Dr. Wright, a psychologist. "Let's try that one."*
>
> *When Paddock had connected with Dr. Wright's office, the lights in Laurie's messy bedroom dimmed, and the images covering the walls transformed it into a cozy three-dimensional virtual office. "And now I bring you a special presentation imaginatively entitled 'For Any Potential New Client,' meaning you," said Paddock, grandly. Laurie saw an ordinary-looking man comfortably seated in an easy chair. He gave the impression of being too 20th century and too educated for Laurie, but he did not appear to be nerdy or pompous. His eyes were sincere, and he had a likable smile. Dr. Wright spoke in a soft voice for several minutes, comprehensively answering many of the questions a new patient might have about starting treatment. Laurie was amused when Dr. Wright mentioned*

---

[1] A familiar is a spirit, usually in the form of an animal, dedicated to helping or guarding a particular person. Paddock is the name of a familiar who calls from offstage in Shakespeare's *Macbeth*.

that he did not offer any money-back guarantees. Talk about an old-fashioned therapist! But maybe that retro touch was a good sign, showing that he was less commercial than most shrinks nowadays.

As the presentation ended and Laurie indicated an interest in speaking with Dr. Wright, Paddock informed her that he would be available in 30 minutes. All she had to do was say, "Yes."

"Yes," Laurie agreed, and the room lights came up. She fetched a soda from her refrigerator, combed her hair, and began to straighten out her room.

Dr. Wright appeared for the virtual intake appointment in 30 minutes, as promised. This time he was actually "there," interacting with Laurie. He apologized for not being available at the moment she first tried to contact him. When he responded to Laurie's gently sarcastic reply in kind, Laurie got the feeling that Dr. Wright might be someone who could tune in to her. He asked whether he could clarify any questions raised by the introductory vignette she had seen, because he needed to have her formal permission on record before he could explore how he might help. After Laurie discussed the virtual preliminary consent form and the Notice of Privacy Policy and endorsed them with her electronic signature gesture, the teleconsultation session officially began.

Laurie agreed to authorize the release of information about her previous health care, to fill out some questionnaires, and to transmit some physiologic data after this preliminary session ended. But first she wanted to talk about her problems.

Under Dr. Wright's skillful questioning, Laurie sketched out her situation, described her moodiness, and outlined her main relationships. Dr. Wright noticed that when she mentioned her father's death, Laurie's eyes reddened, she changed her posture, and she began complaining about her boyfriend.

Dr. Wright asked her about her apparent emotion. They discussed her sadness about her father and her boyfriend, the similarities between the two men, and the feelings she has for each of them. Dr. Wright explained how he was putting together some homework for Laurie to go through before their next appointment. In addition to writing about her feelings for her father and her boyfriend, Dr. Wright wanted her to consider the rationale for, and implications of, his tentative DSM-V diagnosis of dysthymia and to read about it and his recommended treatments on his Web site. They agreed to meet twice during the next week to fill in the outline of the treatment plan Dr. Wright had just assembled. Those sessions would allow Dr. Wright to obtain a detailed personal history and to make a thorough assessment. In a gentle but firm tone, Dr. Wright said it was time to end their first session.

Dr. Wright's office then disappeared and Laurie was again sitting in her room with Paddock and her soda. Paddock informed her that a batch of patient handouts was finished printing, along with a link to Dr. Wright's Web site, other recommended Web sites, and a preliminary action plan. Her PDF suggested that Laurie might do a few laps on her treadmill, eat the blueberry yogurt due to expire tomorrow, and then put in half an hour working on the assignment from Dr. Wright before showering and getting ready for a 2 o'clock pedicure that Paddock had arranged for her down at Tosies.

Too futuristic? Difficult to say. Some of this vignette can already be implemented with today's technology. It's only a matter of economics—offering superbroadband transmission channels to the public, mass producing lightening-quick computer processors, and rounding up enough programmers to create the software. In other words, given the current economic climate, spoken conversation with a computer assistant may have to wait for another decade (Dvorac, 2002).

The advancing and converging fields of affective computing and virtual reality aim to enable computers to sense tone and emotion, unscramble idioms and slang, interpret gestures and fleeting facial expressions, and deduce complex thought processes and then to respond in a convincing social manner. Laurie's personal computer network was able to learn about her personality traits, coordinate with the insurance company, connect with her primary care physician, and help choose a suitable psychotherapist at her spoken request. Dr. Wright's office was projected as a high-resolution 3-D image into Laurie's room. Such personalized and immersive virtual reality interactions may make computer-bridged communication more convenient, fluent, and satisfactory. In particular, electronically mediated mental health services may surpass current in-person methods in both efficiency and effectiveness by being accessible on demand, multimodal, readily amenable to computer support and to a team approach, more continuous and integrated from provider to provider, more open to research and administrative control, and ultimately less expensive.

Current technologies applied to long-acknowledged needs will create the scenarios this book has been discussing. It is safe to assume that some of these predictions will come true. Now let's try to describe how emerging technologies may affect how practitioners will deliver mental health care in a decade or two.

NATURAL INTERFACING

Move over, movable type. The dominance of the printed word that began with Johannes Gutenberg's innovation and his 1453 Mazarin Bible may end during the Information Age. The greatest deficit in handheld PDAs (personal digital assistant computers) is the need for an incongruously large keyboard or an awkward writing pad and stylus for data entry. The second inconvenience is the small viewing screen. *Natural interfacing* promises to free users from these limitations by allowing human–computer interaction to mimic two people conversing.

Watch Your Language

In addition to his solo private practice as a child psychiatrist in New Rochelle, New York, Daniel Sabbeth, M.D., regularly provides psychiatric assessments for the New York City Board of Education. In addition, attorneys retain him several times each year to evaluate a litigant in an injury or custody case. Dr. Sabbeth's repeat business indicates that people are very satisfied with the quality of his reports. However, Dr. Sabbeth is a terrible typist.

Dr. Sabbeth depends on IBM's Via Voice program (http://www-3.ibm.com/software/speech) installed on his high-speed, high-memory Macintosh computer. Initially, he invested 2 hours to familiarize the program with his way of speaking. Now, when Dr. Sabbeth dictates into the machine, it automatically keeps improving its speech recognition performance and adds new psychiatric terms to its vocabulary. Accuracy is very high, and Dr. Sabbeth's chronic wrist problems are gone.

—Daniel Paul Sabbeth, Ph.D., M.D.
Assistant Professor of Psychiatry
Albert Einstein College of Medicine

Speech and Language Recognition.   Making sense of what is being said, considering context, and applying common sense rules are essential to knowing what people are communicating. Increasingly, computers are applying expert knowledge to speech recognition and need less training to accurately pick out words and sentences from continuously streaming speech.[2] Context is frequently used to distinguish among such homonyms as *their, there,* and *they're.* However, the *artificial intelligence* involved in speech recognition has wider applications. The Kelsey Group estimates that, by 2006, speech-based technologies may produce revenue of more than $2 billion (Advanced Systems Group, 2002).

Automated Backtalk. Computers have long been able to generate speech from text. Actual understanding of text can enhance instantaneous, automatic, simultaneous translation to and from a foreign language, a valuable substitute for today's usual mental health emergency service. Asking important questions, such as "Do you want to kill yourself?" is crucial yet complicated when evaluating a non-English-speaking client through computers.

Understanding sentences may allow computers to talk with meaningful inflection, rhythm, and emphasis. Products that can mimic the voice and speech of specific people, such as one's therapist, may soon be on the market. This ability would allow computers to interact with clients and supplement their direct contact with professionals more convincingly. Technologies that change text to speech may allow e-mail messages to be read to a client with the same tone, cadence, and inflection as a client's therapist. The robotic sounds of today's computer speech may easily be replaced with natural-sounding speech (Advanced Systems Group, 2002).

Similarly, a computer may be able to display and control a moving image of the professional, making it seem as if the therapist rather than a virtual puppet was conversing with the client. Of course, the high abuse potential of such technology may call for such protections as watermarking the voice and image with imperceptible codes, letting the client's computer authenticate the fact that the apparent therapist is a legitimate digital agent of the actual therapist and not a fake perpetrated by a prankster, con artist, or enemy. These protections will also protect therapists from allegations of violating Medicare fraud and abuse laws by letting their digital agents do the talking while they charge their normal rate for person-to-person treatment. In any case, these technologies are potentially rich areas for further exploration and research by the mental health investigators.

Actions Speak Louder than Words

Psychotechnologies may allow mental health care professionals to bypass speech and even cognition in assessing a client's physiological processes. As we describe in chapter 7, PDAs are being pressed into service to let psychiatric clients keep symptom diaries. In addition, physiologic sensors are being interfaced with PDAs to record physiological and behavioral data for subsequent readout and interpretation by a professional. Rather than wait for the next in-person session, a client can e-mail monitored data to the therapist.

The percentage of the U.S. population with direct access to wireless e-mail through PDAs is expected to increase from 2% in 2001 to nearly 59% by 2007 (Nee, 2001).

---

[2] OpenCyc (http://www.opencyc.org) has codified tens of thousands of commonsense rules (such as "always keep the open side of the cup facing up when carrying your coffee") that can carry this trend to the next step—useful interpretation of natural spoken language—so that a computer can respond intelligently. Already, the Travelocity Web site (http://www.travelocity.com) uses advanced Ask Jeeves technology (see http://www.askjeeves.com) to interpret the visitor's request and to perform a satisfactory search.

Immediate accessibility will allow clients to send their behavioral samples, thought records, and other reports to the therapist quickly while on the road or walking down the street—and perhaps to receive a reassuring response or suggestion within minutes.

Constant Comment

Most PDAs and mobile phones take time to boot up and connect. An always-on system, implemented by neighborhood wireless networking or through the convergence of PDAs and mobile phones, will allow convenient and continuous two-way streaming of data and control signals between the client's body and the professional's remote computer system.[3] Constant virtual attachment between professionals and clients will bring new meaning to the concept of continuity of care and a new edginess to the concept of invasion of privacy. These uses of wireless technology are likely to increase and to provide another rich avenue of research. They could also have the unfortunate effect of providing wholly superfluous encouragement to lawyers in search of litigation opportunities.

An example of how wireless technology can be applied to a mental health practice comes from psychiatrist Giovanni Torello, who often receives mobile telephone calls from patients. He states that São Paulo, Brazil, traffic regularly immobilizes drivers for 20 minutes at a time before they can inch ahead one or two car lengths. Patients experiencing or anticipating a panic attack during such situations can call him using their mobile phone. He uses the opportunity for in vivo desensitization sessions or in situ psychoanalytic exploration (G. Torello, personal communication, April 26, 2002).

The continuous monitoring and direction provided by a professional's computer system are well suited to exposure therapy. A professional, for instance, could remotely guide an agoraphobic client through a course of anxiety-provoking places and situations while continuously recording pulmonary and cardiac functioning for current analysis or later discussion with the patient. Likewise, professionals could use their computers to help addicted patients deal with people, places, and things in real life; to provide assertiveness training to socially phobic businesspeople; and to help parents deal with a child's sleep problem. Although all these uses involve talking, remote physiological monitoring enables therapy to move beyond words. Future applications will undoubtedly be more pervasive.

Advances in telecommunication technologies may significantly improve telemonitoring rehabilitation projects. For example, data sensors installed in a client's house may be able to monitor the client's activities throughout the day. For a client suffering from an eating disorder, the sensors could send a message each time the client opens the refrigerator door; the receiving computer could analyze the results and report to the therapist.

Wearable Computers and Smart Clothing

Currently, going through the day with a Holter Monitor recording one's cardiac function feels like a major life event. Soon, it may be as fashionable to wear an entire computer as it is to wear eyeglasses (see http://www.media.mit.edu/wearables/lizzy/

---

[3] Software from Televital (http://www.televital.com) supports an array of physiological measurements with a typical real-time streaming delay of less than 1 second when transmission is over a 56K modem. This speed is fast enough for many biofeedback paradigms that can be effected over cellular connections.

timeline.html), a wristwatch, or a mobile phone. Now, a man can buy Dockers Mobile Pants to hold today's necessary equipment—PDA, MP3 player, radio, laptop computer, cellular phone, power supply with adaptors, surge protector, portable printer, travel mouse, spare batteries, memory cards, digital camera, minikeyboard, keychain USB storage, business card reader, headset, and dangling microphone. The market is ready for an all-in-one integrated *wearable computer* that does away with the necessity for these pants or for the competing 10-pocket Scott eVest v2.0.

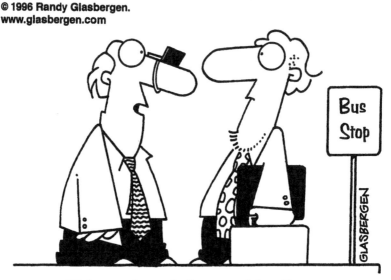

© 1996 Randy Glasbergen.
www.glasbergen.com

**"I introduced the world's first
nose-top computer 18 months ago.
Sales are slower than originally anticipated."**

For some time, computers have been controlled by simple voice commands. Once computers are able to understand complex sentences, put words into context, apply common sense ("Accept only emergency phone calls in the middle of the night"), and respond with succinct speech, it may no longer be necessary to hold, look at, or manipulate a portable computer. A wearable computer may become part of everyone's everyday wardrobe.

Some wearable computer prototypes interface with the user through a small single-handed keyboard, some kind of headphone, and special image projection gear (Affective Computing, n.d.). These wearable computers provide a constant wireless connection to the Internet and potentially to the standard cell telephone network. Future devices may be much more comfortable and low-key. A tiny video camera concealed in the hair may enable face recognition. By recording pictures of the environment, this camera could serve as a memory aid and perhaps be used as legal proof or to resolve the "I said, you said" arguments. People are notoriously inaccurate when recalling what they have witnessed, especially in the case of events that they feel are important (Wald, 2002). The frequency with which criminal defendants are wrongly convicted on the basis of eyewitness testimony supports this assertion. On the other hand, the privacy implications of being filmed by numerous passers-by are numerous. As for sound, the only piece of equipment showing may be a nearly invisible hearing aid–like ear canal speaker (or a person chould choose to have a speaker implanted in the middle ear).[4]

A wearable computer designed for a mental health client may include an array of sensors for skin conductance, temperature, heart rate and EKG pattern, blood oxygenation, brain electrical activity (EEG), the positions of various joints, muscle activation (EMG), and walking speed and distance (see the discussion of the LifeShirt in chapter 7). Clients may be able to record spoken messages for their therapists and could make gestures that mark where and when something of significance occurred. For example, patients' crossed fingers could reveal to practitioners correlations among a rise in blood pressure, indicators of stress in a voiceprint, and fibbing.

From a liability perspective, the expected benefits from improved care must be weighed against the risks. If the mental health professional has patients' electrocardiograms, for example, lawyers will not hesitate to assert that such professionals have a duty to interpret them or to have them interpreted. Given the risks involved in certain dysrhythmias and the urgent need for their recognition and treatment, do practitioners want to have this kind of information?

AnthroTronix is developing wearable electronics to track children's movements and gestures, allowing automated reinforcement of desired behaviors (see http://www.anthrotronix.com/currentprojects.html). Although the purpose of this equipment is to motivate disabled children to engage in prescribed physical rehabilitation exercises, the system could be programmed to extinguish undesired habits. Less controversially, such wireless technologies can help people with certain cognitive impediments function more efficiently. Some courts are already requiring parolees to wear signal-emitting anklets to facilitate tracking their movements.

Full-scale wearable computers, such as the Poma (see http://www.xybernaut.com), have been developed for physicians making hospital rounds and also for workers who fill customer orders by selecting items from bins and racks in a stockroom. This equipment may get its first major use on the battlefield. The advance line would not contain military personnel dressed in special intelligent clothing (a powered exoskeleton bedecked with sensors); rather, a cockroach, outfitted with sensors and chips, would be deployed to scout out the presence of chemical and biological hazards and transmit appropriate warnings (R. Satava, personal communication, October 28, 2002).

CYBORG THEORY

The carpal tunnel syndrome caused by excessive pounding on keypads and headaches arising from prolonged squinting at a computer screens are fueling the fantasy that computer users will be able to bypass today's clumsy user interface in favor of direct access to their electronic equipment. Instead of speakers and monitors, sounds and images may be transmitted straight into our brains and our instructions will be actualized without lifting a finger. Once we become able to merge seamlessly with our machines, the new, often permanent attachments to our physicality will dramatically extend our power and hasten our evolution.

---

[4] The U.S. Food and Drug Administration (FDA) has approved and is considering various kinds of middle-ear implants. Inner-ear (cochlear) implants carry this one level deeper. Intracerebral chips are already a reality but not for casual use.

Appalling as this prospect may seem in many respects, such fusion of carbon-based life-forms with convenient and highly responsive silicon-based electronic gadgets is already well underway. In fact, science-fiction stories about *cyborgs* (composed of feedback-controlled *cybernetic* mechanisms and living *organisms*) are old hat.

It is not simply a matter of the user interface becoming easier. There can be little doubt that our growing facility and intimacy with intelligent machinery will result in important changes in our own psychology, perhaps even some fundamental transformations.

- To what extent is a professional transformed when armed with physiological monitoring equipment and remote tracking technology?
- Where exactly is the professional when a synthetic emulator is responding to a client according to the professional's instructions and using the professional's voice and physical appearance?
- Social constructs of interpersonal contact, relationships, and community must be reworked if they are to continue to shield us from nature's actual chaos as we extend our existence into cyberspace (see the Principia Cybernetica Web site, http://pespmc1.vub.ac.be). The challenges to our sense of identity that have arisen from new biological insights (LeDoux, 2002) and advances in cloning (Brock, 2002) pale before the prospect of becoming cyborgs.

At Rockland State Hospital in Orangeburg, New York, psychiatrist Nathan S. Kline and engineer Manfred Clynes, having implanted an osmotic pump into a rat, dubbed the new animal–machine hybrid a cyborg (Clynes & Nathan, 1960). Today, some people anticipate having an interactive cardiac pacemaker installed. However, our transformation into psychological cyborgs does not require the implantation of physical prostheses or computer chips holding our complete medical history (Haraway, 1991). Sherry Turkle (1995) wrote:

> As human beings become increasingly intertwined with the technology and with each other via the technology, old distinctions between what is specifically human and specifically technological become more complex. Are we living life on the screen or life in the screen? Our new technologically enmeshed relationships oblige us to ask to what extent we ourselves have become cyborgs, transgressive mixtures of biology, technology, and code. (p. 21)

Beyond even this, one parody suggests that a growing dependence on routine access to massive amounts of shared information may produce an intelligent macroorganism, a kind of hive composed of networked human beings. (Williams, 1996). In chat rooms worldwide, people are taking on multiple identities possessing various imagined attributes as they forge intense and sometimes long-lasting relationships with other consciously made-up identities.

Mental health professionals have written about the advantages and disadvantages of using technology to mediate and create relationships (Maheu & Subotnik, 2001; Suler, 1999c, 2000a). A sociology researcher depictes a typical Internet-related problem viewed in terms of cyborg theory:

> Rebecca, a young woman, "may be becoming a cyborg because her sex life is undeniably tied to and dependent upon AOL chat rooms. All her sexual activities involving partners are online." Although she has had cyber-sex and telephone sex with many men through

AOL, Rebecca has not physically had sex with a partner since she began using the service. Rebecca does not practice casual sex in the real world because she does not believe it to be moral or safe. "Rebecca's sex life is undeniably tied to her computer and the telecommunications system it is connected to." (Hamman, 1996)

Saying that people are turning into cyborgs may seem either alarmist or trivial. However, *transhumanism* is a serious interdisciplinary academic and philosophical pursuit, involving "genetic engineering, information technology, and pharmaceuticals, as well as anticipated future capabilities, such as *nanotechnology* (involving microscopic-scale sensors and machines), machine intelligence, uploading, 'paradise-engineering,' and space colonization" (see the Web site of the World Transhumanist Association, http://www.transhumanism.org). Some academics have queried whether a computer may have legally cognizable rights (M. Rothblatt, personal communication, 2001), and it is fairly well established that an organism can be patented.

Today's adolescents and young adults are likely to extend their fascination with technology to the point of implanting chips into their bodies; these chips would cue internal pumps to emit hormones, neurotransmitters, and even junk food into their systems. Similar implanted devices may keep the present generation alive for extended periods.

THE VIRTUE OF VIRTUALITY

Virtual reality (VR) has limitless potential for imaginative applications. For example, it could allow a professional and a client to meet over the Internet in a *virtual office*. A virtual environment can vividly reproduce a client's problem, such as not being able to urinate when within the hearing of other people (see http://www.paruresis.org). Virtual 3-D chat rooms can add a new personal dimension to existing Internet support groups. Professionals may conduct biofeedback within virtual environments to promote generalization of the relaxation response. Professionals also may use virtual 3-D games for social skills training and other therapeutic goals. The improvement of existing virtual technology will probably continue to be driven by pornography and gaming.

Virtual Assessment

HMOs are increasingly interested in objective markers of psychological distress and dysfunction, both before treatment (to assign the most efficient intervention) and after treatment (to assess the outcome). Virtual reality could contribute to a test battery that assesses a patient in a new and more accurate way than current assessment tools. For example the most straightforward virtual reality testing could enable practitioners to determine the cues that trigger various components of a patient's phobic response. A series of potentially phobic environments (high places, a car on the freeway, a party or social gathering, for example) can be presented quickly to clients, who rate their anxiety as sensors monitor their physiologic states. When a particular screening situation elicits a response, the virtual reality software could then branch deeper into situations of the appropriate category until it pinpoints the specific stimuli that are provoking anxiety. These situations could then be used in virtual reality exposure treatment and desensitization. Coupling virtual reality software with biofeedback and/or facial expression analysis technology could fully automate the diagnostic process.

In the realm of assessment, computers of the future could conduct diagnostic interviews while monitoring a patient's physiologic reactions. When the computer senses a reaction, it could immediately probe more deeply, or it could return to the sensitive topic after a digression. The computer could then forward the information to a clinician to assist in rendering an appropriate diagnosis.

Similarly, once video transmissions become more reliable, video recordings might be compared to norms of auditory and visual information for various clinical groups. Through a text box on a video screen, an interviewer could receive automatic and immediate feedback about the patient's number of words spoken per minute; voice inflection; number, type, and size of head, neck, and body movement; and other audible and visible criteria. This feedback also would contain possible diagnoses for the clinician to rule out during the ongoing interview. A flashing light or other computer device could signal the interviewer that the patient's behavior has met minimal clinically relevant criteria. Video assessments might also supply the remote interviewers with drop-down menus of valid and reliable questions to ask to enable the interviewers to rule out possible diagnoses when the computer signals the interviewer that visual and auditory criteria warrant more specific questioning.

Virtual assessment could eventually encompass all the uses discussed. Virtual assessment could immerse the patient in a virtual world and then monitor physiologic response, ask automatic questions, send a report to the clinician, and, finally, allow the clinician to conduct a fully informed clinical interview at the optimal time during the session.

Virtual Support Groups

One way to optimize the social interaction aspect of Internet support groups may be to immerse participants in 3-D chat rooms. Today, many people are visiting online chat rooms to discuss common issues. This resurgence of casual communal gatherings is paving the way for and supporting the development of the technology for formal virtual reality self-help and professionally sponsored mental health support groups.

Virtual Biofeedback

Advanced biofeedback using virtual reality displays may be more helpful than traditional biofeedback in a clinical setting. Alan Pope, a NASA psychologist, has developed VISCEREAL. This system displays a virtual realistic image of a subject's ongoing physiological function, such as a heart pumping or a blood vessel pulsing (see http://www.dif.org/News_Articles/virtual.shtml).

Patients with impaired blood flow, such as many people with diabetes mellitus, are learning to increase fingertip perfusion by visualizing the state of their arterioles even after being disconnected from the biofeedback apparatus. The graphic depiction can be supplemented by such sounds as pumping blood and also could be superimposed on scenery that promotes relaxation, such as a forest or a beach. Commercial versions of this technology could be available in a few years if research results are positive.

Virtual 3-D Therapeutic Games

Of all the revolutions kindled by the personal computer, electronic entertainment has the brightest future. Computer games offer interactivity, realism, and unpredictability—factors that can stimulate people to learn new ways to think and behave. In the next decade, 3-D computer graphics will be many, many times faster. Computer-generated images may be indistinguishable from live ones.

Of relevance to clinicians is that the new technologies developed for 3-D games will undoubtedly stimulate therapeutic applications. As seen in the virtual reality applications discussed in chapters 6 and 7, these game scenarios both entertain and engage clients while exposing them to therapeutic behavioral scenarios.

Some games have potential therapeutic value. For example, the Sims series, a popular set of sophisticated simulations of real-life environments, could help certain clients with schizophrenia learn to cope better with daily social demands.

The therapeutic applications of these games are becoming increasingly lifelike, engaging, and personalized. They also can be expected to become more therapeutically effective.

AFFECTIVE COMPUTING

Affective computing is becoming a reality. Professor Rosalind Picard and colleagues at the MIT Multimedia Group (http://affect.media.mit.edu) are constructing an intellectual framework for giving computers emotional intelligence. They are trying to enable a computer to sense human emotions. Their long-term goal is to make computers genuinely intelligent, enabling them to interact naturally with human beings by being able to recognize, understand, and express emotions. Computer programs that use the therapist's image and voice to assemble and deliver material to mental health patients will eventually enhance the patients' experience with congruent emotional expressivity, similar to Laurie in the vignette introduced at the beginning of this chapter.

Clinicians can recognize human emotions in four ways. One is through an analysis of prosody (the pattern of pitch, melody, intonation, amplitude, speed, rhythm, and other facets of speech). The difficult process of automating the extraction of information carried by prosody is being energetically pursued by American defense agencies (Shriberg & Stolcke, 2002).

A second way of detecting emotion is by listening to vocabulary (especially foul language and odd synonym choice), repetition of words, and dysfluencies (false starts, "ums and ers," and stammering). A third approach is to study the play of facial expression and body language. The fourth way to recognize emotion is for sensors to pick up physiological indicators of emotion. Equipping a client with sensors is the most straightforward method to use and has the most promise of extending a therapist's ability to see into the client. The first three methods can make up for some of the disadvantages of remote treatment; physiological sensing is applicable even in in-person sessions.

The other side of recognizing emotions is exhibiting them. Current systems that use recorded voices to convey information seem unfriendly and mechanical. Also, misunderstandings can occur. For example, one may hear the command "Don't! Go to the bridge!" as "Don't go to the bridge!" and end up letting the ship sink (Shriberg & Stolcke, 2002).

Automated speech will have much more impact when a computer can understand sentence structure, assign proper emphasis to the components of a phrase or sentence, and know when to be jocular or when to speak with reverent tones or in a whisper. Similarly, the virtual puppets that now deliver e-mail with a small selection of facial expressions and gestures (see http://www.lifefx.com) may eventually be able to emulate real people.

In general, information about a person's emotional state and attitudes is conveyed more rapidly and specifically by facial expression than by other physiological responses. Reading a client's face can be essential for counseling and psychotherapy. Assuming a certain facial expression can be an effective way for clinicians to feed information back and change the client's mood.

Some clinicians say that current technology does not adequately transmit facial expression during therapy at a distance. Even the ordinary television is not usually satisfactory in this respect. High-bandwidth connection is needed for the high-quality video that would let two people see each other's expressions.

In time, increased computer processing power will enable computers to decipher the emotions that underlie a person's play of facial expressions. Eventually, facial expressions themselves may be reduced to code, efficiently transmitted, and then convincingly recreated in a virtual reality model of the original person. Some airports use continuous face recognition software into an effort identify terrorists. Psychotherapists might eventually use the same type of recognition software to identify clients and to collect additional data to make inferences about body language.

As usual, the development of applicable statutes lags behind the science. Questions that the law will need to address include these: What right do citizens have to decline to be recognized? What rights do citizens have to discover who has catalogued their image? To object to being so catalogued? To inspect the image? To inspect the images of their children or other loved ones? To delete those images? To demand that certain precautions be taken to protect the images and to limit their use? What right has the custodian of these images to maintain them? To compare them? To sell them?

Because computerized analysis of facial expressions requires complex image analysis and is computationally expensive, it thus is not yet feasible in real-time communication (Calder, Burton, Miller, Young, & Akamatsu, 2001). In addition, computers cannot adiquately capture the dynamics of an emotional expression sequence as it unfolds, because the expression may manifest mixed emotions. More immediately feasible for the therapist to use is automated monitoring of eye movement as a patient is planning and producing speech and trying to comprehend the therapist's interventions. The close correlation between eye movement and cognitive processing (Dahan, Magnuson, & Tanenhaus, 2001) will provide new insights into the psychotherapy process and may make eye tracking a standard part of treatment.

One relatively straightforward application of technology for the recognition of emotional states from facial expression would be for clinicians to use it to tailor a computerized intervention session's content and pace to the client's moods and emotions. Another use would be in the computerized diagnostic assessment of psychological disorders before and after treatment.

HUMAN VERSUS COMPUTER THERAPIST

To share a virtual world over the Internet, people use compression techniques, as discussed in chapter 2. The most efficient approach involves establishing a parallel virtual world in the computer of each linked user. What is communicated between users is neither a new replica of the entire world for each time slice (the method used in cinema) nor a replica of the changes that occur between time slices (essentially the MPEG technique). What is communicated is a set of coordinates for movements. Each user's computer must perform all necessary calculations locally and render images and sounds in accordance with both the state of the world and the characteristics of each user (viewpoint, etc.). In a sense, then, the objects in the virtual world in each user's computer are puppets whose strings are being pulled via transmissions sent over the Internet.

In this scheme, a therapist would be depicted through control signals that activate a model of the therapist operated on the patient's machine. These control signals can produce facial expressions. In a similar manner, speech can be rendered as separately coded collections of phonemes, pitch and timbre, and accent. Pulse Entertainment, Inc., a maker of 3-D animation software (http://www.pulse3d.com), has taken a first step in synthesizing facial expressions.

Within 5 minutes of obtaining a two-dimensional photo, this technology may make it possible to create 3-D virtual clones of people, complete with lip-synching and text-to-speech capabilities.

There are distinct advantages to transmitting the meaning of an audio communication rather than a depiction of the waveform. First, the compression may be greater. The compression also facilitates synchronizing the audio with the visual and tactile components of the virtual reality experience. Furthermore, the implications (the meaning in a human sense) of material that has been analyzed in terms of phonemes and timbre lend themselves to research and to automated classification and interpretation. Similarly, fully automated electronic therapists can more easily generate realistic speech in the manner described than they can seamlessly assemble waveform sound bites from a library.

It is difficult to predict when psychotherapists will be able to use such a remotely synthesized virtual world. Within this kind of a virtual reality, the therapist and the client could assume any identity by selecting a speaking and moving avatar most appropriate to their therapeutic goals. Different types of psychotherapists may select images of their strongest protagonists: Sigmund Freud for psychoanalysis, Milton H. Erickson for hypnotherapy, Aaron Beck for cognitive therapy, and David Barlow for cognitive-behavior therapy might be popular choices.

When live therapists are not present, clients could interface with their preferred synthetic avatar in order to report progress, have homework exercises checked, and/or leave messages. The client would know that the real therapist would eventually pick up a transcript of the session and that the computer therapist was used to make it easier for the client to enter information into the system.

Therapists could incorporate existing specialized psychoeducational treatment modules into virtual reality easily to optimize training their clients in specific skills. These modules might inclule cognitive-behavioral treatment packages for social skills training, communication training, systematic desensitization, exposure to phobic stimuli, and/or habit-reversal training. Therapists also could use modules for treating computer phobia or Internet dependence! Within the next decade, an expert system could be programmed that includes all the empirically tested interventions for a wide range of psychological disorders.

Modern artificial intelligence (AI) methods may even allow creation of a sophisticated computer program capable of conducting therapy, especially if the machine is highly structured (Wagman, 1999) and has good conversational skills. A 3-D animated graphic representation of a therapist enhanced by facial expression technology and a realistically modulated voice would be fairly easy to create. The virtual therapist could have its own personality that reflects its history, memory, and experiences with the client in the virtual world. Each successive encounter with the client may add personality to the therapist. With more interactions, the virtual therapist would seem more humanlike. In fact, such digital therapists might become synthetic friends, advisers, or assistants to the live therapist.

Another aspect of AI could involve the clinician's use of robots. Robots with effector features (the equivalent of limbs and muscles) could engage in action, going beyond basic social support and therapeutic skills to assist clients in their daily functioning.

Some day, there may be a double-blind comparative study of real therapists and virtual therapists working with clients in a virtual reality environment. Such a study might find that the clients prefer the virtual therapists. Clients might view them as more effective and less expensive. However, there is a limit to how well a machine can hold a patient's hand, both literally and figuratively. Moreover, such a study might be ethically impossible. How does a researcher justify a double-blind approach in these circumstances?

Although these scenarios might appear threatening to some professionals, computerized therapy programs will not replace psychotherapists anytime soon. Despite the relative simplicity of building more human qualities into her, ELIZA does not have a big following and will remain nothing more than a game. The development of an interactive humanlike entity may receive funding from the adult entertainment industry, but no funding will be forthcoming from health care foundations.

The old science fiction vision of anthropoid general-purpose robots has given way to the reality of machines optimally configured for specialized tasks. Serious work on providing mental health through a simulated therapist may be based on highly structured and active treatment paradigms. The computer therapist may guide the client to sequentially attain specific graded objectives. There will be little, if any, support for efforts to replace human therapists with mechanical equivalents. Economic competition may lead to the gradually emergent superiority of the machine in cost–benefit analyses. Rather than wholesale replacement of psychotherapists with computers, developers in the next decade will focus on piecemeal improvements in the human–computer interface. These improvements will be adjunctive tools and will rarely replace the psychotherapist's soothing or challenging presence. Speaking on the telephone might be the next best thing to being there, but it is not the same as being there.

Now that this final chapter has detailed a number of possible future directions, the epilogue points to specific ways to get started. The epilogue discusses essential issues and provides checklists to address the professional's needs.

Epilogue: Immediate Steps—A Checklist

This epilogue is devoted to practical matters. After focusing on essential issues, the epilogue provides action checklists and suggestions to help professionals implement immediate change. However slight such changes might be, they can have far-reaching implications for recipients of mental health services.

SUMMARY OF RISK MANAGEMENT ISSUES

As discussed throughout much of the text, mental health professionals, particularly those in private practice need to minimize their legal risks in a number of areas. Private practitioners work in a highly litigious environment, with very few protections from action taken by third party carriers on one side and patients on the other side. Gone are the days when risk management can be left to paying for professional association membership and malpractice insurance. When using any of the psychotechnologies the essential ingredients of risk management include:

- Professional training.
- Supervision.
- Referral processes and authenticating client identity.
- Anticipating threat assessment and duty-to-warn situations.
- Client education, including reasonable risks involved with psychotechnologies.
- Patients matched with the appropriate psychotechnology.
- Security: safeguarding privacy and confidentiality.
- Informed-consent agreement, including duty-to-warn obligations that address potential technical problems and traditional topics covered by these agreements.
- Legal issues: old and new.
- Licensure.
- Ethical breaches.
- Emergency backup.
- Awareness of local conditions when communicating from a distance.
- Cultural and linguistic competence.
- The protection of children.
- Professional standards and guidelines (including, where appropriate, meeting proposed standards where none have been adopted).

- Documentation of efforts to:
  - Obtain relevant education and supervision.
  - Supply emergency clinical backup.
  - Maintain security.
  - Repair damage in case of privacy breaches.
  - Obtain consultation.
- Contracts with dot-com or other commercial entities to provide clinical services and/or other professional work.
- Considerations for partnering with employers, labor unions, and employees.
- Cautious use of marketing materials.
- Dealing with mass media.
- Disclosures of referral sources, where appropriate.

Even though previous chapters detail many of these risk management issues, we now highlight key action items related to the following:

- Security.
- The protection of children.
- Dealing with mass media.
- Considerations for partnering with employers, labor unions, and employees.

The goal in drawing attention to these issues is to advance the adoption of the psychotechnologies while protecting both the public and the practitioner.

Security

Computers crash, disks degrade, networks go down, viruses invade, power fails, and carrier services have outages. To the extent that personal financial health and patients' health and welfare depend on a computer, mental health professionals need strategies to continue functioning despite a balky information system. Professionals should be sure to have:

- The latest security patches for software.
- A virus protection program (e.g., Norton *AntiVirus* or McAfee *ViruScan*) that includes:
  - Screening e-mails and downloaded material.
  - Regular scans of existing files.
  - Frequent updates.
- Licenses, reinstallation disks, and activation codes for all software.
- A paper file of contracts and printouts of instructions from the vendors of antivirus programs and firewall software and devices in use.
- Backup equipment and gear (including blank disks).
- Regularly tested and implemented backup procedures.
- A frequently refreshed system recovery disk.
- Surge protectors guarding power lines.
- Power supply backup.

- A paper or diskette file of log-in information, passwords, encryption keys, and key Internet addresses kept in a locked drawer or file in the office or at home.
- Instructions for staff, coworkers, family, members, heirs, and assignees on how to access vital clinical and financial data in one's absence.

Safeguarding Patient Information. Additional precautions that practitioners can take with patient information stored in a computer system include:

- A written office standard operating procedure for data security (whether required by HIPAA or not).
- A log of activities relevant to security measures, as well as documentation of reasonable measures taken to protect sensitive data from theft, loss, unauthorized alteration, and corruption.
- Encryption of all stored patient data.
- Hiding sensitive files, if allowed by the computer.
- Required password when turning computer on.

Inevitably, some mental health professionals and patients engaged in online treatment will be harmed by accidents, viruses, and/or hackers. Although thoroughly documented informed consent mitigates liability, there is an implied expectation that professionals will do everything appropriate to maintain security and data integrity. Professionals should be prepared to demonstrate a diligent and consistent effort. Every level of security professionals implement strengthens their defense in court when being tried for an accidental breach of patient confidentiality. Remember: There is no such thing as being too secure.

Protective Measures. Malicious code (viruses, worms, Trojan horses, etc.) can be introduced into a computer in many ways. For example, on September 30, 2002, the Bugbear worm entered the sent-mail folders in e-mail programs, then copied and transmitted old messages it found, possibly including patients' names and addresses and confidential clinical information. The worm struck without warning, even when no e-mail program was open. Encrypting e-mail as it was being sent out afforded no protection, because Bugbear went after the stored file, not the encrypted transmission stream. Bugbear also recorded keystrokes in order to capture passwords and keys to encryption schemes. It opened a back door in the infected computer so that when the machine was online, an outsider using a Web browser could inspect everything in it and corrupt the file content (Roberts, 2002).

The dispersion of this worm was not an isolated incident. Viruses are continually being created and spread throughout the Internet. By the time professionals are informed of each new virus, it may already be too late for their computers.

E-mail attachments have been the most prominent avenue of infection, but browsing a Web site also can precipitate a computer disaster. Some sites inject program scripts into the browser. On execution, these scripts carry out a series of operations, such as delivering the pop-up advertisements that invite the reader to click on various portions to execute further commands. Professionals can configure their browsers not to obey the script's instructions or to do so only under restricted conditions. Professionals surfing the Web should consult the browser's instructions and set up appropriate protections.

Many pornography sites use scripts to cause a browser to begin spawning multiple windows showing other porn sites, which in turn, can bring up others. A quick shutdown of the computer may be the only recourse to eliminate these sites. However, computer shut down may result in, damage to or loss of any open files or unsaved data. (On a personal computer using a Microsoft operating system, however, manually ending the program through the Windows Task Manager may be attempted first.) Scripts can do more than create a nuisance. The most malicious scripts can invade a browser and create an opening for a hacker to control the computer.

Internet Explorer also allows behavioral helper objects (BHOs), a special type of add-in to the Web browser, to be installed when downloading programs from the Internet. Not all BHOs are malicious, but some may send sensitive information (e.g., transmit keystrokes) to advertisers. Installing a program that identifies and deactivates harmful BHOs, such as BHO Cop (http://www.pcmag.com/article2/0,4149,270,00.asp), may further secure a professional's computer and may also reduce the number of pop-up ads (Philippot, 2002).

Professionals are advised to do the following:

- Consult the instructions that came with the browser to set up appropriate restrictions.
- Experiment with the e-mail program and use its features to block harmful input and identify and isolate questionable material.
- Open e-mail attachments from known sources only.
- Ask the sender of an unknown e-mail attachment to resend the message but to put the material in the body of the e-mail message, if possible.
- Confirm that the sender's computer is not infected if it is necessary to accept a file in e-mail, on a disk, or from a Web site.
- Automatically delete strange-looking e-mail (e.g., with a blank Subject: line, with the recipient's name missing or misspelled, or with an inappropriate name in the From: field).
- Use firewalls.

Not only e-mail and Web pages but also other files entering a computer can deliver a harmful payload. This material includes files on floppy disks, CD-ROMs, and DVDs. Professionals should scrutinize such material for risk. A disk with a pirated copy of Mozart's greatest works may contain malicious hidden programs. Installing illegal software or bootlegged media may cause more harm than good.

A laptop may become infected in the user's home or during travel and, when reattached to the office local area network, infect other computers in the network. A virus spread this way will bypass the firewall, which stops malicious material from entering only from outside the network. An infected disk loaded onto a computer also skirts firewall protection.

In case of infection, professionals may want to look for effects that may not be immediately obvious. When a computer has been infected, the professional could:

- Thoroughly disinfect the computer, following instructions in the virus protection program or gleaned from antivirus Web sites.
- Run virus scans on all network computers.
- Change all log-ins and passwords.

- Inspect all computers on the network for damage by hacker intrusion.
- Document all measures taken to reestablish security, minimize harm, and prevent future attacks.

Professional practices that are large enough to justify the expense should hire an information technology expert to install and maintain needed equipment, answer questions, put out fires, fight viruses, and so on. Hiring an expert enables the professionals to communicate electronically or use a computer for other office-related activities while knowing little about the offenses and defenses discussed here. If the expense can be justified, an information technology expert allows mental health professionals to focus on the activities for which they have been trained.

Children and the Web

An important ethical imperative for professionals operating a Web site is to protect children. Children can potentially access every Web site, and effective barriers are difficult to create. Legally, sites are not considered attractive nuisances (like an unfenced swimming pool), but for commercial sites that specifically target children, Federal Trade Commission guidelines call for the following:

- Clear notice of information collection and use practices.
- Obtainment of verifiable offline parental consent before collecting and using personal information.
- Provision of parental access to children's personal information.
- Prevention of further use of children's personal information by unauthorized sources.

Note that these requirements include all personal information, not just health data. Should a health care Web site serve children directly? Many clinics for safe sex, resources for suicidal children, campaigns to discourage chemical abuse, and other efforts to assist and inform children and adolescents are designed to bypass parents and authorities. To provide similar support over the Internet, professionals could learn how real-world entities have met objections to such practices raised by prosecutors, parents, and pressure groups.

Impressing the Press

It is important for mental health practitioners to expand their roles by becoming advocates for mental health and the mental health community. Although training does not usually address advocacy techniques, training in this area is becoming more crucial for securing needed attention, funding, and resources for professionals and their patients.

Many journalists have little idea of what the psychotechnologies involve. Just as they may tend to conflate the various mental health disciplines, journalists may also tend to lump psychotechnologies together and to oversimplify the issues down to basic questions of privacy, alienation, disregard for the individual, or gimmickry. However, descriptions of advances in the psychotechnologies and reports of research findings can be catchy columns in a hometown paper and interesting human interest segments on television during a slow news day.

Clinicians can aid in the publication of psychotherapy-sensitive and -relevant information by engaging with the media whenever possible. We offer the following tips for promoting the psychotechnologies effectively.

When discussing a particular psychotechnology in an article or interview, be sure to specify the type of technology used and the venue (without being too technical): chat room, e-mail, videoconferencing over low-bandwidth (POTS) or high-bandwidth (ISDN, DSL) carrier systems, or any combination. Then, using whatever latitude the interviewer or reporter offers, emphasize the following:

- The value of professionalism in delivering care via the psychotechnologies.
- The importance of ethical protections.
- Limiting the scope of practice to one's area of competence and licensure.
- Adequate training, supervision, and experience.
- A background in theory and general clinical work but absence of extravagant claims of proficiency.
- Peer support.
- Availability of emergency backup and consultation.
- Continuing professional education.
- Having clinical backup in case of emergency, clinician unavailability, or any other reason.
- The necessity of providing a high quality of service to patients even for initial tentative contacts and seemingly minor issues.
- The importance of respecting each patient's individuality.
- How the psychotechnologies promote patient empowerment.
- The ability of the psychotechnologies to enhance collaboration with the patient.
- How the psychotechnologies can help reach people who have not dealt with their mental health issues because of:
  - Stigma.
  - Inaccessibility.
  - Cost.
  - Misunderstanding of mental health care.
- The potential cost savings that some psychotechnologies offer.
- The ability of the psychotechnologies to make it easier for the patient, therapist, and other people to understand, track, aggregate, and analyze what is taking place in treatment (known as *transparency*).
- The ability of the psychotechnologies to improve rather than degrade security and privacy, depending on legislation and government regulations.

Partnering with Employers, Labor Unions, and Employees

Stress reduction through the psychotechnologies is appropriate in the workplace, particularly when on-the-job stress has been shown to be a potential workplace killer (Aptel & Cnockaert, 2002). Employers, labor unions, and employees could become valuable allies for enhancing delivery of mental health care with the psychotechnologies. Some employers that have the funds to afford creative approaches are willing to experiment. For instance, Nigel Bryson, the director of health and environment for

GMB, Britain's general workers union, complained that "many employers are bringing in masseurs, having lunchtime yoga sessions and even bringing in clowns for employees who are working in stressful environments" (GMB, 2002). Although many employers recognize the advantage of having a mental health care program associated with their firm, the success of such programs can be enhanced by recruiting the active support of labor unions to create within the enterprise a culture that encourages people to seek competent help appropriately.

RESEARCH

> Substantial, quality research is needed in order to address the real impact of psychology applications using telehealth technologies (Rabasca, 2000).

The Internet is filled with claims for miracle cures for any physical or psychological problem under the sun, and it is difficult for clients to know which technology-based approach is empirically supported. Because people tend to focus on the dramatic case, they can be led down the wrong path by anecdotal evidence of dozens of supposedly successful treatments. As professionals learn in college and graduate school, only scientific study and comparison with established treatments can substantiate the use of a new approach when offered as a clinical service rather than as an experiment. It is the licensed professional's responsibility to distinguish between experimental treatments (and to obtain approval for the experiment by an appropriate academic review board or human subjects committee) and clinical services.

A number of issues arise when performing research on psychotechnologies. For instance, unless high tech–supported therapies are tested in the client population for whom they are intended (e.g., on people with social phobia or pedophilia rather than on healthy college students), there is the possibility of overgeneralizing a program's successful outcome. Valuable time, resources, and consumer confidence can all be lost. The following sections outline how research may address immediate and future needs for developing and testing behavioral e-health applications that will soon be available. Optimal treatment dissemination by Internet-enabled technologies requires a multidisciplinary initiative to focus the talents, energy, and creativity of behavioral and social scientists.

Immediate Needs

Several controlled studies have found that computer-aided interventions can be effective in treating depression and anxiety and in helping with weight regulation (see chapter 6 and appendix A). Overall, however, few long-term controlled studies have focused on the use of the psychotechnologies with specific clinical populations.

Where might the reasonable researcher begin? First, researchers must recognize that a wide gap exists between practitioners and scientists and that the psychotechnologies have acted both to decrease and to increase this gap. On one hand, researchers have demonstrated a keen interest in developing the psychotechnologies, and have helped produce a wide range of psychotechnologies available to the professional. On the other hand, the Internet has generated a small movement of behavioral e-health therapists who have neither formal training nor a scientific basis for their behavioral e-health services but who nonetheless these services deliver to unknown, unseen, and undiagnosed Internet users worldwide.

Fortunately, some telehealth and telemedicine programs evince a strong interest in mental health practice. For several decades, mental health professionals have been practicing remotely, using sophisticated telecommunication technologies, and have set precedents for referral systems and working alliances between multidisciplinary groups of practitioners. Mental health is likely to continue to be the most well-funded, meaningful, and efficacious avenue for the interested researcher or practitioner to follow.

Translation of current structured in-person interventions into Internet-based multimedia technology should start with interventions that have strong empirical validation in the literature. Many current cognitive-behavioral interventions (e.g., Barlow, 2001) are appropriate for this translation process, and the empirical evidence of their safety and effectiveness is sufficient to justify their place among the initial interventions used for Internet study. Tested behavioral medicine programs for smoking cessation or weight loss should also remain effective after migration to the Internet. School-based prevention programs aimed at smoking, recreational drug use, and alcoholism, as well as safe-sex programs, also need to be evaluated. Initial research at Stanford University indicates that interactive multimedia technology may help reduce the incidence of eating disorders among young people, which could be of great public health importance (Taylor, Winzelberg, & Celio, 2001).

The highly structured, systematic, and reproducible therapy provided through computers is of great advantage for scientific study, which requires methodological rigor and reproducibility. The computer can record log-on times and interactions with a moderator or other participants. Professionals can then analyze the data to profile compliance rates or typical usage patterns and to identify programs that are not frequented sufficiently. Professionals can analyze text exchanges to determine the degree of emotional disclosure and other psychologically relevant variables during the course of therapy and how these variables are related to treatment outcome.

After research has shown that some basic structured in-person interventions translate well to Internet-based multimedia, other applications of this technology can be explored. Maintenance of treatment gains and prevention of relapse can potentially be effectively accomplished by providing Internet-based information and e-mail contact with a professional or paraprofessional. A combined approach to helping clients transition to health through the Web could be ideal. For example, regular in-person intervention could increasingly be supported by Internet-based information. At the end of treatment, the client could be introduced to a community of people who are recovering from the same disorder, such as is available at several large mental health community Web sites. Additionally, automatic instructions or reminders by mobile phone or e-mail could help clients in their transition from therapy. This model can be applied to many disorders, but it appears especially potent for the treatment of anxiety, substance abuse, and dependency.

A combined approach could also be used with a variety of psychopharmacological interventions, which could be phased out while psychoeducation and social support are phased in to promote long-term success. Pharmacological therapy could be supported by online checkups and reminders. An important medical application of Internet-based psychosocial support would be in the prevention of significant and lasting mood changes after surgery, which can increase mortality and interfere with rehabilitation efforts (Rozanski, Blumenthal, & Kaplan, 1999).

The Internet is an ideal technology for studying the treatment of rare disorders. Some psychological disorders are so rare that it is difficult to conduct systematic research on them in a single geographic area. Researchers could develop and test

Internet-based treatments by accumulating cases from health care providers across the United States or the rest of the world. Furthermore, for targeted populations, the Internet allows the development and study of social support groups that would normally reach insufficient size within one geographic area. For example, a 30-year-old patient who is struggling with trichotillomania and who lives in an isolated area in the U.S. Midwest may benefit from being part of an Internet-based, moderated support group that includes other such patients from around the world.

Research data gathered from such a group may help develop specialized programs that could be translated into various languages and offered to the mental health community as a resource for practitioners to use with their clients. Similarly, two gay fathers raising a family of three children may find it difficult to discuss parenting issues without the support and input of other gay parents. If these fathers were part of an online community of gay parents, they could access resources and feel the support of other people who share similar extended family, neighborhood, school, and health care situations. Research conducted in such groups would be of benefit to other gay or lesbian parents.

In addition to pursuing computer-aided research on and developing interventions for a wider variety of disorders, professionals should try to streamline and optimize these interventions. For example, professionals could adapt an intervention to the needs of specific users by monitoring their usage patterns and progress. Clients with problematic usage characteristics, such as insufficient time spent with self-help programs, can be automatically identified and can receive a specific motivational intervention.

The integration of new technologies also needs to be tested. For example, translation of PC-based interventions to cellular personal digital assistants (PDA) could be useful because PDAs are always available. The much smaller PDA screen requires the information to be delivered in small, usable chunks, however. It is not known whether this approach would be effective. PDA-based interventions might be well suited for psychoeducational programs that promote healthy behavior, such as programs that deliver medication use reminders or help with food regulation or exercise regimens.

Telehealth research would be helpful in exploring these issues:

- How telehealth interventions affect various clinical groups.
- What effect telehealth has on therapeutic relationships.
- Whether practitioners and consumers find telehealth interventions accessible and desirable.
- How socioeconomic status, ethnicity, culture, geographic location, age, and sex affect patient access to and acceptance of telehealth.
- How to most effectively educate consumers and practitioners in the use of telehealth.

For an extensive list of research related to the use of PDAs in health care, readers can review bibliographies online. One bibliography is available through the Arizona Health Sciences Library Web site at http://educ.ahsl.arizona.edu/pda/art.htm.

Journal Resources

Over the past decade, some journals have included special issues or occasional articles about telemedicine, telehealth, and e-health. Other journals have developed specifically to address these topics, and some are devoted exclusively to mental health. Readers can start their search for anecdotal discussions, pilot, or empirical research from these sources:

- American Psychological Association (http://www.apa.org/journals).
  - *American Psychologist.*
  - *Journal of Applied Psychology.*
  - *Journal of Consulting and Clinical Psychology.*
  - *Monitor on Psychology* (http://www.apa.org/monitor).
  - *Professional Psychology: Research and Practice.*
  - *Psychotherapy: Theory/Research/Practice/Training.*
- Association for Advancement of Behavioral Therapy (http://www.aabt.org/publication).
  - *The Behavior Therapist.*
  - *Behavior Therapy.*
- Mary Ann Liebert, Inc. (http://www.liebertpub.com).
  - *Cyberpsychology and Behavior.*
  - *Telemedicine Journal and E-health.*
- Various Publishers.
  - *Interacting with Computers* (http://www.elsevier.nl/locate/intcom).
  - *Journal of American Health Information Management Association* (http://www.ahima.org).
  - *Journal of Computer-Mediated Communication* (http://www.ascusc.org/jcmc).
  - *Journal of Medical Internet Research* (http://www.jmir.org).
  - *Journal of Telemedicine and Telecare* (http://www.coh.uq.edu.au/jtt).
  - *Open Minds* (http://www.openminds.com).
  - *Telemedicine Today* (http://www.telemedtoday.com).

Additional Information Sources

Professionals interested in mental health may want to affiliate with general telehealth programs, both regionally and internationally. Such programs are evolving so rapidly that it is difficult for professionals to separate marketing hype from valid program features and benefits. Some large professional associations and agencies have addressed the need for guidance. Assistance is available from a number of credible clearinghouses. Resources for information about ethical statements, initiatives, funding, programs or projects include:

- American Counseling Association (http://www.counseling.org).
- American Psychiatric Association (http://www.psych.org).
- American Psychological Association (http://www.apa.org).
- American Telemedicine Association (http://www.atmeda.org).
- Association of Telehealth Service Providers (http://www.atsp.org).
- Health Resources and Services Administration (http://www.hrsa.gov).
- International Society for Telemedicine (http://www.isft.org).

- National Institute on Disability and Rehabilitation Research (http://www.ed. gov/about/offices/list/osers/nidrr/index.html).
- National Institutes of Mental Health (http://www.nimh.nih.gov).
- Office for the Advancement of Telehealth (http://telehealth.hrsa.gov).
- RUS Distance Learning and Telemedicine Grant Program (http://www.usda. gov/rus/telecom/dlt/dlt.htm).
- Telemedicine Information Exchange (http://tie.telemed.org).
- Telemedicine Information Service (http://www.tis.bl.uk).
- Robert Wood Johnson Foundation (http://www.rwjf.org).
- Small Business Innovation Research Program (http://grants1.nih.gov/grants/ funding/sbir.htm).
- Small Business Technology Transfer (http://www.sba.gov/sbir).
- United States National Library of Medicine (http://www.nlm.nih.gov).

GENERAL SUGGESTIONS

As a final effort, we respectfully submit the following suggestions:

- Practitioners could encourage colleagues to learn about and become active with the psychotechnologies. Learning about and assisting colleagues to overcome resistance to using technology is something all practitioners can do. Practitioners helping and empowering one another could be a transformative, grass-roots approach to mobilizing the professions.
- National, state, and local resources for research and project development could be obtained and allocated (e.g., NIH, NIMH, and private grants). Practitioners might learn how to better position themselves to obtain such funding for new areas of research and practice related to technology.
- Professional associations should consider calling for research in all areas related to the psychotechnologies.
- Graduate schools should authorize graduate training in all areas of behavioral telehealth to equip students with skills for the future and to provide the research base for making sound, empirically based decisions related to ethics, assessment, interventions, and the law.
- State licensing groups could encourage practitioners to gain proficiency in the psychotechnologies by offering continuing education credits for telehealth training.
- Professionals might create and encourage patients to take courses designed for a lay audience on the benefits and risks of using e-mail in health care.
- Practitioners might participate with state governing boards and professional organizations to help develop reasonable procedures for protecting consumers and practitioners.
- Practitioners might seek ways to participate in developing technology to help authenticate the identity of clients and practitioners using electronic media.
- Practitioners might foster the development of a new vocabulary to fully communicate the dynamics of behavioral telehealth.

- Practitioners should push for practitioner procedure codes in states in which tele-health laws have mandated insurance payment but in which billable insurance codes do not exist.
- Practitioners should address the need for a clear, operational definition of psychotherapy that includes ethical, legal, and clinical considerations. This definition would address the special problems of psychological practice using e-mail, chat rooms, newsgroups, Web-based audio streams, interactive video equipment, computer-based programs and devices, as well as the next generation of telecommunication technology.
- Practitioners can offer research to evaluate risks and benefits of various forms of electronic consultation and can define suggested target populations and at-risk populations.
- Practitioners could work with legal consultants to develop text-based, graphic, audio, and video statements about training, competence, licensure, confidentiality, risk management, scope of practice, and other factors. These statements should be designed to educate both practitioners and consumers.
- Practitioners could become active in developing electronic referral systems to other practitioners who use the psychotechnologies.
- Minimal requirements for a nationwide (and worldwide) emergency backup system should be delineated for mental health patients. Funds and resources to support the backup system should be allocated. This system needs to be responsive to differing needs of both patients and practitioners operating under different conditions (e.g., combination of remote and in-person sessions versus exclusively remote, cross-national, or cross-cultural, trauma victims, disaster zones).
- Practitioners and security engineers could collaborate in building tools to safeguard clients' communications and records.
- Ultimately, as technological tools advance, mental health practitioners need to determine whether and when in-person treatment is a necessary component of a treatment plan for a particular patient. Practitioners need to make research-based and ethical decisions about which technological tools to use, with which patient, at which point in the treatment process, and why.

CONCLUDING REMARKS

However uncertain any forecasting may be, there is no question that technology is changing health care. It is both advantageous and crucial for mental health professionals to become active at this formative stage. Pressure from patients and health care organizations will force professionals to overcome their fears of being overwhelmed with electronic messages, liability problems, and breaches in security (Eysenbach & Diepgen, 1998; Spielberg, 1998). Mental health programs can prosper in this new arena but only if visionary professionals answer the call.

There are many ways help the development of behavioral telehealth and behavioral e-health. With determination, mental health practitioners can improve quality while providing safe and reliable services for patients through the use of technology. It is for the betterment of the professions and services that professionals educate their peers, the public, and policymakers on issues of technology. Ways for professionals to assist the adoption of the new technologies in mental and behavioral health include the following:

- Learn as much as practical about the psychotechnologies.
- Educate colleagues about the use of any of the psychotechnologies.
- Support the writing and administration of grants to develop and deliver services to underserved clinical populations.
- Supervise, advise, or directly conduct research.
- Engage in the publication of research.
- Influence the development of specific guidelines and ethical codes.
- Develop and conduct surveys to determine how well ethical guidelines are being followed.
- Take an active role in local, state, and national professional associations to bring about legislative change through legislation, including tort reform.
- Educate the public about using the psychotechnologies safely.
- Seek employment in existing telehealth sites, such as schools, hospitals, military, and correctional and other facilities, with the goal of participating in behavioral telehealth.
- Develop and/or evaluate programs for telehealth delivery projects, with special focus on outcomes as well as on ethical and legal issues, particularly issues concerning privacy, confidentiality, security, and data integrity.
- Develop appropriate content for distribution through Web sites.
- Work with technology companies to responsibly develop products that add value to practitioners, patients, and the therapeutic relationship.
- Work with insurance companies to protect practitioner and patient rights, as well as the principles underlying the integrity of mental health care.

The reader undoubtedly has noticed that we have repeatedly cautioned against jumping too quickly into unknown waters. This conservative approach may seem overly cautious, but as technology buffs, we have seen some mental health professionals blithely sail into online clinical practice without adequate forethought. We hope that by considering the issues this book presents, the eager professional will proceed while managing the risks for patients, practitioners, and sponsoring organizations.

As the barriers and risks involved in providing online clinical services are resolved, we are excited by the possibilities for enhanced effectiveness, an enlarged client population, as well as high practitioner and client satisfaction in mental health care. We hope that this books strikes a reasonable balance between enthusiasm and professionalism. As professionals, we all have the opportunity to change mental health care by shaping and embracing the psychotechnologies for the respective disciplines.

Appendix A

Comparative Studies of Psychotechnologies

Modalities, Clinical Condition, or Patient Population Studied	Study Synopsis (N)	Findings
Telephone (Napolitano, 1999)	Lung transplantation (71). For 8 consecutive weeks, experimental subjects received a weekly phone call delivering supportive and cognitive-behavioral therapy; a randomized control group received no phone calls or special mental health care.	Experimental subjects showed greater increases than did controls in general well-being, quality of life, and social support.
Networked and locally stored computer support program (Schneider, Walter, & O'Donnell, 1990)	Tobacco dependency (1,158). In 2 × 2 design, subjects were randomly allowed access to networked and/or locally stored computerized supplementary support during course of in-person treatment.	Higher abstinence and lower dropout if subjects had both networked and local computer access; worst outcome if neither.
Internet program (Winzelberg et al., 2000)	Concern about weight (60). Subjects given access to Internet health education program compared with unsupported random control subjects.	Significant improvement in body image and drive for thinness in experimental subjects over controls.
Internet program, informational Web site (Tate, Wing, & Winett, 2001)	Obesity (65). Overweight subjects participated in a structured behavioral e-mail-based program; overweight control subjects accessed an educational Web site.	E-mail behavioral therapy group lost more weight and waist size than did controls.
Internet, person to person (Cohen & Kerr, 1998)	Anxiety (24). Impact of online counseling compared with in-person counseling using the State-Trait Anxiety Inventory, the Counselor Rating form, the Session Evaluation Questionnaire, and a computer use survey.	Significant comparable decreases in anxiety were reported by subjects using each modality. Counselor ratings were similar for each modality.

Cont.

Modalities, Clinical Condition, or Patient Population Studied	Study Synopsis (N)	Findings
Internet program (Gustafson et al., 1999)	HIV (184). Experimental subjects completed trial of Comprehensive Health Enhancement Support System (CHESS) for 3 to 6 months at home; randomized controls received no intervention. Self-report surveys on quality of life and medical service use were completed before and during experiment and at 2, 5, and 9 months follow-up.	Users reported better quality of life, less time spent on ambulatory care visits, and reduced hospitalization compared with control subjects. High user satisfaction.
Interactive voice response system (Osgood-Hynes et al., 1998)	Mild to moderate depression (28). Treatment booklets supplemented by touch-tone-activated interactive voice response telephone calls recommended self-help strategies based on information entered by clients; outcome evaluated by HAMD and by Work and Social Adjustment ratings.	Significant improvement in Depression, Work and Social Adjustment scores, with 64% of completers achieving more than 50% reduction in HAMD scores.
Interactive voice response (IVR), paper and pencil, live telephone (Baer, Brown-Beasley, Sorce, & Henriques, 1993)	Obsessive-compulsive disorder (18). Randomized order of administration of the YBOCS by 3 methods in each session for each subject.	Very high agreement of all modalities. Interactive computer–telephone system was rapid and well accepted by subjects.
Interactive voice response (IVR), person to person (Kobak, Greist, Jefferson, Katzelnick, & Mundt, 2001)	Psychiatric patients (113). HAMD was clinician-administered in person or by computer over the telephone.	Psychometric properties of IVR version of the HAMD were like standard. Patients preferred the clinicians but were less embarrassed with IVR.
Interactive voice response (IVR), person to person (Kobak et al., 2001)	Psychiatric patients (74). HAMA was clinician-administered in person or by computer over the telephone.	Psychometric properties of IVR version of the HAMA were like standard. Patients preferred the clinicians but were less embarrassed with IVR.
Interactive voice response (IVR), person to person (Mundt et al., 1998)	Ambulatory psychiatric clinic patients (367). HAMD in full or short forms was clinician-administered in person or by computer over the telephone.	Scores obtained by IVR were similar to clinicians' scores.
Interactive voice response (IVR), telephone (Kobak et al., 1997b)	Ambulatory psychiatric clinic patients (105). PRIME-MD, IVR-PRIME-MD, and a computer version of modified modules of the SCID were administered to each patient.	For screening purposes, each instrument performed equally well in each modality, except that the IVR-PRIME-MD diagnosed more dysthymia.
Videophone (May et al., 2001)	Depression and anxiety (22). Extensive interviews probed subjective reactions to mental health sessions conducted by videophone.	Users reported that videophone communication was difficult and interfered with therapeutic relationships.

Cont.

Modalities, Clinical Condition, or Patient Population Studied	Study Synopsis (N)	Findings
Narrow-bandwidth videoconferencing, person to person (Baer et al., 1995)	Obsessive-compulsive disorder (26). YBOCS, HAMD, and HAMA administered to 16 in-person subjects and 10 videoconferencing subjects.	No degradation in excellent interrater reliability using videoconferencing. Good satisfaction expressed by both patients and raters.
Low-cost videoconferencing, person to person (Ball, Scott, & McLaren, & Wotson 1993)	Schizophrenia, depression, and movement disorder (11). MMSE administered in person, then repeated in modified version via videoconferencing.	High correlation between ratings for in-person and videoconferencing administration.
Videoconferencing at high and low bandwidths, person to person (Zarate et al., 1997)	Schizophrenia (45). Scores on BPRS, SAPS, and SANS obtained by high- or low-bandwidth videoconferencing and compared with previous in-person ratings.	Reliability of all modalities was equal for BPRS and SAPS, but SANS fared worse under low-bandwidth condition. Acceptability was good.
Videoconferencing, telephone, person to person (Glueckauf et al., 2002)	Epilepsy (22). Six sessions of videoconferencing, speakerphone, or office-based counseling. Measured the severity and frequency of the problem, Social Skills Rating System, modified Working Alliance Inventory, and adherence to treatment.	No difference in adherence or initial treatment outcomes across all 3 modalities, while significant reductions in problem severity and frequency in all 3 conditions were reported.
Videoconferencing, telephone, person to person (Day, 2000)	Psychotherapy alliance (48). Each of the 16 subjects in each modality completed 5 videotaped cognitive-behavioral treatment sessions subsequently rated for Therapist Exploration, Client Participation, and Client Hostility.	No differences found in the working alliance, suggesting that technology can be used among various patient groups to provide therapy.
Videoconferencing, person to person (Gammon, Sørlie, Bergvik, & Hoifodt, 1998; Sørlie, Gammon, Bergvik, & Sexton, 1999)	Psychotherapy supervision (12). Alternating videoconferencing and in-person sessions more than 6 months gathered information on the benefits and drawbacks of videoconferencing for supervising psychiatry residents.	Supervisors and trainees expressed satisfaction.
Videoconferencing, person to person (Brodey, Claypoole, Motto, Arias, & Goss, 2000)	Psychiatric symptoms (43). Incarcerated psychiatric patients were interviewed in person or by videoconferencing and rated on the Global Severity Index of the BSI.	Group means were comparable, as was the moderate level of expressed satisfaction in both groups.
Videoconferencing, person to person (Dongier, Tempier, Lalinec-Michaud, & Meunier, 1986)	Psychiatric clinic and hospital patients (85). Questionnaire rating opinions about psychiatric interviews completed by patients, therapists, and consultants involved in either in-person or videoconferencing sessions.	Mean ratings for videoconferencing were almost as good as for in-person interviewing.

Cont.

Modalities, Clinical Condition, or Patient Population Studied	Study Synopsis (N)	Findings
Videoconferencing, person to person (Menon et al., 2001)	Depression and cognitive status (24). Subjects assessed with the GDS short version, the HAMD, and the SPMSE. A second interviewer repeated this assessment either in person or by low-bandwidth videophone.	Videophone assessment results were close to in-person results, but subjects preferred the former modality to a 2-hour trip to the clinic.
Videoconferencing, person to person (Pollard & LePage, 2001)	Psychiatric therapeutic relationship (35). Patients usually seen using in-person methods were interviewed after their first videoconferencing session.	Twenty-seven patients felt that the physician understood them at least as well in the videoconference, and 22 considered that modality the same as or better than in-person contact. Five were unwilling to use videoconferencing again.
Videoconferencing, person to person (Rhein, 2001)	Depressive disorders (90). Course of psychotherapy delivered either remotely or in person.	There was no interaction of treatment modality with the observed adverse impact of personality disorders on treatment outcome.
Videoconferencing, person to person (Tang, Chiu, Woo, Hjelm, & Hui, 2001)	Psychiatric assessments (45). Psychiatric assessments of veterans by videoconferencing.	Videoconferencing was highly feasible, acceptable to all participants, and cost-effective, as compared with in-person visits.
Videoconferencing, person to person (Schopp, Johnstone, & Merrell, 2000)	Interpersonal factors (98). Experimental subjects interviewed by videoconferencing; control subjects interviewed in person.	No group differences in ratings of interpersonal factors between modalities. Cost of video was less and subjects preferred it, but psychologists preferred in-person interviewing.
Videoconferencing, person to person (Baigent et al., 1997)	Psychiatric disorders (63). One psychiatrist conducted semistructured interviews, and a second psychiatrist observed either remotely or in same room.	Interrater reliability of diagnoses was the same in both settings, but "degree of concern" for the patient and frequency of certain symptoms were lower with videoconferencing.
Videoconferencing, person to person (Ruskin et al., 1998)	Psychiatric disorders (30). Two psychiatrists conducted SCID interviews with each subject, either both in person or one by videoconferencing.	Reliability for each diagnosis was the same for in-person and different-location comparisons.
Videoconferencing, person to person (Montani et al., 1996)	Geriatric patients (10). MMSE and clock-face test given in person and through videoconferencing.	Subjects performed slightly worse with remote administration, possibly because of difficulty with hearing.
Videoconferencing, person to person (Stevens, Doidge, Goldbloom, Voore, & Farewell, 1999)	Psychotic and nonpsychotic psychiatric patients (40). California Psychotherapy Alliance Scale and a special Interview Satisfaction Scale were completed by subjects randomly assigned to in-person or high-bandwidth videoconferencing unstructured 90-minute psychiatric assessment and treatment-planning interviews.	Alliance scores were the same for both modalities, and satisfaction was good, but the psychiatrists preferred in-person interviewing.

Cont.

Modalities, Clinical Condition, or Patient Population Studied	Study Synopsis (N)	Findings
Videoconferencing, person to person (Bouchard et al., 2004)	Panic with agoraphobia (21). Cognitive behavior therapy (CBT).	Videoconference was reported to be as effective as person to person treatment.
Videoconferencing (Simpson et al., 2003)	Eating Disorders (12). Psychological and nutritional services offered to patients in remote areas of Scotland.	Informal study demonstrated various benefits to video-based services.
Videoconferencing, person to person (Nelson, Barnard & Cain, 2003)	Childhood depression (28). Random assignment. Various measures used to screen and assess progress after 8 week cognitive behavior therapy.	Treatment was effective across both conditions.
Virtual reality, person to person (Garcia-Palacios, Hoffman, See, Tsai, & Botella, 2001)	Arachnophobia (1,423). Undergraduate students completed a survey that contained explanations of the two treatment procedures and provided ratings of their willingness to participate in each procedure.	Eighty-one percent chose virtual reality over in-person treatment.
Virtual reality, person to person (Perpina et al., 1999)	Eating disorders (13). Subjects were randomly assigned to either the standard body image treatment or virtual reality condition and then assessed using psychotherapy, ED, and BI measures.	ED measures showed no differences. The virtual reality condition showed greater improvement in depression, anxiety, and various BI measures.

Note. BPRS = Brief Psychiatric Rating Scale (Overall & Gorham, 1962). BSI = Brief Symptom Inventory (Derogatis & Melisarators, 1983). California Psychotherapy Alliance Scale (Gaston, 1991). Counselor Rating form (Barak & Lacrosse, 1975). GDS = Geriatric Depression Scale short version (Yesavage et al., 1982). HAMA = Hamilton Anxiety Rating Scale (Hamilton, 1959). HAMD = Hamilton Depression Rating Scale (Hamilton, 1960). IVR-PRIME-MD = computer version of PRIME-MD. MMSE = Mini-Mental Status Examination (Folstein, Folstein, & McHugh, 1975). PRIME-MD = Primary Care Evaluation of Mental Disorder (Spitzer et al., 1994). SANS = Scale for the Assessment of Negative Symptoms (Andreasen, 1984a). SAPS = Scale for the Assessment of Positive Symptoms (Andreasen, 1984b). SCID = Structured Clinical Interview for DSM-IV (Spitzer, Williams, Gibbon, & First, 1990). Session Evaluation Questionnaire (Stiles, 1980). SPMSE = Short Portable Mental Status Exam (Pfeiffer, 1975). State-Trait Anxiety Inventory (Spielberger, Sydeman, Owen, & Marsh, 1999). YBOCS = Yale-Brown Obsessive Compulsive Scale (Goodman et al., 1989).

Appendix B

Sample Listserv Guidelines

The following guidelines should be available to all subscribers on a professional listserv. These guidelines have proved to be useful and necessary through the years when dealing with complex situations that demand well-considered professional responses.

The guidelines can be easily modified for consumer listservs as well. This listing is by no means all-inclusive. Rule of thumb: If it concerns psychology and the Internet, it is a relevant topic. The guidelines are divided into these name sections:

    I. Agreement for Participating.
    II. Topics to Be Discussed on the NetPsy List.
    III. Deciding to Participate.
    IV. NetPsy Policy Statements.
    V. Enforcing List Rules.
    VI. Listserv How To.
    VII. Netiquette.
    VIII. Disclaimers.
    IX. NetPsy Web Page.

I. AGREEMENT FOR PARTICIPATING

NetPsy is a loose sounding board for professionals interested in applications of psychology with the Internet. Subscribers agree to adhere to the following guidelines as a condition of the subscription. For example: No patient identifiers may be used. Privacy is not ensured. In fact, there is probably little chance that, in case of a claim, most courts would shield from discovery statements made here. No subscriber may disclose the name of any other subscriber to nonsubscribers or other people.

II. TOPICS TO BE DISCUSSED ON THE NetPsy LIST

NetPsy is a place to discuss the theory and practice of using the Internet for such psychological applications as therapy and counseling, crisis intervention, testing, research, and support groups, for example.

List members are not permitted to use NetPsy to seek clients or therapists for personal reasons. That is, professionals can not try to market their services, and list members can not seek the professional services of another member on the NetPsy list. Such exchanges are considered to be off topic.

Some examples of relevant topics include:

- Interpersonal effects of current and evolving forms of online technology.
- New behavioral patterns evolving in online environments; manifestation of traditional human interactions as they occur online, such as e-mail behavior, chat room behavior, and their foci, such as professional discussion, romance, or grieving.
- Influences of the online community in the daily offline and online lives of users.
- Limitations and benefits of visual or auditory feedback in interpersonal communications (both group and individual).
- Use of the Internet as a vehicle for psychotherapy, crisis counseling, and other professional interventions, including those related to disaster.
- Ethical and legal issues related to behavioral health care online.
- Online behavioral health care demographics.
- Research related to all aspects of psychology and the Internet, or the psychology of Internet use.
- Funding sources for Internet research.
- Technological advances affecting behavioral health care on the Internet.
- Innovative uses of online technology to treat disorders as classified in *DSM-IV*.
- Online behavioral health care terminology and symbols.
- Reviews of online behavioral health care resource sites, lists, newsletters, and so on.
- Self-help, support, and moderated lists for group therapy.
- Online group dynamics.
- Financial aspects of professionals offering services online.
- Credentialing issues for professionals online.

III. DECIDING TO PARTICIPATE

Trained mental health professionals are not the only people allowed to participate on this list; all points of view are encouraged. However, professionals should not say that they are practicing clinicians, either by implication or, by omission of fact, unless they are so credentialed. On the other hand, credentialed professionals should not withhold that information.

Participants should post a short introduction stating how they would like to be addressed, what they do, what they would like to be doing, and what they are seeking from this list. Giving the specifics of credentials, training, years in practice, and the exact nature of the service delivered is required.

If possible, professionals should develop and use an e-mail signature file that includes the state or country from which they work, their license number, if any, and their full name and e-mail address. Any license number must be posted in the signature.

Signature files should be no more than six lines. Professionals who are unable to use a signature file should include their name and credentials at the end of each post.

IV. NetPsy POLICY STATEMENTS

All new members will be placed on probationary status, which may include being placed on moderated status until their subscriptions are approved by the list owner or administrator. Probationary members who consistently ignore or violate common Netiquette as outlined in Section VII will be denied membership.

Members must clearly identify themselves. They should create a signature file as described in section III or include their name and credentials with each post. Members are not permitted to use an alias or otherwise conceal their identity. Doing so will result in immediate removal from the list.

Any member using the NetPsy subscriber list to bypass the listserv in order to send private e-mail to the list subscribers for any purpose at any time will be subject to immediate and irrevocable removal from this list. People on moderated status who resubscribe under another name and address to circumvent the moderated status, regardless of their motive, will be permanently unsubscribed. Baiting, taunting, name calling, and general disrespect for the points of view of other subscribers will not be tolerated and will be grounds for immediate removal from this list.

V. ENFORCING LIST RULES

To facilitate respectful discussion, essential Netiquette policies will be enforced in the following manner at the sole discretion of the list owner:

- First, members will receive a courtesy warning from the list owner or administrator and possibly will be asked to refrain from posting to the list for a week. Members who continue to post will be permanently removed from the list.
- A member who, for any reason, posts a public complaint about the courtesy warning, however veiled, will be permanently removed from the list.
- Members who are asked to refrain from posting for a week and comply may begin posting to the list again. However, members who repeat the unacceptable behavior will be permanently excluded from participation in the list without further warning.

VI. LISTSERV HOW TO

It is important to understand the difference between the two listserv e-mail addresses. Messages that are intended for the list to read are sent to NETPSY@MAELSTROM. STJOHNS.EDU. Messages intended to send commands to the listserver are sent to LISTSERV@MAELSTROM.STJOHNS.EDU

Read the following carefully:

- **How to post to the Group:** Send an e-mail message to NETPSY@MAELSTROM. STJOHNS.EDU.

- **How to Send a Command to the Listserv:** Send an e-mail message to LISTSERV@MAELSTROM.STJOHNS.EDU.
- **How to Unsubscribe:** Send an e-mail message to LISTSERV@MAELSTROM. STJOHNS.EDU. In the body of the message, type "SIGNOFF NETPSY".
- **How to Tell Friends to Subscribe:** Send an e-mail message to LISTSERV@MAELSTROM.STJOHNS.EDU. In the body of the message, type "SUB NETPSY <firstname lastname>".
- **How to Set Listserv Options:** Send an e-mail message to LISTSERV @MAELSTROM.STJOHNS.EDU.

Information on LISTSERV commands can be found in the LISTSERV Reference Card, which can be retrieved by sending an INFO REFCARD command to the Listserv at LISTSERV@MAELSTROM.STJOHNS.EDU.

VII. NETIQUETTE

Holding a discussion online is very different from a face-to-face discussion. The lack of facial expressions, body language, and vocal inflections makes it easy to misinterpret a comment that is read. This list uses guidelines called Netiquette to help make messages come across as intended—polite. All participants should adhere to these guidelines.

- *Format:* Be informal but thoughtful. A note's contents and header should be carefully reviewed before being sent. The note should be correctly addressed, free of typos, and mean what it says.
- *Sensitivity:* Remember that human beings with feelings are reading the messages.
- *Subject line:* Give the message a meaningful and accurate subject line descriptor. Doing so will eliminate the need for subscribers not drawn to a topic to sort through mail.
- *Forwarding mail:* Make sure that the list from which you draw postings allows them to be reposted.
- *Using humor:* Without accompanying nonverbal cues and voice tone, subtle humor in messages can easily be interpreted as searing sarcasm.
- *Copyright:* The issue of copyright is still being hotly debated, so messages signed with a copyright notice may not in fact be copyrighted. Participants should not post trade secrets. All files on this listserv are owned by Pioneer Development Resources and are publicly accessible through various Web sites online. PDR will not protect an individuals copyright under any circumstances. Any extensive or sensitive information to be shared should be posted on a Web page and list readers referred to that page.

    You are responsible for own communications, and for the consequences of their posting. Therefore, participants should do not do any of the following:
  - Transmit material that is copyrighted unless you are the copyright owner or have the permission of the copyright to post it.
  - Send material that infringes on any other intellectual property rights of other people or on the privacy or publicity rights of other people.

- Send material that is obscene, defamatory, threatening, harassing, abusive, hateful, and/or embarrassing to another user or to any other person or entity.
- Send sexually explicit images.
- Send advertisements or solicitations of business.
- Send chain letters or pyramid schemes.
- Impersonate another person.

- *Context and quotes:* Include the points to which you are responding in the text of your reply by quoting a little of the original in your mail reader or by summarizing. Our list is housed by St. Johns University. Its resources are stretched with more than 750 lists. Therefore, please delete all but the critical portions of mail you are citing. Please quote only as much as is germane to your reply, and do not repost an entire message. Write private notes when you need to agree with or apologize to a specific list member, don't post to the entire list. Use professional guidelines in citing references. Also, be aware that any individual can send only four e-mails to the list in a 24-hour period. Therefore, plan postings carefully if you are involved in a discussion.

- *Attachments:* Please do not send attachments to the group; not all e-mail programs are able to handle attachments, and some programs will crash.

- *Response time:* If you choose to participate, please check and respond to your e-mail regularly.

- *Respect others:* Be respectful of differences. This list consists of nonprofessionals and professionals; of givers and receivers of psychotherapy; of U.S. and non-U.S. citizens; of individuals with English and other languages as a first language; and of a multitude of professionals with various professional designations who answer to different ethics codes, state laws, and federal laws (and in some cases laws of other governments) and who are all experimenting with the multitude of nuances possible in a global community.

  Not everyone thinks as you do, so don't expect the list to agree with everything you say. Differing opinions will surface. Respect the opinions of other people even if you do not agree with them.

- *Debate:* Use logic, and feel free to challenge other people's logic. If other people are using non sequiturs, let them know. Stick to the facts, cite someone's words and respond to them, not to your own assumptions about what the person is saying or implying. Do so in a professional and nonconfrontational manner.

- *Observe e-mail behavior:* Use your clinical sense when observing e-mail behavior. Even though much e-mail discussion is standard interaction, this new medium does involve new behavioral possibilities. Feel free to comment on such behavior, but be respectful.

- *Forgive and acknowledge errors:* Sometimes, what may look like distortions are simply errors in assumption. Be aware that repeated errors in assumption can be damaging to a colleague in e-mail; much as with the so-called telephone effect, distortions of any nature can eventually be considered fact.

  Putting anyone in a position of having to write additional posts to defend or correct misinformation you presented as fact is disrespectful and can lead to your removal from this list. Check your facts before responding to posts criticizing a colleague's position.

- *Doubt:* If in doubt about a colleague's position, please ask for clarification. In the absence of answers to questions, ask again; if no answer is forthcoming, respect other people enough to disengage from the topic publicly. Answering e-mail is a choice, not an obligation.   .

- *Flaming:* Flamers on this list will be subject to removal. Accept full responsibility for your participation. Even if you get flamed, you will live and can continue to contribute. If you are upset by someone's posting, sleep on it, talk it over with a few colleagues, and then decide what to do. If you decide to respond, present facts, not attacks. One way to avoid such unpleasantness is to comment on issues, not on people. Use basic psychological principles of communication—being polite is the first rule.

- *Spamming:* This term refers to the sending of unsolicited e-mail, generally an advertisement. Spamming can also take the form of soap box. No member may use the list of NetPsy members to send unsolicited e-mail (spam). The list is private, and all members expect that their NetPsy subscription will not expose them to unwanted e-mail. Members found to be spamming will immediately be removed from this list and possibly also removed from all lists hosted by St. John's University.

- *Professionalism:* Thousands of people may eventually see your messages as archived for future decades. These people may include individuals you know, clients, and/or someone you may employ or may seek employment from in the future. One or more of these people could also, conceivably, be your adversary at law. Information posted blindly or impulsively may come back to haunt you.

VIII. DISCLAIMERS

No Practice of Psychology or Medicine or Nursing

In creating and maintaining this listserv, we are not providing health care services to you; nor are we practicing psychology, medicine, nursing, or any other branch of the healing arts. By creating and maintaining this listserv, we do not enter into a provider–patient relationship with you. We cannot diagnose any health or mental or emotional problem you may have or treat you for any such condition; nor do we attempt to do so. If you wish to be diagnosed or treated, contact your psychologist or physician. If you believe that you or someone you are concerned about is in danger or is facing a real or potential emergency, leave this site and contact your doctor or 911 immediately.

As a condition of participation, you must accept responsibility for your own reactions and related behavior, regardless of what you read from this list. Do not rely on any statement made here as though it were professional advice. Base no decisions on the contents of the list.

This list is not intended to be a replacement for professional consultation or supervision; nor is it a professional publication. Individuals seeking professional journal references should seek information in traditionally recognized sources.

Information distributed is not checked for accuracy. We do not warrant that the listserv will operate error-free or that the listserv and its server are free of computer viruses or other harmful material. If your use of the listserv or the listserv's material results in the need for servicing or replacing equipment or data, we shall not be responsible for those costs.

This listserv and its material are provided on an as-is basis, without any warranties of any kind. We and our affiliates, to the fullest extent permitted by law, disclaim all warranties, express or implied, including the warranty of merchantability, noninfringement of third parties' rights, and the warranty of fitness for particular purpose. Neither we nor our affiliates make any warranties about the accuracy, reliability, completeness, or timeliness of the material, services, software, text, graphics, and links on our listserv.

Limitation of Liability

In no event shall we or our owners, administrators, assistants, or their delegates be liable for any damages whatsoever (including, without limitation, incidental, consequential, or punitive damages, lost profits, or damages resulting from lost data or business interruption) resulting from the use or inability to use material on this listserv, whether based on warranty, contract, tort, or any other legal theory, whether or not we and/or any affiliate is advised of the possibility of such damages.

Indemnity

By using this listserv, you agree to defend, indemnify, and hold harmless us, our owners, administrators, assistants, or their delegates, and our officers, directors, employees, and agents, from and against any and all losses, claims, damages, costs, and expenses (including reasonable legal and accounting fees) that we may become obligated to pay arising or resulting from your use of the listserv or your breach of these guidelines. We reserve the right to assume or participate, at your expense, in the investigation, settlement, and defense of any such action or claim.

IX. NetPsy WEB PAGE

NetPsy has a Web page. There, you will find these guidelines, as well as listserv commands, the SJU list owner policy statement, and access to the NetPsy archives. The URL is http://www.shpm.com/ppc/netpsy/index.shtml.[1]

---

[1] NetPsy List is owned by Pioneer Development Resources, Inc.

Appendix C

Addendum to Patient Consent Agreement

This addendum discusses risks and benefits of telehealth videoconferenced consultation. Please have your attorney review it carefully.

Patient Name:

I, the undersigned, or his or her designee(s), agree to participate in videoconferenced consultation with ——————————. This means that I authorize information related to my medical and mental health care to be electronically transmitted in the form of images and data through an interactive video connection to and from the above-named mental health care provider, other persons involved in my health care, and the staff operating the consultation equipment. I understand that I will be informed of the identities of all parties present during the consultation and of their purpose for attending the consultation.

My health care provider has explained how the telehealth consultation(s) is performed and how it will be used for my treatment. My health care provider has also explained how the consultation(s) will differ from in-person services, including but not limited to emotional reactions that may be generated by the technology. In brief, I understand that my mental health care provider ("provider") will not be physically in my presence. Instead, we will see and hear each other electronically. Some information my provider would ordinarily get in fact-to-face consultation may not be available in teleconsultation. My provider will be unable to touch me or to render any emergency assistance. I understand that telehealth consultation(s) are a new form of treatment, in an area not yet fully validated by research, and that they have potential risks, including the possibility that the technology will fail before or during the consultation, that the transmitted information in any form will be unclear or inadequate for proper use in the consultation(s), and that the information will be intercepted by an unauthorized party(s).

I understand that a physical examination may be performed by individuals at my location at the request of the consulting provider. I authorize the release of any information pertaining to me determined by the above-named health care providers or by my insurance carrier to be relevant to the consultation(s) or processing of insurance claims, including but not limited to my name, Social Security number, birth date, and clinical or medical record information.

I understand that at any time, the consultation(s) can be discontinued either by myself or by my designee or by my health care providers. I further understand that I do not have to answer any question that I feel is inappropriate or answer to which I do not wish persons present to hear, that any refusal to participate in the consultation(s) will not affect my continued treatment, and that no action will be taken against me. I acknowledge, however, that diagnosis depends on information, and treatment depends on diagnosis, so if I withhold information, I assume the risk that a diagnosis might not be made or might be made incorrectly. Were that to happen, my treatment might be less successful than it otherwise would be, or it could fail entirely. I have had the alternatives to the consultation(s) explained to me, and I understand that I can still pursue in-person consultations. I understand that the telehealth consultation(s) does not necessarily eliminate my need to see a specialist in person, and I have received no guarantee as to the consultation's effectiveness.

I understand that my telehealth consultation(s) may be recorded and stored electronically as part of my medical records. I understand that consultations, test results, and disclosures will be held in confidence subject to state and/or federal law. I understand that I am ordinarily guaranteed access to my medical records and that copies of records of consultation(s) are available to me on my written request. I also understand, however, that if my provider, in the exercise of professional judgment, concludes that providing my records to me could threaten the safety of a human being, myself or another person, he or she may rightfully decline to provide them. If such a request is made and honored, I understand that I retain sole responsibility for the confidentiality of the records and that I may have to pay a fee to get a copy. Additionally, I understand that my records may be used for telehealth program evaluation, education, and research and that I will not be personally identified if such a use occurs. I hereby authorize these disclosures to take place without prior written consent. I understand that I am not entitled to royalties or to other forms of compensation for participation in the telehealth consultation(s).

I have received a copy of my health care provider's contact information, including his or her name, telephone number, pager and/or voice mail number, business address, mailing address, and e-mail address (if applicable). I have also been provided with a list of local support services in case of an emergency. I am aware that my health care provider may contact the proper authorities in the case of an emergency. I acknowledge, however, that if I am facing or if I think I may be facing an emergency situation that could result in harm to me or to another person, I am not to seek a telehealth consultation. Instead, I will seek care immediately through my own local provider or at the nearest hospital emergency department or by calling 911.

These are the names and telephone numbers of my local emergency contacts (including local physician; crisis hotline; trusted family, friend, or adviser).

Name   Telephone Number

Name   Telephone Number

Name   Telephone Number

I unconditionally release and discharge _____ (name of organization), its affiliates, agents, employees; _____ (name of consulting organization), its affiliates, agents, and employees; my health care provider and his or her designees from any liability in connection with my participation in the remote consultation(s).

I have read this document carefully and fully understand the benefits and risks. I have had the opportunity to ask any questions I have and have received satisfactory answers. With this knowledge, I voluntarily consent to participate in the telehealth videoconference consultation(s), including but not limited to any care, treatment, and services deemed necessary and advisable, under the terms described herein.

_____   _____
Patient's Signature   Date and Time

_____   _____
Social Security Number   Witness

The above release is given on behalf of _____ because the patient is a minor or has been determined to be incompetent to give medical consent for the following reasons: _____ .

_____   _____
Parent or Legal Guardian   Date and Time

_____
Witness

Appendix D

Draft International Convention on Telemedicine and Telehealth

The State Parties to the Convention,

Inspired by recent advances in the provision of health care and medical education through the use of technology,

Recognizing the common interest of all mankind in the health and welfare of the peoples of the world,

Believing that the promotion of telemedicine and telehealth will contribute to the availability and quality of medical services to those in need, and hence to significant alleviation of human suffering and to improvement of health care and the quality of life for mankind,

Believing that these telemedical services should be available for the benefit of all peoples,

Recognizing that discrimination in the provision of health care services on the basis of race, color, descent, national or ethnic origin, sex or creed would be inconsistent with the principles established in the International Convention on the Elimination of All Forms of Racial Discrimination of March 7, 1966,

Recognizing the right to privacy and confidentiality in health matters,

Desiring to contribute to broad international cooperation in the scientific, legal, and ethical aspects of the use of telemedicine,

Believing that such cooperation will contribute to the development of mutual understanding and to strengthening of friendly relations between States and peoples,

Encouraging continued support for the advancement of telemedicine and its applications,

Convinced that a convention on telemedicine and telehealth will further the goal of providing all people with the highest practicably attainable standard of health care,

Have agreed as follows:

Article 1

TELEMEDICINE AND TELEHEALTH DEFINITIONS

For purposes of this Convention and unless otherwise indicated in a provision of this Convention or required by the Context the terms below shall have the following meanings:

1. *Health care information* is information or data, from whatever source, in any communicable form or medium, obtained in the course of the diagnosis, treatment or care of a patient, that either identifies or can readily be identified to that patient and that relates to the patient's health care or condition.

2. *Telehealth* refers to a diverse group of health-related activities, including health professional education, community health education, public health, research, and administration of health services.

3. *Telehealth information* means information used in the course of delivering health care and related services via electronic media.

4. *Telemedicine* means clinical or supportive medical practice delivered across distances via telecommunications and interactive video technology, performed by licensed or otherwise legally authorized individuals.

5. A *telemedicine physician* is a physician licensed by the appropriate body to provide health care through a telemedicine medium.

Article 2

GENERAL PRINCIPLES

1. The Convention shall be binding in all cases of telemedicine and telehealth delivered across state boundaries:
   a. when the States are Contracting States; or
   b. when the rules of private international law lead to the application of the law of the Contracting State.

2. For purposes of this convention, the State Parties agree that, whenever possible health care delivered through electronic means, regardless of form, shall be treated no differently from health care delivered face to face, directly between health care worker and patient. This Article includes, but is not limited to, issues of financial reimbursement that may arise in relation to this convention.

3. The State Parties shall take reasonable steps to ensure the protection and confidentiality of intellectual property developed to facilitate telemedicine, including, but not limited to, the provision of patenting or other formal recognition in accordance with national laws and international treaties.

4. State Parties shall undertake, with appropriate protection of intellectual property rights:
   a. to foster international dissemination of scientific knowledge concerning telemedicine and telehealth equipment and associated information for the purposes of research and of provision of medical services;
   b. to develop and implement telemedicine and telehealth technology safely and efficiently, particularly in remote, under-served or developing areas; and
   c. to foster scientific and cultural cooperation, particularly between industrialized and developing countries.

5. No provision of this convention may be used by any State, group or person to ends contrary to the principles set forth herein.

6. Each State Party will emphasize and encourage infrastructure development.

7. Each State Party shall ensure, through legislation or other means as appropriate, that all telemedicine and telehealth research carried on within its jurisdiction is

conducted in accordance with internationally accepted medical, scientific and bioethical standards.

8. Each State Party shall endeavor to prohibit and bring to an end, by all appropriate means, discrimination by any persons, group or organization in the provision of health care services on the basis of race, color, descent, national or ethnic origin, sex or creed.

9. The singular includes the plural and the masculine includes the feminine within the text of this Convention.

Article 3

REGULATION OF TELEMEDICINE AND TELEHEALTH; AUTHORIZATION TO PRACTICE

1. *State Licensure.* Each State Party shall ensure that its health and medical licensing boards provide for reasonable opportunity for [full and unrestricted] licensure to physicians and other health care providers who wish to provide telehealth services.

   Where sub-jurisdictions of State Parties regulate licensure requirements within the State Party's general jurisdiction, the State Party shall require such sub-jurisdictions to comply with the provisions of this Convention and ensure that sub-jurisdiction's licensure procedures are no more onerous or time consuming than is contemplated below.

2. *License.* No health care professional shall practice telemedicine or those activities of telehealth which would otherwise require licensure within the State Party's jurisdiction unless he has obtained an authorization to practice issued by the competent authority of the State Party or organization recognized by the State Party to grant licensing authorization.

3. *License Application.* To obtain authorization to practice telehealth as provided for in Article 3.2 the applicant shall apply to the competent authority of the State Party, or to an internationally recognized organization whose standards are recognized by the State Party concerned. Each State Party shall ensure that the competent authority is clearly set out by the State Party. The following particulars and documents shall accompany the application by the applicant:
   a. the name and permanent residence address of the applicant;
   b. the address of the applicant's place of practice;
   c. a certified copy of the professional diploma or other professional certification;
   d. certification of good standing with the applicant's current professional body in the jurisdiction in which the applicant is currently practicing or a proof of inscription on the list of the Order of Physicians;
   e. description of the experience or expertise, if any, which the applicant has in the delivery of the applicant's services via telecommunications media;
   f. description of the area or practice specialty, if any, which the applicant wishes to pursue;
   g. not less than two professional references; and
   h. description of the means of communication, including, but not limited to, software to be used to practice telehealth.

4. *Types of Licenses.* Except as limited by the provision of this convention, each State Party may establish categories of license for telehealth professionals, and may define the scope of practice applicable to each.

5. *Approval Timing.* Each State Party shall take all appropriate measures to ensure that the procedure for reviewing and making a determination with respect to the telehealth care license application is completed within thirty (30) days from the date on which the applicant's submission is complete. Each State Party shall ensure that incomplete applications are noted to the applicant within thirty (30) days of the date of submission of the application. Each State Party shall be entitled to extend the thirty (30) day period for a further fifteen (15) days upon notice to the applicant provided such notice is given to the applicant prior to the expiry of the thirty (30) day review period. A State Party may authorize telehealth practice at a level lower than that applied for. Refusal to grant the higher level may be appealed in the same manner and to the same extent as the State Party provides for applicants for licensure to practice conventional health care.

6. *License Refusal.* Authorization provided for in Article 3.2 may be refused if:

   a. the applicant has not provided the competent authority the requirement particulars and documents set out in Article 3.3; or

   b. after verification of the particulars and documents set out in Article 3.3, the competent authority of the State Party reasonably determines that the applicant cannot provide for the safety of patients in the State Party's jurisdiction in accordance with the standards of the State Party and the reasons for such a conclusion are set out in writing.

7. *License Refusal Disputes.* The World Health Organization may establish a non-binding mediation service to help resolve disputes regarding license refusal and/or suspension or revocation.

8. *Compliance with Rules.* Each State Party shall take all appropriate measures to ensure that the holder of an authorization complies with all the medical, health, legal and disciplinary rules on the practice of medicine, other health practices or telehealth as such may apply in the State Party's jurisdiction.

9. *Liability.* Remedies prescribed by this Convention are not intended to deal with other potential disputes between a patient and a telemedical physician, such as claims arising out of misuse of patient records or claims for payment for services where no dispute exists as to the quality of the services.

10. *Term of License.* Authorizations granted by the competent authority of the State Party shall be valid for a period of not less than three (3) years and may be renewed for further three (3) year periods on application by the holder not less than three (3) months before expiration of the then current authorization. Notwithstanding the term, the State Party may require an annual report by the holder to confirm the particulars of the holder and the holder's activities in the preceding year.

11. *Suspension or Revocation of License.* The competent authority of the State Party may suspend or revoke an authorization to practice granted by such competent authority where:

   a. it is found that the applicant/holder no longer possesses the qualifications set out in Article 3.3;

   b. the particulars and documents supporting the application under Article 3.3 are found to be false or materially incorrect;

      c. where the applicant/holder is, in the reasonable determination of the competent authority, not able to conduct a practice in a reasonably safe manner or without adversely affecting the health of patients; or without adversely affecting the health of patients; or

      d. where the applicant/holder has breached any professional, disciplinary or legal rules relating to the practice being undertaken.

12. *License Appeals*. Each State Party shall ensure that processes are available to an applicant/holder that will allow the applicant/holder to know in detail and in writing the determination and reasons for any negative determination relating to an application, renewal, suspension or revocation. Each State Party shall inform applicants of the remedies available to him/her under the laws of the State Party and of any time limits allowed for the exercise of such remedies.

13. *Mutual Recognition*. In the absence of an international licensing system, each State Party agrees to utilize a combination of consulting, mutual recognition and full licensure with the goal of moving toward mutual recognition. No State Party shall impose documentation or other requirements upon applicants beyond those reasonably necessary to ensure a reasonable standard of care for the people of the State.

14. *Hospital Credentialing*. Those State Parties that require specific authorization to be granted by the health care facility where telehealth care will be provided before a health care provider may provide that care in the facility will ensure that such facilities treat telehealth care providers in a manner similar to that applied to those providers whose practice brings them physically into the facility. It is the express intention of this provision that no one be treated differently solely because he is providing health care at a distance with the assistance of electronic media.

15. *Prescriptions*. Health care workers providing services through electronic means shall have the same authority to prescribe medications as a similar type/category of health care worker in the State Party in which the patient receiving care is located.

16. *Common Standards and Guidelines*. Each State Party shall work with other State Parties and with the World Health Organization to establish and implement international standards, guidelines and protocols for licensure for telehealth and telemedicine professionals, organizations, technology providers and suppliers of goods and services.

17. *Harmonization*. To the extent permitted by national and political norms, each State Party shall encourage the harmonization of its rules and regulations of telehealth and licensure with those of other State Parties. Further, each State Party shall encourage harmonization of the rules and regulations relating to telehealth and licensure within the sub-jurisdictions of such State Party.

Article 4

EQUIPMENT

1. All medical devices used in provision of telehealth services will be subject to the laws and regulations of the State Party in which they are located.

2. In order to reduce exposure to liability and ensure adequate delivery of tele-medicine, each State Party shall require providers of telemedical services to identify and document:

    a. all equipment (both hardware and software) used for telemedicine;

    b. the owners and parties responsible for maintaining the equipment;

    c. the format for transmitting medical information;

    d. what studies are to be interpreted; and

    e. the frequency and format of reports.

3. Each State Party will require that transmission verification procedures be developed at both local and remote sites. This may involve:

    a. establishing well-defined procedures for confirming the receipt of the transmission;

    b. verifying that there are no errors or omissions in the transmission or conversion of the data; and

    c. verifying that the images received are appropriate for evaluation and rendering a diagnosis.

4. No State Party will unreasonably withhold approval of devices that promote the safe and effective delivery of telehealth care services, nor treat such devices differently from any others used in health care there solely on the basis that the subject device is to be used in telehealth.

Article 5

CONFIDENTIALITY OF RECORDS

1. Each State Party shall ensure that, except in limited circumstances, information regarding a person's physical condition, psychological condition, healthcare and treatment shall not be released without his consent.

2. To minimize the risk of, among other things, possible interception by third parties, and if intercepted, to reduce the probability that the intercepting party will be able to use or understand the information, each State Party shall ensure that transmission of medical information, including, but not limited to, electronic transmissions of telemedical records to and from telemedical facilities, is done in an internationally acceptable manner.

3. Each State Party shall make the referring physician responsible to take reasonable steps to provide for safe storage and/or transmission of the patient's records by utilizing an adequate encryption system. Each State Party shall make the referring physician responsible to take reasonable steps to prevent anyone other than himself and his accredited colleagues from obtaining the encryption key. Each State Party shall make the referring physician and the telemedicine physician responsible to advise the patient that no medical record, paper or electronic, is completely confidential and that security breaches may occur with either.

4. Each State Party shall prohibit unauthorized access to telemedical records and patient information by all appropriate means, including legislation as required by circumstances.

5. For purposes of medical research and training, and when the identity of the person to whom the information relates cannot be determined, health care information may be divulged without his express consent. All other existing and subsequent International Agreements governing the use of Human Subjects in medical research will be followed.

6. Each State Party agrees that telecommunications used **exclusively** for treatment of the sick or wounded during armed conflict will be protected in ways similar to those afforded hospitals and medical transports. Such transmissions will not be encrypted, thereby allowing adversaries and others to determine the nature of the transmission, and to determine that these non-combatant communication links pose no threat to the State Party's security. Except for the purposes identified in this paragraph, the duty of confidentiality remains binding upon anyone who may come to learn of health care information.

Article 6

COMPLIANCE

1. Each State Party shall annually report and publish its progress in complying with the terms of this Convention.

2. Each State Party agrees to support efforts on behalf of national law associations, in consultation with scientific, medical and other relevant organizations, independently to collect information concerning worldwide compliance with the provisions of this Convention.

3. Each State Party agrees to support its national law associations to participate in meetings of the World Health Organization and the International Bar Association dedicated to assessing worldwide compliance with the provisions of this Convention.

Each State Party agrees to provide due consideration to biennial reports and recommendations of the World Health Organization and the International Bar Association with regard to worldwide compliance with the provisions of this Convention.

Article 7

SIGNATURE, RATIFICATION AND ACCESSION

1. This Convention shall be open to all States for signature. Any State that does not sign this Convention before its entry into force in accordance with paragraph 3 of this Article may accede to it at any time.

2. This Convention shall be subject to ratification by signatory States. Instruments of ratification and instruments of accession shall be deposited with the Governments of [INSERT COUNTRIES], which are hereby designated the Depositary Governments. This Convention shall enter into force upon the deposit of instruments of ratification by five Governments, including the Governments designated as Depositary Governments under this Convention.

3. For States whose instruments of ratification or accession are deposited subsequent to the entry into force of this Convention, it shall enter into force on the date of the deposit of their instruments of ratification or accession.
4. The Depositary Governments shall promptly inform all signatory and acceding States of the date of each signature, the date of deposit of each instrument of ratification of and accession to this Convention, the date of its entry into force and other notices.
5. This Convention shall be registered by the Depositary Governments pursuant to Article 102 of the Charter of the United Nations.

Article 8

AMENDMENTS

Any State Party to this Convention may propose amendments to this Convention. Amendments shall enter into force for each State Party to the Convention accepting the amendments upon their acceptance by a majority of the State Parties to the Convention and thereafter for each remaining State Party to the Convention on the date of acceptance by it.

Article 9

PERIODIC REVIEW

Ten years after the entry into force of this Convention, the question of the review of this Convention shall be included in the provisional agenda of the United Nations General Assembly in order to consider, in light of past application of the Convention, whether it requires revision. The International Bar Association and other relevant international organizations are invited to produce reports and recommendations on the subject of any necessary revisions. At any time after the Convention has been in force for five years, however, and at the request of one third of the State Parties to the Convention, and with the concurrence of the majority of the State Parties, a conference of the State Parties shall be convened to review this Convention. The World Health Organization, the International Bar Association, and other relevant international organizations, shall be invited to attend this conference in the role of expert advisors to the State Parties.

Article 10

WITHDRAWAL

Any State Party to this convention may give notice of its withdrawal from the Convention one year after its entry into force by written notification to the Depositary Governments. Such withdrawal shall take effect one year from the date of receipt of this notification.

Article 11

LANGUAGES

This Convention, of which the texts in other languages are equally authentic, shall be deposited in the archives of the Depositary Governments. Duly certified copies of this Convention shall be transmitted by the Depositary Governments to the Governments of the signatory and acceding States.

Vignette Contributors

Merrick Alpert
E-Ceptionist
2000 Bagby, Suite 5442
Houston, TX 77002
Tel: (713) 520-6688
Fax: (603) 308-6179
merrick@e-ceptionist.com

Greg Alter, Ph.D.
Teleotech Systems
1300 Quarry Court #311
Pt. Richmond, CA 94801
Tel: (510) 307-4321
alter@teleotech.com
http://www.teleotech.com

Page Anderson, Ph.D.
2450 Lawrenceville Highway, Suite 101
Decatur, GA 30033
Tel: (404) 634-3400
Fax: (404) 634-3482
Anderson@virtuallybetter.com

Jodi Aronson, Ph.D.
CIGNA Behavioral Health
11095 Viking Drive, Suite 350
Eden Prairie, MN 55344
Tel: (952) 996-2021
Fax: (952) 996-2659
jodi.aronson@cignabehavioral.com

Sandra J. Beinar
Arizona Telemedicine Program
PO Box 245105
Tuscon, AZ 85724-5105
Tel: (520) 626-2493

beinars@u.arizona.edu
http://www.telemedicine.arizona.edu

Larry E. Beutler, Ph.D.
Pacific Graduate School of Psychology
904 East Meadow Drive
Palo Alto, CA 94303
Tel: (805) 570-0123
Fax: (650) 494-7446
lbeutler@pgsp.edu

Michael Bollini, Ph.D.
ValueOptions
3110 Fairview Park Drive
Falls Church, VA 22042
Tel: (703) 208-8831
Fax: (703) 205-6749
michael.bollini@valueoptions.com

Pamela G. Clark, Ph.D.
INTEGRIS Jim Thorpe Rehabilitation
  Center
4219 South Western
Oklahoma City, OK 73109
Tel: (405) 644-5343
Fax: (405) 951-8851
clarpg@integris-health.com

Susan E. Coldwell, Ph.D.
Dental Public Health Sciences
University of Washington
Box 357475
Seattle, WA 91895-7475
Tel: (206) 616-3087
Fax: (206) 685-4258
scoldwel@u.washington.edu

Stephen J. Cozza, M.D.
11524 Gauguin Lane
Potomac, M.D. 20854
Tel: (206) 782-5950
Fax: (202) 782-2282
Stephen.cozza@na.amedd.army.mil

Susan X. Day, Ph.D.
Clinical Research Faculty
University of Houston
10055 S. Shepherd Drive, Suite
  804
Houston, TX 77014
Tel: (713) 303-7195
sxday@iastate.edu

Claude H. Dennery, Psy.D.
Psychology Department
FCI Fairton
PO Box 280
Fairton, NJ 08320
Tel: (856) 453-4098
Fax: (856) 453-4188
chdennery@bop.gov

Ruth Eldon
The Committee on Law and Medicine
Section on Legal Practice, International
  Bar Association
271 Regent Street
London, England W1B 2AQ
Tel: +44 (0)20 7629 1206
Fax: +44 (0)20 7409 0456
http://www.ibanet.org

Gregory A. Gahm, Ph.D., LTC
Psychology Department
Madigan Army Medical Center
Tacoma, WA 98431
Tel: (253) 968-2700
Fax: (253) 968-3731
Gregory.gahm@nw.amedd.army.mil
http://mamc.amedd.army.mil/bhd/
  Psychology/deptpsychology.asp

Dale John Giolas, M.D.
Catalyst Integrations
1995 Hicks Road
Rolling Meadows, IL 60008
Tel: (847) 359-9125

Fax: (847) 359-9263
dale.giolas@psychwise.com
http://www.psychwise.com

Randy Glasbergen
randy@glasbergen.com
http://www.glasbergen.com

Robert L. Glueckauf, Ph.D.
Center for Research on Telehealth and
  Healthcare Communications
Department of Clinical and Health
  Psychology
University of Florida
PO Box 100165
Gainesville, FL 32610-0165
Tel: (352) 265-0680 ext. 46880
Fax: (352) 265-0468
http://www.hp.ufl.edu/chp/telehealth
http://www.floridatelecare.com

Marybeth Goulet-Connolly, APRN, CS
Acadia Healthcare
Enfield Road
Lincoln, ME 04457
Tel: (207) 794-8471
mgouletconnolly@EMH.org

Kevin Grold, Ph.D.
2923 Sandy Point #6
Del Mar, CA 92014
Tel: (858) 481-1515
Fax: (858) 481-5143
grold@aol.com

Sandra Haber, Ph.D.
211 West 56 Street, Suite 21 H
New York, NY 10019
Tel: (212) 246-6057
Fax: (718) 768-4851
DrSHaber@aol.com
http://www.DrHaber.com

Tim Hodgens, Ph.D.
18 Lyman Street
Westborough, MA 01581
Tel: (508) 836-9595
Fax: (508) 836-9898
hodgenstim@aol.com
http://www.paniccoach.com

Norman G. Hoffmann, Ph.D.
Evince Clinical Assessments
PO Box 17305
Smithfield, RI 02917
Tel: (401) 231-2993
Fax: (401) 231-2055
evinceassessment@aol.com
http://www.evinceassessment.com

Larry C. James, Ph.D., ABPP
Department of Psychology
Walter Reed Army Medical Center
Washington, DC 20307
Tel: (202) 782-5922
Fax: (202) 782-7165
Larry.James@NA.AMEDD.
  ARMY.MIL

Leigh W. Jerome, Ph.D.
Pacific Telehealth and
  Technology
Tripler Army Base
150 Hamajua #426
Kailua, HI 96724
Tel: (808) 433-1483
Leigh.Jerome@haw.tamc.amedd.
  army.mil

Edward R. Jones, Ph.D.
Pacific Behavioral Health
5990 Sepulveda Boulevard,
  Suite 400
Van Nuys, CA 91411
Tel: (818) 623-5723
Fax: (818) 623-5789
Edward.jones@phs.com

Warren B. Karp, Ph.D., DMD
Medical College of Georgia
766 Faircloth Commons
  Road
Evans, GA 30809
Tel: (404) 978-1260, ext. 7685
Fax: (706) 721-6276
wkarp@onebox.com
wkarp@mail.mcg.edu

Cleo Kiernan
Route 3, Box 172-1
Pawnee, OK 74058

Tel: (918) 762-3239
Fax: (918) 762-3293
scout@skally.net

Sunkyo Kwon, Ph.D.
Free University Berlin
Health Psychology Department
Habelschwerdter Allee 45,
  14195
Berlin, Germany
Tel: 4930-838.55977
Fax: 4930-838.55634
contact@sunkyo-kwon.net
http://www.kwon.ws

Chao-Cheng Lin
91 Hsing-Hsin Street
Yu-Li, Hualien County
Taiwan, 981
Tel: (886) 3-8886752
Fax: (866) 3-8880474
psyjkjk@mail2000.com.tw

Paulo J. Negro, M.D., Ph.D.
University of Maryland Hospital
22 South Greene Street, Box 351
Baltimore, M.D. 21201
Tel: (410) 328-6610
pjnegro@pol.net

Monica E. Oss
OPEN MINDS
163 York Street
Gettysburg, PA 17325-2301
Tel: (717) 334-1329
Fax: (717) 334-0538
monicaoss@openminds.com
http://www.openminds.com

Les Posen, Ph.D.
PO Box 1229
St. Kilda South, Australia 3182
Tel: 61 (0) 413 040 747
Fax: 61 (3) 9504 8338
lesposen@mac.com
http://homepage.mac.com/lesposen

Dana E. Putnam, Ph.D.
PO Box 181
Morro Bay, CA 93443

Tel: (805) 772-7602
drputnam@onlinesexaddict.org
http://www.onlinesexaddict.org

Gerald Quimby, M.A. NCC,
  LMHC
444 Luna Lino Home Road # 605
Honolulu, Hawaii 96825
Tel: 808-284-6445
jerry@jquimby.com

Harry Rhodes, M.B.A. RHIA
American Health Information
  Management Association
233 N. Michigan Avenue, Suite
  2150
Chicago, IL 60601-5800
Tel: (312) 233-1100
Fax: (312) 233-1500
info@ahima.org
http://www.ahima.org

Daniel Paul Sabbeth, Ph.D., M.D.
72 Overlook Road
New Rochelle, NY 10804-4139
Tel: (914) 636-2745
dsabbeth@aol.com

Sherri Scherf
PO Box 576
Blanchard, OK 73010
Tel: (405) 222-5324
dscherf@earthlink.net

Henry A. Smith, L.C.S.W.
Cumberland Mountain Community
  Services
PO Box 810
Cedar Bluff, VA 24609
Tel: (540) 964-6702
Fax: (540) 964-5669
hsmith@cmcsb.com
http://www.cmcsb.com

Duffy Soto
Executive Director of Technology
  and Innovation
Lake City Community College
Route 15, Box 3146
Lake City, FL 32024

Tel: (386) 754-4241
Fax: (386) 752-4790
sotod@lakecitycc.edu
http://www.lakecity.cc.fl.us

Agnes T. Spadafora, RDH, BSDH
Department of Dental Public Health
  Sciences
University of Washington
HSB Box 357475
1959 NE Pacific Street
Seattle, WA 98195-7475
Tel: (206) 543-2034
Fax: (206) 685-4258
aspad@u.washington.edu

Rob Sprang, M.B.A.
Kentucky Telecare
University of Kentucky
K117 KY Clinic
740 S. Limestone
Lexington, KY 40536-0284
Tel: (859) 257-6404
Fax: (859) 257-2811
rsprang@pop.uky.edu
http://kytelecare.uky.edu

B. Hudnall Stamm
Institute of Rural Health
Campus Box 8174
Pocatello, ID 83209-8174
Tel: (208) 282-4436
Fax: (208) 282-4074
bhstamm@isu.edu

John Suler, Ph.D.
Psychology Department
Rider University
Lawrenceville, NJ 08648
Tel: (215) 340-0525
suler@mindspring.com
http://www.rider.edu/users/suler/
psycyber/psycyber.html

Roxy Szeftel, M.D.
8730 Alden Drive
Los Angeles, CA 90048
Tel: (310) 423-3566
Fax: (310) 423-1044
roxy.szeftel@cshs.org

David Tener, M.B.A.
3086 State Route 160
Gallipolis, OH 45631
Tel: (740) 446-5550
Fax: (740) 441-4402
execdirwci@mindspring.com
http://wci.centersite.org

Giovanni Torello, M.D.
Rua Tucuma 141
São Paulo, Brazil 01455-010
Tel: 55 11 3812 0050
Fax: 55 11 3819 4566
Giovanni@polbr.med.br

Tom Trabin, Ph.D., MSM
5820 Barrett Avenue
El Cerrito, CA 94530
Tel: (510) 236-6868
Fax: (510) 234-1925
tom@trabin.com

Ken Weingardt, Ph.D.
Program Evaluation Resource Center
VA Palo Alto Health Care System and
  Stanford University School of Medicine

795 Willow Road (152-MPD)
Menlo Park, CA 94025
Tel: (650) 493-5000, ext. 22846
Fax: (650) 617-2736
kenweingardt@hotmail.com

Andy J. Winzelberg, Ph.D.
Department of Psychiatry and Behavioral
  Sciences
Stanford University School of
  Medicine
401 Quarry Road
Stanford, CA 94305-5717
Tel: (650) 723-6627
Fax: (650) 723-9807
winzel@stanford.edu

Joel Yager, M.D.
Department of Psychiatry
University of New Mexico School of
  Medicine
2400 Tucker, NE
Albuquerque, NM 87131-5326
Tel: (505) 272-5416
Fax: (505) 272-4639
jyager@unm.edu

References

Administration on Aging. (2001, June 21). *Profile of older Americans: 2000.* Retrieved July 27, 2001, from http://www.aoa.gov/aoa/stats/profile/default.htm#figure1

Advanced Systems Group. (2002, July). Just say the word. *IT Solutions and Strategies, 5*(7), 1–8.

Affective Computing. (n.d.). *Wearable computer systems for affective computing.* Retrieved March 18, 2002, from http://affect.media.mit.edu/AC_research/wearables.html

Agency for Healthcare Research and Quality. (2001). *Telemedicine for the Medicare population* (Evidence Report/Technology Assessment No. 24 01-E012). Washington, DC: Agency for Healthcare Research and Quality.

Agras, W. S., Taylor, C. B., Feldman, D. E., & Losch, M. (1990). Developing computer-assisted therapy for the treatment of obesity. *Behavior Therapy, 21*(1), 99–109.

Alcatel. (2000). *Internet speed record smashed: KPNQwest & Alcatel quadruple top speed for data transfer.* Retrieved May 9, 2000, from www.alcatel.nl/html/nieuws/pers/20000508.shtml

Alessi, N. (2001). Information technology and child and adolescent psychiatry: Ethical issues. *Drug Benefit Trends, 13*(9), 24–27.

Alexander, G. (1999, December). *Telehealth: Regulation of interstate psychology.* Retrieved September 11, 2002, from http://telehealth.net/articles/regulation.html

Alexander, G. (2000, August 6). *Licensure and cyberpsych.* Paper presented at the American Psychological Association, Washington, DC.

Allen, A. (1998). A review of cost effectiveness research. *Telemedicine Today, 6*(5), 10–12, 14–15.

Allen, A., & Wheeler, T. (1998, April). Telepsychiatry background and activity survey. *Telemedicine Today, 6*(2), 34–37.

Allen, D. H. (1984). The use of computer fantasy games in child therapy. In M. D. Schwartz (Ed.), *Using computers in clinical practice* (pp. 329–334). New York: Haworth.

Allen, J., Harmon-Jones, E., & Cavender, J. (2001). Manipulation of frontal EEG asymmetry through biofeedback alters self-reported emotional responses and facial EMG. *Psychophysiology, 38*(4), 685–693.

Allen, L., & Green, P. (2002, September 20). *Equivalence of the computerized and orally administered Word Memory Test effort measures.* Retrieved October 10, 2002, from http://home.earthlink.net/~rkmck/vault/allengreen/WMT.pdf

Alpers, G. W., Wilhelm, F. H., & Roth, W. T. (1999). *Psychophysiological changes during exposure therapy.* Paper presented at the 19th National Conference of the Anxiety Disorders Association of America, San Diego, CA.

Alpert, D., Pulvino, C. J., & Lee, J. L. (1985). Computer applications in counseling: Some practical suggestions. *Journal of Counseling and Development, 63*(8), 522–523.

AMA Member Communications. (2002, May 24). *New online consultation introduced. American Medical Association.* Retrieved June 6, 2002, from http://www.ama-assn.org/ama/pub/article/1615-6042.html

American Academy of Child and Adolescent Psychiatry. (2000, June 16). *American Academy of Child Psychiatry guidelines for psychiatric standards of care.* Retrieved March 5, 2002, from http://www.familymentalhealth.com/aacapguide_p.htm

American Accreditation HealthCare Commission. (2001, July 27). *Health Web site standards.* Retrieved August 31, 2001, from http://www.urac.org/v1-0.PDF

American College of Physicians. (2003, March). *The changing face of ambulatory medicine—Reimbursing physicians for computer-based care.* Retrieved April 17, 2003, from http://www.acponline.org/hpp/e-consult.pdf

American Counseling Association. (1999, October). *Ethical standards for Internet on-line counseling.* Retrieved August 24, 2001, from http://www.counseling.org/gc/cybertx.htm

American Educational Research Association, American Psychological Association, and National Council on Measurement in Education. (1999). *The standards for educational and psychological testing.* Washington, DC: AERA Publications.

American Health Information Management System. (n.d.). *Advanced IT/IM applications: Building the CPR.* Retrieved October 25, 2002, from http://www.ahimacampus.org/demos/Hisdemo/part4/intro.htm

American Medical Association. (1998). *H-140.989 informed consent and decision-making in health care.* Retrieved October 3, 2002, from http://www.ama-assn.org/apps/pf_online/pf_online?f_n=browse&doc=policyfiles/HOD/H-140.989.HTM

American Medical Association. (2002, July 17). *AMA study: Physicians' use of Internet steadily rising.* Retrieved April 21, 2003, from http://www.ama-assn.org/ama/pub/article/1616-6473.html

American Medical Association. (2003, August 8). *New guidelines help physicians ensure safe and secure Internet prescribing.* Retrieved November 20, 2003, from http://www.ama-assn.org/ama/pub/article/1615-7814.html

American Medical Association House of Delegates. (1999). *Creation of AMA data bank on interstate practice of medicine.* Retrieved October 22, 2001, from http://www.ama-assn.org/meetings/public/annual99/reports/refcomm/rtf/ref123.rtf

American Nurses Association. (1995, November). *Position paper on computer-based patient record standards.* Retrieved May 23, 2003, from http://www.nursingworld.org/readroom/position/joint/jtcpri1.htm

American Psychiatric Association. (1998a). *APA resource document on telepsychiatry via videoconferencing.* Retrieved May 23, 2003, from http://www.psych.org/pract_of_psych/tp_paper.cfm

American Psychiatric Association. (1998b). *The principles of medical ethics with annotations especially applicable to psychiatry.* Washington, DC: Author.

American Psychiatric Association. (2000a). *Diagnostic and statistical manual of mental disorders: Text revision (DSM-IV-TR).* Washington, DC: Author.

American Psychiatric Association. (2000b, November 27). *Telepsychiatry likely to become prevalent form of treatment.* Retrieved April 16, 2001, from http://www.newswise.com/articles/2000/11/TELEPSYC.APA.html

American Psychiatric Association. (2002). *Practice guideline development process.* Retrieved March 13, 2003, from http://www.psych.org/pract_guide/qrg/guidelinedevprocess91802.pdf

American Psychological Association. (1990). *APA guidelines for providers of psychological services to ethnic, linguistic, and culturally diverse populations.* Retrieved July 8, 2002, from http://www.apa.org/pi/oema/guide.html

American Psychological Association. (1992). *Ethical principles of psychologists and code of conduct.* Retrieved October 3, 2002, from http://www.apa.org/ethics/code.html#1.24

American Psychological Association. (1997, November 5). *APA statement on services by telephone, teleconferencing, and Internet.* Retrieved August 24, 2001, from http://www.apa.org/ethics/stmnt01.html

American Psychological Association. (1999a). *Standards for educational and psychological testing.* Washington, DC: Author.

American Psychological Association. (1999b). Test security: Protecting the integrity of tests. *American Psychologist, 54*(12), 1078.

American Psychological Association. (2000). *APA Council of Representatives adopt guidelines for the treatment of gay, lesbian, and bisexual clients.* Retrieved October 28, 2002, from http://www.apa.org/releases/guidelinesgay.html

American Psychological Association. (2001, June). *APA ethics code draft 5, June 2001, for comment.* Retrieved August 27, 2001, from http://anastasi.apa.org/draftethicscode/draftcode.cfm#intro

American Psychological Association. (2002a). *Ethical principles of psychologists and code of conduct.* Retrieved October 28, 2002, from http://www.apa.org/ethics/code2002.pdf

American Psychological Association. (2002b). *Getting ready for HIPAA: A primer for psychologists.* Washington: Author.

American Psychological Association Task Force on Self-Help Therapies. (1978). *Task force report on self-help therapies.* Unpublished manuscript.

American Telemedicine Association. (2001). *Memorandum: Credentialing of specialists providing teleconsultations.* Retrieved March 5, 2002, from http://www.atmeda.org/news/credprivstandards3.2.html

Anderson, A., Newlands, A., & Mullin, J. (1996). Impact of video-mediated communication on simulated service encounters. *Interactive Computing, 8*(2), 193–206.

Anderson, K. (1998, January 19). The digital bubble: Waking up from the new media pipe dream. *The New Yorker, 73*(43), 30.

Anderson, P. L., Rothbaum, B. O., & Hodges, L. (2000). Virtual reality: Using the virtual world to improve quality of life in the real world. *Bulletin of the Menninger Clinic, 65*(1), 78–91.

Andreasen, N. C. (1984a). *Scale for the Assessment of Negative Symptoms (SANS).* Iowa City: University of Iowa.

Andreasen, N. C. (1984b). *Scale for the Assessment of Positive Symptoms (SAPS).* Iowa City: University of Iowa.

Andress, M. (2001, May 28). Biometrics at work? *InfoWorld,* 73–75. Retrieved March 12, 2003, from http://archive.infoworld.com/articles/tc/xml/01/05/28/010528tcbiom.xml

Aneshensel, C. S., Frerichs, R. R., Clark, V. A., & Yokopenic, P. A. (1982). Telephone versus in-person surveys of community health status. *American Journal of Public Health, 72*(9), 1017–1021.

Aptel, M., & Cnockaert, J. C. (2002, September). Stress and work-related musculoskeletal disorders of the upper extremities. *TUTB Newsletter, 19,* 50–56.

Architectural and Transportation Barriers Compliance Board. (2000). Electronic information technology accessibility standards: Final rule. *Federal Register.* Washington, DC: Government Printing Office.

Arlington, S., Barnett, S., Hughes, S., & Palo, J. (n.d.). *Pharma 2010: The threshold of innovation.* IBM. Retrieved April 18, 2003, from http://www-1.ibm.com/services/strategy/e_strategy/pharma_2010.html

Asso, A. E. (Ed.). (1999). *Standards for educational and psychological testing 1999.* Washington, DC: American Educational Research Association.

Association of State and Provincial Licensing Boards. (n.d.). *Psychology licensure.* Retrieved November 13, 2001, from http://www.asppb.org

Association of Telehealth Service Providers. (1999). *Highlights of ATSP 1999 Report on U.S. Telemedicine Activity.* Retrieved April 11, 2003, from http://www.atsp.org/survey/reports/1999_highlights.asp

Association of Test Publishers. (2000). *Guidelines for computer-based testing.* Washington, DC: Author.

Attree, E. A., Brooks, B. M., Rose, F. D., Andrews, T. K., Leadbetter, A. G., & Clifford, B. R. (1996, July). Memory processes and virtual environments: I can't remember what was there, but I can remember how I got there: Implications for people with disabilities. In P. Sharkey (Ed.), *Proceedings of the First European Conference on Disability, Virtual Reality and Associated Technology* (pp. 117–121). Maidenhead, United Kingdom.

Australian Psychological Society. (1999). *Considerations for psychologists providing services on the Internet.* Retrieved August, 2000, from http://www.psychsociety.com.au/about/internet.pdf

Ax, R. K., Fagan, T. J., & Holton, S. (2003). Individuals with serious mental illnesses in prison: Rural perspectives and issues. In B. H. Stamm (Ed.), *Rural behavioral health care: An interdisciplinary guide* (pp. 203–215). Washington, DC: American Psychological Association.

Baer, L., Brown-Beasley, M. W., Sorce, J., & Henriques, A. I. (1993). Computer-assisted telephone administration of a structured interview for obsessive-compulsive disorder. *American Journal of Psychiatry, 150*(11), 1737–1738.

Baer, L., Cukor, P., & Coyle, J. (1997). Telepsychiatry: Application of telemedicine. In R. L. Bashshur, J. H. Sanders, & G. W. Shannon (Eds.), *Telemedicine: Theory and practice* (pp. 265–290). Springfield, IL: Thomas.

Baer, L., Cukor, P., Jenike, M., Leahy, L., O'Laughlen, J., & Coyle, J. (1995). Pilot studies of telemedicine for patients with obsessive-compulsive disorder. *American Journal of Psychiatry, 152*(9), 1383–1385.

Baer, L., Elford, D. R., & Cukor, P. (1997). Telepsychiatry at forty: What have we learned? *Harvard Review of Psychiatry, 5*(1), 7–17.

Baigent, M. F., Lloyd, C. J., Kavanagh, S. J., Ben-Tovim, D. I., Yellowlees, P. M., Kalucy, R. S., & Bond, M. J. (1997, June). Telepsychiatry: "Tele" yes, but what about the "psychiatry"? *Journal of Telemedicine and Telecare, 3*(Suppl. 1), 3–5.

Baker, T. (2002). *Telepsychiatry clinic meets needs of future psychiatrists and patients.* Medical College of Georgia. Retrieved March 13, 2002, from http://www.mcg.edu/telemedicine/TelepsychResRot.htm

Baldwin, G. (2001, April). Physicians bring color and flare to their Web sites. *Internet Health Care.* Retrieved July 13, 2001, from http://www.internethealthcaremag.com/html/current/CurrentIssueStory.cfm?DID=5307

Ball, C. J., McLaren, P. M., Summerfield, A., Lipsedge, M., & Watson, J. P. (1995). A comparison of communication modes in adult psychiatry. *Journal of Telemedicine and Telecare, 1*(1), 22–26.

Ball, C. J., Scott, N., McLaren, P. M., & Watson, J. P. (1993). Preliminary evaluation of a low-cost videoconferencing (LCVC) system for remote cognitive testing of adult psychiatric patients. *British Journal of Clinical Psychology, 32*(Pt. 3), 303–307.

Ballie, R. (2001, November). Medicare will now cover some telehealth psychotherapy services. *Monitor on Psychology, 32*(10), 84.

Banisar, D. (2002). *Pricacy & human rights 2002: An international survey of privacy laws and developments.* Retrieved April 13, 2003, from http://www.privacyinternational.org/survey/index2000.html

Barak, A. (1999). Psychological applications on the Internet: A discipline on the threshold of a new millennium. *Applied and Preventive Psychology, 8*(4), 231–246.

Barak, A. (2002, August 24). *SAHAR: Emotional support and prevention for suicidal people via the Internet.* Paper presented at the American Psychological Association, Chicago.

Barak, A., & Lacrosse, M. B. (1975). Multidimensional perception of counselor behavior. *Journal of Counseling Psychology, 22*(6), 471–476.

Barak, A., & Wander-Schwartz, M. (1999, August). *Empirical evaluation of brief group therapy through an Internet chat room.* Retrieved April 29, 2001, from http://construct.haifa.ac.il?~azy/cherapy.htm

Bard, M. (2000, January). *The future of eHealth.* Retrieved September 8, 2000, from http://www.cyberdialogue.com

Bard, M. (2002, July 1). *Benefits abound if you can move customer service online.* Retrieved December 13, 2002, from http://www.managedhealthcareexecutive.com/mhe/article/articleDetail.jsp?id=25502

Bardone, A. M., Krahn, D. D., Goodman, B. M., & Searles, J. S. (2000). Using interactive voice response technology and timeline follow-back methodology in studying binge eating and drinking behavior: Different answers to different forms of the same question? *Addictive Behaviors, 25*(1), 1–11.

Barker, G. L., & Alessi, N. E. (2001). Webcasting and video streaming basics: Applications in telepsychiatry. *Telemedicine Journal and e-Health, 7*(2), 149.

Barkham, M., Margison, F., Leach, C., Lucock, M., Mellor-Clark, J., Evans, C., Benson, L., Connell, J., Audin, K., & McGrath, G. (2001). Service profiling and outcomes benchmarking using the CORE-OM: Toward practice-based evidence in the psychological therapies: Clinical outcomes in routine evaluation-outcome measures. *Journal of Consulting and Clinical Psychology, 69*(2), 184–196.

Barlow, D. H. (1988). *Anxiety and its disorders: The nature and treatment of anxiety and panic.* New York: Guilford.

Barlow, D. H. (Ed.). (2001). *Clinical handbook of psychological disorders: A step-by-step treatment manual* (3rd ed.). New York: Guilford.

Barlow, D. H., Craske, M. G., Cerny, J. A., & Klosko, J. S. (1989). Behavioral treatment of panic disorder. *Behavior Therapy, 20,* 261–282.

Barlow, J., Peter, P., & Barlow, L. (2002). *Smart videoconferencing: New habits for virtual meetings.* San Francisco: Berrett-Koehler.

Barnett, D. (1982). A suicide prevention incident involving the use of a computer. *Professional Psychology: Research & Practice, 13*(5), 565–570.

Barrett, L., & Gross, J. (2001). Emotional intelligence: A process model of emotion representation and regulation. In T. Mayne & G. Bonanno (Eds.), *Emotions: Current issues and future directions* (pp. 286–310). New York: Guilford.

Barrett, R. (2002, December 3). *Speedier Internet 2 could revolutionize world of medicine.* Retrieved August 18, 2003, from http://www.jsonline.com/bym/news/dec02/100685.asp

Bartlett, M., Sterne, J., & Egger, M. (2002, July 13). What is newsworthy? Longitudinal study of the reporting of medical research in two British newspapers. *British Medical Journal, 325*(7355), 81–84.

Bashshur, R. A. (1997). Telemedicine and the health care system. In R. L. Bashshur, J. H. Sanders, & G. W. Shannon (Eds.), *Telemedicine: Theory and practice* (pp. 5–35). Springfield, IL: Thomas.

Bashshur, R. A. (2001, Winter). Where are we in telemedicine/telehealth, and where do we go from here? *Telemedicine Journal and e-Health, 7*(4), 273–278.

Baur, C., & Doering, M. (2000, September 26). *Proposed frameworks to improve the quality of health Web sites.* Retrieved August 25, 2001, from www.medscape.com

Bayer, R., & Colgrove, J. (2002, September 13). Public health vs. civil liberties. *Science, 297*(5588), 1811.

Beahrs, J. O., & Gutheil, T. G. (2001). Informed consent in psychotherapy. *American Journal of Psychiatry, 158*(1), 4–10.

Beck, A. T., Ward, C. H., Mendelson, M., Mock, J., & Erbaugh, J. (1961). An inventory for measuring depression. *Archives of General Psychiatry, 4*(6), 561–571.

Bedell, J., Hunter, R., & Corrigan, P. (1997). Current approaches to assessment and treatment of persons with serious mental illness. *Professional Psychology: Research & Practice, 28*(3), 217–228.

Behavioural Medicine Institute of Australia. (2002). *Telehealth and biofeedback.* Retrieved November 18, 2003, from http://www.behavioural-medicine.com/articles/telebio/001.html

ben Maimon, M. (1956). *Guide for the perplexed* (2nd ed.; M. Friedlander, Trans.). New York: Dover.

Benarde, M. A. (2002). *You've been had!: How the media and environmentalists turned America into a nation of hypochondriacs.* Piscataway, NJ: Rutgers University Press.

Bennett, M. (2001). *Simply sectors: Wireless technology and the future of 3G.* Retrieved March 28, 2001, from http://google.yahoo.com/bin/query?p=wireless+technology+future&hc=0&hs=3

Benschoter, R. A. (1971, October). CCTV-Pioneering Nebraska Medical Center. *Educational Broadcasting,* 1–3.

Benschoter, R. A., Wittson, C. L., & Ingham, C. G. (1965, March). Teaching and consultation by television. *Mental Hospital, 16*(3), 99–104.

Benson, B. (2001, April 6). Virtual housecall. *Praxis Post.* Retrieved July 23, 2001, from http://praxispost.com/post/trends/040401

Berger, A. M., Portenoy, R. K., & Weissman, D. E. (Eds.). (2002). *Principles and practice of palliative care and supportive oncology* (2nd ed.). Philadelphia: Lippincott Williams & Wilkins.

Bergvik, S., & Gammon, D. (1997, September 26). Video conferencing in group training of psychiatric nurses. Paper presented at the Proceedings of the 6th International Congress on Nursing Informatics, Stockholm, Sweden.

Berland, G. K., Elliott, M. N., Morales, L. S., Algazy, J. I., Kravitz, R. L., Broder, M. S., Kanouse, D. E., Muñoz, J. A., Puyol, J.-A., Lara, M., Watkins, K. E., Yang, H., & McGlyn, E. A. (2001). Health information on the Internet: Accessibility, quality, and readability in English and Spanish. *Journal of the American Medical Association, 285*(20), 2612–2621.

Berman, J., & Bruckman, A. S. (2000, September 27). *The Turing game: An examination of cultural identity in online environments.* Retrieved July 10, 2002, from http://www.cs.berkeley.edu/~danyelf/cscw2000/bermanbruckman.htm

Berman, J., & Bruckman, A. S. (2001). The Turing game: Exploring identity in an online environment. *Convergence, 7*(3), 83–102.

Bernard, S. (2000). Consolidation and convergence of the eHealth space. In P. Joyce Florey (Ed.), *Internet healthcare strategy guide* (pp. 127–128). Santa Barbara, CA: COR Health.

Beutler, L. E., & Clarkin, J. F. (1990). *Systematic treatment selection: Toward targeted therapeutic interventions.* New York: Brunner/Mazel.

Beutler, L. E., Clarkin, J. F., & Bongar, B. (2000). *Guidelines for the systematic treatment of the depressed patient.* New York: Oxford University Press.

Beutler, L. E., & Groth-Marnat, G. (2003). *Integrative assessment of adult personality* (2nd ed.). New York: Guilford.

Beutler, L. E., & Harwood, T. M. (2000). *Prescriptive therapy: A practical guide to systematic treatment selection.* New York: Oxford University Press.

Beutler, L. E., & Williams, O. B. (1995). Computer applications for the selection of optimal psychosocial therapeutic interventions. *Behavioral Healthcare Tomorrow, 4*(4), 66–68.

Bier, M. C., Sherblom, S. A., & Gallo, M. A. (1996). Ethical issues in a study of Internet use: Uncertainty, responsibility, and the spirit of research relationships. *Ethics and Behavior, 6*(2), 141–151.

Biofeedback. (2001, Spring). Retrieved February 27, 2003, from http://www.aapb.org/public/articles/index.cfm?Cat=18

Black, N. B., Balun, D. A., & Cozza, S. (2002). Comparison of parental therapeutic alliances before and after initial psychiatric interviews. *Telemedicine Journal and e-Health, 8*(2), 207.

Blade, R. A., & Padgett, M. L. (2002). Virtual environments standards and terminology. In K. M. Stanney (Ed.), *Handbook of virtual environments: Design, implementation, and applications* (pp. 15–27). Mahwah, NJ: Lawrence Erlbaum Associates.

Blair, R. (2001, February). Psychotherapy online. *Health Management Technology, 22*(2), 24–27.

Bloom, J. W. (1998). The ethical practice of WebCounseling. *British Journal of Guidance and Counselling, 26*(1), 53–59.

Blum, D., & Knudson, M. (Eds.). (1998). *A field guide for science writers.* New York: Oxford University Press.

Board on Behavioral Cognitive and Sensory Sciences and Education, & Committee on National Statistics. (2003). *The polygraph and lie detection.* Washington, DC: National Academies Press.

Board of Psychology. (2002, March). Statement on medication. *BOP Update, 9*, 9.

Bondmass, M., Bolger, N., Castro, G., & Avitall, B. (2000, March 27). The effect of physiologic home monitoring and telemanagement on chronic heart failure outcomes. *Internet Journal of Advanced Nursing Practice, 3*(2). Retrieved March 12, 2003, from http://www.ispub.com/ostia/index.php?xmlFilePath=journals/ijanp/vol3n2/chf.xml

Bongar, B. (1991). *The suicidal patient: Clinical and legal standards of care.* Washington, DC: American Psychological Association.

Borkovec, T. D., & Costello, E. (1993). Efficacy of applied relaxation and cognitive-behavioral therapy in the treatment of generalized anxiety disorder. *Journal of Consulting and Clinical Psychology, 61*(4), 611–619.

Borowitz, S., & Wyatt, J. (1998). The origin, content, and workload of e-mail consultations. *Journal of the American Medical Association, 280*(15), 1321–1324.

Bouchard, S., Paquin, B., Payeur, R., Allard, M., Rivard, V., Fournier, T., Renaud, P., & Lepierre, J. (2004). Delivering cognitive-behavior therapy for panic disorder with agoraphobia in videoconferencing. *Telemedicine Journal and e-Health, 10*(1), 3–25.

Bracken, P., & Thomas, P. (2001). Postpsychiatry: A new direction for mental health. *British Medical Journal, 322*(7288), 724–727.

Brandt, M. (1996). *Practice guidelines for managing health information* (American Health Informatics Management Association Practice Brief, Document 406). Chicago: American Health Informatics Management Association.

Breuer, J., & Freud, S. (1955). On the psychical mechanism of hysterical phenomena: Preliminary communication. In J. Strachey (Ed., & Trans.). *Studies on hysteria* (Vol. 2, pp. 4–21). London: Hogarth Press.

British Standards Institution. (2001). *A code of practice for the use of information technology for the delivery of assessments.* London: Author.

Brittin, A. (2001). Protecting electronic data and managing risk by adopting best practices. In J. Mack & A. Wittel (Eds.), *The new frontier: Exploring ehealth ethics* (pp. 117–121). Washington, DC: URAC and the Internet Healthcare Coalition.

Broadhurst, J. (2000, November 7). Multilingual content translates into international success. *InternetContent.net.* Retrieved October 12, 2002, from http://www.internetcontent.net/Newsletters/Newsletter110/Newsletter110.html

Brock, D. W. (2002, April 12). Human cloning and our sense of self. *Science, 296*(5566), 314–316.

Brodey, B. B., Claypoole, K. H., Motto, J., Arias, R. G., & Goss, R. (2000). Satisfaction of forensic psychiatric patients with remote telepsychiatric evaluation. *Psychiatric Services, 51*, 1305–1307.

Brown, D., & Wilson, J. (1995). LIVE: Learning in virtual environments. *Ability: The Journal of British Computer Society Disability Group, 15*, 24–25.

Brown, F. (1977). Answer. In F. Brown (Ed.), *The best of Frederic Brown.* New York: Ballantine.

Brown, T. M. (2000, May 24). The growth of George Engel's biopsychosocial model. *Free Associations: Psychoanalysis and the public sphere.* Retrieved October 21, 2002, from http://www.human-nature.com/free-associations/engel1.html

Brown, W. M., Palameta, B., & Moore, C. (2003). Are there nonverbal cues to commitment? An exploratory study using the zero-acquaintance video presentation paradigm. *Evolutionary Psychology, 2003*(1), 42–69. Retrieved April 3, 2003, from http://human-nature.com/ep/articles/ep014269.html

Brown-Connolly, N. (1999). *Telemedicine: Operations manual Blue Cross of California.* Chicago: Author.

Brown-Connolly, N. (2001a, October). *Rural Telemedicine Demonstration Project: Summary results.* Paper presented at the Blue Cross Blue Shield Association Best of Blue Awards in Pharmacy and Medical Management, Health Services Research, Chicago.

Brown-Connolly, N. (2001b, October). *Health services research: Blue Cross of California Rural Telemedicine Demonstration Project.* Chicago: Blue Cross Blue Shield Association.

Brown-Connolly, N. (2002a). Patient satisfaction with telemedical access to specialty services in rural California. *Journal of Telemedicine and Telecare, 8*(2), 7–10.

Brown-Connolly, N. (2002b). *Reimbursement, funding and economic outlook.* Paper presented at Telehealth 2002, online broadcast.

Bruckman, A. (1996). Finding one's own space in cyberspace. *Technology Review, 99*(1), 48–54.

Burke, M. J., & Normand, J. (1987). Computer psychological testing: Overview and critique. *Professional Psychology: Research and Practice, 18*(1), 42–51.

Burton, D. (1997). Report of an active telehealth project: Kentucky advances mental health services through Kentucky Telecare and the state mental health network. *TelehealthNews.* Retrieved January 11, 1999, from http://telehealth.net/telehealth/newslettr_2.html

Burton, D., & Huston, J. (1998). Use of video in the informed consent process. *Journal of Telemedicine and Telecare, 4*(1), 38–40.

Bushe, G. R. (1995, Fall). Advances in appreciative inquiry as an organization development intervention. *Organization Development Journal, 13*(3), 14–22.

Bushnell, J. A., Wells, J. E., Hornblow, A. R., Oakley-Browne, M. A., & Joyce, P. (1990). Prevalence of three bulimia syndromes in the general population. *Psychological Medicine, 20*(3), 671–680.

Byron, E. (2001, November 5). The Web @ work/Astra Zeneca: A weekly case study. *The Wall Street Journal.* Retrieved November 16, 2001, from www.wsj.com

Cabaniss, K. (2001). *Counseling and computer technology in the new millennium: An Internet delphi study.* Unpublished doctoral dissertation, Virginia Polytechnic Institute and State University.

Calder, A., Burton, A., Miller, P., Young, A., & Akamatsu, S. (2001). A principal component analysis of facial expressions. *Vision Research, 41*(9), 1179–1208.

California Business and Professions Code: Section 2052. (n.d.). Retrieved November 26, 2003, from http://www.leginfo.ca.gov/cgi-bin/waisgate?WAISdocID=8886249865+0+0+0&WAISaction=retrieve

California Business and Professions Code: Section 2903. (n.d.). Retrieved August 10, 2002, from http://www.leginfo.ca.gov/calaw.html

California Business and Professions Code: Section 4980.02. (n.d.). Retrieved September 10, 2002, from http://www.leginfo.ca.gov/cgi-bin/waisgate?WAISdocID=70023315204+4+0+0&WAISaction=retrieve

California Business and Professions Code: Section 4996.9. (n.d.). Retrieved September 10, 2002, from http://www.leginfo.ca.gov/cgi-bin/waisgate?WAISdocID=70023315204+0+0+0&WAISaction=retrieve

California Department of Consumer Affairs Board of Psychology. (2004, January). Psychological services and the Internet. *BOP Update, 11,* 6–7.

California Healthcare Foundation. (1999, January 28). *Americans worry about the privacy of their computerized medical records.* Retrieved July 29, 2001, from http://www.chcf.org/press/view.cfm?itemID=362

California Healthline. (1999, April 21). *Medical privacy: Agreement, but a long way to go.* Retrieved March 21, 1999, from http://www.chcf.org/press/viewpress.cfm?itemID=362

California Healthline. (2001). *More health plans look into reimbursing physicians for e-mail consultations.* Retrieved December 10, 2001, from http://ehealth.chcf.org/view.cfm?section=eHealth&itemID=4660

California Telehealth/Telemedicine Coordination Project. (1997). *Telehealth and telemedicine: Taking distance out of caring.* Sacramento: Author.

Calle, E. E., Thun, M. J., Petrelli, J. M., Rodriguez, C., & Heath, C. W., Jr. (1999). Body-mass index and mortality in a prospective cohort of U.S. adults. *New England Journal of Medicine, 341*(15), 1097–1105.

Cameron, S. (2002, Summer). Learning to write case notes using the SOAP format. *Journal of Counseling and Development, 80*(3), 286–292.

Cap Gemini Ernst & Young U.S. LLC. (2002, October). *How health plans are using the Internet to reach customers.* Retrieved December, 2002, from http://www.us.cgey.com/downloadlibrary/files/Health_2002PayorWebSite_v2.pdf

Carlbring, P., Forslin, P., Willebrand, M., Ljungstrand, P., Strandlund, C., Ekselius, L., & Andersson, G. (2002). Is the Web-administered CIDI-SF equivalent to a human SCID-interview? *European Psychiatry, 17*(1), 151–152.

Carnes, P. (Ed.). (2001). *In the shadows of the Net: Breaking free of compulsive online sexual behavior.* Center City, MN: Hazelden.

Carr, A., Ghosh, A., & Marks, I. (1988). Computer-supervised exposure treatment for phobias. *Canadian Journal of Psychiatry, 33*(2), 112–117.

Carroll, J. (2003, March). *Getting schooled.* Retrieved April 8, 2003, from http://www.healthleaders.com/magazine/feature1.php?contentid=43024&categoryid=152

Cassidy, J., Easton, M., Capelli, C., Singer, A., & Bilodeau, A. (1996). Cognitive remediation of persons with severe and persistent mental illness. *Psychiatric Quarterly, 67*(4), 313–321.

Cavanagh, K., Zack, J., & Shapiro, D. (2003). Empirically supported computerized psychotherapy. In R. Wooton, P. Yellowlees, & P. McLaren (Eds.), *Telepsychiatry and e-Mental Health* (pp. 273–290). London, England: Royal Society of Medicine Press.

CEA. (2002, June 16). *Workplace becoming the locale of choice for online shopping.* Retrieved July 13, 2002, from http://www.ce.org/press_room/press_release_detail.asp?id=9971

Center for Devices and Radiological Health. (1996, July 11). *Telemedicine related activities.* Retrieved November 7, 2001, from http://www.fda.gov/cdrh/telemed.html

Center for Medicare and Medicaid Services. (1996). Health Insurance Portability and Accountability Act. Retrieved October 3, 2002, from http://cms.hhs.gov/hipaa

Center for Medicare and Medicaid Services. (1998, November 2). *Payment for teleconsultations in rural health professional shortage area.* Retrieved December 1, 2003, from http://tie.telemed.org/legal/medic/medicare_rules.asp

Center for Research on Telehealth and Healthcare Communications. (2002). *National Institute on Disability and Rehabilitation Research (NIDRR) videocounseling for rural teens with seizures project.* Retrieved February 26, 2002, from http://www.hp.ufl.edu/chp/telehealth/projectsr.html#

Cepelewicz, B. (1998, October 8). *Telemedicine and strategies to minimize risks of liability.* Paper presented at the Telemedicine National Conference on Legal and Policy Developments, Washington, DC.

Ceridian Corporation. (2002). *First-ever study finds employees highly motivated to use online EAP and work-life services.* Retrieved August 29, 2002, from http://www.ceridian.com/corp/content/0,1336,914-2167,00.html

Chambless, D. L., Caputo, G. C., Hasin, S. E., Gracely, E. J., & Williams, C. (1985). The mobility inventory for agoraphobia. *Behaviour Research and Therapy, 23*(1), 35–44.

Chambless, D. L., & Ollendick, T. H. (2001). Empirically supported psychological interventions: Controversies and evidence. *Annual Review of Psychology, 52,* 685–716.

Children's Online Privacy Protection Act. (1998). Retrieved October 3, 2002, from http://www.ftc.gov/ogc/coppa1.htm

Childress, C. (1998). Potential risks and benefits of online psychotherapeutic interventions. Retrieved July 27, 2001, from http://www.ismho.org/issues/9801.htm

Chin, T. (2001, January 29). Security breach: Hacker gets medical records. *American Medical News*. Retrieved August 29, 2001, from http://www.ama-assn.org/sci-pubs/amnews/pick_01/tesa0129.htm

Chin, T. (2002, September 23/30). *Investors say $70 million in MedUnite is now worth zero*. amednews.com. Retrieved November 21, 2003, from http://www.ama-assn.org/amednews/2002/09/23/bisc0923.htm

Clarke, B., & Schoech, D. (1983). A computer-assisted therapeutic game for adolescents: Initial developments and comments. In M. D. Schwartz (Ed.), *Using computers in clinical practice* (pp. 335–353). New York: Haworth.

Clarke, B., & Schoech, D. (1994). A computer-assisted therapeutic game for adolescents: Initial development and comments. *Computers in Human Services, 11*(1–2), 121–140.

Clarkson, P. (1996). Researching the therapeutic relationship in psychoanalysis, counselling psychology and psychotherapy: A qualitative analysis. *Counselling Psychology Quarterly, 9*(2), 143.

Clawson, V., Bostrom, R., & Anson, R. (1993). The role of the facilitator in computer-supported meetings. *Small Group Research, 24*(4), 547–565.

Clear and simple: Developing effective print materials for low-literate readers. (1995). Washington, DC: National Cancer Institute.

Clynes, M. E. K., & Nathan, S. (1960, September). Cyborgs and space. *Astronautics, 14*(9), 26–27, 74–75.

Code of Ethics of the National Association of Social Workers. (1999). Retrieved August 24, 2001, from http://www.naswdc.org/Code/ethics.htm

Cohen, G. E., & Kerr, B. A. (1998). Computer-mediated counseling: An empirical study of a new mental health treatment. *Computers in Human Services, 15*(4), 13–26.

Colby, K. M., Gould, R. L., & Aronson, G. (1989). Some pros and cons of computer-assisted psychotherapy. *Journal of Nervous and Mental Disease, 177*(2), 105–108.

Colby, K. M., Watt, J. B., & Gilbert, J. P. (1966). A computer method of psychotherapy: Preliminary communication. *Journal of Nervous and Mental Disease, 142*(2), 148–152.

Coldwell, S. E., Getz, T., Milgrom, P., Prall, C. W., Spadafora, A., & Ramsay, D. S. (1998). CARL: A LabView 3 computer program for conducting exposure therapy for the treatment of dental injection fear. *Behaviour Research and Therapy, 36*(4), 429–441.

Coley, S. M., & Scheinberg, C. A. (1990). *Proposal writing*. Newbury Park, CA: Sage.

Colón, Y. (1996). *Chatter(er)ing through the fingertips: Doing group therapy online*. Retrieved August 27, 2001, from http://www.echonyc.com/~women/Issue17/public-colon.html

Colón, Y. (1999). Digital digging: Group therapy online. In J. Fink (Ed.), *How to use computers and cyberspace in clinical practice of psychotherapy* (pp. 66–81). Northvale, NJ: Jason Aronson.

Combs v. PayPal, No. C024227 (N.D. Cal. 2002).

Computer-Based Patient Record Institute. (1999). *CPRI toolkit: Managing information security in health care*. Bethesda, MD: Author.

Cooper, A. (1998). Sexuality and the Internet: Surfing into the new millennium. *CyberPsychology and Behavior, 1*(2), 181–187.

Cooper, A. (Ed.). (2002). *Sex and the Internet: A guide book for clinicians*. Bristol, PA: Taylor & Francis.

Cooper, A., Boies, S., Maheu, M., & Greenfield, D. (2000). Sexuality and the Internet: The next sexual revolution. In L. Szuchman & F. Muscarella (Eds.), *Psychological perspectives on human sexuality* (pp. 519–545). New York: Wiley.

Cooper, A., McLoughlin, I., & Campbell, K. (2000). Sexuality in cyberspace: Update for the 21st century. *CyberPsychology and Behavior, 3*(4), 521–536.

Cooper, A., Morahan-Martin, J., Mathy, R. M., & Maheu, M. (2002). Toward an increased understanding of user demographics in online sexual activities. *Journal of Sex and Marital Therapy, 28*(2), 105–129.

Cornish, P. A., Church, E., Callanan, T., Bethune, C., Robbins, C., & Miller, R. (2003). Rural interdisciplinary mental health team building via satellite: A demonstration project. *Telemedicine Journal and e-Health Spring, 9*(1), 63–71.

Corrigan, J. M., Greiner, A., & Erickson, S. M. (Eds.). (2002). *Fostering rapid advances in healthcare: Learning from system demonstrations*. Washington, DC: Institute of Health Care.

Couchman, G., Forjuoh, S., & Rascoe, T. (2001, May). E-mail communications in family practice: What do patients expect? *Journal of Family Practice, 50*(5), 414–418.

Council on Accreditation. (2002). *The employee assistance program standards and self-study manual* (2nd ed.). New York: Author.

Council on Competitiveness. (1996). *Highway to health: Transforming U.S. health care in the information age*. Washington, DC: Author.

Counselman, E. F., & Weber, R. L. (2002). Changing the guard: New leadership for an established group. *International Journal of Group Psychotherapy, 52*(3), 373–386.

Cromby, J. J., Standen, P. J., & Brown, D. J. (1996). The potentials of virtual environments in the education and training of people with learning disabilities. *Journal of Intellectual Disability Research, 40*(6), 489–501.

Croweroft, J. (1997). Supporting videoconferencing on the Internet. In K. E. Finn, A. J. Sellen, & S. B. Wilbur (Eds.), *Video-mediated communication: Computers, cognition, and work* (pp. 519–540). Mahwah, NJ: Lawrence Erlbaum Associates.

Cukor, P., Baer, L., Willis, B. S., Leahy, L., O'Laughlen, J., Murphy, M., Withers, M., & Martin, E. (1998). Use of videophones and low-cost standard telephone lines to provide a social presence in telepsychiatry. *Telemedicine Journal, 4*(4), 313–321.

Cummings, N. (1996). Now we're facing the consequences. *The Scientist Practitioner, 6*(1), 9–13.

Cummings, N., Budman, S., & Thomas, J. (1998). Efficient psychotherapy as a viable response to scarce resources and rationing of treatment. *Professional Psychology: Research & Practice, 29*(5), 460–469.

Cummins, C., & Spagat, E. (2002, September 5). At Williams Cos., two trendy bets yield snake eyes. *The Wall Street Journal*, p. 1.

Cyber Dialogue. (2000, July 12). *Online healthcare consumers focused on privacy.* Retrieved September 18, 2001, from www.cyberdialogue.com/news/releases/2000/07-12-cch-privacy.html

CyberEdge Information Systems. (n.d.). *The virtual lexicon.* Retrieved July 10, 2002, from http://www.cyberedge.com/4a1.html

Daft, R., & Lengel, R. (1986). Organizational information requirements, media richness and structural design. *Management Science, 32*(5), 554–571.

Dahan, D., Magnuson, J. S., & Tanenhaus, M. K. (2001). Time course of frequency effects in spoken-word recognition: Evidence from eye movements. *Cognitive Psychology, 42*(4), 317–367.

Dakins, D., & Jones, E. (1996). Cream of the crop: Ten outstanding telemedicine programs. *Telemedicine and Telehealth Networks, 2*(11), 24–41.

D'Angelo, N. (2002, November 20). *Consumer use of hospital and health plan Web sites has tripled in the last year.* Retrieved February 14, 2003, from http://www.manhattanresearch.com/11-20-02%20Press%20Release.pdf

Datamonitor. (2002, June 13). *Psychiatrists and the Internet.* Retrieved October 25, 2002, from http://www.datamonitor.com/~645f299ac35b4646bb067815254eb466~/all/reports/product_summary.asp?pid=DMHC1798

Davidson, R. J. (1993). The neuropsychology of emotion and affective style, *Handbook of emotions* (pp. 143–154). New York: The Guilford Press.

Davies, S. (1997). Re-engineering the right to privacy: How privacy has been transformed from a right to a commodity. In P. Agro & M. Rotenberg (Eds.), *Technology and privacy: The new landscape* (pp. 149–165). Cambridge, MA: MIT Press.

Day, S. X. (2000). *Psychotherapy using distance technology: A comparison of face-to-face, video, and audio treatments.* Urbana: University of Illinois at Urbana–Champaign.

Day, S. X., & Schneider, P. (2000). The subjective experiences of therapists in face-to-face, video, and audio sessions. In J. W. Bloom & G. R. Garry (Eds.), *Cybercounseling and cyberlearning: Strategies and resources for the millennium* (pp. 203–218). Alexandria, VA: American Counseling Association.

DeGuzman, M., & Ross, W. M. (1999). Assessing the application of HIV and AIDS relates education and counseling on the Internet. *Patient Education and Counseling, 36,* 209–228.

DeLeon, P. (2000). The critical need for licensure mobility. *Monitor on Psychology, 31*(4), 9.

DeLeon, P., Folen, R., Jennings, F., & Willis, D. (1991). The case for prescription privileges: A logical evolution of professional practice. *Journal of Clinical Child Psychology, 20*(3), 254–267.

DeLeon, P., Sammons, M., Frank, R., & VandenBos, G. (1998). Changing health care environment in the United States: Steadily evolving into the 21st century. In A. S. Bellak and M. Hersen (Eds.), *Comprehensive clinical psychology* (pp. 394–409). Oxford, England: Permagon Press.

DeLeon, P., & Wiggins, J. (1996). Prescription privileges for psychologists. *American Psychologist, 51*(3), 225–229.

Derogatis, L. R., & Melisaratos, N. (1983). The Brief Symptom Inventory: An introductory report. *Psychological Medicine, 13*(3), 595–605.

Dertouzos, M. (1997). *What will be: How the new world of information will change our lives.* New York: HarperCollins.

Desmond, D. W., Tatemichi, T. K., & Hanzawa, L. (1994). The telephone interview for cognitive status (TICS): Reliability and validity in a stroke sample. *International Journal of Geriatric Psychiatry, 9*(9), 803–807.

Dick, R. S., Steen, E. B., & Detmer, D. E. (Eds.). (1997). *The computer-based patient record: An essential technology for health care* (Committee on Improving the Patient Record, Institute of Medicine, National Academy of Science). Washington, DC: National Academy Press.

Diener, A., O'Brien, B., & Gafni, A. (1998). Health care contingent valuation studies: A review and classification of the literature. *Health Economics, 7*(4), 313–326.

Diener, E. (1984). Subjective well-being. *Psychological Bulletin, 95*(3), 542–575.

Diener, E. (1996, Spring). Works on subjective well-being. *Journal of Macromarketing, 16*(1), 135.

Ditton, P. (1999, July). *Bureau of Justice statistics: Special report.* Retrieved March 30, 2001, from http://www. ojp.usdoj.gov/bjs/pub/pdf/mhtip.pdf

Dongier, M., Tempier, R., Lalinec-Michaud, M., & Meunier, D. (1986). Telepsychiatry: Psychiatric consultation through two-way television: A controlled study. *Canadian Journal of Psychiatry, 31*(1), 32–34.

Dow Jones & Company Inc v. Gutnick. (2002, December 10). High Court of Australia. Retrieved April 11, 2003, from http://www.austlii.edu.au/au/cases/cth/high_ct/2002/56.html

Doze, S., Simpson, J., Hailey, D., & Jacobs, P. (1999). Evaluation of a telepsychiatry pilot project. *Journal of Telemedicine and Telecare, 5*(1), 38–46.

Drewnowski, A., Yee, D. K., Kurth, C. L., & Krahn, D. D. (1994). Eating pathology and DSM-III-R bulimia nervosa: A continuum of behavior. *American Journal of Psychiatry, 151*(8), 1217–1219.

D'Souza, D. (2002, January). *Tele-health in improving treatment adherence and logitudinal outcomes in patients with serious mental illness: A case control study in the use of a tele-psycho educational service for patients and families.* Paper presented at the TeleMed '02, Telemedicine and e-Health Forum, London.

D'Souza, R., & Hawker, F. (1998). *A pilot study of outcomes and satisfaction with the use of tele-consultation liaison psychiatry.* Retrieved October 2, 2001, from www.adelaide.net.au/~telmed/abstract1.htm

Dunn, K., & Viegas, S. (1998). *Telemedicine: Practicing in the information age.* Philadelphia: Lippincott Williams & Wilkins.

Dvorac, J. C. (2002, June 17). E-Mac, i-Mac, no Mac. *PC Magazine.* Retrieved June 20, 2002, from http://www. pcmag.com/article2/0,4149,1885,00.asp

Dwyer, T. (1973). Psychiatric consultation by interactive television. *American Journal of Psychiatry, 130*(8), 865–869.

Dyson, E. (1998). *Release 2.1: A design for living in the digital age.* New York: Broadway Books.

Ebenezer, C. (2003). Use of the Internet in psychiatry and clinical psychology. In R. Wooton, P. Yellowlees, and P. McLaren (Eds.), *Telepsychiatry and e-Mental Health* (pp. 217–229). London, England: Royal Society of Medicine Press.

Edwards, J. (1997). Military contributions to digital radiology and networking. In G. Segre (Ed.), *Telemedicine source book, 1998* (pp. 212–216). New York: Faulkner & Gray.

Egloff, B., Wilhelm, F. H., Neubauer, D. H., Mauss, I. B., & Gross, J. (2002). Implicit anxiety measure predicts cardiovascular reactivity to an evaluated speaking task. *Emotion, 2*(1), 3–11.

E-Health-Media. (2002, July 25). *Telemedicine helps babies, parents and staff in neonatal ICUs.* Retrieved August 12, 2002, from http://www.babycarelink.com/news.asp?fn=n38&f=

Eichel, S. K. (2002). *Credentialing: It may not be the cat's meow.* Retrieved July 16, 2002, from http://users. snip.net/~drsteve/Articles/Dr_Zoe.htm

Eisenberg, D. M., Davis, R. B., Ettner, S. L., Appel, S., Wilkey, S., Van Rompay, M., & Kessler, R. C. (1998). Trends in alternative medicine use in the United States, 1990–1997: Results of a follow-up national survey. *Journal of the American Medical Association, 280*(18), 1569–1575.

Eissa, M. A., Poffenbarger, T., & Portman, R. J. (2001). Comparison of the actigraph versus patients' diary information in defining circadian time periods for analyzing ambulatory blood pressure monitoring data. *Blood Pressure Monitoring, 6*(1), 21–25.

Electronic Communications Privacy Act of 1986. Retrieved October 3, 2002, from http://floridalawfirm. com/privacy.html.

Electronic Information Technology Accessibility Standards: Final Rule, 65 Fed. Reg. 80499–80528 (2000).

Electronic Privacy Information Center. (2002). *Privacy and human rights: An international survey of privacy laws and developments.* Washington, DC: Author.

Elias, M. (2001, May 22). Online therapy clicks: Practice is expanding, along with concerns. *USA Today,* pp. 1D–2D.

Ellen, E. F. (2002, August). Identifying and treating suicidal college students. *Psychiatric Times, 191*(8), 1.

Ellenberger, H. F. (1974). Psychiatry from ancient to modern times. In S. Arieti (Ed.), *The foundations of psychiatry* (2nd ed.; Vol. 1; p. 1270). New York: Basic Books.

Eng, T. (2001). *The ehealth landscape: A terrain map of emerging information and communication technologies in health and health care.* Robert Wood Johnson Foundation. Retrieved December 1, 2003, from http://www. rwjf.org/publications/publicationsPdfs/eHealth.pdf

Erdman, H. P., Greist, J. H., Gustafson, D. H., & Taves, J. E. (1987). Suicide risk prediction by computer interview: A prospective study. *Journal of Clinical Psychiatry, 48*(12), 464–467.

Erdman, H. P., Klein, M. H., Greist, J. H., & Skare, S. S. (1992). A comparison of two computer-administered versions of the NIMH Diagnostic Interview Schedule. *Journal of Psychiatric Research, 26*(1), 85–95.

Erlanger, D. M., Kaushik, T., Broshek, D., Feldman, D., & Festa, J. (2002). Development and validation of a Web-based screening tool for monitoring cognitive status. *Journal of Head Trauma Rehabilitation, 17*(5), 458–476.

European Commission. (2001, June 18). *Data protection: Commission approves standard contractual clauses for data transfers to non-EU countries.* Retrieved November 13, 2001, from http://europa.eu.int/comm/internal_market/en/dataprot/news/clauses2.htm

European Health and Telematics Association. (n.d.). *EHTEL Mission Statement.* Retrieved November 24, 2003, from http://www.ehtel.org/SHWebClass.ASP?WCI=ShowDoc&DocID=309

European Union. (1998a). *Data protection.* Retrieved November 13, 2001, from http://europa.eu.int/comm/internal_market/en/dataprot/index.htm

European Union. (1998b). *International market.* Retrieved November 13, 2001, from http://europa.eu.int/comm/dg15/en/media/dataprot/index.htm

Ewalt, D. M. (2003, February 26). Rescue specialist's mission: Calm frantic data losers. *Information Week.* Retrieved February 28, 2003, from http://www.informationweek.com/story/IWK20030225S0007

Eysenbach, G., & Diepgen, T. (1998). Responses to unsolicited patient e-mail requests for medical advice on the World Wide Web. *JAMA, 280*(15), 1333–1335.

Fahey, A., Day, N. A., & Gelber, H. (2003). Tele-education in child mental health for rural allied health workers. *Journal of Telemedicine and Telecare, 9*(2), 84–88.

Fahrenberg, J., & Myrtek, M. (1996). *Ambulatory assessment: Computer-assisted psychological and psychophysiological methods in monitoring and field studies.* Gottingen, Germany: Hogrefe & Huber.

Fairburn, C. G., & Beglin, S. J. (1990). Studies of the epidemiology of bulimia nervosa. *American Journal of Psychiatry, 147*(4), 401–408.

Falling through the Net. (2001). Retrieved February 18, 2002, from http://digitaldivide.gov/about.htm

Farrell, S. P., & McKinnon, C. R. (2003). Technology and rural mental health. *Archives of Psychiatric Nursing, 17*(1), 20–26.

Faulkner, A., & Thomas, P. (2002). User-led research and evidence-based medicine. *British Journal of Psychiatry, 180*(1), 1–3.

Federal Trade Commission. (n.d.). *Frequently asked questions about the Children's Online Privacy Protection Rule.* Retrieved November 13, 2001, from http://www.ftc.gov/privacy/coppafaqs.htm

Federal Trade Commission. (2002, June 26). *FTC warns consumers about online gambling and children.* Retrieved July 13, 2002, from http://www.ftc.gov/opa/2002/06/onlinegambling.htm

Federal Trade Commission & Department of Commerce (2001, June). Section 101(c)(1)(C)(ii) Electronic Signatures in Global and National Commerce Act. Retrieved March 17, 2003, from http://www.ftc.gov/os/2001/06/esign7.htm

Federation of State Medical Boards. (1995, August). *Draft model act to regulate the practice of medicine across state lines.* Retrieved March 14, 2003, from http://www.netreach.net/~wmanning/fsmb.htm

Fekken, G. C., & Holden, R. R. (1992). Response latency evidence for viewing personality traits as schema indicators. *Journal of Research in Personality, 26*(2), 103–120.

Fekken, G. C., & Jackson, D. N. (1988). Predicting consistent psychological test item responses: A comparison of models. *Personality and Individual Differences, 9*(5), 873–882.

Fenichel, M., Suler, J., Barak, A., Zelvin, E., Jones, G., Munro, K., Meunier, V., & Walker-Schmucker, W. (2002). Myths and realities of online clinical work. *CyberPsychology & Behavior, 5*(5), 481–497.

Fenig, S., Levav, I., Kohn, R., & Yelin, N. (1993). Telephone vs. face-to-face interviewing in a community psychiatric survey. *American Journal of Public Health, 83*(6), 896–898.

Ferguson, T. (1998). Digital doctoring: Opportunities and challenges in electronic patient–physician communication. *Journal of the American Medical Association, 280*(15), 1361–1362.

Fernandes, L., Brandt, M., Casey, D., Fletcher, D., Grant, K., Petrosky, C., Postal, S., Skeens, M., Wheatley, V., & Winter, T. (1997, July/August). Master Patient (Person) Index (MPI): Recommended core data elements. *Journal of American Health Informatics Management Association, 68*(7). Retrieved March 12, 2003, from http://library.ahima.org/xpedio/groups/public/documents/ahima/pub_bok1_000073.html

Finn, J. (1995). Computer-based self-help groups: A new resource to supplement support groups. *Social Work with Groups, 18*(1), 109–117.

Finn, J. (1996). Computer-based self-help groups: On-line recovery for addictions. *Computers in Human Services, 13*(1), 21–41.

Finn, J., & Lavitt, M. (1994). Computer-based self-help groups for sexual abuse survivors. *Social Work with Groups, 17*(1–2), 21–46.

Finn, K. E., Sellen, A. J., & Wilbur, S. B. (Eds.). (1997). *Video-mediated communication (computers, cognition, and work).* Mahwah: Lawrence Erlbaum Associates.

First Consult Group. (2002, December). *Rural health care delivery: Connecting communities through technology.* Retrieved December 11, 2002, from http://www.chcf.org/documents/ihealth/RuralHealthCareDelivery.pdf

First, M. B., Spitzer, R. L., Gibbon, M., & Williams, J. B. W. (1995). *Structured clinical interview of DSM IV axis I disorders.* New York: Biometrics Research Department.

Fisher, C. (2001). *Psychology, the Internet, and the new APA ethics code.* Paper presented at the American Psychological Association, Washington, DC.

Fisher, D., Beutler, L. E., & Williams, O. B. (1999). Making assessment relevant to treatment planning: The STS Clinician Rating Form: Systemic treatment selection. *Journal of Clinical Psychology, 55*(7), 825–842.

Florey, J. (2001a, March). Consumer expectations to reshape providers' Net strategies. *Internet Healthcare Strategies, 3*(3), 10–11.

Florey, J. (2001b, April). Jupiter analysts predict strong future for physician Web sites. *Internet Healthcare Strategies, 3*(4), 13–14.

Folstein, M. F., Folstein, S. E., & McHugh, P. R. (1975). "Mini-mental state": A practical method for grading the cognitive state of patients for the clinician. *Journal of Psychiatric Research, 12*(3), 189–198.

Fowler, R. D. (1985). Landmarks in computer-assisted psychological assessment. *Journal of Consulting and Clinical Psychology, 53*(6), 748–759.

Fox, J., Merwin, E., & Blank, M. (1995). De facto mental health services in the rural South. *Journal of Health Care for the Poor and Underserved, 6*(4), 434–468.

Frabotta, D. (1998). People addicted to the Internet: Psychologists link Internet use and depression. *The Digital Kent Stater.* Retrieved May 29, 2003, from http://www.stater.kent.edu/stories_old/98fall/112498/f6a.html

Freedman, J., & Combs, G. (2002). *Narrative Therapy with Couples . . . and a whole lot more: A collection of papers, essays and exercises.* Adelaide, South Australia: Dulwich Centre Publications.

French, C. C., & Beaumont, J. G. (1989). A computerized form of the Eysenck Personality Questionnaire: A clinical study. *Personality and Individual Differences, 10*(10), 1027–1032.

Freud, S. (1923). Lecture XXXI: Anxiety and instinctual life. In J. Strachey (Ed., & Trans.), *New introductory lectures on psychoanalysis and other titles* (Vol. 22; pp. 57–80). London: Hogarth Press.

Freudenheim, M. (2002, August 31). Health insurers still struggling with a service on the Internet. *The New York Times,* pp. B1, B3.

Fridhandler, B. (2002, September–October). HIPAA and *therapist* privacy: An idea worth defending. *The California Psychologist, 35*(5), 9.

Fussell, S., & Benimoff, I. (1995). Social cognitive processes in interpersonal communications: Implications for advanced telecommunications technologies. *Human Factors, 37*(2), 228–250.

Futterman, A., & Shapiro, D. (1986). A review of biofeedback for mental disorders. *Hospital Community Psychiatry, 37*(1), 27–33.

Gale, S. (1992). Desktop video conferencing: Technical advances and evaluation issues. *Computer Communication, 15*(8), 517–526.

Galegher, J., Sproull, L., & Kiesler, S. (1998, October). Legitimacy, authority, and community in electronic support groups. *Written-Communication, 15*(4), 493–530.

Galinsky, M. J., Schopler, J. H., & Abell, M. D. (1997). Connecting group members through telephone and computer groups. *Health & Social Work, 22*(3), 181–188.

Gallo, J. J., & Breitner, J. C. S. (1995). Alzheimer's disease in the NAS-NRC registry of ageing twin veterans: IV. Performance characteristics of a two-stage telephone screening procedure for Alzheimer's dementia. *Psychological Medicine, 25*(6), 1211–1219.

Gammon, D., Sørlie, T., Bergvik, S., & Hoifodt, T. S. (1998). Psychotherapy supervision conducted by video-conferencing: A qualitative study of users' experiences. *Journal of Telemedicine and Telecare, 4*(Suppl. 1), 33–35.

Gammon, D., Svendsen, G. B., Jenssen, M. A., & Bergvik, S. (2003). The Internet, social isolation, and mental health: Future perspectives. In R. Wooton, P. Yellowlees, & P. McLaren (Eds.), *Telepsychiatry and e-mental health* (pp. 317–326). London, England: Royal Society of Medicine Press.

Garber, P. M. (2000). *Famous first bubbles: The fundamentals of early manias.* Cambridge, MA: MIT Press.

Garcia, B. E. (2002, May 11). Medical chips implanted. *Miami Herald.* Retrieved October 5, 2002, from http://www.miami.com/mld/miami/business/3240630.htm

Garcia-Palacios, A., Hoffman, H. G., See, S. K., Tsai, A., & Botella, C. (2001). Redefining therapeutic success with virtual reality exposure therapy. *CyberPsychology and Behavior, 4*(3), 341–348.

Gaston, L. (1991). Reliability and criterion-related validity of the California Psychotherapy Alliance Scales—Patient version. *Psychological Assessment, 3*(1), 68–74.

Gates, B., Myhrvold, N., & Rinearson, P. (1995). *The road ahead.* New York: Viking.

Geertz, C. (1973). *The interpretation of cultures: Selected essays.* New York: Basic Books.

George, M. S., & Skinner, H. A. (1990). Using response latency to detect inaccurate responses in a computerized lifestyle assessment. *Computers in Human Behavior, 6*(2), 167–175.

George, T. (2002, October 21). Communication gap. *InformationWeek*. Retrieved November 21, 2003, from http://www.informationweek.com/story/showArticle.jhtml?articleID=6503753

Gezairy, H. A. (2001, November 11–13). *Opening presentation*. Paper presented at the Regional Conference on Medical Librarianship: Building the Virtual Health Sciences Library of the Eastern Mediterranean region, Teheran, Iran.

Ghosh, G., McLaren, P., & Watson, J. (1997). Evaluating the alliance in video-link teletherapy. *Journal of Telemedicine and Telecare, 3*(1), 33–35.

Gibson, S. (2000). *Telepsychiatry in northern Arizona*. Phoenix, AZ: American Telemedicine Association.

Gilbert, A. (2002). Is Dr. Koop taking care of privacy? *ZDNet News*. Retrieved September 13, 2002, from http://zdnet.com.com/2100-1106-941028.html

Glantz, K., Durlach, N. I., Barnett, R. C., & Aviles, W. A. (1996). Virtual reality (VR) for psychotherapy: From the physical to the social environment. *Psychotherapy: Theory, Research, Practice, Training, 33*(3), 464–473.

Glueckauf, R. L. (2002). Telehealth and chronic disabilities: New frontier for research and development. *Rehabilitation Psychology, 47*(1), 3–7.

Glueckauf, R. L., Fritz, S. P., Ecklund-Johnson, E. P., Liss, H. J., Dages, P., & Carney, P. (2002). Videoconferencing-based family counseling for rural teenagers with epilepsy: Phase 1 findings. *Rehabilitation Psychology, 47*(1), 49–72.

Glueckauf, R. L., Nickelson, D. W., Whitton, J., & Loomis, J. S. (2003). Telehealth and chronic illness: Emerging issues and developments in research and practice. In T. Boll, J. Baum, & R. Frank (Eds.), *Handbook of clinical psychology* (Vol. 1). Washington, DC: American Psychological Association.

Glueckauf, R. L., Whitton, J., Baxter, J., Kain, J., Vogelgesang, S., Hudson, M., & Wright, D. (1998). Videocounseling for families of rural teens with epilepsy: Project update. *TelehealthNews*. Retrieved September 5, 2000, from http://tele-health.net/subscribe/newslettr_3.html

GMB. (2002, August 13). Workplace stress kills—don't trivialise it. Retrieved October 12, 2002, from http://www.gmb.org.uk/press_office/display.asp?id=194

Go, R. C., Duke, L. W., Harrell, L. E., Cody, H., Bassett, S. S., Folstein, M. F., Albert, M. S., Foster, J. L., Sharrow, N. A., & Blacker, D. (1997). Development and validation of a Structured Telephone Interview for Dementia Assessment (STIDA): The NIMH Genetics Initiative. *Journal of Geriatric Psychiatry and Neurology, 10*(4), 161–167.

Gold, M. (2003). Can managed care and competition control Medicare costs? *Health Affairs*. Retrieved April 11, 2003, from http://www.healthaffairs.org/WebExclusives/Gold_Web_Excl_040203.htm

Goldberg, A. I. (1997). Tele-home healthcare on call: Trends leading to the return of the housecall. *Telemedicine Today, 5*(4), 14–15.

Goldfield, G. S., & Boachie, A. (2003). Delivery of family therapy in the treatment of anorexia nervosa using telehealth: A case report. *Telemedicine Journal and e-Health, 9*(1), 111–114.

Goldman, J., Hudson, Z., & Smith, R. (2000, January). *Report on the privacy policies and practices of health Web sites*. Retrieved September 18, 2001, from http://www.informatics-review.com/thoughts/policy.htm

Gonsalves, A. (2002, March 20). Software pulls collaboration tools into single secure workspace. *Information-Week*. Retrieved March 23, 2002, from http://www.informationweek.com/story/IWK20020320S0010

Gonzalez, G. M., Costello, C. R., La Tourette, T. R., Joyce, L. K., & Valenzuela, M. (1997). Bilingual telephone-assisted computerized speech-recognition assessment: Is a voice-activated computer program a culturally and linguistically appropriate tool for screening depression in English and Spanish? *Cultural Diversity and Mental Health, 3*(2), 93–111.

Goode, E. (2000). How culture molds habits of thought. *The New York Times*. Retrieved March 29, 2003, from http://www.nytimes.com/library/national/science/health/080800hth-behavior-culture.html

Goodman, W. K., Price, L. H., Rasmussen, S. A., Mazure, C., Fleischmann, R. L., Hill, C. L., Heninger, G. R., & Charney, D. S. (1989). The Yale-Brown Obsessive Compulsive Scale: I. Development, use, and reliability. *Archives of General Psychiatry, 46*(11), 1006–1011.

Gotlib, I. H., & Neubauer, D. L. (2000). Information-processing approaches to the study of cognitive biases in depression. In S. L. Johnson, A. M. Hayes, T. M Field, N. Schneiderman, & P. McCabe (Eds.), *Stress, coping, and depression* (pp. 117–143). Mahwah, NJ: Lawrence Erlbaum Associates.

Gould, R. L. (1990). The Therapeutic Learning Program. In J. Mezirow (Ed.), *Fostering critical reflection in adulthood: A guide to transformative and emancipatory learning* (pp. 134–156). San Francisco: Jossey-Bass.

Gould, R. L. (1996a). Development, problem solving, and generalized learning: The Therapeutic Learning Program (TLP). In M. Miller, and K. Hammond, & M. Hile (Eds.), *Computers and medicine: Mental health computing*. New York: Springer.

Gould, R. L. (1996b). The use of computers in therapy. In T. Trabin & M. Freeman (Eds.), *The computerization of behavioral healthcare* (pp. 39–62). San Francisco: Jossey-Bass.

Gould, R. L. (1978). *Transformations: Growth and change in adult life*. New York: Simon & Schuster.

Gould, R. L. (1990). The Therapeutic Learning Program (TLP): Computer-assisted short-term therapy. In G. Gumpert & S. L. Fish (Eds.), *Talking to strangers: Mediated therapeutic communication* (pp. 184–199). Stamford, CT: Ablex.

Gould, R. L. (2001). A feedback-driven computer program for outpatient training. In L. L'Abate (Ed.), *Distance writing and computer-assisted interventions in psychiatry and mental health* (pp. 93–111). Westport, CT: Ablex.

Graber, M. A., Roller, C. M., & Kaeble, B. (1999, January). Readability levels of patient education material on the World Wide Web. *Journal of Family Practice, 48*(1), 58–61.

Greenemeier, L. (2000). Gateway turns display models into revenue generator. *InformationWeek*. Retrieved December 11, 2002, from http://www.informationweek.com/story/IWK20021211S0011

Greenemeier, L. (2002, September 30). Utility computing's payoff. *InformationWeek*. Retrieved November 21, 2003, from http://www.informationweek.com/story/showArticle.jhtml?articleID=6503224

Greenwald, A. G., Banaji, M. R., Rudman, L. A., Farnham, S. D., Nosek, B. A., & Mellott, D. S. (2002). A unified theory of implicit attitudes, stereotypes, self-esteem, and self-concept. *Psychological Review, 109*(1), 3–25.

Greist, J. H., Gustafson, D., Stauss, F., Rowse, G., Laughren, T., & Chiles, J. (1973). A computer interview for suicide-risk prediction. *American Journal of Psychiatry, 130*(12), 1327–1332.

Greist, J. H., Jefferson, J. W., Wenzel, K. W., Kobak, K., Bailey, T., Katzelnick, D., Hagerson, S., & Dottl, S. (1997). Telephone assessment program: Efficient patient monitoring and clinician feedback. *MD Computing, 14*(5), 382–387.

Greist, J. H., Klein, M. H., Erdman, H. P., & Bires, J. K. (1987). Comparison of computer- and interviewer-administered versions of the Diagnostic Interview Schedule. *Hospital and Community Psychiatry, 38*(12), 1304–1311.

Griffiths, M. (2001). Online therapy: A cause for concern? *The Psychologist, 14*(5), 244–248.

Grigsby, B. (1997). *ATSP report on U.S. telemedicine activity*. Retrieved August 30, 1998, from http://www.atsp.org

Grigsby, B., & Brown, N. (2000). *The 1999 ATSP report on U.S. telemedicine activity*. Portland, OR: Association of Tele-health Service Providers.

Grohol, J. (1999, May 14). *Best practices in e-therapy: Definition and scope of e-therapy*. PsychCentral. Retrieved October 9, 2002, from http://psychcentral.com/best/best3.htm

Grohol, J. (2001, May 2). Best practices in e-therapy: Clarifying the definition. *Psych Central*. Retrieved October 9, 2002, from http://psychcentral.com/best/best5.htm

Grohol, J. (2002). *The insider's guide to mental health resources online*. New York: Guilford.

Gross, C. P., Anderson, G. F., & Powe, N. R. (1999). The relation between funding by the National Institutes of Health and the burden of disease. *New England Journal of Medicine, 340*(24), 1881–1887.

Grossman, L. (2001, May 17). *Consumers want more assurance of the reliability of health care Web sites new survey shows*. Retrieved August 24, 2001, from http://www.urac.org/010517ws.htm

Groth-Marnat, G., & Schumaker, J. (1989). Computer-based psychological testing: Issues and guidelines. *American Journal of Orthopsychiatry, 59*(2), 257–263.

Gruber, K., Moran, P. J., Roth, W. T., & Taylor, C. B. (2001). Computer-assisted cognitive behavioral group therapy for social phobia. *Behavior Therapy, 32*(1), 155–165.

Guerin Gue, D. (2003). *The HIPAA Security Rule (NPRM): Overview*. HIPAAdvisory. Retrieved May 23, 2003, from http://www.cms.hhs.gov/regulations/hipaa/cms0003-5/0049f-econ-ofr-2-12-03.pdf

Gustafson, D. H., Bosworth, K., Chewning, B., & Hawkins, R. (1987). Computer-based health promotion: Combining technological advances with problem-solving techniques to effect successful health behavior changes. *Annual Review of Public Health, 8*, 387–415.

Gustafson, D. H., Bosworth, K., Hawkins, R., Boberg, E., & Bricker, E. (1992, November). *CHESS: A computer-based system for providing information, referrals, decision support and social support to people facing medical and other health-related crises*. Paper presented at the 16th Annual Symposium on Computer Applications in Medical Care, Baltimore.

Gustafson, D. H., Hawkins, R., Boberg, E., Bricker, E., Pingree, S., & Chan, C. (1994). *The use and impact of a computer-based support system for people living with AIDS and HIV infection*. Madison: University of Wisconsin at Madison.

Gustafson, D. H., Hawkins, R., Boberg, E., Pingree, S., Serlin, R. E., Graziano, F., & Chan, C. L. (1999). Impact of a patient-centered, computer-based health information/support system. *American Journal of Preventive Medicine, 16*(1), 1–9.

Gustafson, D. H., Wise, M., McTavish, F., Taylor, J. O., Wolberg, W., Stewart, J., Smalley, R. V., & Bosworth, K. (1993). Development and pilot evaluation of a computer-based support system for women with breast cancer. *Journal of Psychosocial Oncology, 11*(4), 69–93.

Gustke, S., Balch, D., West, V., & Rogers, L. (2000). Patient satisfaction with telemedicine. *Telemedicine Journal*, 6(1), 5–13.

Haas, L. J., Benedict, J. G., & Kobos, J. C. (1996). Psychotherapy by telephone: Risks and benefits for psychologists and consumers. *Professional Psychology: Research and Practice*, 27(2), 154–160.

Hagel, J., III, & Armstrong, A. (1997). *Net.gain: Expanding markets through virtual communities*. Boston: Harvard Business School Press.

Hagland, M. (2003, January). Doctor's orders. *Healthcare Informatics*, 39, ff.

Halverson, D. (2001, September). *Rural Wisconsin Health Cooperative virtual private network feasibility and design study*. Retrieved August 16, 2002, from http://www.rwhc.com/papers/VPN.Report.pdf

Hamilton, L. K. (2003, May). Seven VoIP lessons from the real world: Trials, deployments yield knowledge you can use now. *Communications Technology*. Retrieved September 17, 2003, from http://www.cableworld.com/ct/archives/0503/0503_telephony.html

Hamilton, M. (1959). The assessment of anxiety states by rating. *British Journal of Medical Psychology*, 32(1), 50–55.

Hamilton, M. (1960). A rating scale for depression. *Journal of Neurology, Neurosurgery and Psychiatry*, 23, 56–62.

Hamman, R. B. (1996). *Cyborgasms: Cybersex amongst multiple-selves and cyborgs in the narrow-bandwidth space of America Online chat rooms*. Retrieved June 4, 2002, from http://www.socio.demon.co.uk/Cyborgasms.html

Hao, S. (2002, March 22). Wireless Web devices debut. *Florida Today*, p. C2.

Hapgood, F. (1998). Iphone. *Wired*, 3(10), 1–6.

Haraway, D. J. (1991). *Simians, cyborgs and women: The reinvention of nature*. New York: Routledge.

Harris Interactive. (2001a, February 19). The coming battle for the hearts and minds of cyberchondriacs. *Harris Interactive Healthcare News*, 1(7), 1–3.

Harris Interactive. (2001b, April 23). eHealth traffic critically dependent on search engines and portals. *Harris Interactive Healthcare News*, 1(13), 1–3.

Harris Interactive. (2001c, February 26). New data show Internet, website, and email usage by physicians all increasing. Retrieved July 30, 2001, from http://www.harrisinteractive.com/about/healthnews/HI_HealthCareNews2001Vol1_iss8.pdf

Harris Interactive. (2001d, March 5). Are ehealth consumers reading your ads? It depends on the site. *Harris Interactive Healthcare News*. Retrieved September 1, 2001, from http://www.harrisinteractive.com/news/healthnews/HI_HealthCareNews2001Vol1_iss9.pdf

Harris Interactive. (2002, May 28). *Four-nation survey shows widespread but different levels of Internet use for health purposes*. Retrieved April 25, 2003, from http://www.harrisinteractive.com/news/newsletters/healthnews/HI_HealthCareNews2002Vol2_Iss11.pdf

Hart, R. R., & Goldstein, M. A. (1985). Computer-assisted psychological assessment. *Computers in Human Services*, 1(3), 69–75.

Hartley, D., Bird, D., & Dempsey, P. (1999). Mental health and substance abuse. In T. Ricketts (Ed.), *Rural health in the United States*. New York: Oxford University Press.

Hausman, K. (2001, June 15). Competing agendas threaten to limit computer privacy. *Psychiatric News*, 36(12), 2.

Hawkins, R. P., Gustafson, D. H., Chewning, B., & Bosworth, K. (1987). Reaching hard-to-reach populations: Interactive computer programs as public information campaigns for adolescents. *Journal of Communication*, 37(2), 8–28.

Hawthorne, N. (1906). *The scarlet letter*. New York: Dutton.

Hayes, S. C., Barlow, D., & Nelson-Gray, R. (1999). *The scientist practitioner: Research and accountability in the age of managed care*. Boston: Allyn & Bacon.

Headlam, B. (2001, April 8). *How to e-mail like a C.E.O.* Retrieved April 10, 2001, from http://www.nytimes.com/2001/04/08/magazine/08WWLN.html?ex=987659573&ei=1&en=aeb585498cc95095

Healinx. (2001, May 9). *Impact of online doctor-patient communication to be studied by University of California Berkeley professors*. Retrieved July 30, 2001, from http://www.healinx.com/Corporate/v/Corporate/news24.asp

Health Care Financing Administration. (1998, November 24). *HCFA Internet security policy*. Retrieved March 5, 2002, from http://www.hcfa.gov/security/isecplcy.htm

Healthcare Informatics. (2004, February). Nine tech trends. Retrieved March 22, 2004 from http://www.healthcare-informatics.com/issues/2002/02_02/cover.htm

Health Internet Ethics. (n.d.). *Ethical principles for offering Internet health services to consumers*. Retrieved August 31, 2001, from http://www.hiethics.com/Principles/index.asp

Health on the Net Foundation. (1998). *Health on the Net Foundation code of conduct for medical and health Web sites*. Retrieved November 18, 1998, from http://www.hon.ch/HONcode/Conduct.html

HealthLeaders. (2001, June). *Online communications can raise liability concerns for providers.* Retrieved July 13, 2001, from http://www.healthleaders.com/magazine/feature1.php?contentid=20035&categoryid=155&CE_Session=84cb2237e8caf9348534ebc1beae5d5b

Heimberg, R. G., Hope, D. A., Dodge, C. S., & Becker, R. E. (1990). DSM-III-R subtypes of social phobia: Comparison of generalized social phobics and public speaking phobics. *Journal of Nervous and Mental Disease, 178*(3), 172–179.

Heinlen, K. T., Reynolds Welfel, E., Richmond, E. N., & Rak, C. F. (2003, Winter). The scope of Web-Counseling: A survey of services and compliance with NBCC Standards for the Ethical Practice of WebCounseling. *Journal of Counseling & Development, 8*(1), 61–69.

Helwig, A., Lovelle, A., Guse, C., & Gottlieb, M. (1999). An office-based Internet patient education system: A pilot study. *Journal of Family Practice, 48*(12), 123–127.

Henkel, J. (2001, March). Buying drugs online: It's convenient and private, but beware of "rogue sites." *FDA Consumer Magazine.* Retrieved March 5, 2002, from http://www.fda.gov/fdac/features/2000/100_online.html

Henker, B., Whalen, C. K., Jamner, L. D., & Delfino, R. J. (2002, June). Anxiety, affect, and activity in teenagers monitoring daily life with electronic diaries. *Journal of the American Academy of Child and Adolescent Psychiatry, 41*(6), 660–670.

Hester, R. K. (1995). Behavioral self-control training. In *Handbook of alcoholism treatment approaches: Effective alternatives* (2nd ed., pp. 148–159). Needham Heights, MA: Allyn & Bacon.

Hester, R. K., & Delaney, H. D. (1997). Behavioral self-control program for Windows: Results of a controlled clinical trial. *Journal of Consulting and Clinical Psychology, 65*(4), 686–693.

Hilty, D. M., Marks, S. L., Urness, D., Nesbitt, T. S., & Yellowlees, P. M. (2004, January). Clinical and educational telepsychiatry applications: A review. *Canadian Journal of Psychiatry, 49*(1), 12–23.

HIPAA Resource Center. (n.d.). *Solution to standards for electronic transmission.* Retrieved August 16, 2002, from http://www.hipaainfo.us/VPNandHIPAA.html

Hobson, J. A., & Leonard, J. (2001). *Out of its mind: Psychiatry in crisis.* Cambridge, MA: Perseus.

Hoffman, H. G., Doctor, J., Patterson, D., Carrougher, G., & Furness, T. (2000). Use of virtual reality for adjunctive treatment of adolescent burn pain during wound care: A case report. *Pain, 85*(1–2), 305–309.

Hoffman, H. G., Patterson, D. R., & Carrougher, G. J. (2000). Use of virtual reality for adjunctive treatment of adult burn pain during physical therapy: A controlled study. *Clinical Journal of Pain, 16*(3), 244–250.

Hoffman, H. G., Patterson, D. R., Carrougher, G. J., Nakamura, D., Moore, M., Garcia-Palacios, A., & Furness, T. A. (2001). The effectiveness of virtual reality pain control with multiple treatments of longer durations: A case study. *International Journal of Human–Computer Interaction, 13*(1), 1–12.

Hoffman, H. G., Patterson, D. R., Carrougher, G. J., & Sharar, S. (2001). The effectiveness of virtual reality based pain control with multiple treatments. *Clinical Journal of Pain, 17*(3), 229–235.

Holden, C. (2000, April 7). Mental health: Global survey examines impact of depression. *Science, 288*(5463), 39–40.

Holland, N. (1996). *The Internet regression.* Retrieved July 30, 2001, from http://www.human-nature.com/free-associations/holland.html

Hsiung, R. C. (Ed.). (2002). *e-Therapy: Case studies, guiding principles, and the clinical potential of the Internet.* New York: Norton.

Hsiung, R. C. (2003). E-therapy: Opportunities, dangers and ethics to guide practice. In R. Wooton, P. Yellowlees, & P. McLaren (Eds.), *Telepsychiatry and e-Mental Health* (pp. 73–82). London, England: Royal Society of Medicine Press.

Hulme, G. V. (2002, December 20). Former UBS PaineWebber systems administrator charged with planting logic bomb. *InformationWeek.* Retrieved December 23, 2002, from http://www.informationweek.com/story/IWK20021220S0007

Hulme, G. V. (2003, January 13). Group releases top 10 Web application development mistakes. *Information Week.* Retrieved January 15, 2003, from http://www.informationweek.com/story/IWK20030114S0003

Hunkeler, E. M., Meresman, J. F., Hargreaves, W. A., Fireman, B., Berman, W. H., Kirsch, A. J., Groebe, J., Hurt, S. W., Braden, P., Getzell, M., Feigenbaum, P. A., Peng, T., & Salzer, M. (2000). Efficacy of nurse telehealth care and peer support in augmenting treatment of depression in primary care. *Archives of Family Medicine, 9*(8), 700–708.

Huston, J., & Burton, D. (1997). Patient satisfaction with multispecialty interactive teleconsultations. *Journal of Telemedicine and Telecare, 3*(4), 205–208.

Hutcherson, C., & Williamson, S. H. (1999, May 31). Nursing regulation for the new millennium: The mutual recognition model. *Online Journal of Issues in Nursing.* Retrieved March 5, 2002, from http://www.nursingworld.org/ojin/topic9/topic9_2.htm

IDC. (2000, October 10). *Email deluge continues with no end in sight.* Retrieved October 11, 2001, from www.idc.com:8080/software/press/PR/SW101000pr.stm

Imperio, W. (2000, November). Online therapy sparks concern. *Clinical Psychiatry News, 28*(11), 1–5.

Institute for Healthcare Improvement. (2002). *One size does not fit all: Think segmentation.* Retrieved October 8, 2002, from http://www.ihi.org/resources/qi/qitips/ci0402tip.asp

Institute of Medicine. (1996). *Telemedicine: A guide to assessing telecommunications in health care.* Washington, DC: National Academy Press.

Institute of Medicine. (1997). *The computer-based patient record: An essential technology for health care.* Washington, DC: National Academy Press.

Integrated school-based mental health and learning evaluations via telepsychiatry: The role of the child psychiatrist. (2000). *Telemedicine Journal, 6*(1), 117.

International Organization for Standardization. (2001). Introduction. Retrieved November 7, 2001, from http://www.iso.ch/iso/en/aboutiso/introduction/index.html

Internet Healthcare Coalition. (2000). *eHealth ethics initiative.* Retrieved August 31, 2001, from http://www.ihealthcoalition.org/ethics/ehealthcode0524.html

Internet Healthcare Strategies. (2001). New research reveals e-health paradox: it's harder to reach patients online than to have an effect on them. *Internet Healthcare Strategies, 3*(7), 10–11.

Jackson, T. (2002, September 14). Both sides now. *British Medical Journal, 325*(7364), 603.

Jacobs, M. K., Christensen, A., Snibbe, J. R., Dolezal-Wood, S., Huber, A., & Polterok, A. (2001). A comparison of computer-based versus traditional individual psychotherapy. *Professional Psychology: Research and Practice, 32*(1), 92–96.

Jaffee v. Redmond. (1996). 518 U.S. 1. Retrieved April 24, 2003, from http://supct.law.cornell.edu/supct/html/95-266.ZS.html

James, B. (1998, March 19). What next in multimedia revolution? Beware predictions. *International Herald Tribune.* Retrieved March 12, 2003, from http://www.iht.com/IHT/BJ/98/bj031998.html

James, L. C. (2001, August). *Duty to warn and emergency back-up.* Paper presented at the American Psychological Association Annual Convention, San Francisco.

Jauhar, S. (2002, July 2). Advice rejoins consent. *The New York Times,* p. F5.

Jean-Louis, G., Zizi, F., Von Gizycki, H., & Hauri, P. (1999). Actigraphic assessment of sleep in insomnia: Application of the Actigraph Data Analysis Software (ADAS). *Physiology and Behavior, 65*(4–5), 659–663.

Jerome, L. (1986). Telepsychiatry. *Canadian Journal of Psychiatry, 31*(5), 489.

Jerome, L. (1993). Assessment by telemedicine. *Hospital and Community Psychiatry, 44*(1), 81–83.

Jerome, L. (1997). E-mail therapy. *Journal of the American Academy of Child and Adolescent Psychiatry, 36*(7), 868.

Jerome, L., & Zaylor, C. (2000). Cyberspace: Creating a therapeutic environment for telehealth applications. *Professional Psychology: Research and Practice, 31*(5), 478–483.

Johnson, D. (2001). Is integration the problem or the solution? A look at how consumers get behavioral health treatment services and what it means for the field. *Open Minds, 13*, 3–5.

Johnston, B., Wheeler, L., Deuser, J., & Sousa, K. (2000, January). Outcomes of the Kaiser Permanente tele-home health research project. *Archives of Family Medicine, 9*(1), 40–45.

Johnston, D., & Jones, B. (2001). Telepsychiatry consultations to a rural nursing facility: A 2-year experience. *Journal of Geriatric Psychiatry and Neurology, 14*(2), 72–75.

Joint Commission on Accreditation of Healthcare Organizations. (2002). *Revisions to selected medical staff standards: Comprehensive accreditation manual for hospitals.* Retrieved March 5, 2002, from http://www.jcaho.org/standard/medicalstaff_rev.html

Jones, E. (1953). *The life and work of Sigmund Freud.* New York: Basic Books.

Jones, S. (1995). *Cybersociety: Computer-mediated communication and community.* Thousand Oaks, CA: Sage.

Jupiter Communications. (2000, January 26). *Internet health commerce to soar to $10 billion, but current offerings don't deliver on consumer convenience.* Retrieved September 19, 2001, from www.jup.com/company/pressrelease.jsp?doc=pr000126

Kaakko, T., Milgrom, P., Coldwell, S., Getz, T., Weinstein, P., & Ramsay, D. (1998). Dental fear among university employees: Implications for dental education. *Journal of Dental Education, 62*(6), 415–420.

Kaiser Family Foundation. (1997, November 5). *Is there a managed care "backlash"?* Retrieved September 19, 2001, from www.kff.org/content/archive/1328/mcarepr.html

Kalb, C. (2001, January 22). Seeing a virtual shrink. *Newsweek.* Retrieved January 22, 2001, from http://www.msnbc.com/news/516029.asp?cp1=1

Kane, B., & Sands, D. (1998). Guidelines for the clinical use of electronic mail with patients. *Journal of the American Medical Informatics Association, 5*(1), 104–111.

Kann, L. K. (1987). Effects of computer-assisted instruction on selected interaction skills related to responsible sexuality. *Journal of School Health, 57*(7), 282–287.

Kanz, J. E. (2001). Clinical-supervision.com: Issues in the provision of online supervision. *Professional Psychology: Research & Practice, 32*(4), 415–420.

Kaplan, E. (1997, Summer). Telepsychotherapy: Psychotherapy by telephone, videotelephone, and computer videoconferencing. *Journal of Psychotherapy Practice and Research, 6*(3), 227–237.

Kassirer, J. P. (2000). Patients, physicians, and the Internet. *Health Affairs, 19*(6), 115–123.

Kenardy, J., Evans, L., & Oei, T. P. (1988). The importance of cognitions in panic attacks. *Behavior Therapy, 19*(3), 471–483.

Kenardy, J., Fried, L., Kraemer, H. C., & Taylor, C. B. (1992). Psychological precursors of panic attacks. *British Journal of Psychiatry, 160*(5), 668–673.

Kendall, C. J. (1998). Directing misperceptions: Researching the issues facing manual-based treatments. *Clinical Psychology: Science and Practice, 5*(3), 396–399.

Kendall, P. C., Marrs-Garcia, A., Nath, S. R., & Sheldrick, R. C. (1999). Normative comparisons for the evaluation of clinical significance. *Journal of Clinical and Consulting Psychology, 67*(3), 285–299.

Kennedy, C., & Yellowlees, P. (2003). The effectiveness of telepsychiatry measured using the Health of the Nation Outcome Scale and the Mental Health Inventory. *Journal of Telemedicine and Telecare, 9*(1), 12–16.

Kernberg, O. F. (1993). Paranoiagenesis in organizations. In H. I. Kaplan & B. J. Sadock (Eds.), *Comprehensive group psychotherapy* (pp. 47–57). Baltimore: Williams & Wilkins.

Kiesler, C. A. (2000). The next wave of change for psychology and mental health services in the health care revolution. *American Psychologist, 55*(5), 481–487.

Kihlstrom, J. F. (1987). The cognitive unconscious. *Science, 237*(4821), 1445–1452.

Kim, P., & Bailey, J. M. (1997). Sidestreets on the information highway: Paraphilias and sexual variations on the Internet. *Journal of Sex Education and Therapy, 22*(1), 35–44.

King, S. A., & Moreggi, D. (1998). Internet therapy and self-help groups: The pros and cons. In J. Gackenbach (Ed.), *Psychology and the Internet: Intrapersonal, interpersonal and transpersonal implications* (pp. 77–109). San Diego, CA: Academic Press.

Kirby, K., Hardesty, P., & Nickelson, D. (1998). Telehealth and the evolving health care system: Strategic opportunities for professional psychology. *Professional Psychology: Research and Practice, 29*(6), 527–535.

Kirkby, K. (1996). Computer-assisted treatment of phobias. *Psychiatric Services, 47*(2), 139–142.

Kirkpatrick, K. (n.d.). Five technologies that can save you money. *Fortune c/net Tech Review.* Retrieved February 15, 2002, from http://fortune.cnet.com/fortune/0-5937473-7-6116125.html?tag=subdir

Kirsch, B. (2002, October). *Salve for the body and mind.* Scientific American. Retrieved November 25, 2003, from http://www.sciam.com/print_version.cfm?articleID=000138DA-66C5-1D7E-90FB809EC5880000

Kirsch, I., Jungeblut, A., Jenkins, L., & Kolstad, A. (1993). *Adult literacy in America: A first look at the results of the National Adult Literacy Survey.* Washington, DC: U.S. Department of Education, National Center for Education Statistics.

Klein, D. F. (1995). Response to Rothman and Michels on placebo-controlled clinical trials. *Psychiatric Annals, 25*(7), 401–403.

Klein, D. F., & Davis, J. M. (1969). *Diagnosis and drug treatment of psychiatric disorders.* Baltimore: Williams & Wilkins.

Klein, J. (2002, August 6). HIPAA and the encryption of protected health information. Retrieved November 14, 2003, from http://nedarc.med.utah.edu/HIPAA/108890.pdf

Kleinmuntz, B., & McLean, R. S. (1968). Diagnostic interviewing by digital computer. *Behavioral Science, 13*(1), 75–80.

Kling, R. (1996). Synergies and competition between life in cyberspace and face-to-face communities. *Social Science Computer Review, 14*(1), 50–54.

Kobak, K. A., Greist, J. H., Jefferson, J. W., & Katzelnick, D. J. (1996). Computer-administered clinical rating scales: A review. *Psychopharmacology, 127*(4), 291–301.

Kobak, K. A., Greist, J. H., Jefferson, J. W., Katzelnick, D. J., & Mundt, J. C. (2001). New technologies to improve clinical trials. *Journal of Clinical Psychopharmacology, 21*(3), 255–256.

Kobak, K. A., Greist, J. H., Jefferson, J. W., Mundt, J. C., & Katzelnick, D. J. (1999). Computerized assessment of depression and anxiety over the telephone using interactive voice response. *MD Computing: Computers in Medical Practice, 16*(3), 64–68.

Kobak, K. A., Taylor, L. H., Dottl, S. L., Greist, J. H., Jefferson, J. W., Burroughs, D., Katzelnick, D. J., & Mandell, M. (1997a). Computerized screening for psychiatric disorders in an outpatient community mental health clinic. *Psychiatric Services, 48*(8), 1048–1057.

Kobak, K. A., Taylor, L. V., Dottl, S. L., Greist, J. H., Jefferson, J. W., Burroughs, D., Mantle, J. M., Katzelnick, D. J., Norton, R., Henk, H. J., & Serlin, R. C. (1997b). A computer-administered telephone interview to identify mental disorders. *Journal of the American Medical Association, 278*(11), 905–910.

Koocher, G., & Morray, E. (2000). Regulation of telepsychology: A survey of state attorneys general. *Professional Psychology: Research and Practice, 31*(5), 503–508.

Kopelman, P. G. (1998, August). Emerging management strategies for obesity. *International Journal of Obesity and Related Metabolic Disorders, 22*(1), S7–11; discussion S12, S42.

Kopelman, P. G. (2000). Obesity as a medical problem. *Nature, 404*(6778), 635–643.

Koran, L. M. (1991). *Medical evaluation field manual.* Stanford, CA: Stanford University Medical Center.

Kordy, H., Hannover, W., & Richard, M. (2001). Computer-assisted feedback-driven quality management for psychotherapy: The Stuttgart-Heidelberg model. *Journal of Consulting and Clinical Psychology, 69*(2), 173–183.

Kramer, P. D. (1993). *Listening to Prozac: A psychiatrist explores antidepressant drugs and the remaking of the self.* New York: Viking.

Kraut, R., Patterson, M., Lundmark, V., Kiesler, S., Mukopadhyay, T., & Scherlis, W. (1998). Internet paradox. A social technology that reduces social involvement and psychological well-being? *American Psychologist, 53*(9), 1017–1031.

Kreuter, M. W., Strecher, V. J., & Glassman, B. (1999, Fall). One size does not fit all: The case for tailoring print materials. *Annals of Behavioral Medicine, 21*(4), 276–283.

Kuhn, T. (1962). *The structure of scientific revolutions.* Chicago: University of Chicago Press.

Kulik, C.-L. C., & Kulik, J. A. (1991). Effectiveness of computer-based instruction: An updated analysis. *Computers in Human Behavior, 7*(1–2), 75–94.

Kuszler, P. C. (2000, September). A question of duty: Common law legal issues resulting from physician response to unsolicited patient email inquiries. *Journal of Medical Internet Research, 2*(3), e17.

L'Abate, L. (Ed.). (2001). Distance writing and computer-assisted interventions on psychiatry and mental health. Westport, CT: Greenwood Press.

L'Abate, L. (2002a). Beyond psychotherapy: Programmed writing and structured, computer-assisted interventions. Westport, CT: Ablex.

L'Abate, L. (2002b). *A guide to self-help workbooks.* Atlanta, GA: Workbooks for Better Living.

LaCoursiere, S. (2001, February 4–6). *Session 137: Online healthcare applications: What do patients care about?* Retrieved December 12, 2001, from http://www.himss.org/content/files/proceedings/2001/sessions/ses137.pdf

Ladd, J. (1991). The quest for a code of professional ethics: An intellectual and moral confusion. In D. G. Johnson (Ed.), *Ethical issues in engineering* (pp. 130–136). Englewood Cliffs, NJ: Prentice-Hall.

Lake, D. (2000, November 20). *E-mail outpaces the Web.* Retrieved March 21, 2001, from http://www.thestandard.com/research/metrics/display/0,2799,20265,00.html

Lamberg, L. (1997). Computers in psychiatry. *Journal of the American Medical Association, 278*(10), 799–801.

Lambert, M. J., & Bergin, A. (1994). The effectiveness of psychotherapy. In A. Bergin & S. Garfield (Eds.), *Handbook of psychotherapy and behavior change* (4th ed., pp. 143–189). New York: Wiley.

Lambert, M. J., Hansen, N. B., & Finch, A. E. (2001). Patient-focused research: Using patient outcome data to enhance treatment effects. *Journal of Consulting and Clinical Psychology, 69*(2), 159–172.

Lambert, M. E., Hedlund, J. L., & Vieweg, B. W. (1990). Computer simulations in mental health education: Current status. *Computers in Human Services, 7*(3–4), 211–229.

Lange, A., van de Ven, J. P., Schrieken, B. A., Bredeweg, B., & Emmelkamp, P. M. (2000). Internet-mediated, protocol-driven treatment of psychological dysfunction. *Journal of Telemedicine and Telecare, 6*(1), 15–21.

Lange, A., van de Ven, J. P., Schrieken, B., & Emmelkamp, P. M. (2001). Interapy, treatment of posttraumatic stress through the Internet: A controlled trial. *Journal of Behavior Therapy and Experimental Psychiatry, 32*(2), 73–90.

Larose, S., Gagnon, S., Ferland, C., & Pepin, M. (1989). Psychology of computers: XIV. Cognitive rehabilitation through computer games. *Perceptual and Motor Skills, 69*(3), 851–858.

Larson, M. A., Rizzo, A. A., Buckwalter, J. G., van Rooyen, A., Kratz, K., Neumann, U., Kesselman, C., Thiebaux, M., & van der Zaag, C. (1999). Gender issues in the application of a virtual environment spatial rotation project. *CyberPsychology and Behavior, 2*(2), 113–124.

Laska, E. M. (Ed.). (1975). *Safeguarding psychiatric privacy: Computer systems and their uses.* New York: Wiley.

Laszlo, V., Esterman, G., & Zabko, S. (1999). Therapy over the Internet? Theory, research and finances. *CyberPsychology and Behavior, 2*(4), 293–307.

Laveman, L. (1994). The multi-level supervision model and the interplay between clinical supervision and psychotherapy. *The Clinical Supervisor, 12*(2), 75–91.

Lavoie, F., Borkman, T., & Gidron, B. (1994). *Self-help and mutual aid groups: International and multicultural perspectives.* Binghamton, NY: Haworth.

Lawrence, G. H. (1986). Using computers for the treatment of psychological problems. *Computers in Human Behavior, 2*(1), 43–62.

Lea, M. (1991). Rationalist assumptions in cross media comparisons of computer-mediated communication. *Behavior and Information Technology, 10*(2), 153–172.

Lea, M., & Spears, R. (1995). Love at first byte? Building personal relationships over computer networks. In J. Wood & S. Duck (Eds.), *Understudied relationships* (pp. 197–233). Thousand Oaks, CA: Sage.

Lebow, J. (1998). Not just talk, maybe some risk: The therapeutic potentials and pitfalls of computer-mediated conversation. *Journal of Marital and Family Therapy, 24*(2), 203–206.

LeDoux, J. (2002). *Synaptic self: How our brains became who we are.* New York: Viking.

Leffert, M. (2002). Analysis and psychotherapy by telephone: Twenty years of clinical experience. *Journal of the American Psychoanalytic Association, 51*(1), 101–130.

Lehrer, P., Carr, R., Sargunaraj, D., & Woolfolk, R. (1994). Stress management techniques: Are they all equivalent, or do they have specific effects? *Biofeedback Self Regulation, 19*(4), 353–401.

Lehrer, P., Carr, R. E., Smetankine, A., Vaschillo, E., Peper, E., Porges, S., Edelberg, R., Hamer, R., & Hochron, S. (1997). Respiratory sinus arrhythmia versus neck/trapezius EMG and incentive inspirometry biofeedback for asthma: A pilot study. *Applied Psychophysiology & Biofeedback, 22*(2), 95–109.

Lehrer, P., Smetankin, A., & Potapova, T. (2000). Respiratory sinus arrhythmia biofeedback therapy for asthma: a report of 20 unmedicated pediatric cases using the Smetankin method. *Applied Psychophysiology and Biofeedback, 25*(3), 193–200.

Leon, A. C., Kelsey, J. E., Pleil, A., Burgos, T. L., Portera, L., & Lowell, K. (1999). An evaluation of a computer assisted telephone interview for screening for mental disorders among primary care patients. *Journal of Nervous and Mental Disease, 187*(5), 308–311.

Lerner, L. (2001, January). Virtual insanity! *Maxim,* 117.

Leslie, R. S. (2002, March 10). *Newsletter of the American Association for Marriage and Family Therapy,* 1.

Levant, R. (n.d.). *The problem of licensure mobility.* Retrieved October 13, 2003, from http://www.drronaldlevant.com/licmob.html

Levant, R. (2003, Winter). Washington update: The problem of licensure mobility. *The Independent Practitioner, 23*(1). Retrieved November 14, 2003, from http://www.division42.org/MembersArea/IPfiles/Wtr_03/advocacy/licensure_mobility.html

Levit, K., Cowan, C., Lazenby, H., Sensenig, A., McDonnell, P., Stiller, J., & Martin, A. (2000). Health spending in 1998: Signals of change. *Health Affairs, 19*(1), 124–132.

Lewis, D. (1999). Computer-based approaches to patient education: A review of the literature. *Journal of the American Medical Informatics Association, 6*(4), 272–282.

Lichstein, K. L. (1988). *Clinical relaxation strategies.* New York, NY: John Wiley & Sons.

Licklider, J. C. R. (1960, March). Man–machine symbiosis. *IRE Transactions on Human Factors in Electronics, HFE-1*(1), 4–11.

Liebson, E. (1997). Telepsychiatry: Thirty-five years' experience. *Medscape Mental Health.* Retrieved November 15, 1997, from http://www.medscape.com/Medscape/MentalHe...02.n07/mh3112.liebson/mh3112.liebson.html

Lièvre, M. (2002, September 14). Alosetron for irritable bowel loss. *British Medical Journal, 325*(7364), 555–556.

Lindberg, D., & Humphreys, B. (1998, October 21). Medicine and health on the Internet: The good, the bad, and the ugly. *Journal of the American Medical Association, 280*(15), 1303–1304.

Lindemann, C. (2001, November 12). Videoconferencing meets the desktop. *VAR Business, 17*(23), 73–76.

Lippeveld, T., Sauerborn, R., & Bodart, C. (Eds.). (2000). *Design and implementation of health information systems.* Geneva: World Health Organization.

Lipsey, M. W., & Wilson, D. B. (1993). The efficacy of psychological, educational, and behavioral treatment. Confirmation from meta-analysis. *American Psychologist, 48*(12), 1181–1209.

Lipton, G., Arends, M., Bastian, K., Wright, B., & O'Hara, P. (2002). The psychosocial consequences experienced by interpreters in relation to working with torture and trauma clients: A West Australian pilot study. *Synergy (Australian Transcultural Mental Health Network), 3,* ff.

Liss, H. J., Glueckauf, R. L., & Ecklund-Johnson, E. P. (2002). Research on telehealth and chronic medical conditions: Critical review, key issues, and future directions. *Rehabilitation Psychology, 47*(1), 8–30.

Loganbill, C. R., Hardy, C. V., & Delworth, U. (1982). Supervision: A conceptual model. *The Counseling Psychologist, 10*(1), 3–42.

Lorden, D., Vorhees, N., & Richards, C. (2002). Telepharmacy offers hope for rural hospitals. *Telemedicine Today, 9*(3), 13–15.

Luborsky, L., Diguer, L., Seligman, D. A., Rosenthal, R., Krause, E. D., Johnson, S., Halperin, G., Bishop, M., Berman, J. S., & Schweizer, E. (1999). The researcher's own therapy allegiances: A "wild card" in comparisons of treatment efficacy. *Clinical Psychology: Science and Practice, 6*(1), 95–106.

Lucas, R. W., Mullin, P. J., Luna, C. B., & McInroy, D. C. (1977). Psychiatrists and a computer as interrogators of patients with alcohol-related illnesses: A comparison. *British Journal of Psychiatry, 131,* 160–167.

Lueger, R. J., Howard, K. I., Martinovich, Z., Lutz, W., Anderson, E. E., & Grissom, G. (2001). Assessing treatment progress of individual patients using expected treatment response models. *Journal of Consulting Clinical Psychology, 69*(2), 150–158.

Lukin, M. E., Dowd, E. T., Plake, B. S., & Kraft, R. G. (1985). Comparing computerized versus traditional psychological assessment. *Computers in Human Behavior*, 1(1), 49–58.

Lynch, D. J., Tamburrino, M. B., & Nagel, R. (1997). Telephone counseling for patients with minor depression: Preliminary findings in a family practice setting. *Journal of Family Practice*, 44(3), 293–298.

Lyons v. Grether, 239 Va. S.E.2d 103 (1977).

Mack, J., & Wittel, A. (Eds.). (2001). *The new frontier: Exploring ehealth ethics*. Washington, DC: URAC and the Internet Healthcare Coalition.

MacLeod, C., Mathews, A., & Tata, P. (1986). Attentional bias in emotional disorders. *Journal of Abnormal Psychology*, 95(1), 15–20.

Maheu, M. (1997a, December). Licensure investigations by the California Board of Psychology: Practitioner beware. *Telehealth.net*. Retrieved September 11, 2002, from http://telehealth.net/articles/licens.html

Maheu, M. (1997b). Will online services for consumer self-help improve behavioral healthcare? *Behavioral Healthcare Tomorrow*, 6(6), 32–38.

Maheu, M. (1999). Virtual private networks. *Telehealth.net*. Retrieved August 16, 2002, from http://telehealth.net/subscribe/newslettr_8.html

Maheu, M. (2001, July). Exposing the risk yet moving forward: A behavioral e-health model. *Journal of Computer-Mediated Communication*. Retrieved September 20, 2001, from http://www.ascusc.org/jcmc/vol6/issue4/maheu.html

Maheu, M., Callan, J., & Nagy, T. (1998). Call to action: Ethical and legal issues for behavioral telehealth including online psychological services. Unpublished manuscript.

Maheu, M., & Gordon, B. L. (2000). Counseling and therapy on the Internet. *Professional Psychology: Research and Practice*, 31(5), 484–489.

Maheu, M., & Subotnik, R. (2001). *Infidelity on the Internet: Virtual relationships and real betrayal*. Naperville, IL: Sourcebooks.

Maheu, M., Whitten, P., & Allen, A. (2001). *E-health, telehealth, and telemedicine: A guide to start-up and success*. San Francisco: Jossey-Bass.

Majeski, T. (2003, January 19). *Web sites help decide which treatment is best*. Retrieved May 5, 2003, from http://seattletimes.nwsource.com/text/134618050_besttreat19.html

Mallen, M. J., Day, S. X., & Green, M. A. (2003, Spring/Summer). Online versus face-to-face conversations: An examination of relational and discourse variables. *Psychotherapy: Theory, Research, Practice, Training*, 40(1–2), 155–163.

Manhal-Baugus, M. (2001). E-therapy: Practical, ethical, and legal issues. *CyberPsychology & Behavior*, 4(5), 551–563.

Mara, J. (1995). *Clear and simple: Developing effective print materials for low-literate readers*. Washington, DC: National Cancer Institute.

Marek, S. (2002, February 4). Satellite survivors spreading broadband's benefits. *Wireless Internet Magazine*. Retrieved June 22, 2002, from http://www.wirelessinternetmagazine.com/news/020204/020204_feature_satellite.htm

Margraf, J., Taylor, C. B., Ehlers, A., Roth, W. T., & Agras, W. S. (1987). Panic attacks in the natural environment. *Journal of Nervous and Mental Disease*, 175(4), 558–565.

Marhula, D. C. (2003, January). Is e-health FACT or FICTION? *Healthcare Informatics*. Retrieved November 17, 2003, from http://www.healthcare-informatics.com/issues/2003/01_03/marhula.htm

Markoff, J. (2002, April 15). *A computer scientist's lament: Has grammar lost its technological edge?* The New York Times. Retrieved April 17, 2002, from http://www.nytimes.com

Marks, I. M. (1978). *Living with fear: Understanding and coping with anxiety*. New York, NY: McGraw-Hill.

Marks, I. M., Blanes, T., & McKenzie, N. (1995). Computerised clinical benefit-cost audit of mental health care: I. Theoretical and practical issues. *Journal of Mental Health (UK)*, 4(1), 63–69.

Marks, I. M., Shaw, S., & Parkin, R. (1998, Summer). Computer-aided treatments of mental health problems. *Clinical Psychology: Science and Practice*, 5(2), 151–170.

Martin, D. (2000, November). The ethical practice of Internet therapy: Can it be done? *The California Psychologist*, 33(6), 32–34.

Masi, D. (2002, August 25). *Telephonic and online services*. Paper presented at the American Psychological Association, Chicago.

Masi, D., & Back-Tamburo, M. (2001, May). *Motivation for the use of an online EAP and work/life product: A study for Ceridian*. Baltimore: University of Maryland Graduate School of Social Work.

Masi, D., & Freeman, M. (1999, June). *Factors that contribute to client's utilization of telephone information/consultation and face-to-face information/consultation: A study for Ceridian Performance Partners*. Baltimore: University of Maryland Graduate School of Social Work.

Masi, D., & Jacobson, J. (2002). *Outcome measurements for Ceridian lifeworks online: A study for Ceridian Lifeworks Services by the University of Maryland*. Baltimore: University of Maryland Graduate School of Social Work.

Matarazzo, J. D. (1986). Computerized clinical psychological test interpretations: Unvalidated plus all mean and no sigma. *American Psychologist, 41*(1), 14–24.

Mathews, S. (1998, March). Protection of personal data: The European view. *Journal of AHIMA, 69*(3). Retrieved March 14, 2003, from http://www.ahima.org/journal/features/feature.9803.html

Matthews, T. J., de Santi, S. M., Callahan, D., & Koblenz-Sulcov, C. J. (1987). The microcomputer as an agent of intervention with psychiatric patients: Preliminary studies. *Computers in Human Behavior, 3*(1), 37–47.

Maxmen, J. (1977). Telecommunications in psychiatry. *American Journal of Psychotherapy, 32*(3), 450–456.

May, C., Gask, L., Atkinson, T., Ellis, N., Mair, F., & Esmail, A. (2001). Resisting and promoting new technologies in clinical practice: The case of telepsychiatry. *Social Science and Medicine, 52*(12), 1889–1901.

Mayfield, D., McLeod, G., & Hall, P. (1974). The CAGE questionnaire: Validation of a new alcoholism instrument. *American Journal of Psychiatry, 131*(10), 1121–1123.

McCarthy, P., Kulakowski, D., & Kenfield, J. (1994). Clinical supervision practices of licensed psychologists. *Professional Psychology: Research and Practice, 25*(2), 177–181.

McClosky-Armstrong, T. (1999). *Telehealth technology guidelines: Mental health.* Retrieved October 7, 2002, from http://telehealth.hrsa.gov/pubs/tech/techhome.htm

McCormick, N., & McCormick, J. (1992). Computer friends and foes: Content of undergraduates' electronic mail. *Computers in Human Behavior, 8*(4), 379–405.

McCoy, W. D. (2002, June 11). *Abundance of "cures" brings ills.* Retrieved March 12, 2003, from http://www.vaccinationnews.com/DailyNews/June2002/AbundanceCuresBringsIlls.htm

McCrone, P. (2003). Health economics of telepsychiatry. In R. Wooton, P. Yellowlees, & P. McLaren (Eds.), *Telepsychiatry and e-Mental Health* (pp. 29–38). London, England: Royal Society of Medicine Press.

McDonald, D. (1999, March). *Telemedicine can reduce correctional health care costs: An evaluation of a prison telemedicine network.* Retrieved August 12, 2002, from http://www.ncjrs.org/telemedicine/toc.html

McDonald, T. (2002, March 18). *Study: Online gamblers may have serious problems.* Retrieved July 8, 2002, from http://www.newsfactor.com/perl/story/16814.html

McGinnis, J., & Foege, W. (1993). Actual causes of death in the United States. *Journal of the American Medical Association, 270*(18), 2207–2212.

McGinnis, J., Williams-Russo, P., & Knickman, J. R. (2002). The case for more active policy attention to health promotion. To succeed, we need leadership that informs and motivates, economic incentives that encourage change, and science that moves the frontiers. *Health Affairs, 21*(2), 78–93.

McLaren, P. M. (2003). Telemedicine and telecare: What can it offer mental health services? *Advances in Psychiatric Treatment, 9*(1), 54–61.

McLaren, P. M., Ahlbom, J., Riley, A., Mohammedali, A., & Denis, M. (2002, January). *The North Lewisham Telepsychiatry Project: Beyond the application project.* Paper presented at TeleMed '02, Telemedicine and e-Health Forum, London.

McLaren, P. M., Ball, C. J., Summerfield, A. B., Lipsedge, M., & Watson, J. P. (1992). Preliminary evaluation of a low cost videoconferencing system for teaching in clinical psychiatry. *Med Teach, 14*(1), 43–47.

McLaren, P. M., Blunden, J., Lipsedge, M., & Summerfield, A. (1996). Telepsychiatry in an inner-city community psychiatric service. *Journal of Telemedicine and Telecare, 2*(1), 57–59.

McLendon, K. (2000). E-commerce and HIM: Ready or not, here it comes. *Journal of the American Health Information Management Association, 71*(1), 22–23.

McLuhan, M. (1964). *Understanding media: The extensions of man.* New York: McGraw-Hill.

McLuhan, M., & Fiore, Q. (1967). *The medium is the message.* New York: Bantam.

McMenamin, J. P. (1996). Telemedicine and the law. *International Legal Practitioner, 21,* 126.

McMenamin, J. P. (1998). Does product liability litigation threaten picture archiving and communication systems and/or telemedicine? *Journal of Digital Imaging, 11*(1), 21–32.

McPeck, P. (2001, August 27). Cross-country nursing. *Nurseweek, 14*(18), 25.

Mechanic, M. (2001, July 30). *Take two aspirin and log on in the morning.* Retrieved August 3, 2001, from http://www.thestandard.com/article/0,1902,28075,00.html

Medem. (2000, November 6). *Latest research reveals that half of physicians interested in using e-mail with patients if reimbursed.* Retrieved March 20, 2001, from http://www.medem.com/Corporate/press/corporate_medeminthenews_press023.cfm

Medicare Telehealth Validation Act of 2003. (2003, May 1). Retrieved November 4, 2003, from http://www.theorator.com/bills108/hr1940.html

Melonas, J. (2002, March 15). Talk not cheap if you lower your guard. *Psychiatric News, 37*(6), 8.

Menon, A. S., Kondapavalru, P., Krishna, P., Chrismer, J. B., Raskin, A., Hebel, J. R., & Ruskin, P. E. (2001). Evaluation of a portable low cost videophone system in the assessment of depressive symptoms and cognitive function in elderly medically ill veterans. *Journal of Nervous and Mental Disease, 189*(6), 399–401.

Metzger, D. S., Koblin, B., Turner, C., Navaline, H., Valenti, F., Holte, S., Gross, M., Sheon, A., Miller, H., Cooley, P., & Seage, G. R., III. (2000). Randomized controlled trial of audio computer-assisted self-interviewing: Utility and acceptability in longitudinal studies: HIVNET Vaccine Preparedness Study Protocol Team. *American Journal of Epidemiology, 152*(2), 99–106.

Meuret, A. E., Wilhelm, F. H., & Roth, W. T. (2001). Respiratory biofeedback assisted therapy for panic disorder. *Behavior Modification, 25*(4), 584–605.

Michaelson, K. (1996). Information, community and access. *Social Science Computer Review, 14*(1), 57–59.

Milholland, D. K., & Reed, G. M. (1998). *Report of the Joint Interdisciplinary Telehealth Standards Working Group.* Washington, DC: American Psychological Association.

Miller, H. (1995, October 17). *The presentation of self in electronic life: Goffman on the Internet.* Retrieved July 5, 2001, from http://www.ntu.ac.uk/soc/psych/miller/goffman.htm

Miller, J., & Gergen, K. (1998). Life on the line: The therapeutic potentials of computer-mediated conversation. *Journal of Marital and Family Therapy, 24*(2), 189–202.

Miller, K. (2001). *Digital divide now has 2 spans.* Retrieved October 17, 2003, from http://www.thestandard.com/article/article_print/0,1153,22407,00.html

Miller, R., & Berman, J. (1983). The efficacy of cognitive behavior therapies: A quantitative review of the research evidence. *Psychological Bulletin, 94*(1), 39–53.

Millstein, S. G. (1987). Acceptability and reliability of sensitive information collected via computer interview. *Educational and Psychological Measurement, 47*(2), 523–533.

Mineka, S., & Sutton, S. K. (1992). Cognitive biases and the emotional disorders. *Psychological Science, 3*(1), 65–69.

Ministry of Health Services. (2002). *Medical Services Plan (MSP) forms for practitioners.* Retrieved December 12, 2002, from https://www.healthservices.gov.bc.ca/exforms/mspprac/#directpayment

Mintz, J., Drake, R., & Crits-Christoph, P. (1996). The efficacy and effectiveness of psychotherapy: Two paradigms, one science. *American Psychologist, 51*(10), 1084–1085.

Mistretta, A. J. (2002). Psychiatrists use video links to treat rural patients. *New Orleans City Business, 23*(8), 28–29.

Mitchell, J., & Mitchell, B. (1994, December). *The challenge to embed telepsychiatry.* Retrieved March 27, 2001, from http://www.jma.com.au/telepsyc.htm

Mitchell, J. E., Wonderlich, S., Crosby, R., Myers, T., Swan-Kremeier, L., & Lancaster, K. (2003). A randomized trial delivering psychotherapy via telemedicine. *Telemedicine Journal and e-Health, 9*(1), 49.

Mohatt, D., & Kirwan, D. (1995). *Meeting the challenge: Model programs in rural mental health.* Rockville, MD: Office of Rural Health Policy.

Mohr, D. C., Likosky, W., Dick, L. P., Van Der Wende, J., Dwyer, P., Bertagnolli, D., & Goodkin, D. E. (2000). Telephone-administered cognitive-behavioral therapy for the treatment of depressive symptoms in multiple sclerosis. *Journal of Consulting and Clinical Psychology, 68*(2), 356–361.

Molitor, A. (2001). *Deploying a dynamic voice-over-IP firewall with IP telephony applications.* Retrieved February 15, 2002, from http://www.brint.com/members/01040530/voip

Moncher, M. S., Parms, C. A., Orlandi, M. A., & Schinke, S. P. (1989). Microcomputer-based approaches for preventing drug and alcohol abuse among adolescents from ethnic-racial minority backgrounds. *Computers in Human Behavior, 5*(2), 79–93.

Montani, C., Billaud, N., Couturier, P., Fluchaire, I., Lemaire, R., Malterre, C., Lauvernay, N., Piquard, J. F., Frossard, M., & Franco, A. (1996). "Telepsychometry": A remote psychometry consultation in clinical gerontology: Preliminary study. *Telemedicine Journal, 2*(2), 145–150.

Montani, C., Billaud, N., Tyrrell, J., & Fluchaire, I. (1997). Psychological impact of a remote psychometric consultation with hospitalized elderly people. *Journal of Telemedicine and Telecare, 3*(3), 140–145.

Monteiro, I. M., Boksay, I., Auer, S. R., Torossian, C., Sinaiko, E., & Reisberg, B. (1998, Spring). Reliability of routine clinical instruments for the assessment of Alzheimer's disease administered by telephone. *Journal of Geriatric Psychiatry and Neurology, 11*(1), 18–24.

Moore, C. (2001, September 7). *Videoconferencing takes control.* InfoWorld. Retrieved November 25, 2003, from http://archive.infoworld.com/articles/fe/xml/01/09/10/010910fevidconf.xml

Moore, N. C., Summer, K. R., & Bloor, R. N. (1984). Do patients like psychometric testing by computer? *Journal of Clinical Psychology, 40*(3), 875–877.

Morgan, A. (2000). *What is narrative therapy?* Adelaide, South Australia: Dulwich Centre Publications.

Motluk, A. (2000, September 30). *Someone to watch over you.* Retrieved May 27, 2003, from http://medg.lcs.mit.edu/projects/ga/NewScientist

Moynihan, R. (2002, September 14). Alosetron: A case study in regulatory capture, or a victory for patients' rights? *British Medical Journal, 325*(7364), 562–565.

Mulder, P., Kenkel, M., Shellenberger, S., Constantine, M., Streiegel, R., Sears, S., Jumper-Thurman, P., Kalodner, M., Danda, C., & Hager, A. (2001). *The behavioral health care needs of rural women.* Washington, DC: American Psychological Association.

Mulligan, K. (2002a, January 4). Medical-record privacy may suffer in post-terrorism backlash. *Psychiatric News, 37*(1), 1, 28.

Mulligan, K. (2002b, September 20). Medicare agrees to reimburse telehealth psychiatric interviews. *Psychiatric News, 37*(18), 2.

Muncer, S., Burrows, R., Pleace, N., Loader, B., & Nettleton, S. (2000, March 1). Births, deaths, sex and marriage . . . but very few presents? A case study of social support in cyberspace. *Critical-Public-Health, 10*(1), 1–18.

Mundell, E. J. (2000). *"Telepsychiatry" brings needed care to rural patients.* Retrieved November 16, 2000, from http://dailynews.yahoo.com/h/nm/20001116/hl/telepsychiatry_1.html

Mundt, J. C., Kobak, K. A., Taylor, L. V., Mantle, J. M., Jefferson, J. W., Katzelnick, D. J., & Greist, J. H. (1998). Administration of the Hamilton Depression Rating Scale using interactive voice response technology. *MD Computing: Computers in Medical Practice, 15*(1), 31–39.

Murphy, C. (2002, September 30). IT confidential: Reasons to stay awake at night. InformationWeek. Retrieved March 14, 2003, from http://www.informationweek.com/story/IWK20020927S0039

Murphy, J. W., & Pardeck, J. T. (1988, Winter). Technology and language use: Implications for computer mediated therapy. *Journal of Humanistic Psychology, 28*(1), 120–134.

Murphy, L., & Mitchell, D. (1998). When writing helps to heal: E-mail as therapy. *British Journal of Guidance and Counselling, 26*(1), 43–52.

Murray, J. D., & Keller, P. A. (1991, March). Psychology and rural America: Current status and future directions. *American Psychologist, 46*(3), 220–231.

Myers, K., Sulzbacher, S., & Melzer, S. M. (2003). Telemedicine for pediatric mental health in rural areas. *Telemedicine Journal and e-Health, 9*(1), 53.

Myers, T. C., & Mitchell, J. E. (2003, September/October). Telemedicine delivery of psychotherapy for bulimia nervosa: Clinical and logistical considerations. *Telehealth Practice Report, 8*(4), 3–8.

Nagel, K. (1995). *The natural life cycle of mailing lists.* Retrieved October 26, 2001, from http://www.catalog.com/vivian/lifecycle.html

Nagoski, E., & Froehle, T. (n.d.). *Counselor responses in online counseling: Toward a research agenda.* Unpublished manuscript.

Nagy, T. F. (2001, August 25). *Does the "e" in etherapy also stand for ethics?* Paper presented at the American Psychological Association Annual Convention, San Francisco.

Napolitano, M. A. (1999). *Telephone-based psychosocial intervention for patients awaiting lung transplantation.* Durham, NC: Duke University.

Narrow, W. E., Rae, D. S., Robins, L. N., & Regier, D. A. (2002, February). Revised prevalence estimates of mental disorders in the United States: Using a clinical significance criterion to reconcile 2 surveys' estimates. *Archives of General Psychiatry, 59*(2), 115–123.

National Archives and Records Administration, 42 C.F.R. §2.32. (2001). Retrieved November 13, 2001, from http://www.access.gpo.gov/nara/cfr/cfr-table-search.html

National Committee for Quality Assurance. (2000). *2000 standards and surveyor guidelines for the accreditation of managed behavioral health organizations.* Washington, DC: Author.

National Emergency Telemedical Communications Act. (2002, June 3). Retrieved November 4, 2003, from http://conrad.senate.gov/~conrad/releases/02/07/2002708B11.html

National Institute of Mental Health. (2001, January). *Mental disorders in America.* Retrieved July 27, 2001, from http://www.nimh.nih.gov/publicat/numbers.cfm

National Mental Health Association. (2001, June 6). *Barriers to diagnoses for common mental illnesses could prolong suffering, according to new national survey.* Retrieved July 27, 2001, from http://www.nmha.org/newsroom/system/news.vw.cfm?do=vw&rid=309

National Mental Health Association & The Jed Foundation. (2002). *Safeguarding your students against suicide: Expanding the safety net.* Retrieved March 14, 2003, from http://www.nmha.org/suicide/report.pdf

National Telecommunications and Information Administration. (1997, January 31). *Telemedicine report to Congress.* Retrieved August 30, 2001, from http://www.ntia.doc.gov/reports/telemed

National Telecommunications and Information Administration. (2000, April). *Advanced telecommunications in rural America: The challenge of bringing broadband service to all Americans.* Retrieved October 11, 2001, from www.ntia.doc.gov/reports/ruralbb42600.pdf

National Work Group on Literacy and Health. (1998). Communicating with patients who have limited literacy skills. *Journal of Family Practice, 46*(2), 168–175.

Naughton, J. (2002, July/August). The coaching boom. *Psychotherapy Networker, 26*(4), 24–31.

Naughton-Travers, J. (2002). MBHO/EAP enrollment reaches 227 million in 2002: Magellan, ValueOptions & United Behavioral Health control 50% of market. *Open Minds, 14*(6), 7–9.

Nee, E. (2001, March 19). *10 tech trends to bet on.* Retrieved April 10, 2001, from http://fortune.com/indexw.jhtml?channel=artcol.jhtml&doc_id=200846&page=9&_DARGS=%2Fartcol.jhtml.3_A&_DAV=artcol.jhtml

Nelson, E.-L., Barnard, M., & Cain, S. (2003). Treating childhood depression over videoconferencing. *Telemedicine Journal and e-Health, 9*(1), 49–55.

Nemeroff, C. B. (2001, January). The development of new technologies in medicine: What will the impact be in psychiatry? *CNS Spectrums, 6*(1), 21.

Nettleman, M., Olchanski, V., & Perlin, J. (1998). E-mail medicine: Dawn of a new era in physician-patient communication. *Clinical Performance and Quality Health Care, 6*(3), 138–141.

Neville, R., Greene, A., McLeod, J., Tracy, A., & Surie, J. (2002, September 14). Mobile phone text messaging can help young people manage asthma. *British Medical Journal, 325*(7364), 600.

New research reveals e-health paradox: It's harder to reach patients online than to have an effect on them. (2001). *Internet Healthcare Strategies, 3*(7), 10–11.

New York Academy of Medicine. (2003, September 12). *Sept. 9 conference revisits the long-lasting mental and physical health impacts from Sept. 11 attacks on World Trade Center.* Retrieved April 21, 2003, from http://www.nyam.org/news/2002/091302.shtml

Newman, B. (1997). The use of online services to encourage exploration of ego-dystonic sexual interests. *Journal of Sex Education and Therapy, 22*(1), 45–48.

Newman, M. G., Consoli, A., & Taylor, C. B. (1997). Computers in assessment and cognitive behavioral treatment of clinical disorders: Anxiety as a case in point. *Behavior Therapy, 28*(2), 211–235.

Newman, M. G., Consoli, A., & Taylor, C. B. (1999). A palmtop computer program for the treatment of generalized anxiety disorder. *Behavior Modification, 23*(4), 597–619.

Newman, M. G., Kenardy, J., Herman, S., & Taylor, C. B. (1996). The use of hand-held computers as an adjunct to cognitive-behavior therapy. *Computers in Human Behavior, 12*(1), 135–143.

Newman, M. G., Kenardy, J., Herman, S., & Taylor, C. B. (1997). Comparison of palmtop-computer–assisted brief cognitive-behavioral treatment to cognitive-behavioral treatment for panic disorder. *Journal of Consulting and Clinical Psychology, 65*(1), 178–183.

The newspaper as a pathological factor. (2001, July 18). *Journal of the American Medical Association, 286*(3), 278.

Newton, H. (1998). *Newton's telecom dictionary.* New York: Flatiron.

Nicholson, B. (2002, October 13). First for online medicine. *The Age.* Retrieved October 23, 2002, from www.theage.com

Nickelson, D. (2002, August 24). *New frontiers of psychology: Legal, ethical, and practical situations.* Paper presented at the American Psychological Association, Chicago.

Nielsen, J. (2001a, October 28). Poor code quality contaminates users' conceptual models. *The Alert Box: Current Issues in Web Usability.* Retrieved October 29, 2001, from http://www.useit.com/alertbox/20011028.html

Nielsen, J. (2001b, July 22). Tagline blues: What's the site about? *The Alert Box: Current Issues in Web Usability.* Retrieved July 21, 2001, from http://www.useit.com/alertbox/20010722.html

Nisbett, R. E. (2003). *The geography of thought: How Asians and westerners think differently . . . and why.* New York: The Free Press.

Nisbett, R. E., Peng, K., Choi, I., & Norenzayan, A. (2001). Culture and systems of thought: Holistic versus analytic cognition. *Psychological Review, 108*(2), 291–310.

Noell, J., & Glasgow, R. E. (1999). Interactive technology applications for behavioral counseling: Issues and opportunities for health care settings. *American Journal of Preventive Medicine, 17*(4), 269–274.

North, M. M., North, S. M., & Coble, J. R. (1995). Effectiveness of virtual environment desensitization in the treatment of agoraphobia. *International Journal of Virtual Reality, 1*(2), 25–34.

North, M. M., North, S. M., & Coble, J. R. (1997). Virtual reality therapy for fear of flying. *American Journal of Psychiatry, 154*(1), 130.

NSW Health. (2001). *What is telehealth?* Retrieved July 11, 2001, from http://www.health.nsw.gov.au/pmd/telehealth/about/about.htm

NUA Internet Surveys. (2003, April). *How many online?* Retrieved October 25, 2002, from http://www.nua.ie/surveys/how_many_online/index.html

Ó hAnluain, D. (2002, September 4). Why text messaging turns ugly. *Wired News.* Retrieved March 21, 2003, from http://www.wired.com/news/school/0,1383,54771,00.html

Oberkirch, A. (2000). *Telepsychiatry in the management of five fragile patients: Improve quality and lower costs.* Phoenix, AZ: American Telemedicine Association.

Office of Technology Assessment. (1990). *Health care in rural America* (OTA-H-434). Washington, DC: Government Printing Office.

O'Leary, D. S. (2000). Accreditation's role in reducing medical errors. *British Medical Journal, 320*(7237), 727–728.

Omanson, R., Lew, G., & Schumacher, R. (1998). Creating content for both paper and the Web. In C. Forsythe, E. Gross, & J. Ratner (Eds.), *Human factors and Web development.* Mahwah, NJ: Lawrence Erlbaum Associates.

Oravec, J. A. (2000). Online counselling and the Internet. Perspectives for mental health care supervision and education. *Journal of Mental Health, 9*(2), 121–135.

Orleans, C. T. (1999). Context, confidentiality, and consent in tailored health communications: A cautionary note. *Annals of Behavioral Medicine, 21*(4), 307–310.

Orleans, C. T., Schoenback, V. J., Wagner, E. H., Quade, D., Salmon, M. A., Pearson, D. C., Fielder, J., Porter, C. Q., & Kaplan, B. H. (1991). Self-help quit smoking intervention: Effects of self-help materials, social support intervention, and telephone counseling. *Journal of Consulting and Clinical Psychology, 59*(3), 439–448.

Orubeondo, A. (2001, September 10). Meeting via video offers big rewards. *InfoWorld.* Retrieved November 25, 2003, from http://archive.infoworld.com/articles/fe/xml/01/09/10/010910fevideo.xml

Orwell, G. (1949). *Nineteen eighty-four.* London: Martin Secker & Warburg.

Osgood-Hynes, D. J., Greist, J. H., Marks, I. M., Baer, L., Heneman, S. W., Wenzel, K. W., Manzo, P. A., Parkin, J. R., Spierings, C. J., Dottl, S. L., & Vitse, H. M. (1998, July). Self-administered psychotherapy for depression using a telephone-accessed computer system plus booklets: An open U.S.–U.K. study. *Journal of Clinical Psychiatry, 59*(7), 358–365.

Oss, M. (1999). *Yearbook of managed behavioral health organization market share in the United States.* Gettysburg, PA: Open Minds.

Oss, M. (2001). Consumer access to new biomedical advances dependent on system reengineering: Benefit plan design and delivery system structure. *Open Minds, 13*(5), 3–5.

Otten, P. J. (2002, September 19). South African companies under attack by a threat more virulent than any traditional virus. *All Africa Global Media.* Retrieved September 26, 2002, from http://allafrica.com/stories/200209190135.html

Overall, J. E., & Gorham, D. R. (1962). The Brief Psychiatric Rating Scale. *Psychological Reports, 10,* 799–812.

Oyston, J. (2000, September). Anesthesiologists' responses to an email request for advice from an unknown patient. *Journal of Medical Internet Research, 2*(3), e16.

Paciello, M. G. (2000). *Web accessibility for people with disabilities.* Gilroy, CA: CMP Books.

Pacific Health Policy Group. (2002). *HIPAA administrative simplification: Tool kit for small group and safety-net providers.* Retrieved March 5, 2002, from http://ehealth.chcf.org/view.cfm?section=Privacy&itemID=4620

Palmer, K., Montgomery, R., & Harland, A. (2003). Emergency telemental health: Canada's first. *Telemedicine Journal and e-Health, 9*(1), 63.

Papp, L. A., Klein, D. F., & Gorman, J. M. (1993). Carbon dioxide hypersensitivity, hyperventilation, and panic disorder. *American Journal of Psychiatry, 150*(8), 1149–1157.

Pappu, R., Recht, B., Taylor, J., & Gershenfeld, N. (2002, September 20). Physical one-way functions. *Science, 297*(5589), 2026–2030.

Parks, M., & Floyd, K. (1996). Making friends in cyberspace. *Journal of Communication, 46*(1), 80–97.

PATH Organization (2002). *Managing consumer health behavior.* Retrieved October 8, 2002, from http://www.pathinstitute.com/Managing.htm

Paulsen, A. S., Crowe, R. R., Noyes, R., & Pfohl, B. (1988). Reliability of the telephone interview in diagnosing anxiety disorders. *Archives of General Psychiatry, 45*(1), 62–63.

Pearn, J. (2003). Children and war. *Journal of Paediatrics and Child Health, 39*(3), 166–172.

Pelletier, M. (2002, August 25). *Psychotherapy via e-mail and videoconferencing: Empirical and future directions.* Paper presented at the American Psychological Association, Chicago.

Pennebaker, J., & Beall, S. (1986). Confronting a traumatic event: Toward an understanding of inhibition and disease. *Journal of Abnormal Psychology, 95*(3), 274–281.

Pennebaker, J., Hughes, C., & O'Heeron, R. (1987). The psychophysiology of confession: Linking inhibitory and psychosomatic processes. *Journal of Personality and Social Psychology, 52*(4), 781–793.

Pennebaker, J., & Susman, J. (1988). Disclosure of traumas and psychosomatic processes. *Social Science and Medicine, 26*(3), 327–332.

Perpina, C., Botella, C., Baños, R., Marco, H., Alcaniz, M., & Quero, S. (1999). Body image and virtual reality in eating disorders: Is exposure to virtual reality more effective than the classical body image treatment? *CyberPsychology and Behavior, 2*(2), 149–155.

Peters, L., & Andrews, G. (1995). Procedural validity of the computerized version of the Composite International Diagnostic Interview (CIDI-Auto) in the anxiety disorders. *Psychological Medicine, 25*(6), 1269–1280.

Peters, L., Clark, D., & Carroll, F. (1998). Are computerized interviews equivalent to human interviewers? CIDI-Auto versus CIDI in anxiety and depressive disorders. *Psychological Medicine, 28*(4), 893–901.

Pew Internet and American Life Project. (2000). *The online health care revolution: How the Web helps Americans take better care of themselves.* Retrieved May 14, 2001, from http://www.pewinternet.com/reports/toc.asp?Report=26

Pew Internet and American Life Project. (2001a, February 18). *Daily Internet activities.* Retrieved July 20, 2001, from http://www.pewinternet.org/reports/chart.asp?img=6_daily_activities.jpg

Pew Internet and American Life Project. (2001b, February 18). *Internet activities.* Retrieved July 20, 2001, from http://www.pewinternet.org/reports/toc.asp?Report=30

Pew Internet and American Life Project. (2001c). Risky business: Americans see greed cluelessness behind dot-coms' comeuppance. Retrieved May 14, 2001, from http://www.pewinternet.com/reports/toc.asp?Report=31

Pew Internet and American Life Project. (2002, June 24). *Broadband users use Net differently.* Retrieved July 30, 2002, from http://www.nua.net/surveys/index.cgi?f=VS&art_id=905358090&rel=true

Pfeiffer, E. (1975). A short portable mental status questionnaire for the assessment of organic brain deficit in elderly patients. *Journal of the American Geriatrics Society, 23*(10), 433–441.

Phelps, E. A., O'Connor, K. J., Cunningham, W. A., Funayama, E. S., Gatenby, J. C., Gore, J. C., & Banaji, M. R. (2000). Performance on indirect measures of race evaluation predicts amygdala activation. *Journal of Cognitive Neuroscience, 12*(5), 729–738.

Philippot, P. (2002). Put an end to Adware. *PC Magazine.* Retrieved December 11, 2002, from http://www.pcmag.com/article2/0,4149,2023,00.asp

Pies, R. (2002). The Internet "expert": Promise and perils. In R. C. Hsiung (Ed.), *e-Therapy: Case studies, guiding principles, and the clinical potential of the Internet* (pp. 24–38). New York: Norton.

Pine, D., Fyer, A., Grun, J., Phelps, E., Szeszko, P., Koda, V., Li, W., Ardekani, B., Maguire, E., Burgess, N., & Bilder, R. (2001). Methods for developmental studies of fear conditioning circuitry. *Biological Psychiatry, 50*(3), 225–228.

Plaut, S. (1997). Online ethics: Social contracts in the virtual community. *Journal of Sex Education and Therapy, 22*(1), 84–91.

Plutchik, R., & Karasu, T. B. (1991). Computers in psychotherapy: An overview. *Computers in Human Behavior, 7*(1), 33–44.

Podesta, J. (2001, September 19). Tools for counterterrorism. *The Washington Post.* Retrieved September 20, 2001, from http://www.washingtonpost.com/wp-dyn/articles/A53161-2001Sep18.html

Poensgen, A., & Larsson, S. (2001). *Patients, physicians, and the Internet: Myth, reality, and implications.* Boston: Boston Consulting Group.

Polauf, J. (n.d.). *E-mail as a modality for crisis intervention.* Retrieved March 20, 2001, from http://www.telehealth.net/articles/email.html

Polauf, J. (1998). *Psychotherapy on the Internet: Theory and technique.* Retrieved February 22, 1999, from http://www.nyreferrals.com/psychotherapy

Pollard, R. (2003). *Strong Connections: A videoconference-based sign language interpreter service for healthcare settings.* Rochester, NY: Northeast Technical Assistance Center, National Technical Institute for the Deaf.

Pollard, S. E., & LePage, J. P. (2001). Telepsychiatry in a rural inpatient setting. *Psychiatric Services, 52*(12), 1659.

Pope, J. (2002, September 16). Firms beef up job of security. *The Los Angeles Times,* p. C3.

Pope, K. S., Tabachnick, B. G., & Keith-Spiegel, P. (1987). *American Psychologist, 42*(11), 993–1006.

Pope, K. S., & Vasquez, M. J. T. (1998). *Ethics in psychotherapy and counseling: A practical guide* (2nd ed.). San Francisco: Jossey-Bass.

Posen, L. (2001, March 20). *Telehealth: Web sites and their scientific boards—trusted sources or paid spruikers!* Retrieved September 17, 2001, from http://telehealth.net/articles/credibility.html

Potts, M. K., Daniels, M., Burnam, M. A., & Wells, K. B. (1990). A structured interview version of the Hamilton Depression Rating Scale: Evidence of reliability and versatility of administration. *Journal of Psychiatric Research, 24*(4), 335–350.

Powell, T. (1998). *Online counseling: A profile and a descriptive analysis.* Retrieved July 30, 2001, from http://www.netpsychology.com/Powell.htm

Prochaska, J. O., DiClemente, C. C., & Norcross, J. C. (1992). In search of how people change: Applications to addictive behaviors. *American Psychologist, 47*(9), 1102–1114.

Prochaska, J. O., Johnson, S. S., & Lee, P. (1998). The transtheoretical model of behavior change. In E. Schron, J. Ockene, S. Schumaker, & W. Exum (Eds.), *The handbook of behavioral change* (2nd ed., pp. 159–184). New York: Springer.

Prussog, A., Mühlbach, L., & Böcker, M. (1994, October 25). *Telepresence in videocommunications*. Paper presented at the Human Factors and Ergonomics Society 38th Annual Meeting, Santa Monica, CA.

Pugnetti, L., Mendozzi, L., Attree, E. A., Barbieri, E., Brooks, B. M., Cazzullo, C. L., Motta, A., & Rose, F. D. (1998). Probing memory and executive functions with virtual reality: Past and present studies. *CyberPsychology and Behavior, 1*(2), 151–161.

Puskin, D., Mintzer, C., & Wasem, C. (1997). Telemedicine: Building rural systems for today and tomorrow. In P. Brennan, S. Schneider, & E. Tornquist (Eds.), *Information networks for community health* (pp. 276–281). New York: Springer.

Quimby, G. R. (1999, January 4). Avatar Process Training Group Project. *SelfhelpMagazine*. Retrieved October 1, 2002, from http://www.shpm.com/ppc/viewpoint/avatar.html

Rabasca, L. (2000, April). Taking telehealth to the next step. *APA Monitor, 31*(4). Retrieved March 14, 2003, from http://www.apa.org/monitor/apr00/telehealth.html

Randolph, C. (2002, April). Neuropsychological testing: Evolution and emerging trends. *CNS Spectrums, 7*(4), 307–312.

Reece, R. L. (2003, April 7). The physician culture and resistance to change Part I: Why physicians stick to the status quo. *HealthLeaders News*. Retrieved April 8, 2003, from http://www.healthleaders.com/news/feature1.php?contentid=43883

Reed, G. M., McLaughlin, C. J., & Milholland, K. (2000). Ten interdisciplinary principles for professional practice in telehealth: Implications for psychology. *Professional Psychology: Research and Practice, 31*(2), 170–178.

Reents, S. (1999, August). *Industry brief: Seizing the Internet health opportunity*. Retrieved September 5, 2000, from http://www.cyberdialogue.com

Rees, C. S., & Gillam, D. (2001). Training in cognitive-behavioral therapy for mental health professionals: A pilot study of videoconferencing. *Journal of Telemedicine and Telecare, 7*(5), 300–303.

Reese, R. J. (2001, February). Client perceptions of the effectiveness and appeal of telephone counseling. *Dissertation Abstracts International: Section B: The Sciences and Engineering, 61*(7-B), 3857.

Reese, R. J., Conoley, C. W., & Brossart, D. F. (2002, April). Effectiveness of telephone counseling: A field-based investigation. *Journal of Counseling Psychology, 49*(2), 233–242.

Regier, D., Farmer, M., Rae, D., Locke, B., Keith, S., Judd, L., & Goodwin, F. (1990). Comorbidity of mental disorders with alcohol and other drug abuse. *Journal of the American Medical Association, 264*(19), 2511–2518.

Reuters. (2002, February 21). *Online casino ads go mainstream*. Retrieved July 13, 2002, from http://www.nua.net/surveys/index.cgi?f=VS&art_id=905357681&rel=true

Rhein, A. N. (2001). *The effect of personality disorder characteristics on live versus remote treatment for veterans with depressive disorder*. Boston: Boston University.

Rheingold, H. (1991). *Virtual reality*. London: Mandarin.

Rheingold, H. (1993). *The virtual community: Homesteading on the electronic frontier*. Reading, MA: Addison-Wesley.

Rhode, L. (2002, July, 25). Cisco, BT launch VoIP service for MSN users. *InfoWorld*. Retrieved July 26, 2002, from http://www.infoworld.com/articles/hn/xml/02/07/25/020725hnciscobt.xml?0725thwebtech_ar.

Rice, R. (1993). Media appropriateness: Using social presence theory to compare traditional and new organizational media. *Human Communication Research, 19*(4), 451–458.

Richards, A. K. (2001). Panel report: Talking cure in the 21st century: Telephone psychoanalysis. *Psychoanalytic Psychology, 18*(2), 388–391.

Richards, T. (2002). Developed countries should not impose ethics on other countries. *British Medical Journal, 325*(796), 1123–1124.

Riemsma, R. P., Kirwan, J. R., Taal, E., & Rasker, J. J. (2003). Patient education for adults with rheumatoid arthritis (Cochrane Review). Chichester, UK: John Wiley & Sons.

Riemsma, R. P., Taal, E., Kirwan, J. R., & Rasker, J. J. (2002). Patient education programs for adults with rheumatoid arthritis. *British Medical Journal, 325*(7364), 558–559.

Right to Financial Privacy Act. (1974). 12 U.S.C. 3401 et seq.

Right to Privacy Act. (1980). Retrieved October 3, 2002, from http://www4.law.cornell.edu/uscode/42/ch21A.html

Riva, G. (1998). Virtual reality in psychological assessment: The Body Image Virtual Reality Scale. *CyberPsychology and Behavior, 1*(1), 37–44.

Riva, G., Alcaniz, M., Anolli, L., Bacchetta, M., Baños, R., Beltrame, F., Botella, C., Galimberti, C., Gamberini, L., Gaggioli, A., Molinari, E., Mantovani, G., Nugues, P., Optale, G., Orsi, G., Perpina, C., & Troiani, R.

(2001). The VEPSY updated project: Virtual reality in clinical psychology. *Cyberpsychology and Behavior,* 4(4), 449–455.

Riva, G., Bacchetta, M., Baruffi, M., Rinaldi, S., & Molinari, E. (1999). Virtual reality based experiential cognitive treatment of anorexia nervosa. *Journal of Behavior Therapy and Experimental Psychiatry,* 30(3), 221–230.

Riva, G., & Galimberti, C. (1997). The psychology of cyberspace: A socio-cognitive framework to computer-mediated communication. *New Ideas in Psychology,* 15(2), 141–158.

Riva, G., & Melis, L. (1997). Virtual reality for the treatment of body image disturbances. In G. Riva (Ed.), *Virtual reality in neuro-psycho-physiology: Cognitive, clinical and methodological issues in assessment and rehabilitation* (pp. 95–111). Amsterdam: IOS Press.

Rizzo, A. A., Buckwalter, J. G., Bowerly, T., McGee, J., van Rooyen, A., van der Zaag, C., Neumann, U., Thiebaux, M., Kim, L., Pair, J., & Chua, C. (2001). Virtual environments for assessing and rehabilitating cognitive/functional performance: A review of projects at the USC Integrated Media Systems Center. *Presence: Teleoperators and Virtual Environments,* 10(4), 359–374.

Rizzo, A. A., Buckwalter, J. G., & van der Zaag, C. (2002). Virtual environment applications for neuropsychological assessment and rehabilitation. In K. Stanney (Ed.), *Handbook of virtual environments* (pp. 1027–1064). Mahwah, NJ: Lawrence Erlbaum Associates.

Rizzo, A. A., Neumann, U., Pintaric, T., & Norden, M. (2001). Issues for application development using immersive HMD 360 degree panoramic video environments. In M. J. Smith, G. Salvendy, D. Harris, & R. J. Koubek (Eds.), *Usability evaluation and interface design* (pp. 792–796). Mahwah, NJ: Lawrence Erlbaum Associates.

Rizzo, A. A., Schultheis, M. T., & Rothbaum, B. O. (2002). Ethical issues for the use of virtual reality in the psychological sciences. In S. Bush & M. Drexler (Eds.), *Ethical issues in clinical neuropsychology* (pp. 243–280). Lisse, The Netherlands: Swets & Zeitlinger.

Rizzo, A. A., Wiederhold, M., & Buckwalter, J. G. (1998). Basic issues in the use of virtual environments for mental health applications. *Virtual environments in clinical psychology and neuroscience: Methods and techniques in advanced patient-therapist interaction* (pp. 21–42). Amsterdam: IOS Press.

Robert E. Nolan Company. (2001, March). *Analysis of HHS cost estimates for the final HIPAA privacy regulation.* Retrieved March 6, 2002, from http://bcbshealthissues.com/relatives/17340.pdf

Roberts, P. (2002, October 2). Bugbear virus spreading rapidly. *InfoWorld.* Retrieved October 7, 2002, from http://www.infoworld.com/articles/hn/xml/02/10/02/021002hnbugbear.xml?s=IDGNS

Robertson, E. B., Ladewig, B. H., Strickland, M. P., & Boschung, M. D. (1987). Enhancement of self-esteem through the use of computer-assisted instruction. *Journal of Educational Research,* 80(5), 314–316.

Robertson, R. M. (2001). Women and cardiovascular disease: The risks of misperception and the need for action. *Circulation,* 103(19), 2318–2320.

Robins, L., & Helzer, J. (1985). *The Diagnostic Interview Schedule Version III-A.* St. Louis, MO: Washington University.

Robinson, P. H., & Serfaty, M. A. (2001). The use of e-mail in the identification of bulimia nervosa and its treatment. *European Eating Disorders Review,* 9(3), 182–193.

Roccaforte, W. H., Burke, W. J., Bayer, B. L., & Wengel, S. P. (1992). Validation of a telephone version of the Mini-Mental State Examination. *Journal of the American Geriatric Society,* 40(7), 697–702.

Roessler, A., Mueller-Spahn, F., Baehrer, S., & Bullinger, A. H. (2000). A rapid prototyping framework for the development of virtual environments in mental health. *Cyberpsychology and Behavior,* 3(3), 359–367.

Roffman, D., Shannon, D., & Dwyer, C. (1997). Adolescents, sexual health, and the Internet: Possibilities, prospects, and challenges for educators. *Journal of Sex Education and Therapy,* 22(1), 49–55.

Rohde, P., Lewinsohn, P. M., & Seeley, J. R. (1997). Comparability of telephone and face-to-face interviews in assessing axis I and II disorders. *American Journal of Psychiatry,* 154(11), 1593–1598.

Rohland, B. (2001). Telepsychiatry in the heartland: If we build it, will they come? *Community Mental Health Journal,* 37(5), 449–459.

Rohland, B., Saleh, S. S., Rohrer, J. E., & Romitti, P. A. (2000). Acceptability of telepsychiatry to a rural population. *Psychiatric Services,* 51(5), 672–674.

Rosen, G. M. (1987). Self-help treatment books and the commercialization of psychotherapy. *American Psychologist,* 42(1), 46–51.

Rosen, L. D. (2000, September–October). Taking a second look at practice management software. *National Psychologist.* Retrieved October 21, 2002, from http://www.technostress.com/tnp32.htm

Rosen, L. D., & Weil, M. M. (1997). *The mental health technology bible.* New York: Wiley.

Rosenman, S., Korten, A., & Levings, C. (1997). Computerised diagnosis in acute psychiatry: Validity of CIDI-Auto against routine clinical diagnosis. *Journal of Psychiatric Research,* 31(5), 581–592.

Rosenman, S., Levings, C., & Korten, A. (1997). Clinical utility and patient acceptance of the computerized Composite International Diagnostic Interview. *Psychiatric Services,* 48(6), 815–820.

Roten, Y. D., Gilliéron, E., Despland, J.-N., & Stigler, M. (2002). Functions of mutual smiling and alliance building in early therapeutic interaction. *Psychotherapy Research, 12*(2), 193–212.

Roth, W. T. (1998). Applying psychophysiology in the clinic. *Psychophysiology, 35*, S9.

Rothbaum, B. O., Hodges, L., Alarcon, R., Ready, D., Shahar, F., Graap, K., Pair, J., Hebert, P., Gotz, D., Wills, B., & Baltzell, D. (1999). Virtual reality exposure therapy for PTSD Vietnam veterans: A case study. *Journal of Traumatic Stress, 12*(2), 263–271.

Rothbaum, B. O., Hodges, L., & Kooper, R. (1997). Virtual reality exposure therapy. *Journal of Psychotherapy: Practice and Research, 6*(3), 219–226.

Rothbaum, B. O., Hodges, L. F., Kooper, R., & Opdyke, D. (1995). Effectiveness of computer-generated (virtual reality) graded exposure in the treatment of acrophobia. *American Journal of Psychiatry, 152*(4), 626–628.

Rothman, K. J., & Michels, K. B. (1994). The continuing unethical use of placebo controls. *New England Journal of Medicine, 331*(6), 394–398.

Royal National Institute for the Blind. (2000, November 12). *Websites that work.* Retrieved August 23, 2001, from http://www.rnib/org/uk/digital/wtw.htm

Roy-Byrne, P. P., Milgrom, P., Khoon-Mei, T., & Weinstein, P. (1994). Psychopathology and psychiatric diagnosis in subjects with dental phobia. *Journal of Anxiety Disorders, 8*(1), 19–31.

Rozanski, A., Blumenthal, J., & Kaplan, J. (1999). Impact of psychological factors on the pathogenesis of cardiovascular disease and implications for therapy. *Circulation, 99*(16), 2192–2217.

Runyon, D., Han, J., Hilty, D. M., Roberts, C., Roach, A., & Connor, M. (2003). Telepsychiatric services for HIV clients in a rural/remote setting. *Telemedicine Journal and e-Health, 9*(1), 117.

Ruskin, P., Reed, S., Kumar, R., Kling, M., Siegel, E., Rosen, M., & Hauser, P. (1998). Reliability and acceptability of psychiatric diagnosis via telecommunication and audiovisual technology. *Psychiatric Services, 49*(8), 1086–1088.

Ryan, E. B. (1994). Memory for Goblins: A computer game for assessing and training working memory skill. *Computers in Human Services, 11*(1–2), 213–217.

Ryle, G. (1968). *The thinking of thoughts: What is "Le Penseur" doing?* Retrieved July 10, 2002, http://lucy.ukc.ac.uk/CSACSIA

Saab, P. G., McCalla, J. R., Coons, H. L., Christensen, A. J., Kaplan, R., Johnson, S. B., Ackerman, M. D., Stepanski, E., Krantz, D. S., & Melamed, B. (2004, March). Technological and medical advances: Implications for health psychology. *Health Psychology, 23*(2), 142–146.

Sacks, O. (1985). *The man who mistook his wife for a hat and other clinical tales.* New York: Summit Books.

Samoilovich, S., Riccitelli, C., Schiel, A., & Siedi, A. (1992). Attitude of schizophrenics to computer videogames. *Psychopathology, 25*(3), 117–119.

Sampson, J., Kolodinsky, R., & Greeno, B. (1997). Counseling on the information highway: Future possibilities and potential problems. *Journal of Counseling and Development, 75*(3), 203–211.

Sampson, J. P. (2000). Using the Internet to enhance testing in counseling. *Journal of Counseling and Development, 78*(3), 348–356.

Sampson, J. P., Jr. (1990). Computer applications and issues in using tests in counseling. In C. E. Watkins & V. L. Campbell (Eds.), *Testing in counseling practice* (pp. 451–474). Hillsdale, NJ: Lawrence Erlbaum Associates.

Sanchez, L. M., & Turner, S. M. (2003). Practicing psychology in the era of managed care: Implications for practice and training. *American Psychologist, 58*(2), 116–129.

Satcher, D. (1999). *Mental health: A report of the Surgeon General.* Retrieved July 27, 2001, from http://www.surgeongeneral.gov/library/mentalhealth/home.html

Saville-Troike, M. (2003). *The ethnography of communication: An introduction* (3rd ed.). Oxford, England: Blackwell.

SB 1875. (2000, September). Minimization of medication-related errors. Chapter 816 (2.05). Retrieved March 6, 2003, from http://www.leginfo.ca.gov/cgi-bin/waisgate?WAISdocID=22723524497+2+0+0&WAISaction=retrieve

Schachter, J. (2002). *Transference: Shibboleth or albatross?* Mahwah, NJ: Lawrence Erlbaum Associates.

Schaefer, C., & Reid, S. E. (2001). *Game play: Therapeutic use of childhood games* (2nd ed.). New York: Wiley.

Schaefermeyer, M., & Sewell, E. (1988). Communicating by electronic mail. *American Behavioral Scientist, 32*(2), 112–123.

Schanz, S. J. (1996). California passes telemedicine development act. *Telemedicine Today, 4*(5), 7–9.

Schanz, S. J., & Cepelewicz, B. B. (Eds.). (2001). *Telemedicine law and practice: Practical guidance: Compendium of federal and state laws.* Kingston, NJ: Civic Research Institute.

Scheidlinger, S. (1993). History of group psychotherapy. In H. I. Kaplan & B. J. Sadock (Eds.), *Comprehensive group psychotherapy* (3rd ed., pp. 2–10). Baltimore: Williams & Wilkins.

Schnarch, D. (1997). Sex, intimacy, and the Internet. *Journal of Sex Education and Therapy, 22*(1), 15–20.

Schneider, C. (1987). Cost effectiveness of biofeedback and behavioral medicine treatments: A review of the literature. *Biofeedback and Self-Regulation, 12*(2), 71–92.

Schneider, J., & Weiss, R. (2001). *Cybersex exposed: Simple fantasy or obsession?* Center City, MN: Hazelden Information Education.

Schneider, P. (1999, August). *Psychotherapy using distance technology: A comparison of outcomes.* Paper presented at the American Psychological Association, Boston.

Schneider, S. J., Walter, R., & O'Donnell, R. (1990). Computerized communication as a medium for behavioral smoking cessation treatment: Controlled evaluation. *Computers in Human Behavior, 6*(2), 141–151.

Schneider, W. (1988). Micro Experimental Laboratory: An integrated system for IBM PC compatibles. *Behavior Research Methods, Instruments and Computers, 20*(2), 206–217.

Schneidman, E., Farberow, N., & Litman, R. (1983). *The psychology of suicide.* New York: Jason Aronson.

Schopp, L., Johnstone, B., & Merrell, D. (2000). Telehealth and neuropsychological assessment: New opportunities for psychologists. *Professional Psychology: Research and Practice, 31*(2), 179–183.

Schreier, P. G. (n.d.). *The dark side of Internet technology.* Retrieved March 21, 2003, from http://www.chipcenter.com/dsp/DSP001026F1.html

Schuemie, M. J., van der Straaten, P., Krijin, M., & van der Mast, C. (2001). Research on presence in virtual reality: A survey. *Cyberpsychology and Behavior, 4*(2), 183–201.

Schwartz, J. (2001, July 8). Dear world: Loose lips sink more than ships. *The New York Times.* Retrieved July 10, 2001, from http://www.nytimes.com

Schwartz, M. S. (Ed.). (1995). *Biofeedback: A practitioner's guide* (2nd ed.). New York: Guilford.

Science Panel on Interactive Communication and Health. (1999, April). *Wired for health and well-being: The emergence of interactive health communication.* US Department of Health and Human Services. Retrieved November 18, 2003, from http://www.health.gov/scipich/pubs/report/wired-pb.pdf

SearchNetworking.com. (2001). *ISDN: Integrated Service Delivery Network.* Retrieved March 13, 2001, from http://www.msic.com/technical/network_protocol/isdn.shtml

Segal, D. L., & Falk, S. B. (1998). Structured interviews and rating scales. In A. S. Bellack & E. Hersen (Eds.), *Behavioral assessment: A practical handbook* (4th ed., pp. 158–178). Boston: Allyn & Bacon.

Seligman, M. E. P. (1998, June 26). Treatment becomes prevention and treatment. *Prevention and Treatment.* Retrieved October 10, 2002, from http://www.journals.apa.org/prevention/volume1/pre0010001e.html

Sellen, A. (1995). Remote conversations: The effects of mediating talk with technology. *Human-Computer Interaction, 10*(4), 401–444.

Selmi, P. M., Klein, M. H., Greist, J. H., Sorrell, S. P., & Erdman, H. P. (1990). Computer-administered cognitive-behavioral therapy for depression. *American Journal of Psychiatry, 147*(1), 51–56.

Shaw, J. (1997). Treatment rationale for Internet infidelity. *Journal of Sex Education and Therapy, 22*(1), 29–34.

Sheahan, B. (2002). Remote communities, child telepsychiatry & primary health care. *Youth Studies Australia, 21*(2), 52.

Shepard, B. (2001). *A war of nerves: Soldiers and psychiatrists in the twentieth century.* Boston: Harvard University Press.

Shields, R. (1996). *Cultures of the Internet: Virtual spaces, real histories, living bodies.* London: Sage.

Shiffman, S. (1993). Assessing smoking patterns and motives. *Journal of Consulting and Clinical Psychology, 61*(5), 732–742.

Shore, M., & Beigel, A. (1996). The challenges posed by managed behavioral health care. *New England Journal of Medicine, 334*(2), 116–119.

Short, J., Williams, E., & Christie, B. (1976). *The social psychology of telecommuncations.* London: Wiley.

Shriberg, E., & Stolcke, A. (2002, February 26). *Harnessing speech prosody for human-computer interaction.* Paper presented at the NASA Intelligent Systems Workshop, Pensacola, FL.

Simon, G. E., Revicki, D., & VonKorff, M. (1993). Telephone assessment of depression severity. *Journal of Psychiatric Research, 27*(3), 247–252.

Simon, G. E., VonKorff, M., Rutter, C., & Wagner, E. (2000). Randomised trial of monitoring, feedback, and management of care by telephone to improve treatment of depression in primary care. *British Medical Journal, 320*(7234), 550–554.

Simmons, S. C., West, V. L., & Chimiak, W. J. (2003). Telecommunications and videoconferencing for psychiatry. In R. Wooton, P. Yellowlees, & P. McLaren (Eds.), *Telepsychiatry and e-Mental Health* (pp. 15–27). London, England: Royal Society of Medicine Press.

Simpson, J. B. (1988). *Simpson's contemporary quotes.* Retrieved November 20, 2003, from http://www.bartleby.com/63/20/3120.html

Simpson, S. (2003). The use of videoconferencing in clinical psychology. Telepsychiatry and e-Mental Health. In R. Wooton, P. Yellowlees, & P. McLaren (Eds.), *Telepsychiatry and e-Mental Health* (pp. 171–182). London, England: Royal Society of Medicine Press.

498   REFERENCES

Simpson, S., Knox, J., Mitchell, D., Ferguson, J., Brebner, J., & Brebner, E. (2003). A multidisciplinary approach to the treatment of eating disorders via videoconferencing in north-east Scotland. *Journal of Telemedicine and Telecare, 9*(1), 37–38.

Skinner, C. S., Strecher, V. J., & Hospers, H. (1994, January). Physicians' recommendations for mammography: Do tailored messages make a difference? *American Journal of Public Health, 84*(1), 12–13.

Slack, W. V., Leviton, A., Bennett, S. E., Fleischmann, K. H., & Lawrence, R. S. (1988). Relation between age, education, and time to respond to questions in a computer-based medical interview. *Computers and Biomedical Research, 21*(1), 78–84.

Sleek, S. (1995, November). On-line therapy services raise ethical questions. *APA Monitor*, p. 9.

Smith, D. (2001, May). Helping psychologists on the move: States and provinces make professional mobility easier for psychologists. *Monitor on Psychology, 32*(5), 73.

Smith, H. (1998). Telepsychiatry. *Psychiatric Services, 49*, 1494–1495.

Smith, H., & Allison, R. (2000, Spring). After five years of telemental health, what have we learned? *Telemedicine Journal, 6*(1), 187.

Smith, M., Glass, G., & Miller, T. (1980). *The benefits of psychotherapy*. Baltimore: Johns Hopkins University Press.

Smith, S., Heffler, S., & Freeland, M. (1999). The next decade of health spending: A new outlook. *Health Affairs, 18*(4), 86–95.

Smyth, J. M. (1998). Written emotional expression: Effect sizes, outcome types, and moderating variables. *Journal of Consulting and Clinical Psychology, 66*(1), 174–184.

Sørlie, T., Gammon, D., Bergvik, S., & Sexton, H. (1999). Psychotherapy supervision face-to-face and by videoconferencing: A comparative study. *British Journal of Psychotherapy, 15*(4), 452–462.

Spalding, L. R., & Hardin, C. D. (1999). Unconscious unease and self-handicapping: Behavioral consequences of individual differences in implicit and explicit self-esteem. *Psychological Science, 10*(6), 535–539.

Spielberg, A. R. (1998). On call and online: Sociohistorical, legal, and ethical implications of e-mail for the patient-physician relationship. *Journal of the American Medical Association, 280*(15), 1353–1359.

Spielberger, C. D., Sydeman, S. J., Owen, A. E., & Marsh, B. J. (1999). Measuring anxiety and anger with the State-Trait Anxiety Inventory (STAI) and the State-Trait Anger Expression Inventory (STAXI). In M. E. Maruish (Ed.), *The use of psychological testing for treatment planning and outcomes assessment* (2nd ed., pp. 993–1021). Mahwah, NJ: Lawrence Erlbaum Associates.

Spitzer, R. L., Williams, J. B. W., Gibbon, M., & First, M. B. (1990). *Structured Clinical Interview for DSM-III-R-Patient Version 1.0 (SCID-P)*. Washington, DC: American Psychiatric Press.

Spitzer, R. L., Williams, J. B. W., Kroenke, K., Linzer, M., deGruy, F. V., Hahn, S. R., Brody, D., & Johnson, J. G. (1994). Utility of a new procedure for diagnosing mental disorders in primary care: The PRIME-MD 1000 study. *Journal of the American Medical Association, 272*(22), 1749–1756.

Squibb, N. (1999). Video transmission for telemedicine. *Journal of Telemedicine and Telecare, 5*(1), 1–11.

Stacy, T. (2000, September 22). *Toward standardization of information security: BS 7799*. Retrieved November 28, 2001, from http://www.sans.org/infosecFAQ/policy/standardization.htm

Stafford, L., Kline, S., & Dimmick, J. (1999, Fall). Home e-mail: Relational maintenance and gratification opportunities. *Journal of Broadcasting and Electronic Media, 43*(4), 659–669.

Stamm, B. (1998). Clinical applications of telehealth in mental health care. *Professional Psychology: Research and Practice, 29*(6), 536–542.

Stamm, B. (2000). Shifting gears: Integrating models of telehealth and telemedicine into current models of mental health care. In L. G. Lawrence (Ed.), *Innovations in clinical practice* (Vol. 17, pp. 385–400). Sarasota, FL: Professional Resource Press.

Stamm, B., & Pearce, F. (1995). Creating virtual community: Telemedicine and self-care. In B. H. Stamm (Ed.), *Secondary traumatic stress: Self-care issues for clinicians, researchers, and educators* (pp. 179–207). Lutherville, MD: Sidran Press.

Standards for Privacy of Individually Identifiable Health Information; Final Rule, 65 Fed. Reg. 82461–82510 (2000).

Standards for Privacy of Individually Identifiable Health Information; Final Rule, 67 Fed. Reg. 53181–53273 (2002).

Stanley, J., & Steinhardt, B. (2003, January). *Bigger monster, weaker chains: The growth of an American surveillance society*. American Civil Liberties Union. Retrieved January 21, 2003, from http://www.aclu.org/Files/OpenFile.cfm?id=11572

Stein, M. B., Millar, T. W., Larsen, D. K., & Kryger, M. H. (1995). Irregular breathing patterns during sleep in patients with panic disorder. *American Journal of Psychiatry, 152*(8), 1168–1173.

Steiner, P. (1993, July 5). On the Internet, nobody knows you're a dog. [Cartoon]. *The New Yorker*. Retrieved May 16, 2003, from http://www.cartoonbank.com

Stevens, A., Doidge, N., Goldbloom, D., Voore, P., & Farewell, J. (1999). Pilot study of televideo psychiatric assessments in an underserviced community. *American Journal of Psychiatry, 156*(5), 783–785.

Stevens, L. (2001). *Informational healthcare Web sites to give way to robust medical Web e-service channels by 2005.* Retrieved August 13, 2001, from http://www.corhealth.com/motn/Sub/CatDetail.asp? STRCategory1_Position=FIL%3AORD%3AABS%3A2KEY%3APAR%3A%40category%3D%27Web+ Trends%27

Stiles, W. B. (1980). Measurement of the impact of psychotherapy sessions. *Journal of Consulting and Clinical Psychology, 48*(2), 176–185.

Still, A., & Velody, I. (Eds.). (1992). *Rewriting the history of madness: Studies in Foucault's Histoire de la folie.* London: Routledge.

Stillman, R., Roth, W. T., Colby, K. M., & Rosenbaum, C. P. (1969). An on-line computer system for initial psychiatric inventory. *American Journal of Psychiatry, 125*(7), 8–11.

Stofle, G. S. (1997). *Thoughts about online psychotherapy: Ethical and practical considerations.* Retrieved August 24, 2001, from http://members.aol.com/stofle/onlinepsych.htm

Stone, A. A., & Shiffman, S. (1994). Ecological momentary assessment (EMA) in behavorial medicine. *Annals of Behavioral Medicine, 16*(3), 199–202.

Stone, T. W., & Jumper, J. M. (2001). Information about age-related macular degeneration on the Internet. *Southern Medical Journal, 94*(1), 22–25.

Stoney, G. (1998). Suicide prevention on the Internet. In R. J. Kosky & H. S. Eshkevari (Eds.), *Suicide prevention: The global context* (pp. 237–244). New York: Plenum.

Strickland, D., Mesibov, G. B., & Hogan, K. (1996). Two case studies using virtual reality as a learning tool for autistic children. *Journal of Autism & Developmental Disorders, 26*(6), 651–659.

Stroem, L., Pattersson, R., & Andersson, G. (2000). A controlled trial of recurrent headache conducted via the Internet. *Journal of Consulting and Clinical Psychology, 68*(4), 722–727.

Suarez-Almazor, M. E., Kendall, C. J., & Dorgan, M. (2001). Surfing the Net—Information on the World Wide Web for persons with arthritis: Patient empowerment or patient deceit? *Journal of Rheumatology, 28*(1), 185–191.

Suler, J. (1996a). *Life at the palace: A cyberpsychology case study.* Retrieved August, 1999, from http://www. rider.edu/users/suler/psycyber/palacestudy.html

Suler, J. (1996b). *One of us: Participant observation research at the palace.* Retrieved August, 1999, from http://www.rider.edu/users/suler/psycyber/partobs.html

Suler, J. (1998). *E-mail communication and relationships.* Retrieved July 20, 2001, from http://www.rider.edu/ users/suler/psycyber/emailrel.html

Suler, J. (1999a, June). *Avatar psychotherapy.* Retrieved October 1, 2002, from http://www.rider.edu/users/ suler/psycyber/avatarther.html

Suler, J. (1999b, April). *The psychology of avatars and graphical space in multimedia chat communities.* Retrieved October 1, 2002, from http://www.rider.edu/users/suler/psycyber/psyav.html

Suler, J. (1999c). *Psychotherapy in cyberspace.* Retrieved August, 1999, from http://www.rider.edu/users/ suler/psycyber/therapy.html

Suler, J. (2000a). *The final showdown between in-person and cyberspace relationships or can I hold you in cyberspace?* Retrieved July 29, 2000, from http://www.rider.edu/users/suler/psycyber/showdown.html

Suler, J. (2000b). *Identity management in cyberspace.* Retrieved July 29, 2000, from http://www.rider.edu/ users/suler/psycyber/identitymanage.html

Suler, J. (2000c). *Psychological dynamics of online synchronous conversations in text-driven chat environments.* Retrieved July 24, 2000, from http://www.rider.edu/users/suler/psycyber/texttalk.html

Suler, J. (2000d). *Psychotherapy and clinical work in cyberspace.* Retrieved July 25, 2000, from http://www. rider.edu/users/suler/psycyber/therintro.html

Sullivan, M. J. (2000–2001). Directorate helps to promote mechanisms for mobility. *Practitioner Focus, 13*(4), 16.

Sussman, R. (2000). Counseling over the Internet: Benefits and challenges in the use of new technologies. *Cybercounseling.* Retrieved July 31, 2000, from http://cybercounsel.uncg.edu/manuscripts/ internetcounseling.htm

Sutter, E., McPherson, R., & Geeseman, R. (2002). Contracting for supervision. *Professional Psychology: Research and Practice, 33*(5), 495–498.

Swenson, W. M., Rome, H. P., Pearson, J. S., & Brannick, T. L. (1965). A totally automated psychological test. *Journal of the American Medical Association, 191*(11), 925–927.

Swinson, R. P., Fergus, K. D., Cox, B. J., & Wickwire, K. (1995). Efficacy of telephone-administered behavioral therapy for panic disorder with agoraphobia. *Behavior Research and Therapy, 33*(4), 465–469.

Szeftel, R. (1999). Comment on "Rural telepsychiatry is economically unsupportable." *Psychiatric Services, 50*(2), 267.

Tallis, F. (2002). *Hidden minds: A history of the unconscious.* London: Profile Books.

Tang, J., & Isaacs, E. (1993). Why do users like video? Studies of multimedia-supported collaboration. *Computer Supported Cooperative Work, 1*(3), 163–196.

Tang, W. K., Chiu, H., Woo, J., Hjelm, M., & Hui, E. (2001). Telepsychiatry in psychogeriatric service: A pilot study. *International Journal of Geriatric Psychiatry, 16*(1), 88–93.

Tanouye, E. (2001, June 13). Mental illness: A rising workplace cost. *Wall Street Journal,* pp. B1, B6.

Tapscott, D. (1998). *Growing up digital: The rise of the Net generation.* New York: McGraw-Hill.

Tate, D. F., Wing, R. R., & Winett, R. A. (2001). Using Internet-based technology to deliver a behavioral weight loss program. *Journal of the American Medical Association, 285*(9), 1172–1177.

Tausig, J. E., & Freeman, E. W. (1988). The next best thing to being there: Conducting the clinical research interview by telephone. *American Journal of Orthopsychiatry, 58*(3), 418–427.

Taylor, C., Winzelberg, A., & Celio, A. (2001). The use of interactive media to prevent eating disorders. In R. Striegel-Moore & L. Smolak (Eds.), *Eating disorders: Innovative directions in research and practice* (pp. 255–269). Washington, DC: American Psychological Association.

Taylor, C. B., Agras, W. S., Losch, M., & Plante, T. G. (1991). Improving the effectiveness of computer-assisted weight loss. *Behavioral Therapy, 22*(2), 229–236.

Taylor, C. B., Fried, L., & Kenardy, J. (1990). The use of a real-time computer diary for data acquisition and processing. *Behavioural Research and Therapy, 28*(1), 93–97.

Taylor, R. J., & Berry, E. (1998). The use of a computer game to rehabilitate sensorimotor functional deficits following a subarachnoid haemorrhage. *Neuropsychological Rehabilitation, 8*(2), 113–122.

TechWeb News. (2002). *RealNetworks promises to plug RealPlayer holes.* Retrieved December 13, 2002, from http://www.informationweek.com/story/IWK20021212S0014

Telecommunications Act. (1996). Retrieved October 3, 2002, from http://www.fcc.gov/telecom.html

Telehealth Improvement and Modernization Act of 2000. (2000, May 4). *S. 2505.* Retrieved December 15, 2000, from http://thomas.loc.gov/cgi-bin/query

Telemedicine helps babies, parents and staff in neonatal ICUs. (2002, July 25). Retrieved August 12, 2002, from http://www.babycarelink.com/news.asp?fn=n38&f=

Telemedicine Information Exchange. (2001). *Telemedicine programs database.* Retrieved June 19, 2001, from http://tie.telemed.org/programs.asp

Telemedicine Information Exchange. (2004). *Telemedicine programs database.* Retrieved April 14, 2004, from http://tie.telemed.org

Telephone Consumer Protection Act. (1991). Retrieved November 18, 2003, from http://www.jmls.edu/cyber/statues/email/tcpa.html

Thalheim, L., Krissler, J., & Ziegler, P. (2001, May 17). Körperkontrolle: Biometrische Zugangssicherungen auf die Probe gestellt. *c't 11,* 114–123.

Thomas, C. R. (2003). Telepsychiatry in a rural women's shelter: Addressing domestic violence. *Telemedicine Journal and e-Health, 9*(1), 53–54.

Thomas, R., Cahill, J., & Santilli, L. (1997). Using an interactive computer game to increase skill and self-efficacy regarding safer sex negotiation: Field test results. *Health Education and Behavior, 24*(1), 71–86.

Thompson, M. (1996, September 25). *The Telemedicine Development Act of 1996.* Sonoma County Physician. Retrieved November 26, 2003, from http://info.sen.ca.gov/pub/95-96/bill/sen/sb_1651-1700/sb_1665_bill_960925_chaptered.pdf

Tingey, R., Lambert, M., Burlingame, G., & Hansen, N. B. (1996). Assessing clinical significance: Proposed extensions to method. *Psychotherapy Research, 6*(2), 109–123.

Towers Perrin. (2002, October 2). *Towers Perrin forecasts 15% increase in health care costs: Highest percentage increase in more than a decade.* Retrieved May 16, 2003, from http://www.towers.com/towers_news/news/news_frame.asp?target=http://www.towers.com/towers_news/news/news_date.htm

Troester, A., Paolo, A., Glatt, S., Hubble, J., & Koller, W. (1995). "Interactive video conferencing" in the provision of neuropsychological services to rural areas. *Journal of Community Psychology, 23*(1), 85–88.

Trott, P., & Blignault, I. (1998). Cost evaluation of a telepsychiatry service in northern Queensland. *Journal of Telemedicine and Telecare, 4*(1), 66–68.

Tunstall, N., Prince, M., & Mann, A. (1997). Concurrent validity of a telephone-administered version of the Gospel Oak instrument (including the SHORT-CARE). *International Journal of Geriatric Psychiatry, 12*(10), 1035–1038.

Turisco, F., & Metzger, J. (2003). *Rural health care delivery: Connecting communities through technology.* First Consulting Group. Retrieved May 1, 2003, from http://www.chcf.org/topics/view.cfm?itemid=20206

Turkle, S. (1995). *Life on the screen: Identity in the age of the Internet.* New York: Touchstone.

Tutty, S., Simon, G., & Ludman, E. (2000). Telephone counseling as an adjunct to antidepressant treatment in the primary care system. A pilot study. *Effective Clinical Practice, 3*(4), 170–178.

University of California Davis Medical Center. (n.d.). *Colorblind study.* Retrieved October 17, 2003, from http://www.ucdmc.ucdavis.edu/pulse/scripts/00_01/colorblind.pdf

University of Rochester Medical Center. (2003). Strong Connections: Telehealth sign language solutions. Retrieved August 18, 2003, from http://www.urmc.rochester.edu/strongconnections/index.html

URAC and Hi-Ethics collaborate on health Web site accreditation. (2001, May 21). Retrieved August 24, 2001, from http://www.urac.org/010521Hi-EthicsURAC.htm

U.S. Department of Commerce. (1997). *Telemedicine report to Congress* (1997-418-626/42023). Washington, DC: U.S. Government Printing Office.

U.S. Department of Health and Human Services. (2000, December 28). Standards for Privacy of Individually Identifiable Health Information; Final Rule. Federal Register, 65(250), 82461–82467. Retrieved May 10, 2004, from http://www.bricker.com/legalservices/practice/hcare/hipaa/privacy1.pdf

U.S. Department of Health and Human Services. (2001a). § 414.65. Centers for Medicare & Medicaid Services. Retrieved November 26, 2003, from http://a257.g.akamaitech.net/7/257/2422/14mar20010800/edocket.access.gpo.gov/cfr_2002/octqtr/pdf/42cfr414.65.pdf

U.S. Department of Health and Human Services. (2001a, June 14). *The new centers for Medicare and Medicaid services (CMS).* Retrieved February 19, 2002, from http://www.os.dhhs.gov/news/press/2001pres/20010614a.html

U.S. Department of Health and Human Services. (2002). *42 CFR 1001.952.* Retrieved December 1, 2003, from http://www.dwt.com/practc/healthcr_compliance/publications/OIG_SmallGroup_Compliance/docs/1001_952D.PDF

U.S. Department of Health and Human Services. (2002). Standards for Privacy of Individually Identifiable Health Information; Final Rule (45 C.F.R. Pts. 160 and 164). *Federal Register, 67*(157), 53181–53273. Retrieved May 29, 2003, from http://www.hhs.gov/ocr/hipaa/privruletxt.txt

U.S. Department of Health and Human Services. (2003, April 17). Standards for Privacy of Individually Identifiable Health Information. Office of Civil Rights. Retrieved November 26, 2003 from http://www.hhs.gov/ocr/combinedregtext.pdf

U.S. Food and Drug Administration. (1997). *Federal Food, Drug and Cosmetic Act.* Retrieved November 26, 2003, from http://www.fda.gov/opacom/laws/fdcact/fdctoc.htm

U.S. General Accounting Office. (1991, April). *Mentally ill inmates: Better data would help determine protection and advocacy needs.* Washington, DC: Author.

U.S. General Accounting Office. (1999, February 24). *Medical records/privacy: Access needed for health research, but oversight of privacy protections is limited* (Publication No. B-280657). Retrieved May 5, 2000, from http://frwebgate.access.gpo.gov

U.S. Public Health Service. (2000). *Report of the Surgeon General's Conference on Children's Mental Health: A national action agenda.* Washington, DC: U.S. Department of Health and Human Services.

VandenBos, G. R., & Williams, S. (2000). The Internet versus the telephone: What is telehealth anyway? *Professional Psychology: Research and Practice, 31*(5), 490–492.

Varney, C. A. (1996). *Consumer privacy in the Information Age: A view from the United States.* Retrieved April 16, 2003, from http://www.ftc.gov/speeches/varney/priv&ame.htm

Varon, C., & Rosenau, J. (1998, January 26). 21st haiku challenge. *Salon.* Retrieved April 9, 2003, from http://www.salon.com/21st/chal/1998/01/26chal.html

Video Development Initiative. (2000, June). *Video conferencing cookbook.* Retrieved February 12, 2002, from http://www.vide.gatech.edu/cookbook2.0

Video Privacy Protection Act. (1988). Retrieved October 3, 2002, from http://www4.law.cornell.edu/uscode/18/2710.html

Virtual Private Network Consortium. (n.d.). *Implications of HIPAA for the VPN industry.* Retrieved August 16, 2002, from http://www.vpnc.org/hipaa.html

Wagenfield, M., Murray, J., Mohatt, D., & DeBruyn, J. (Eds.). (1994). *Mental health and rural America: An overview and annotated bibliography, 1978–1993.* Washington, DC: U.S. Government Printing Office.

Wagman, M. (1980). PLATO DCS: An interactive computer system for personal counseling. *Journal of Counseling Psychology, 27*(1), 16–30.

Wagman, M. (1982). A computer method for solving dilemmas. *Psychological Reports, 50*(1), 291–298.

Wagman, M. (1988). *Computer psychotherapy systems: Theory and research foundations.* Amsterdam, Netherlands: Gordon and Breach Publishers.

Wagman, M. (1999). *The human mind according to artificial intelligence: Theory, research, and implications.* Westport, CT: Praeger Publishers/Greenwood Publishing Group.

Wald, M. L. (2002, June 23). For air crash detectives, seeing isn't believing. *The New York Times.* Retrieved June 24, 2002, from http://www.nytimes.com

Waller, N. G., & Reise, S. P. (1989). Computerized adaptive personality assessment: An illustration with the Absorption scale. *Journal of Personality and Social Psychology, 57*(6), 1051–1058.

Walther, J. (1996). Computer-mediated communcation: Impersonal, interpersonal, and hyperpersonal interaction. *Communication Research, 23*(1), 3–43.

Walther, J., Anderson, J., & Park, D. (1994). Interpersonal effects in computer-mediated interaction: A meta-analysis of social and anti-social communication. *Communication Research, 21*, 460–487.

Wann, J. P., Rushton, S. K., Smyth, M., & Jones, D. (1997). Virtual environments for the rehabilitation of disorders of attention and movement. In G. Riva, *Virtual reality in neuro-psycho-physiology: Cognitive, clinical and methodological issues in assessment and treatment* (pp. 157–164). Amsterdam: IOS Press.

Wasson, J., Gaudette, C., Whaley, F., Sauvigne, A., Baribeau, P., & Welch, H. G. (1992). Telephone care as a substitute for routine clinic follow-up. *Journal of the American Medical Association, 267*(13), 1788–1793.

Waters, J., & Finn, E. (1995). Handling client crises effectively on the telephone. In A. R. Roberts (Ed.), *Crisis intervention and time-limited cognitive treatment* (pp. 251–289). Thousand Oaks, CA: Sage.

Waters, R. (1999, April 18–21). *Telemedicine: Establishing care links around the world.* Paper presented at the National Conference on Legal and Policy Developments, Salt Lake City, UT.

Weil, M., & Rosen, L. (1997). *TechnoStress: Coping with technology @work @home @play.* New York: Wiley.

Weinberg, H. (2001, July). Group process and group phenomena on the Internet. *International Journal of Group Psychotherapy, 51*(3), 361–378.

Weinberg, N., Uken, J., Schmale, J., & Adamek, M. (1995). Therapeutic factors: Their presence in a computer-mediated support group. *Social Work with Groups, 18*(4), 57–69.

Weinrich, J. (1997). Strange bedfellows: Homosexuality, gay liberation, and the Internet. *Journal of Sex Education and Therapy, 22*(2), 58–66.

Weisband, S., & Kiesler, S. (1996, April 13–18). *Self-disclosure on computer forms: Meta-analysis and implications.* Paper presented at the Conference on Human Factors in Computing Systems, Vancouver, British Columbia, Canada.

Weizenbaum, J. (1966). ELIZA: A computer program for the study of natural language communication between man and machine. *Communications of the Association for Computing Machinery, 9*(1), 36–45.

Weizenbaum, J. (1976). *Computer power and human reason.* San Francisco: Freeman.

Wellman, B., & Gulia, W. (1995). Net surfers don't ride alone: Virtual communities as communities. In P. Kollock & M. Smith (Eds.), *Communities in cyberspace* (pp. 167–194). Berkeley: University of California Press.

Wells, K. B., Burnam, M. A., Leake, B., & Robins, L. N. (1988). Agreement between face-to-face and telephone-administered versions of the depression section of the NIMH Diagnostic Interview Schedule. *Journal of Psychiatric Research, 22*(3), 207–220.

Werner, A., & Anderson, L. E. (1998). Rural telepsychiatry is economically unsupportable: The Concorde crashes in a cornfield. *Psychiatric Services, 49*(10), 1287–1290.

Whatis.com. (2001a). Retrieved October 9, 2001, from http://whatis.techtarget.com

Whatis.com. (2001b). *Fast guide to DSL.* Retrieved March 13, 2001, from http://whatis.techtarget.com/WhatIs_Definition_Page/0,4152,213915,00.html

Whatis.com. (2001c). *XML.* Retrieved October 1, 2001, from http://searchmiddleware.techtarget.com/sDefinition/0,,sid26_gci213404,00.html

White, M. (2000). *Reflections on narrative practice.* Adelaide, South Australia: Dulwich Centre Publications.

Whittaker, S. (1995). Rethinking video as a technology for interpersonal communication: Theory and design implications. *International Journal of Human–Computer Studies, 42*(5), 501–529.

Whittaker, S., & O'Conaill, B. (1997). The role of vision in face-to-face and mediated communication. In A. Sellen & S. Wilbur (Eds.), *Video-mediated Communication* (pp. 23–49). Mahwah, NJ: Lawrence Erlbaum Associates.

Whitten, P., & Franken, E. A. (1995). Telemedicine for patient consultation: Factors affecting use by rural primary-care physicians in Kansas. *Journal of Telemedicine and Telecare, 1*(3), 139–144.

Whitten, P., & Mair, F. (2000, June 3). A systematic review of telemedicine patient satisfaction studies: Research which yields more questions than answers. *British Medical Journal, 320*(7248), 1517–1520.

Whitten, P., Zaylor, C., & Kingsley, C. (2000). An analysis of telepsychiatry programs from an organizational perspective. *CyberPsychology and Behavior, 3*(6), 911–915.

Wiederhold, B. K., & Wiederhold, M. D. (2002, April). Advanced technologies prove useful in mental health applications. *San Diego Psychologist, 11*(4), 1.

Wilhelm, F. H., Alpers, G. W., Meuret, A. E., & Roth, W. T. (2001). Respiratory pathophysiology of clinical anxiety outside the laboratory: Assessment of end-tidal pCO2, respiratory pattern variability, and transfer function RSA. In J. Fahrenberg (Ed.), *Progress in ambulatory assessment* (pp. 313–343). Göttingen: Hogrefe & Huber.

Wilhelm, F. H., Gerlach, A. L., & Roth, W. T. (2001). Slow recovery from voluntary hyperventilation in panic disorder. *Psychosomatic Medicine, 63*(4), 638–649.

Wilhelm, F. H., Gevirtz, R., & Roth, W. T. (2001). Respiratory dysregulation in anxiety, functional cardiac, and pain disorders: Assessment, phenomenology, and treatment. *Behavior Modification, 25*(4), 513–545.

Wilhelm, F. H., & Roth, W. T. (1998). Taking the laboratory to the skies: Ambulatory assessment of self-report, autonomic, and respiratory responses in flying phobia. *Psychophysiology, 35*(5), 596–606.

Wilhelm, F. H., & Roth, W. T. (2001). The somatic symptom paradox in DSM-IV anxiety disorders: Suggestions for a clinical focus in psychophysiology. *Biological Psychology, 57*(1–3), 105–140.

Wilhelm, F. H., Trabert, W., & Roth, W. T. (2001a). Characteristics of sighing in panic disorder. *Biological Psychiatry, 49*(7), 606–614.

Wilhelm, F. H., Trabert, W., & Roth, W. T. (2001b). Physiological instability in panic disorder and generalized anxiety disorder. *Biological Psychiatry, 49*(7), 596–605.

Williams, D. (1996, April). The human macro-organism as fungus. *Wired*. Retrieved May 16, 2003, from http://www.wired.com/wired/archive/4.04/viermenhouk.html

Williams, M. A. (1994). The Chicago study at a glance. *Contemporary Sexuality, 28*(11), 2.

Wilson, F. R., Genco, K. T., & Yager, G. G. (1985). Assessing the equivalence of paper-and-pencil vs. computerized tests: Demonstration of a promising methodology. *Computers in Human Behavior, 1*(3–4), 265–275.

Wilson-Steele, G. (2000). The next-generation healthcare organization Web site. In J. Florey (Ed.), *Internet healthcare strategy guide 2001* (pp. 33–35). Santa Barbara, CA: Cor Health.

Winchell, C., & Wilbright, W. A. (2003). Telemedical mental health services for a juvenile correctional population. *Telemedicine Journal and e-Health, 9*(1), S124.

Winker, M. A., Flanagin, A., Chi-Lum, B., White, J., Andrews, K., Kennett, R. L., DeAngelis, C. D., & Musacchio, R. A. (2003, July 25). *Guidelines for medical and health information sites on the Internet.* Retrieved November 20, 2003, from http://www.ama-assn.org/ama/pub/category/1905.html

Winn, D. L., & Angelocci, T. (2002). What are you waiting for? The "tops" total office paperless solution. *e-MDs*. Retrieved March 5, 2002, from http://www.e-mds.com/emds/benefits/index.html

Winzelberg, A. J., Eppstein, D., Eldredge, K. L., Wilfley, D., Dasmahapatra, R., Dev, P., & Taylor, C. B. (2000). Effectiveness of an Internet-based program for reducing risk factors for eating disorders. *Journal of Consulting and Clinical Psychology, 68*(2), 346–350.

Winzelberg, A. J., Taylor, C. B., Sharpe, T., Eldredge, K. L., Dev, P., & Constantinou, P. S. (1998). Evaluation of a computer-mediated eating disorder intervention program. *International Journal of Eating Disorders, 24*(4), 339–349.

Witmer, L. (1907). Clinical psychology. *Psychological Clinic, 1*, 1–9.

Wittchen, H. (1994). Reliability and validity studies of the WHO-Composite International Diagnostic Interview (CIDI): A critical review. *Journal of Psychiatric Research, 28*(1), 57–84.

Wittson, C., & Benschoter, R. (1972). Two-way television: Helping the medical center reach out. *American Journal of Psychiatry, 129*(5), 624–627.

Woloshin, S., & Schwartz, L. M. (2002, June 5). Press releases: translating research into news. *Journal of the American Medical Association, 287*(21), 2856–2858.

Wood, A. F., & Smith, M. J. (2001). *Online communication: Linking technology, identity, and culture.* Mahwah, NJ: Lawrence Erlbaum Associates.

Wooton, R., & Blignault, I. (2003). Guidelines for telepsychiatry and e-mental health. In R. Wooton, P. Yellowlees, & P. McLaren (Eds.), *Telepsychiatry and e-Mental Health* (pp. 293–304). London, England: Royal Society of Medicine Press.

World Health Organization. (1990). *International Classification of Diseases for Oncology, fourth edition.* Geneva: Author.

World Health Organization. (1998). *Directory of health technology assessment organizations worldwide.* Washington, DC: Medical Technology and Practice Patterns Institute.

World Health Organization. (2001). World health report 2001. Retrieved July 25, 2002, from http://www.who.int/whr/2001/main/en/media/disorders.htm

Yager, T. (2002, December 9). *Software goes extinct.* InfoWorld. Retrieved November 26, 2003, from http://www.infoworld.com/article/02/12/06/021209opestrat_1.html

Yarnall, K., Pollak, K., Østbye, T., Krause, K., & Michener, J. (2003). Primary care: Is there enough time for prevention? *American Journal of Public Health, 93*(4), 635–641.

Yellowlees, P. (2003). E-mental health in the future. In R. Wooton, P. Yellowlees, & P. McLaren (Eds.), *Telepsychiatry and e-mental health* (pp. 305–316). London, England: Royal Society of Medicine Press.

Yellowlees, P. (2003). The use of information technologies to assist in psychiatric diagnosis. *Telemedicine Journal and e-Health, 9*(1), 66.

Yellowlees, P. M. (n.d.). E-therapy: Your guide to mental health in cyberspace. *MightyWords*. Unpublished manuscript.

Yesavage, J. A., Brink, T. L., Rose, T. L., Lum, O., Huang, V., Adey, M., & Leirer, V. O. (1982). Development and validation of a geriatric depression screening scale: A preliminary report. *Journal of Psychiatric Research, 17,* 37–49.

Young Lawyers Division, Health Care Law Committee. (1998). *Recommendation and report to the assembly of the Young Lawyers Division, American Bar Association,* Cincinnati, OH.

Zarate, C., Jr., Weinstock, L., Cukor, P., Morabito, C., Leahy, L., Burns, C., & Baer, L. (1997). Applicability of telemedicine for assessing patients with schizophrenia: Acceptance and reliability. *Journal of Clinical Psychiatry, 58*(1), 22–25.

Zarr, M. L. (1984). Computer-mediated psychotherapy: Toward patient-selection guidelines. *American Journal of Psychotherapy, 38*(1), 47–62.

Zaylor, C. (1999). Clinical outcomes in telepsychiatry. *Journal of Telehealth and Telecare, 5*(1), 59–60.

Zaylor, C. (2000). *Telepsychiatry services to a rural jail.* Phoenix, AZ: American Telemedicine Association.

Zaylor, C., Spaulding, A., & Cook, D. (2003). Mental health correctional telemedicine. In R. Wooton, P. Yellowlees, & P. McLaren (Eds.), *Telepsychiatry and e-Mental Health* (pp. 137–147). London, England: Royal Society of Medicine Press.

Zaylor, C., Whitten, P., & Kingsley, C. (1999, December). Telemedicine services to a county jail. *Journal of Telemedicine and Telecare, 6*(1), 93–95.

Ziglin, A. L. (1995). *Confidentiality and the appropriate uses of data.* Rockville, MD: Department of Health and Human Services.

Zilboorg, G. (1967). *A history of medical psychology.* New York: Norton.

Author Index

Numbers in italics indicate the page where the complete reference is given.

A

Abell, M. D., 59, 73, *478*
Ackerman, M. D., 7
Adamek, M., 72, *501*
Adey, M., 437, *503*
Administration on Aging, 21, *467*
Advanced Systems Group, 408, *467*
Affective Computing, 410, *467*
Agency for Healthcare Research and Quality, 126, *467*
Agras, W. S., 163, 180, 188, *467*, *487*, *499*
Ahlbom, J., 122, *488*
Akamatsu, S., 416, *472*
Alarcon, R., 189, *495*
Albert, M. S., 117, *479*
Alcaniz, M., 189, 437, *492*, *494*
Alcatel, *467*
Alessi, N. E., 138, 268, *467*, *470*
Alexander, G., 316, 317, *467*
Algazy, J. I., 96, *471*
Allard, M., 437
Allen, A., 8, 84, 114, 120, 152, 206, 223, 292, 327, 339, 342, 344, 388, 390, *467*, *487*
Allen, D. H., 179, *467*
Allen, J., *467*
Allen, L., *467*
Allison, R., 40, 132, *497*
Alpers, G. W., 194, *467*, *502*
Alpert, D., 177, *467*
AMA Member Communications, *467*
American Academy of Child and Adolescent Psychiatry, 242, *467*
American Accreditation HealthCare Commission, 95, 265, 270, 281, 340, *467*
American College of Physicians, 372, *467*
American Counseling Association, 340, *468*
American Educational Research Association, *468*
American Health Information Management System, *468*
American Medical Association, 3, 217, 275, *468*
American Medical Association House of Delegates, 256, *468*
American Nurses Association, 217, *468*

American Psychiatric Association, 120, 218, 264, 278, 335, 348, *468*
American Psychological Association, 155, 160, 161, 229, 253, 259, 263, 270, 277, 303, 305, 308, 335, 339, 352, 370, *468*
American Psychological Association Task Force on Self-Help Therapies, 254, *468*
American Telemedicine Association, *468*
Anderson, A., 121, 139, *468*
Anderson, E. E., 168, *486*
Anderson, G. F., 4, 14, *480*
Anderson, J., 70, 71, *501*
Anderson, K., 252, *468*
Anderson, L. E., 372, *501*
Anderson, P. L., 189, *469*
Andersson, G., 158, 473, *498*
Andreasen, N. C., 437, *469*
Andress, M., 396, *469*
Andrews, G., 158, *492*
Andrews, K., 275, 311, *502*
Andrews, T. K., 189, *469*
Aneshensel, C. S., 117, *469*
Angelocci, T., 199, *502*
Anolli, L., 189, *494*
Anson, R., 298, *474*
Appel, S., 192, *476*
Aptel, M., 424, *469*
Architectural and Transportation Barriers Compliance Board, 103, *469*
Ardekani, B., 39, *492*
Arends, M., 307, *486*
Arias, R. G., 435, *472*
Arlington, S., 193, *469*
Armstrong, A., 97, *480*
Aronson, G., 179, *474*
Asso, A. E., *469*
Association of State and Provincial Licensing Boards, *469*
Association of Telehealth Service Providers, 148, *469*
Association of Test Publishers, *469*
Atkinson, T., 434, *487*
Attree, E. A., 189, *469*, *493*
Audin, K., 168, *470*

505

H

Subject Index

A

Abstracting service, 2
Acceptance, barriers, 122
Access
    electronic practice management, 204, 210, 210, 212
    influence of psychotechnologies, 10
    managing risk for Web site owners, 365
    notes and HIPAA Privacy Rule, 231
    store-and-forward technology, 42
    telephonic and videoconferencing technologies, 115–116
    Web site components, 102
Accession, 457–458
Accountability, 16, 67, 365
Accounts, outstanding, 199
Accreditation standards, 263
Acculturation process, 58
Acculturation scales, 307
Accuracy, interviews, 161, *see also* Internet
Actigraph, 194
Ad out, 76
Add-on vocabulary program, 208
Address, e-mail, 56, *see also* E-mail
Address lists, e-mail, 78, *see also* E-mail
Administrative services, 356
Administrative standards, 280–283
Adolescents, 185–186, 268
Adoption, criteria, 199, *see also* Electronic practice management
Advertising/promotion, 96, 323
Advice, e-mail, 359, *see also* Direct care
Advocacy, 220, 377–379
Aethra, 135–136
Affect, barriers, 121
Affective computing, 415–416
Affordability, barriers, 123–125
Age, standards of online conduct, 268
Agency for Healthcare Research and Quality (AHRQ), 125–126
Aging population, 21
Agreements, Online Clinical Practice Management, 335–345
AHRQ, *see* Agency for Healthcare Research and Quality

AI, *see* Artificial intelligence
Alcoholism, 182
ALERT, *see* Algorithms for Effective Reporting and Treatment
Algorithms for Effective Reporting and Treatment (ALERT), 154–155
Alienation, 139, 175
Alterative therapies, 305–306
Always-on systems, 409
Alzheimer's Caregiver Support Online, 42–43
AMA, *see* American Medical Association
Ambiguities, 351–352
Ambulatory monitoring, 193–195
Amendments, draft international convention, 458
America Online (AOL), 50, 90
American Accreditation Health Care Commission (URAC), 97, 265–266, 270, 280–282, 400
American Medical Association (AMA), 22, 217, 256, 370
American National Standards Institute (ANSI), 284
American Nurses Association (ANA), 217
American Psychiatric Association, 218
American Psychological Association (APA), 63, 253, 370
American Telemedicine Association (ATA), 284
ANA, *see* American Nurses Association
Analog mode, confidentiality, 296
Animation, 103
Annual reunions, 69
Anonymity, referrals, 326–327
ANSI, *see* American National Standards Institute
Antidepressant therapy, 118
Anxiety disorders, 26, 181–182, 189–190, 187
AOL, *see* American Online
APA, *see* American Psychological Association
Appeal, Web sites, 90
Appearance, masking, 349
Application service providers (ASP), 205, 395–396
Appointment
Appointments, 129
    confirmations, 344
    scheduling, 344–345
Archiving, 68
Arizona Telemedicine Program, 6–7
Artificial intelligence (AI), 417–418
ASP, *see* Application service provider

521

Printed at Repro India Limited, India